A Case Approach to Medical-Psychiatric Practice

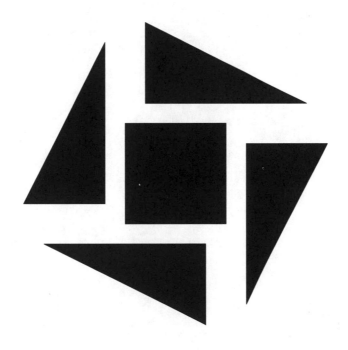

A Case Approach to Medical-Psychiatric Practice

Antoinette Ambrosino Wyszynski, M.D.
Clinical Assistant Professor of Psychiatry
Faculty, Psychoanalytic Institute
New York University Medical Center
and

Bernard Wyszynski, M.D.
Assistant Professor of Psychiatry and of Neurology
Associate Director, Division of Neuropsychiatry
Montefiore Medical Center,
Albert Einstein College of Medicine,
Bronx, New York

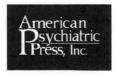

American Psychiatric Press, Inc.

Washington, DC
London, England

Note: The authors have worked to ensure that all information in this book concerning drug dosages, schedules, and routes of administration is accurate as of the time of publication and consistent with standards set by the U.S. Food and Drug Administration and the general medical community. As medical research and practice advance, however, therapeutic standards may change. For this reason and because human and mechanical errors sometimes occur, we recommend that readers follow the advice of a physician who is directly involved in their care or the care of a member of their family.

Books published by the American Psychiatric Press, Inc., represent the views and opinions of the individual authors and do not necessarily represent the policies and opinions of the Press or the American Psychiatric Association.

Copyright © 1996 Antoinette A. Wyszynski and Bernard Wyszynski
ALL RIGHTS RESERVED
Manufactured in the United States of America on acid-free paper
99 98 97 96   4 3 2 1
First Edition

American Psychiatric Press, Inc.
1400 K Street, N.W., Washington, DC   20005

Library of Congress Cataloging-in-Publication Data
Wyszynski, Antoinette Ambrosino, 1954-
     A Case Approach to medical-psychiatric practice / by Antoinette Ambrosino Wyszynski and Bernard Wyszynski.
          p.   cm.
     Includes bibliographical references and index.
     ISBN 0-88048-530-2
     1.   Consultation-liaison psychiatry—Case studies.   I. Wyszynski, Bernard, 1954-   II.   Title.
     [DNLM: 1.   Psychiatry—case studies.   2.   Referral and Consultation—case studies.   3.   Mental Disorders—drug therapy—case studies.   4.   Psychotropic Drugs—therapeutic use—case studies. WM40 W995c 1996]
     RC455.2.C65W97   1996
     616.89—dc20
     DNLM/DLC   95-24976
     for Library of Congress   CIP

British Library Cataloguing in Publication Data
A CIP record is available from the British Library.

This book is dedicated to our parents, Salvatore V. Ambrosino, M.D., Claudia Mazza Ambrosino, Charles M. Wyszynski, the late Margaret Wyszynski; and to the memory of George L. Ginsberg, M.D., Professor of Psychiatry, New York University Medical Center.

Contents

Introduction x

Acknowledgments xi

Chapter 1 **The Cardiovascular Patient** 1

Mr. Doe: The Depressed Cardiovascular Patient 4

Mr. Smith: The Depressed, Post-Myocardial Infarction Patient 35

Ms. Anderson: The Manic Patient With Heart Disease and Hypertension 51

Chapter 2 **The Patient With Pulmonary Disease** 65

Mr. Davis: The Patient With Delirium and Lung Cancer 68

Mrs. Alberts: The Anxious, Depressed Asthmatic Patient 93

Chapter 3 **The Delirious Alcoholic Patient With Cirrhosis** 117

Chapter 4 **The Patient With Kidney Disease** 141

Mrs. Freed: The Manic Patient in Renal Failure on Dialysis 144

Mr. Barry: The Depressed Renal Patient and Transplantation 159

Chapter 5 **The Patient on Steroids** 193

Chapter 6 **The HIV-Infected Patient** 213

Mr. Lowe: The Depressed HIV Patient 216

Ms. Newman: The Female HIV Patient 247

Chapter 7 **The Patient With Gastrointestinal Distress and Psychiatric Symptoms** 275

Chapter 8 **The Obstetrics Patient** 299

Ms. Wright: The Anxious, Depressed Pregnant Patient 302

Ms. Sawyer: The Psychotic, Bipolar Pregnant Patient 324

Chapter 9 **The Gynecology/Oncology Patient** 343

Mrs. Reid (Part I): Menopause, Chronic Pelvic Pain, and Hysterectomy 346

Mrs. Reid (Part II): Breast Cancer 370

Appendix A   A Consultation-Liaison Guide to DSM-IV 392

Appendix B–1   Mini–Mental State Examination 398

Appendix B–2   Statistical Distribution of Trail Making Test Scores by Age 399

Appendix C   Guide to Treating Delirium With Haloperidol and Lorazepam 400

Appendix D   Managing Insomnia and Restlessness in Delirium 402

Appendix E   Differential Diagnosis of the Delirious Psychotic Patient With Cirrhosis 403

Appendix F   A Mini-Outline of Competency and Informed Consent 404

Appendix G   Neuropsychiatric Effects of Electrolyte and Acid-Base Imbalance 409

Appendix H   The Use of Psychotropics in Renal Failure 412

Appendix I   Definitional Criteria for HIV-1–Associated Dementia (HAD) Complex and Cognitive Impairment—American Academy of Neurology AIDS Task Force 415

Appendix J   Revised HIV Classification System for Adolescents and Adults (Centers for Disease Control and Prevention 1993) 416

Appendix K   Management Strategies for the Patient With HIV-Associated Minor Cognitive-Motor Impairment and AIDS Dementia Complex (ADC) 417

Appendix L   The Questions Patients Ask: A Pretest of Countertransference 418

Appendix M   Effects of Psychotropics During Pregnancy 421

Appendix N   Guidelines for Using Psychotropics During Pregnancy 435

Appendix O   Notes on the "New" Antidepressants in the Medical Setting 437

Appendix P   Practical Suggestions for Bedside Manner in the General Hospital Setting 441

Index 443

Introduction

Even for the dedicated psychiatrist, medical knowledge atrophies easily with disuse. Our aim in *A Case Approach to Medical-Psychiatric Practice* is to reclaim consultation psychiatry's medical roots. Case presentations and questions are our starting point. We have sought to revive some of the pathophysiological basics by using the organ system approach, with literature reviews on the interface between selected medical topics and psychiatry. Note that although we have deferred discussion of many psychosocial issues, this does not imply that we feel they are dispensable or unimportant (as witnessed by the copious references, which we hope the interested reader will pursue). Rather, we have tried to offer a resource on the contribution of medical information to the practice of consultation-liaison (C-L) psychiatry. We do not intend our discussions as comprehensive practice guidelines for approaching the patient; they are too unilaterally biological. This integrated perspective is readily available, however, in several masterful texts listed below (see "Recommended Reading"). This book unabashedly attempts to reintegrate C-L psychiatry as one of the *medical* disciplines, and is written as a *teaching tool* rather than a comprehensive textbook.

In the spirit of capturing clinical dilemmas, which respect neither medical-psychiatric boundaries, levels of training, nor test-taking strategies, we simulate the problem-oriented bedside world of consultation-liaison psychiatry in the cases and exercises, rather than Board exam preparation. To stem the book's potential for encyclopedic proportions, neurological issues will be published as a separate *Casebook of Neuropsychiatry* in the future.

Instead of aiming for comprehensiveness, we have presented *selected* topics; consequently, several important areas—for example, many women's health issues (notably, abortion, infertility, and late luteal phase disorder), personality disorders, somatoform disorders, psychoanalytic perspectives on psychosomatics, and pain management—must await another book. (Refer to the excellent texts listed below, especially the recent scholarly works of Stoudemire and Fogel.) New psychotropic medications have multiplied faster than the literature can keep pace with them; we review those that have been studied in medical patients, so our list is more selective than complete.

Use the questions following each case as an exercise before or after—or as a companion to—reading the literature reviews. They were constructed to highlight certain issues for review and discussion. The referencing system is unconventional but practical: in-text citations are numerical to minimize distractions from text content, whereas the bibliographies are alphabetical for easy future reference. They are intended to supplement what we do not cover in the text.

We hope the text will be challenging to psychiatrists at many stages of experience, from the resident new to the consultation-liaison service to the seasoned attending psychiatrist who regularly collaborates with medical and surgical colleagues. There are no standardized scores or percentiles, no answer patterns or strategies—just the patient, the problem, the literature, and your ingenuity and judgment. We are sometimes picky, sometimes obvious; yet always, we hope, as thought-provoking as the patients we describe, who have, in turn, challenged us.

Antoinette Ambrosino Wyszynski, M.D.
Bernard Wyszynski, M.D.
New York City, 1995

Recommended Reading

Breitbart W, Holland J (eds): Psychiatric Aspects of Symptom Management in Cancer Patients. Washington, DC, American Psychiatric Press, 1993

Briggs G, Freeman R, Yaffe S: Drugs in Pregnancy and Lactation, 3rd Edition. Baltimore, MD, Williams & Wilkins, 1990

Cassem N (ed): Massachusetts General Hospital Handbook of General Hospital Psychiatry, 3rd Edition. St. Louis, MO, Mosby Year Book, 1991

Craven J, Rodin G (eds): Psychiatric Aspects of Organ Transplantation. Oxford, UK, Oxford University Press, 1992

Holland J, Rowland J (eds): Handbook of Psychooncology. New York, Oxford University Press, 1990

Kellner R: Psychosomatic Syndromes and Somatic Symptoms. Washington, DC, American Psychiatric Press, 1991

Salzman C: Clinical Geriatric Psychopharmacology, 2nd Edition. Baltimore, MD, Williams & Wilkins, 1992

Stewart D, Stotland N (eds): Psychological Aspects of Women's Health Care: The Interface Between Psychiatry and Obstetrics and Gynecology. Washington, DC, American Psychiatric Press, 1993

Stoudemire A, Fogel B (eds): Medical-Psychiatric Practice, Vol 1. Washington, DC, American Psychiatric Press, 1991

Stoudemire A, Fogel B (eds): Medical-Psychiatric Practice, Vol 2. Washington, DC, American Psychiatric Press, 1993

Stoudemire A, Fogel B (eds): Medical-Psychiatric Practice, Vol 3. Washington, DC, American Psychiatric Press, 1995

Stoudemire A, Fogel B (eds): Psychiatric Care of the Medical Patient. New York, Oxford University Press, 1993

Acknowledgments

This book would not have been possible without the help of the following colleagues, whose generous comments and feedback greatly enhanced the relevance, readability, and scholarship of these chapters:

- **Cardiology:** Drs. Salvatore V. Ambrosino, Jonathan Easton, Robin Freedberg, and Alan Stoudemire
- **Pulmonary disease:** Drs. Jonathan Easton, Stewart Fleishmann, Patrick McKegney, Jan Samet, and Veva Zimmerman
- **Liver disease:** Drs. Robert Cancro, Michael D. Leibowitz, Alan H. Lockwood, Paula T. Trzepacz, and Joel Wallach
- **Renal disease:** Drs. Gregory Fricchione, Richard Friedman, and Paula T. Trzepacz
- **HIV infection:** Drs. Chuck Davis, Jonathan Easton, Stewart Fleischmann, Mary Alice O'Dowd, Sharon Sagemen, Bruce Klutchko, and Victoria Wolfson
- **Gastrointestinal illness:** Drs. David Frank, R. Bruce Lydiard, Kevin W. Olden, and Thomas Wise
- **Obstetrics:** Drs. Lee S. Cohen, Luciano Lizzi, Laura Miller, Darlene Osipuk, and Nada Stotland
- **Gynecology:** Drs. Naomi Bravman, Leslie Gise, Stanley Grossman, Steven Katz, Luciano Lizzi, Nada Stotland, and Mary Jane Massie

Special thanks go to Drs. Matthew Menza and Paula Trzepacz, whose reading of early drafts led to crucial organizational suggestions that were implemented throughout the book. We are grateful to Dr. Karen Brewer's tireless staff at the Frederick L. Ehrman Medical Library at New York University Medical Center—especially the Document Delivery Service and Mr. Richard Faraino, who heroically conducted the massive literature searches. Finally, we would like to thank the psychiatric residents of the New York University–Bellevue program for their enthusiasm, invaluable advice, and editorial help on all of the chapters, especially Drs. Cristina Profumo, Ranu Boppana, Kristin Beizai, Gerald Dariah, Peter Goertz, Adarsh Gupta, David Krakow, Ann Maloney, Danni Michaeli, and Elyse Weiner.

The Cardiovascular Patient

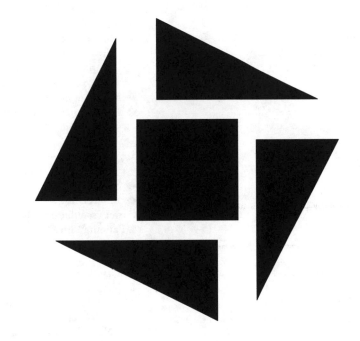

CHAPTER 1

CONTENTS

■ Introduction to Chapter 1 3
■ Case Presentation: Mr. Doe: The Depressed
   Cardiovascular Patient 4
■ Questions 4
■ Answers 7
■ Discussion 8
  ◆ The Psyche and Cardiac Morbidity 8
    Major Depression and Heart Disease 8
      DSM-IV, Medical Illness, and the
        Problem of Depression 8
        Farewell "organic versus
          functional" 9
    Anxiety Disorders and Heart Disease 9
      Mitral Valve Prolapse 10
      Chronic Chest Pain of Unknown Etiology . . . 10
      The Pacemaker Syndrome Versus
        Panic Disorder 10
      "Things That Go Bang in the Night" 11
    Heart and Mind 11
      Stress and Ischemia 11
      Hostility and Type A 11
      Stress and Painless (Silent) Ischemia 12
        Comment: the therapist's dilemma . . . 13
      Sudden Cardiac Death 13
      Job Strain and the Heart 14
      Social Support and Cardiac Morbidity 14
  ◆ Treatment 15
    Psychotherapy 15
      Countertransference 16
    Anxiolytic Pharmacotherapy 16
      Beta-Blockers 17
      Benzodiazepines 17
        Alprazolam 17
        Clonazepam 17
        Buspirone 17
    Antidepressant Pharmacotherapy 17
      Selective Serotonin Reuptake Inhibitors . . . 17
        SSRIs, isoenzymes, and secondary
          cardiovascular toxicity 17
        SSRIs and warfarin 18
        Fluoxetine 18
        Sertraline 20
        Paroxetine 20
      Miscellaneous Agents 20
        Bupropion 20
        Psychostimulants 21
    Electroconvulsive Therapy 22
      Pacemakers and ECT 23
  ◆ Summary 23
  ◆ References 24
■ Case Presentation: Mr. Smith: The Depressed,
   Post-Myocardial Infarction Patient 35
■ Questions 35
■ Answers 38
■ Discussion 39

◆ Tricyclic Antidepressants 39
  Adverse Cardiovascular Effects 39
    Conduction and Rhythm 39
      Doxepin 40
    Electrocardiogram Changes 40
    Orthostatic Hypotension 41
    Cardiotoxicity and Drug Metabolism 41
  Specific Cardiac Conditions 42
    Myocardial Infarction 42
    Heart Block 42
    Congestive Heart Failure 43
    Sick Sinus Syndrome 44
    Atrial Fibrillation 44
◆ Miscellaneous Agents 44
  Trazodone 44
  Maprotiline 44
  Amoxapine 44
◆ Monoamine Oxidase Inhibitors 44
◆ Psychiatric Side Effects of Cardiac Drugs 45
  Quinidine 45
  Lidocaine 45
  Digoxin 45
  Drug Interactions 46
◆ Summary 46
◆ References 47
■ Case Presentation: Ms. Anderson: The Manic
   Patient With Heart Disease and Hypertension . . 51
■ Questions 51
■ Answers 53
■ Discussion 54
◆ Neuroleptics and the Heart 54
  Neuroleptics and the Electrocardiogram 54
  Thioridazine 54
  Neuroleptics, Antidepressants, and the Heart . 55
◆ Antimanic Agents and the Heart 55
  Lithium 55
    Congestive Heart Failure 55
    Post–Myocardial Infarction 55
    Drug Interactions 55
      Increase cardiac toxicity 55
      Induce manic states 55
      Increase lithium toxicity 55
      Decrease lithium levels 56
  Carbamazepine 56
  Valproic Acid 56
◆ Psychological Factors Affecting Hypertension . . 56
  Antihypertensive-Induced Depressive Disorder . 57
    Reserpine, Methyldopa, and Propranolol 57
    Miscellaneous Agents 57
    Drug Interactions 58
◆ Delirium and the Cardiac Patient 58
  After Cardiotomy 58
  Intraaortic Balloon Pump 59
◆ Summary 59
◆ References 59

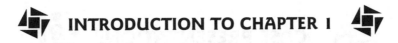

The psychosocial literature on the cardiac patient is extensive and makes for fascinating reading. Compared with the medical writings on the subject, we find this literature more easily accessible than the difficult physiological and pharmacological topics, which often fall into disuse in psychiatric practice. We feel that the latter are worth emphasis because they compose the biological underpinnings of effective psychosocial intervention in the cardiac population.

The case writeups have been intentionally simplified for this purpose. Some organizational decisions were inevitably arbitrary; for example, psychotropic side effects and drug interactions appear in this chapter because they have the most serious adverse effects on the heart. (Other side effects are discussed in the pulmonary, hepatic, and renal chapters [Chapters 2, 3, and 4, respectively].) To repeat, our aim is to highlight the medical perspective rather than aspire to the comprehensiveness of other consultation-liaison texts.[289] References are provided to the psychosocial literature, which is skimmed.

We have purposely *avoided* modeling question-and-answer strategies based on the board examinations. Instead, the questions raise issues in the literature, which the reader is encouraged to evaluate based on his or her knowledge. The questions are not intended to resemble an examination; the options present facts and, consequently, there may be more than one correct answer. The questions may be used before, after, or as a companion to reading the text.

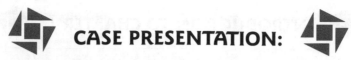

CASE PRESENTATION:
Mr. Doe: The Depressed Cardiovascular Patient

Mr. Doe is a 61-year-old patient with one previous episode of major depression while in his 20s. He has a history of ischemic heart disease and was admitted 1 week ago in congestive heart failure. Furosemide (Lasix) and nitroglycerin are his only medications. He is medically stable.

Psychiatric consultation is requested to evaluate the patient's depression. Over the past 3 weeks, his family has noted progressive loss of interest in his usual activities, pervasive sadness, hopelessness, anergy, and tearfulness.

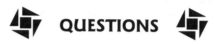

QUESTIONS

Choose all that apply.

1. The staff taking care of Mr. Doe is concerned because he has lost his appetite and does not want to eat. Which of the following are *least* helpful in diagnosing depression in *medically ill* patients?
    a. Vegetative symptoms
    b. Low self-esteem
    c. Guilt
    d. Autonomy of mood

2. Which of the following are true regarding major depression in the setting of coronary artery disease?
    a. There are *medical,* as well as psychiatric, hazards of leaving it untreated.
    b. The *most serious* adverse consequence of deferring psychopharmacological intervention is psychosocial disability.
    c. Untreated major depression *statistically* predicts additional cardiac events.
    d. It tends to be overdiagnosed.

3. The medications that have been evaluated *specifically* in the cardiovascular population include . . .
    a. Fluoxetine (Prozac).
    b. Sertraline (Zoloft).
    c. Bupropion (Wellbutrin).
    d. Paroxetine (Paxil).
    e. Psychostimulants.

4. Mrs. Doe has heard that fluoxetine (Prozac) "makes people go crazy," and does not want her husband to take it. She knows that sertraline (Zoloft) and paroxetine (Paxil) "are in the Prozac family," which further overwhelms Mr. Doe, who is upset that his cardiologist thinks he is "nuts." He asks you to leave him alone in peace to die. Electroconvulsive therapy (ECT) is "out of the question." Which of the following would be true about using psychostimulants for a patient like Mr. Doe?
    a. Psychostimulants would be effective in major depression but not for an adjustment disorder with depressed mood.
    b. They are not effective for depression accompanying medical conditions.
    c. Tolerance tends to develop early.
    d. Worsening anorexia secondary to stimulants like methylphenidate (Ritalin) is a frequent complication.
    e. The effects of psychostimulants on heart rate and blood pressure are minimal.

5. How would you advise the internist regarding psychostimulants for Mr. Doe?
    a. Their abuse potential appears to be low in medical patients.
    b. They are relatively contraindicated in elderly depressed patients.
    c. The high incidence of adverse side effects limits their usefulness for cardiovascular patients.
    d. Clinical response to the psychostimulants is rapid (usually within the first 2 days).
    e. There is a high rate of depressive relapse on these medications.

6. Which of the following are correct statements about psychostimulants in the medical setting?
    a. Dosing should be on a three-times-a-day schedule, with meals.
    b. The initial starting dose in fragile cardiovascular patients is 2.5 mg of either dextroamphetamine (Dexedrine) or methylphenidate (Ritalin).
    c. Failure to respond to the first few psychostimulant doses predicts nonresponse to higher doses.
    d. Provided that vital signs are not adversely affected, the medication should be increased until demonstrable effects are reported by the patient.

7. Many seriously ill patients cannot swallow medications. Which of the stimulants can be used in this setting?
    a. Methylphenidate (Ritalin)
    b. Dextroamphetamine (Dexedrine)
    c. Pemoline (Cylert)
    d. None of the above
    e. Choices a, b, and c are true

8. Which of the psychostimulants magnifies analgesic requirements for patients with chronic pain?
    a. Methylphenidate (Ritalin)
    b. Dextroamphetamine (Dexedrine)
    c. Pemoline (Cylert)
    d. None of the above
    e. Choices a, b, and c are true

9. Mr. Doe cannot tolerate methylphenidate because of jitteriness. He is still quite depressed. He and his family steadfastly refuse ECT. The social worker has a good alliance with Mrs. Doe, who has begun to relent a bit in her stance on fluoxetine. She's been told that it is one of the most widely prescribed antidepressants with few adverse side effects in healthy patients. What are some of the rare adverse cardiovascular effects associated with fluoxetine?
    a. Patients with adverse cardiac side effects uniformly had a prior cardiac history.
    b. Patients with adverse cardiac side effects invariably were taking more than 60 mg/day.
    c. Adverse cardiac effects have been reported almost exclusively in elderly patients.
    d. Syncope and orthostatic hypotension have not yet been reported.
    e. It may destabilize anticoagulation regimens.

10. Selective serotonin reuptake inhibitors (SSRIs) are most likely to have adverse cardiovascular effects through their impact on . . .

    a. Cytochrome P450-2D6.
    b. The HIS bundle.
    c. Sodium currents.
    d. Calcium channels.
    e. None of the above.

11. Fluoxetine (Prozac) and sertraline (Zoloft) cause Mr. Doe severe headache and gastrointestinal upset, and have to be discontinued. Paroxetine (Paxil) makes him too somnolent, even in reduced doses. Mr. Doe continues to refuse ECT, stating that he would rather find a less painful way to commit suicide. What are some of the characteristics of bupropion (Wellbutrin) that you could discuss with the cardiologist?
    a. It does not significantly affect pulse rate in cardiovascular patients.
    b. It has been associated with a decline in supine blood pressure in a majority of cardiovascular patients.
    c. The incidence of orthostatic hypotension is comparable to that with nortriptyline (Pamelor, Aventyl).
    d. It does not significantly prolong cardiac conduction in patients with preexisting bundle branch block.

12. The cardiologist is intrigued by this side-effect profile and asks, "Where's the catch?" You respond . . .
    a. Bupropion has been found to exacerbate preexisting arrhythmias.
    b. It has been associated with inducing higher degrees of atrioventricular (AV) block in patients with preexisting bundle branch block.
    c. Patients with preexisting hypertension may experience hypertensive exacerbations secondary to bupropion.
    d. The main noncardiovascular adverse effect is central nervous system (CNS) depression.

13. Mr. Doe tolerates bupropion well, but his depression does not respond. Meanwhile, he receives a permanent ventricular demand pacemaker without incident. Subsequently, his wife convinces him to try ECT. Three days before his first scheduled treatment, however, he experiences several episodes of shortness of breath, chest pain, and lightheadedness. He is extremely apprehensive that he is having a heart attack and will die momentarily. Repeated 24-hour ambulatory Holter monitoring during the episodes reveals normal sinus rhythm with minimal rate changes, ranging between 70 and 80 beats per minute. Brief periods of paced rhythm show normal

capture and sensing. Premature beats and tachyarrhythmias are absent. Mr. Doe becomes even more agitated and fearful, convinced that his pacemaker is "broken" and that the "electric shock" of ECT will further damage it; he withdraws consent for ECT "so I can die in peace." What are some of the management considerations at this point?

    a. His symptoms are probably due to erratic functioning of the pacemaker.

    b. He probably is having panic attacks.

    c. He probably is having further arrhythmic events.

    d. ECT is temporarily contraindicated in this setting.

14. You emphasize to the patient that pacemakers can withstand the electrical current used in ECT and will not damage the heart. You advise the cardiologist that:

    a. Improper grounding is the main risk of using ECT in pacemaker patients.

    b. Mr. Doe's pacemaker should be converted to fixed-mode operation during the seizure.

    c. Mr. Doe's pacemaker should be converted to demand-mode operation during the seizure.

    d. A temporary pacemaker would be substantially less risky during ECT than Mr. Doe's permanent one.

15. ECT is deferred for the time being. Mr. Doe is given clonazepam (Klonopin) 0.5 mg orally, two times a day, with rapid resolution of his panic attacks. His wife reports that he has "always been a 'hyper' guy" and that she has "learned to ignore it." What facts would be important regarding the relationship between Mr. Doe's emotional stress and potential episodes of myocardial ischemia?

    a. *Mental* stress induces more ischemic episodes than *physical* activities of daily living in coronary patients.

    b. Benzodiazepines are palliative, but are unlikely to affect physiological reactions to exercise-induced stress, such as the catecholamine response.

    c. Ischemia and ST-segment depression associated with psychological stress usually occur without pain.

    d. As long as psychological stress does not increase heart rate to exertional levels, myocardial ischemia is rare.

16. Which of the following are true regarding sudden cardiac death?

    a. Coronary artery disease and the predisposition to sudden cardiac death can be predicted by the same risk factors.

    b. Psychotherapy (*without* medication) is effective in decreasing the chances for recurrent myocardial infarction (MI).

    c. The incidence of sudden death appears to vary independently of life stressors.

    d. Untreated major depressive episodes increase the risk for sudden cardiac death.

17. The component(s) of type A behavior most highly correlated with coronary artery disease is/are

    a. Hostility

    b. Ambition

    c. Competitiveness

    d. Hard-driving behavior

    e. Time urgency

    f. Impatience

    g. Perfectionism

18. Hostility and its variants (e.g., anger, expressed and unexpressed hostility) have been positively correlated with which of the following?

    a. The extent of coronary artery disease as measured by angiography

    b. Alcohol consumption

    c. Smoking cigarettes

    d. Mortality secondary to coronary events

    e. All of the above

19. Factors that have been shown to increase the risk of developing heart disease include . . .

    a. Shift work.

    b. Monotony of work.

    c. Few growth possibilities at work.

    d. Number of children at home.

    e. All of the above.

20. Factors associated with increased mortality include all of the following *except* . . .

    a. Living alone.

    b. Widowhood.

    c. Higher educational level.

    d. Lack of social support.

21. Living alone confers an increased risk for cardiac mortality for post-MI patients. This effect has been shown to be mediated by . . .

    a. The severity of myocardial damage.

    b. The degree of ventricular ectopy.

    c. Correlations with gender.

    d. Differences in drug compliance.

    e. As-yet-undefined factors.

22. Mr. Doe finally consents to treatment with ECT with the support of his family. Which of the following are *not* associated with ECT?
    a. Hypertension
    b. Hypotension
    c. Transient tachycardia
    d. Transient bradycardia
    e. Heart block

Answers

1. Answer: a (pp. 8–9)
2. Answer: a, c (p. 8)
3. Answer: c, e (pp. 20–21)
4. Answer: e (p. 21)
5. Answer: a, d (pp. 21–22)
6. Answer: b, d (p. 22)
7. Answer: c (p. 22)
8. Answer: d (p. 21)
9. Answer: e (pp. 18–20)
10. Answer: a (pp. 17–18)
11. Answer: a, d (pp. 20–21)
12. Answer: c (pp. 20–21)
13. Answer: b (pp. 10–11)
14. Answer: a, b (pp. 22–23)
15. Answer: a, c (pp. 11, 12, 17)
16. Answer: b, d (p. 13)
17. Answer: a (pp. 11–12)
18. Answer: e (p. 12)
19. Answer: e (p. 14)
20. Answer: c (pp. 14–15)
21. Answer: e (p. 14)
22. Answer: e (pp. 22–23)

◄▲► THE PSYCHE AND CARDIAC MORBIDITY

The literature on cardiac morbidity and psychiatry is divided into several areas: 1) the repercussions of psychiatric syndromes, such as depression and anxiety disorders, on cardiac morbidity; 2) the effect of personality or coping style on cardiac morbidity; 3) the impact of acute situational disturbance on factors such as sudden death, ventricular arrhythmias, and myocardial ischemia; and 4) the consequence of sociocultural factors, such as work "overload," life stress, and interpersonal factors (e.g., social support). We will provide a brief survey.

Major Depression and Heart Disease

Most psychiatrists are wary of medicating post–myocardial infarction (MI) or other cardiac patients. We usually think in terms of the adverse effects of psychotropics on the heart; it may come as a surprise that *failure to treat psychiatric syndromes contributes to morbidity in this population.* Physiologically, one's psychological state is thought to interact with cardiovascular morbidity by affecting sympathetic and cardiovascular reactivity.[182,184] This effect is not limited to anxiety disorders but also holds true for major depression, which predicts higher morbidity regardless of cardiac status.[12,45,83] A quick glance at some data easily demonstrates the medical hazards of leaving depression untreated:

◆ Booth-Kewley and Friedman's 1987 meta-analysis[36] of several extant studies concluded that depression is related to coronary heart disease outcomes (i.e., MI, angina, cardiac death) with an effect size that was higher than even that for the type A behavior pattern. When they separately analyzed the six *prospective* studies, the strong correlational link between depression and coronary artery disease (CAD) outcome was maintained.
◆ Untreated depression has been correlated with
  • Failure to maintain modified behavior patterns learned during cardiac rehabilitation.[93]
  • Failure to return to normal functioning after the acute cardiac illness.[93]
  • Failure to comply with medical care and follow-up.[35]
  • Increased mortality after cardiac surgery.[174,301]

  • More than doubled risks of mortality secondary to cardiovascular disease.[239]
  • More frequent adverse medical events, including higher rates of mortality and morbidity.[5a,113,132a,168,269,283]
  • At least a fivefold higher mortality rate among depressed MI survivors, with the impact of depression remaining after controlling for left-ventricular dysfunction and previous depression.[100]

Finally, Carney et al.[44] found that major depression was the best predictor of major cardiac events in CAD patients, such as a second MI, death, need for angioplasty or coronary bypass surgery. This effect was independent of both cardiac and smoking status. Depressed patients are also more likely to experience ventricular tachycardia[43] and angina pectoris,[193] and have more difficulty giving up smoking[193] than do their nondepressed counterparts. Other investigators have recently corroborated the adverse impact of depressed affect and hopelessness on ischemic heart disease.[11]

*These data show that **failure to treat** may be more harmful than intervening,*[64,120,120a,253] *and this possibility creates a powerful mandate for psychiatric intervention.*

DSM-IV, Medical Illness, and the Problem of Depression

The incidence of major depression in cardiac patients has been estimated to be about 18%.[44,103,269] Despite the impressive evidence about the impact of depression on medical outcome, it is alarming that depressive disorders go largely undiagnosed in this population and therefore untreated.[100]

◆ For example, one study showed that for a cohort meeting criteria for depression, only 20% had been identified as depressed before the study.[44,46]
◆ Another study showed that a mere 10% of depressed MI patients had received psychiatric treatment.[269]

In a recent editorial, Williams and Chesney[316] called for more aggressive behavioral interventions and psychopharmacological treatment for post-MI patients.

Unfortunately, this raises the issue of accurate psychiatric diagnosis in medical patients.[104,215] Difficulties include

- The effects of impaired cognitive functioning[250]
- The assumption that depression is a "normal" and appropriate response to a life-threatening illness, rather than a distinct syndrome
- The prominence of realistic threats during recovery[28,267]
- The ambiguous significance of vegetative symptoms (e.g., weight loss, fatigue, weakness, anorexia) as discriminators of major depression versus the physical illness and its treatments[159]

Scales like the Beck Depression Inventory[24] and the Hamilton Depression Rating Scale[126] are not particularly useful for diagnosing depression in medically ill people.[159] The 1994 publication of DSM-IV[8] allowed greater specificity in describing psychiatric symptomatology in the setting of medical illness, but still did not clarify the problem of diagnosing depression in the medically ill. (See Appendix A, "A Consultation-Liaison Guide to DSM-IV.")

Over the years, several writers have offered suggestions for modifying the criteria for depression in the medically ill. Two of these recommendations follow:

1. More than 10 years ago, Endicott[81] advised substituting the following for the "classic" vegetative symptoms (e.g., change in appetite or weight, sleep disturbances, fatigue or loss of energy, diminished ability to think or concentrate, or indecisiveness):
   - *Tearfulness/depressed appearance*
   - *Social withdrawal/decreased talkativeness*
   - *Brooding/self-pity/pessimism*
   - *Lack of reactivity to environmental events*

   Although this approach is controversial,[54] others have found it helpful.[159,243]

2. More recently, Cavanaugh[51] suggested additional criteria that would render the DSM-IV diagnosis of major depression more useful for medically ill individuals:
   - Hopelessness, helplessness, not caring any more
   - Loss of interest, particularly in people
   - Feeling bad about oneself, not the situation; feeling that illness is a punishment for wrongdoing
   - Diminished ability to think or concentrate not easily explained by delirium, dementia, physical illness, or treatments
   - Recurrent thoughts of death not related to wishing to be dead to end physical suffering, but temporally related to affective and cognitive symptoms of depression
   - Vegetative changes (significant weight, sleep, and/or appetite changes; anergia) not easily explained by physical illness, treatments, or hospital environment
   - Psychomotor agitation or retardation not easily explainable by delirium, dementia, physical illness, or treatments
   - Assessment of patient's sphere of functioning extended to include participation in medical care. Patient is not participating in medical care in spite of his or her ability to do so, is not progressing despite improved medical condition, and/or is functioning at a lower level than the medical condition warrants.

Farewell "organic versus functional." A glance at Appendix A shows that several DSM-III-R[7] terms—organic delusional disorder, organic hallucinosis, organic mood disorder, organic anxiety disorder, and organic personality disorder—have been eliminated in DSM-IV. Two new general categories allow the clinician to specify whether the disorder is due to a general medical condition or is induced by a substance (e.g., medication). The conceptualization of mental illness as "organic versus functional" has become obsolete:

> [The DSM-III-R] differentiation of "organic" mental disorders as a separate class implied that "nonorganic" or "functional" mental disorders were somehow unrelated to physical or biological factors or processes. DSM-IV eliminates the term *organic* and distinguishes those mental disorders that are due to a general medical condition from those that are substance induced and those that have no specified etiology. The term *primary mental disorder* is used as a shorthand to indicate those mental disorders that are not due to a general medical condition and that are not substance induced.[8] (p. 165)

Most of the research presented in this book used previous editions of the DSM. For consistency, we will report the diagnostic terminology as it appeared in the literature, and offer DSM-IV alternatives when appropriate.[287a,289b]

Anxiety Disorders and Heart Disease

Chest pain is one of the most frequent chief complaints at medical clinics, with the medical workup often negative.[187] As many as 30% of patients with chest pain simulating CAD are found to have normal coronary arteries.[195] The data on these patients are intriguing:

- They have high rates of generalized anxiety[201] and panic disorder.[23,25,47,53,62,160,224,251,320]
- They are more likely to have first-degree relatives with panic disorder than are normal (i.e., no panic disorder, no CAD) control subjects.[190]
- Those patients with chest pain as a symptom of panic disorder demonstrate significant psychosocial disability.[26]

Fortunately, it appears that panic disorder patients *with* cardiac symptoms are no more likely to have cardiac disease than those *without* prominent cardiac symptoms.[149,161] In addition to simulating symptoms of CAD, panic disorder does also occur in patients with documented heart disease:[155]

- In patients with angiographically proven CAD, 6% also had a diagnosis of panic disorder.[162]
- Approximately 6% of patients in a cardiology practice were found to have panic disorder, with 40%–60% of these patients also suffering from ischemic heart disease.[119]
- One study[119] described two types of panic disorder in cardiac outpatients. *Long-duration panic disorder* generally predated the cardiac illness, occurred before age 30, and followed a chronic course. *Short-duration panic disorder* was associated with the onset of cardiac disease and was posited to be either a misinterpretation of cardiac symptoms or a form of anxiety response to the threat of cardiac illness. (*Duration* referred to the course of the disorder, not to the length of individual panic episodes.)
- Grafing et al.[121] reported a case of CAD associated with continuing chest pain that was not responsive to antianginal therapy; improvement occurred when the patient was treated with clonazepam for a presumptive diagnosis of panic disorder.
- Carter et al.[48] found that panic disorder was quite common in a sample of chest pain patients referred for cardiac workup who had no previously documented CAD. (More than half of the patients had panic disorder, while only a minority had objective signs of heart disease.)

The prospective study by Kawachi et al.[166] showed that the risk of fatal coronary heart disease (and the risk of sudden cardiac death) had a strong association with the level of "phobic anxiety" (as measured by a standard questionnaire).

A vicious cycle may ensue of panic episodes eliciting ischemic pain, which then intensifies anxiety and leads to further panic attacks.[161] In cardiac patients for whom tricyclics are contraindicated or not well tolerated, benzodiazepines are the medications of choice for panic disorder.[161] We discuss treatment at greater length below.

Note that posttraumatic stress disorder (PTSD)–like reactions may be an underrecognized problem for some individuals who sustain an MI or undergo coronary artery bypass surgery.[73,302b]

Mitral Valve Prolapse

Also impressive are the results of Coplan et al.,[61] which showed improved mitral valve prolapse on echocardiogram after patients were successfully treated for panic disorder. (Treatments were a heterogeneous combination of benzodiazepines, tricyclic antidepressants [TCAs], and monoamine oxidase inhibitors [MAOIs].) Mitral valve prolapse patients without psychiatric disorder served as a comparison group. The authors concluded that the prolapse associated with panic disorder may result from autonomic overdrive, leading to temporary deformation in the mitral valve or desynchrony in ventricular contraction. They posited that antipanic treatment may attenuate autonomic overdrive, and thus ameliorate prolapse.

Chronic Chest Pain of Unknown Etiology

Even more perplexing is the patient with chronic chest pain not explained by either cardiac disease or panic disorder.[22,51a,213a] Bradley and colleagues[37] noted the importance of psychosocial factors on the pain behavior of these patients (i.e., pain-coping strategies, the spouse's responses to the patient's pain behaviors, pain thresholds, and the like). These findings imply that psychological variables may potentially differentiate chronic chest pain patients from healthy control subjects or those with other chronic pain disorders. For example, Kisely et al.[176] found that patients with nonspecific chest pain experienced significantly more psychiatric disorders than those with ischemic heart disease. Imipramine (Tofranil) in low doses (25–50 mg) has been found to reduce the frequency of chest pain in some patients with angina-like chest pain and normal coronary angiograms.[42]

The Pacemaker Syndrome Versus Panic Disorder

The *pacemaker syndrome* is in the differential diagnosis of panic-like symptoms occurring in pacemaker patients. Patients with this syndrome present with postural hypotension, dizziness, syncope, dyspnea, chest pain, neck pulsations, lassitude, and weakness.[169]

- The symptoms are attributable to a loss of atrial contribution to ventricular systole; a vasodepressor reflex initiated by atrial contractions against a closed tricuspid valve; and systemic and pulmonary venous regurgitation due to atrial contraction against a closed atrioventricular (AV) valve.[151] Sinus activity and atrial contraction occur at the same time as ventricular pacing and ventricular contraction, producing symptoms and requiring adjustments in the programming of the pacemaker.

◆ Low cardiac output produces lightheadedness, lethargy, hypotension, diaphoresis, apprehension, and palpitations.[14,222]

The diagnosis is made by correlating symptoms with abnormal findings on Holter monitoring. *There is considerable overlap between symptoms of the pacemaker syndrome and panic disorder.*

◆ For example, a 29-year-old woman received a ventricular demand pacemaker for autonomic hyperactivity with secondary carotid sinus hypersensitivity and later developed symptoms misattributed to pacemaker syndrome.[237] Repeated Holter monitoring was normal, however, like Mr. Doe's. There was no correlation between her symptoms and pacemaker activation or dysfunction. The patient nevertheless secluded herself in her home, fearing an attack in public, and was convinced that her spells were of cardiac origin. The psychiatric consultant made the diagnosis of panic disorder with agoraphobia. Clonazepam 1 mg orally three times a day rapidly eliminated her symptoms. Psychotherapy was aimed at cognitive redirection of the anxiety-provoking events that had resulted in her panic attacks. The authors summarized evidence for the theory that panic may be triggered by a phobic reaction to real or imagined unpleasant internal bodily sensations.[237] For example, panic can be induced in anxiety-prone patients (but not in anxiety-free individuals) by convincing them that they are experiencing an abrupt increase in heart rate, when in fact none has occurred.[79]

The lack of temporal association between Mr. Doe's subjective symptoms and documentable cardiovascular abnormalities argues against a diagnosis of pacemaker syndrome and in favor of panic disorder.

"Things That Go Bang in the Night"

There is a growing literature on the adverse psychological effects of implantable cardioverter-defibrillators (ICDs) in patients who have malignant ventricular arrhythmias.[60,75,105,153,171,181,204,205,303] These reactions have been described as anxiety, depression, and severe sleep disorders, including phantom shocks that occur at night without evidence of ICD discharge.

Heart and Mind

Stress and Ischemia

Ischemia occurs when myocardial oxygen demands exceed the capacity of diseased coronary arteries to deliver blood, or when coronary vasoconstriction critically impairs blood flow to certain cardiac areas.[82] The role of mental stress in myocardial ischemia is well recognized.[66,130,228,272] The growing literature on the repercussions of psychological phenomena on cardiac functioning is sobering.[68b,116,117,120b,140a,166a,184,195a,214,235,263,280,282,323] For example:

◆ Barry et al.[19] followed the daily activities of coronary patients and found ST-segment depressions during *most* activities (i.e., sleep, reading, watching television, work, relaxation, and mental stress). Remarkably, after correcting for the amount of time per day spent in each activity, *intervals of **mental stress** demonstrated the **highest** concentration of ischemic episodes.*

Additional highlights follow.

Hostility and Type A

The type A behavior pattern is an action-emotion complex elicited by certain environmental events. It includes

◆ Impatience
◆ Aggressiveness
◆ An intense achievement drive
◆ A sense of time urgency
◆ A desire for recognition and advancement

Type A behavior is fostered by Western culture,[191] which rewards those who can think, perform, and communicate more aggressively than their peers.[258] The type B behavior pattern is described as type A's opposite.[107]

Not all components of type A behavior have been equally associated with coronary risk. Measuring global type A behavior patterns has been replaced by identifying the specific components that are most strongly associated with heart disease. *Hostility* and *anger*—particularly when unexpressed—appear to have more robust correlations to increased cardiovascular risk than do competitiveness, excessive drive, and time urgency.[67,70,137,208,213,217a,219,295a,315] Anger and hostility may trigger malignant arrhythmias[97,122,152,233,247,296] and ischemia,[130] and also predict mortality. Moreover, subsets of individuals may have specific vulnerabilities to psychological stress or physiological propensities to arrhythmia.[246]

◆ Three prospective studies found that hostility (as measured by the Cook-Medley Hostility Inventory[59]) was predictive of CAD.[15,16,273] This inventory, which is derived from the Minnesota Multiphasic Personality Inventory (MMPI),[126a] aims at assessing suspiciousness, resentment, frequent anger, and cynical mistrust of others (rather than overtly aggressive behavior or general emotional distress).[279] Individuals with high scores are less hardy, display more anger, experience more frequent and severe "hassles," and have fewer psychological supports.[279]

◆ Almada et al.[6] found that an MMPI-derived cynicism scale predicted coronary death and total mortality. They also noted that increased hostility was related to more cigarette smoking and alcohol consumption, which also may contribute to heightened mortality.

◆ The "potential for hostility" is a behavioral rating derived from the Structured Interview,[257] an instrument that uses a trained interviewer to ask questions in a deliberately challenging manner so as to elicit type A behaviors. It measures thought content, facial expressions, gestures, and speech characteristics. A high "potential for hostility" rating is reflected in hostile content of the respondent's answers, assays intensity of hostile responses, and shows a hostile style of interaction with the interviewer.[71] Several studies showed that the potential for hostility correlated with cardiovascular disease *independently* of other risk factors.[70,128,179,206,208,212]

◆ An inner sense of insecurity[238b] may underlie the time urgency and hostility characteristic of type A behavior.

The mechanism for hostility's impact on cardiovascular disease is not yet precisely known. Musante and colleagues[226] found that measures of hostility were positively correlated to animal fat intake in women, cigarette smoking and sugar intake in men, and cholesterol intake and vigorous physical activity in both. Hostility may be mediated through other risk behaviors, such as smoking or alcohol consumption. It has also been associated with certain demographic factors, such as low socioeconomic status, nonwhite race, male gender, and low level of education.[18,268] Finally, hostility and anger probably produces repeated and excessive activation of neuroendocrine and cardiovascular responses that predispose to cardiac disease.[17,69,118,182,184,185,208,278,294,309]

◆ One classic study[297] reported a moderate correlation ($r = .40$) between life stress and catecholamines in patients with severe coronary heart disease. Increases in life stress were associated with myocardial ischemia, experienced as anginal pain.

◆ Ironson and colleagues[139] examined the comparative potency of psychological stressors versus exercise in eliciting myocardial ischemia. Twenty-seven subjects underwent both exertional (bicycling) and psychological stressors (e.g., performing mental arithmetic, recalling an incident that elicited anger, giving a short speech defending oneself against a charge of shoplifting). *Anger recall impaired ejection fraction more than did exertion or the other psychological stressors*—further evidence of this affect's power to induce myocardial ischemia.

◆ Dracup et al.[76] studied a group of 134 patients with symptoms of advanced heart failure. They found that self-reported functional status, depression, and hostility significantly influenced patients' psychosocial adjustment to illness. Several *objective* measures of cardiac function significantly correlated with *subjective* psychosocial adjustment.

Stress and Painless (Silent) Ischemia

Anginal pain is frightening and disruptive, but signals that "something is wrong" and prompts intervention. Unfortunately, not all myocardial ischemia triggers pain. *Silent myocardial ischemia* is defined as ST-segment depression in the absence of anginal chest pain. It is a dangerous phenomenon, conferring an increased risk of coronary events, such as sudden death or MI.[271]

◆ *At least 75% of patients with known coronary disease have episodes of ischemia, and most of these episodes are without warning and* **silent.**[120b,183,262,317] Disturbingly, these events occur at mundane times, such as during one's usual daily activities.[271] Patients who experience silent ischemic episodes may also have reduced sensitivity to pain and other bodily sensations.[102]

◆ Myocardial ischemia secondary to mental stress occurs at much *lower* heart rates than exertional (exercise-induced) ischemia in CAD patients,[262,317] with personally relevant mental stress (such as public speaking) most likely to provoke ischemia.

◆ Denial appears to variably influence the occurrence of silent ischemia.[20,21,141–143,170,249,314]

The progression of atherosclerosis and CAD relative to psychological stress is hypothetically mediated by sympathetic nervous system activation.[185,207,208] Despite the dearth of well-designed human studies,[173,265] the indirect data linking psychological states and cardiovascular disease are disconcertingly consistent.[172,191]

Comment: the therapist's dilemma. Think about the implications of these findings: *Cardiac inpatients or outpatients are at ongoing physiological risk from their emotional states whether or not they are alerted by chest pain.* This poses a dilemma for psychotherapists. Although the more structured cognitive/behavioral techniques are the most researched in this population, many cardiac outpatients benefit from exploring issues of self-esteem, relationships, sexuality, and the ubiquitous tension between fantasy and fact. How does the therapist help the patient titrate the anxiety that inevitably arises in insight-oriented therapy, given that it may have silent, physiological effects? Are patients with cardiac illness to be disqualified from an insight-oriented approach? Clearly, chest pain is unreliable in signaling that the material is—psychologically and physiologically—"too much." However, a laissez faire, "do nothing" approach that skims the psychological surface of an anguished patient or produces pharmacological passivity is no answer, either. As reviewed earlier, "benign neglect" of psychological disorders is risky, exposing cardiac patients to physiological peril and predisposing to further morbidity and mortality.

As always, gauging the appropriate level of a psychiatric intervention is partly science, often art—largely a matter of clinical judgment regarding dosing, timing, and tact. When intense emotional content emerges in psychotherapy, it must be thoughtfully managed with an eye on the cardiophysiological effects of discussing or not discussing it. Adding anxiolytic medication or behavioral relaxation strategies may buffer some of the physiological impact, allowing the therapy to progress more safely.

Sudden Cardiac Death

Sudden cardiac death accounts for one-half to one-third of all deaths from CAD, and is estimated to cause 400,000 deaths per year in the United States.[57] *Disturbingly, the classic risk factors for CAD (hypertension, smoking, and hypercholesterolemia) do not identify those at risk for sudden cardiac death.*[189] Its course and precipitants remain difficult to define.

◆ Sudden cardiac death may be the first and only manifestation of heart disease, sometimes accompanied by few acute pathomorphological changes and without obvious pathological cardiac lesions.[98]

◆ The definitive trigger is unknown, nor is sudden cardiac death correlated with activity or physical exertion.[98]

◆ There is evidence that left ventricular dysfunction, frequent ventricular ectopic activity, nonsustained ventricular tachycardia, and late potentials may be markers for increased risk.[275]

A correlation between sudden death and acute, disturbing life events has been established by several authors.[74,106,122,154,227,247,277,296] For example:

◆ Marked elevations in life stresses were found during the 6 months before sudden cardiac death, compared with the same interval 1 year earlier.[241]

◆ Emotional triggers have been identified as precipitating malignant ventricular arrhythmias.[247]

◆ Stress-induced sympathetic arousal is arrhythmogenic in patients with the long-QT syndrome (a condition that increases vulnerability to malignant arrhythmias).[270]

◆ Distress during hospitalization for MI has been correlated with ventricular arrhythmias on ambulatory electrocardiogram (ECG) during the subsequent year.[97]

◆ Experimentally induced stress increased the number of ventricular premature beats, as well as lowered thresholds for ventricular fibrillation, in patients with preexisting ventricular arrhythmias.[203,296]

Although these results are compelling, the literature is not without its inconsistencies.

◆ For example, a 1990 study conducted by Follick et al.[96] in a sample of post-MI patients found no significant relationship between psychological measures and ventricular arrhythmias assessed at 3, 6, and 13 months after entry into the study.

There are few studies[97] that prospectively operationalize the measurement of psychological precipitants relative to ventricular arrhythmias or sudden death. Several model mechanisms have been proposed. In Lown's[202] model, ventricular electrical instability, psychological states (e.g., depression, type A behavior pattern), and trigger events (e.g., emotional incidents, automobile driving) interact to produce the malignant arrhythmia. Kamarck and Jennings[154] propose that psychological and autonomic activation induce sudden death by promoting CAD (e.g., atherosclerosis); by influencing factors such as coronary vasospasm, platelet aggregation, and plaque rupture; and by directly triggering lethal arrhythmias.

Lachar[191] has written,

> [The current evidence] suggests that coronary-prone behavior is a reality and that behavioral and psychosocial factors are demonstrably related to CHD [coronary heart disease]. The coronary-prone patient is no longer conceptualized as the achievement-oriented, overburdened workaholic. Instead, coronary-prone behavior appears to include physiological and emotional reactivity to challenging situations. This reactivity appears to be associated with anger, cynicism, mistrust, and suppressed or expressed hostility. These behavioral characteristics may now be considered potent psychosocial risk factors for CHD, but more research is recommended to extend results to females and to additional ethnic and racial populations. (p. 149)

Job Strain and the Heart

The "job strain" model of coronary risk was proposed by Karasek et al.[157,158] to describe high-risk occupations marked by very demanding work with few opportunities to control the job situation. Several cross-sectional and prospective studies support the correlation between job strain and risk of CAD.[4,5,127,147,157,192] Factors such as shift work, monotony, hectic pace, few growth possibilities, and low social support positively correlate with the risk of developing heart disease. Self-reported incapacity to relax after work was also associated with an increased risk of ischemic heart disease.[293]

♦ A finding relevant to the growing number of two-income families was that employed women with three or more children are twice as likely to develop coronary heart disease as working women with no children—especially clerical workers with less child-care help.[127]

More research is needed into cardiac illness and risk factors for women.[79a]

Social Support and Cardiac Morbidity

Finally, many studies[264] (but not all[29,217]) have found that low levels of social support appear to increase the risk for CAD events by interacting with life stress, job strain, and components of type A behavior pattern.

♦ For example, type A subjects with low levels of social support suffered more severe CAD than type A subjects with high levels of social support; type B subjects showed no such relationship.[32]

♦ A 10-year prospective study of 150 middle-aged Swedish men found that lack of social support or social isolation independently predicted mortality in type A but not type B men—suggesting that social support confers some protective effect in individuals with the type A personality pattern.[234]

♦ Five large prospective studies have shown that a poor social network is associated with an unexplained, several-fold increase of all-cause mortality,[30,58,136,299,312] and for cardiac mortality in a postinfarction population.[264] Previous studies had also noted an inverse relationship between the number of persons in the household and all-cause mortality in a general population,[312] and a higher all-cause mortality in widowed individuals who live alone.[131]

♦ In a prospective study by Case et al.[49] of social integration and subsequent morbidity, it was found that living alone predicted a recurrent major cardiac event *independently* of educational level, severity of myocardial damage, degree of ventricular ectopy, gender, drug compliance, beta-blocker therapy, subsequent angioplasty, or bypass grafting. (Disrupted marriage was not found to be an independent risk factor.) The recurrent cardiac event and death rates were much lower in those living with others, leading the authors to suggest that this condition provides a protective effect. The mechanism is unclear; it may be as simple as quicker availability of medical assistance or as complex as neurohumoral responses to human contact.[136]

♦ Gerin et al.[115] postulated that social support modulates cardiovascular reactivity, which in turn influences heart disease and hypertension. They conducted an experiment in which each of 40 subjects was verbally attacked in a discussion of a controversial issue. In each session, one subject and three confederates participated. Two of the confederates argued with the subject; in half the groups, a third confederate defended the subject's position (social support condition); in the other half, the third confederate sat quietly (no-support condition). Subjects in the social support condition showed significantly smaller increases in cardiovascular measures (blood pressure, heart rate) than those in the no-support condition.

♦ Hedblad et al.[129] studied the influence of psychosocial factors, such as social network and social support, on the cardiac event rate in 98 men with one or more episodes of ischemic-type ST-segment depression. A higher risk was found among men with less emotional support. Moreover, this association held *independently* of previous ischemic heart disease or other known risk factors for MI.

◆ Never underestimate the importance of including families as partners in cardiac health care.[132,175,188] Fleury[95] found that the social network could inhibit desired behavioral change for cardiac rehabilitation subjects. Expectably, doubt and discouragement from social network members "caused patients to question their ability to successfully manage the change process . . . . [This] often decreased the individual's sense of autonomy and responsibility in sustaining lifestyle change. Patients did not feel empowered to create self-determined performance criteria and explore alternatives to achieving desired health outcomes" (p. 142).

The interested reader should refer to several other reviews of this fascinating literature.[98,120,120a,154,223,230,230a]

⚜ TREATMENT

Type A counseling significantly reduces factors such as hostility, time urgency, and impatience, as well as depression and anger, while increasing social support and well-being.[220] Psychotherapy is helpful in dealing with these[34] and other issues such as sexuality[255a] in cardiac patients. Most of the literature on psychotherapy describes interventions to modify type A behavior, based on the premise that these behaviors heighten cardiovascular and neuroendocrine reactivity.

Psychotherapy

Interventions aimed at modifying type A behavior have been the most widely studied psychotherapeutic approach in cardiac patients. They have been quite effective in reducing self-reported[146,261] and overt[33] type A behaviors, as well as improving medical outcome.[245,260,295] Some specifics follow:

◆ Nunes et al.[231] conducted a meta-analysis of 18 controlled studies on the psychological treatment of type A behavior. Treatments reduced type A behavior by about half a standard deviation—a substantial effect compared with the psychiatric treatment intervention literature as a whole. There was only a mar-

ginally significant treatment effect on coronary events and mortality at 1 year. In contrast, two of the studies that collected 3-year follow-up data reported a 50% reduction in coronary events.

◆ The work of Friedman et al.[108–110] has shown that post-MI patients who received counseling for type A behavior in addition to cardiac counseling had a 44% lower MI recurrence rate after 3 years than did those receiving cardiac counseling alone. (The cardiac counseling consisted of instruction regarding regimens for medication, diet, and exercise.) The protective effects of type A counseling endured after 4.5 years.

◆ High stress *without* psychosocial intervention produced an almost *threefold* increased cardiac mortality over 5 years and an approximately 1.5-fold increased risk of reinfarction over the same period. A group of highly stressed patients who took part in a 1-year program of stress monitoring and intervention did not show the same risk for reinfarction.[99] These data extended the results of a previous study,[101] which showed that a stress-reduction intervention group had a 47% lower mortality rate over the first post-MI year, and a 70% lower mortality rate for the initial 4 months after discharge.

The techniques of type A counseling, which are based on cognitive and behavioral strategies, would compose a book in themselves. The work of Roskies[259] is particularly detailed and helpful. Excerpts (pp. 52–53) of her operational objectives and program structure are shown in Table 1–1; interested readers should examine the original volume.[259]

We could find no controlled studies comparing type A counseling with other forms of psychotherapy. It appears that general psychological interventions that were not specifically geared toward modifying type A behavior have also been variably effective, including group[2,138,221,232,242] and individual[123,194,298] psychotherapy. However, the cognitive-behavioral, "stress management" approach has become the standard for cardiac rehabilitation.[27,180,300,302a] It is the most carefully studied technique in this population and appears highly effective.

Countertransference. As will be discussed in subsequent chapters, countertransference reactions on the part of the psychiatrist, cardiologist, and staff may interfere with appropriate management. Sometimes such reactions inadvertently provoke the patient. Levenson[198] has written,

Physicians old enough to be at risk for coronary disease will tend to identify with some of their cardiac patients. Although this could potentially enhance their ability to empathize with patients, it may instead lead them to distance themselves. If patients are very frightened by their heart disease, physicians may withdraw to avoid their own resonant anxiety. If patients are strong deniers, physicians unconsciously worried about their own mortality may collude in the denial, distancing themselves not only from the patients but from the disease as well. (p. 541)

Countertransference reactions to cardiac illness are by no means limited to physicians with gray hair:

Younger physicians are more likely to err in the other direction. Enthusiastically launching an attack on risk factors, they may become almost messianic in their approach to the patient. Concerned over some patients' denial of illness, they may try to directly overcome their defenses. Benevolently, even feeling morally obligated to do

so, the physician may attempt to "reason with" (i.e., scare) the patient by reciting a litany of disastrous consequences if the patient will not stop smoking, lose weight, and so on. This usually increases the patient's anxiety, in turn increasing the need to deny illness. Frustrated, the physician may then become angry, communicating (sometimes nonverbally) to the patient that the disease is self-induced, the result of an indulgent, undisciplined, self-destructive lifestyle.[198] (p. 542)

We discuss countertransference in more detail in Chapter 9.

Anxiolytic Pharmacotherapy

It is important to allow patients to verbalize their concerns without necessarily "jumping" to a medication. Be sure to assess the patient's need for control; some will resist taking medications, particularly antianxiety medications, because they fear losing control.[240]

◆   One patient's anxiety was actually increased by the recommendation of diazepam.[276] (The patient was

---

Table 1–1.   Roskies' techniques for type A counseling

Operational Objectives
1. Increased *awareness* of the many levels—physiological, behavioral, emotional, and cognitive—and of the many situations in which dysfunctional responses are occurring.
2. *Acquisition* of multiple new coping strategies—via learning of new coping techniques and mobilization of existing ones—for evaluating and responding to potential stressors.
3. Ability to *evaluate* the effect of different coping strategies on mental and physical well-being.
4. Repeated *practice* of new coping patterns in an ever-widening variety of situations until these new patterns themselves become habitual.

Program Structure
1. Introduction to the program
2. *Relax:* Learning to control physical stress responses. Skills taught: self-monitoring of physical and emotional tension signs; progressive muscular relaxation.

3. *Control yourself:* Learning to control behavioral stress responses. Skills taught: self-monitoring of behavioral signs of tension; incompatible behaviors; delay; communication skills.
4. *Think productively:* Learning to control cognitive stress responses. Skills taught: self-monitoring of self-talk; cognitive restructuring.
5. *Be prepared:* Learning to anticipate and plan for predictable stress situations. Skills taught: identification of recurrent stress triggers; stress inoculation training.
6. *Cool it:* Learning emergency braking in unpredictable stress situations. Skills taught: identification of signs of heightened tension; application of physical, behavioral, and cognitive controls; anger control.
7. *Building stress resistance:* Learning to plan for rest and recuperation. Skills taught: identification of pleasurable activities; problem solving.
8. *Protect your investment:* Stress management as a lifelong investment. Skills taught: relapse prevention.

Source.   Adapted from Roskies[259], pp. 52–53.

being admitted to the coronary care unit with severe chest pain, tachycardia, and fears about dying.) The patient thought that an anxiolytic would diminish his ability to cope with life-threatening events, and refused any medication.

Beta-Blockers

Beta-blockers such as propranolol should *not* be used as antianxiety agents in patients with congestive heart failure (CHF), because they decrease cardiac contractility and worsen failure.

Benzodiazepines

Benzodiazepines play an important role in reducing morbidity in coronary patients. Williams[317] has emphasized that the potential clinical benefits of benzodiazepines in this population may derive not only from their nonspecific anxiolytic effects but also by muting direct *physiological* responses to stress.

Alprazolam.   For example, alprazolam (Xanax) produces more than symptomatic relief; it *physiologically* mitigates the effects of the stress response:

◆ Alprazolam decreases the usual catecholamine responses that occur during exertional stress,[291,304] producing a 70% reduction in silent ischemia duration in a small sample of coronary patients.[274]

◆ The mechanism of alprazolam's effects—whether due to reduced stress hormone levels, to the drug's anti–platelet activating factor action,[178] or to increased parasympathetic tone—remains unknown.

◆ The addition of alprazolam to propranolol therapy may improve anginal relief among patients with symptomatic coronary disease.[218]

Alprazolam is well tolerated, is unassociated with orthostatic hypotension or anticholinergic side effects, and does not cause increased heart rate, blood pressure, or decreased cardiac vagal tone in subjects with generalized anxiety disorder.[150,216] Disadvantages include short duration of action, interdose rebound anxiety, and difficulties with withdrawal.[186] Patients must be warned not to skip doses and may require a gradual withdrawal regimen using clonazepam (Klonopin) in order to end treatment.[236]

◆ It is unclear whether alprazolam's effects on the catecholamine stress response are unique. Most consultation-liaison authors advise using lorazepam (Ativan) or oxazepam (Serax) in the medical setting, as

will be extensively reviewed later. These medications are well tolerated, have no active metabolites, and may be administered parenterally (lorazepam). Alprazolam still has a following, however, among psychiatrists treating oncological and human immunodeficiency virus (HIV)–infected patients[88,133,211,244] because of its combined antidepressant and anxiolytic properties.[307]

Clonazepam.   Recently, a case report of coexisting panic disorder and CAD documented significant relief with clonazepam of chest pain that had been unresponsive to antianginal therapy.[121] The patient was a 61-year-old woman with a 4-year history of stable CAD who complained of as many as six chest pain episodes per week over 6 months. In addition, the patient was experiencing episodes of dizziness, numbness and tingling, fear of dying, nausea, and tachycardia. When given a double-blind crossover trial of placebo and clonazepam (Klonopin), her chest pain and panic symptoms disappeared on 2.5 mg/day of clonazepam.

Buspirone.   Buspirone (BuSpar) was recently found to be effective in an open-label, 8-week trial of 10 middle-aged men with CAD, without Axis I mental disorder, but with type A behavior pattern.[200] Patients ingested an average of 42 mg/day without adverse cardiac effects. Measures such as time urgency, anxiety, and perceived stress were significantly reduced; hostility was reduced on some—but not all—assessment scales. Although these are promising results, placebo-controlled, double-blind studies are needed to corroborate these findings.

Antidepressant Pharmacotherapy

Selective Serotonin Reuptake Inhibitors

The selective serotonin reuptake inhibitors (SSRIs) are now the first-line agents prescribed by psychiatrists, internists, and cardiologists for depression in cardiac patients.[86,287a] So far, early clinical experience with these medications has been favorable,[137a] with only few cases of cardiovascular complications. However, we await controlled clinical trials with appropriate cardiovascular monitoring before calling any agent "safer" in patients with preexisting cardiac disease (see Appendix O).

SSRIs, isoenzymes, and secondary cardiovascular toxicity.   Most relevant to the issue of cardiotoxicity and the SSRIs, however, have been the findings regarding SSRIs and cytochromes.[289a] Cytochromes are a group of hepatic enzymes that are important in oxidative drug metabolism. Several subgroups (isoenzymes) of cytochrome P450 have been identified; two of them—cytochrome P450-2D6 and cytochrome P450-3A4—may be inhibited by medications commonly used in both psychiatric and medical practice. Table 1–2 is an abridged adaptation of a recent article by Stoudemire and Fogel,[289a] which detailed the relevance of the isoenzyme research to the practice of psychopharmacology in medical patients.

Several crucial points should be noted:

◆ The SSRIs are potent inhibitors of cytochrome P450-2D6 and, to a lesser degree, of cytochrome P450-3A4.

◆ Most psychotropics (including the potentially cardiotoxic tricyclic antidepressants) and many cardiac medications (several antiarrhythmics and beta-blockers) are metabolized by these isoenzymes.

◆ "Poor metabolizers" (i.e., enzyme-deficient patients) are at risk for heightened toxicity, particularly if enzyme activity is further inhibited (e.g., by adding an SSRI to an antiarrhythmic agent or a tricyclic antidepressant).

◆ "Extensive metabolizers" (i.e., individuals who have normal enzyme activity) may be pharmacologically "converted" to poor metabolizers by medications that inhibit cytochrome P450-2D6.

◆ *Most sanguine reports on the SSRIs' freedom from direct cardiovascular toxicity neglect this mode of potential secondary toxicity.*

SSRIs and warfarin.   Variable reports have appeared regarding the impact of SSRIs on anticoagulant control when they are added to previously stable regimens of warfarin (Coumadin).[26a,55,126a,317a,319] The exact mechanism is unclear. Conservative practice would be to monitor clotting parameters (e.g., prothrombin time [PT] and partial thromboplastin time [PTT]) for patients receiving an SSRI on warfarin.

Fluoxetine.   Fluoxetine (Prozac) continues to have a very favorable cardiac side-effect profile: a 1993 tally of *all* cardiovascular events contained in Lilly Research Laboratories' Table of Spontaneous Reports of Adverse postmarketing Events was remarkably low, at 0.04%. In medically healthy individuals, fluoxetine causes mild slowing of heart rate with no significant changes in PR and QRS intervals.[94]

◆ For example, fluoxetine was used safely in a 56-year-old man with a history of several overdose attempts on tricyclics and ECG abnormalities on trazodone (bigeminy, multifocal premature ventricular contrac-

tions [PVCs]) that persisted even after discontinuing trazodone.[321] He also had short episodes of ventricular tachycardia on Holter monitoring. He tolerated fluoxetine well and was without Holter monitor changes, although doses were not specified. Procainamide was eventually started to control the patient's underlying arrhythmias.

However, fluoxetine has not yet been *systematically* tested in patients with cardiovascular disease; individuals with unstable heart disease or recent MI were excluded from the clinical trials. Several case reports indicate that adverse cardiovascular effects—although infrequent—*cannot* be predicted by age, dose, or cardiac history.

◆ A 54-year-old woman with no prior personal or family history of heart disease presented to the emergency department complaining of dizziness, a sensation of pressure in her throat, and shortness of breath.[112] She was 3 weeks into a course of fluoxetine 20 mg/day, with estrogen replacement therapy her only other medication. The symptoms had appeared suddenly 1½ hours earlier and had progressively worsened. ECG showed supraventricular tachycardia at a rate of approximately 200. Her blood pressure was 98/60 mg Hg. Thyroid panel was negative. Fluoxetine was discontinued, a 6-week course of verapamil (Calan) was started, and she remained free of all cardiac symptoms in the subsequent 25 months.

◆ An 87-year-old woman with a history of mild, stable angina (but no history of MI or arrhythmias except for rare premature ventricular contractions) developed atrial fibrillation with rapid ventricular response 1 hour after receiving her second 20-mg dose of fluoxetine.[40] After conversion back to sinus rhythm, another 20-mg dose of fluoxetine given 14 days later elicited atrial fibrillation again. She was treated with a permanent pacemaker, digoxin, and quinidine. A third reintroduction proceeded without adverse cardiac events but also without therapeutic response. The patient was subsequently treated with nortriptyline with no further cardiac toxicity.

There have also been reports of fluoxetine-associated faintness, syncope, bradycardia, and orthostatic hypotension in three relatively young patients *without* cardiac histories, ranging in age from 35 to 42 years, with doses from 20 to 80 mg/day.[80,85]

◆ Bradycardia also occurred in a fluoxetine-pimozide[3] and a fluoxetine-metoprolol interaction.[305]

Table 1–2. Inhibition of Isoenzyme Drug Metabolism: A Potential Hazard of Selective Serotonin Reuptake Inhibitors (SSRIs)

	Medications used in		Notes	Metabolism inhibited by
	Psychiatric practice	General medical practice		
Isoenzyme-2D6	Many neuroleptics Clozapine Fluphenazine Haloperidol Perphenazine Risperidone Thioridazine Trifluperidol TCAs Amitriptyline Clomipramine Desipramine Imipramine Nortriptyline MAOIs SSRIs Fluoxetine Paroxetine	Beta-blockers Alprenolol Bufuralol Metoprolol Propranolol Timolol Antiarrhythmics Encainide Flecainide Mexiletine Propafenone Opiates Codeine Dextromethorphan Ethylmorphine	There is genetic variability (genetic polymorphism), with 5% of the Caucasian population lacking CyP450-2D6. Poor metabolizers (i.e., enzyme-deficient patients) are at risk for heightened toxicity from inadequately metabolized medications, particularly if enzyme activity is further inhibited pharmacologically. Extensive metabolizers (i.e., patients with normal enzyme activity) may be pharmacologically "converted" to poor metabolizers by inhibitors of cytochrome-2D6.	◆ SSRIs (paroxetine > fluoxetine > sertraline) ◆ Quinidine ◆ Thioridazine
Isoenzyme-3A4	Benzodiazepines Alprazolam Midazolam Triazolam Antidepressants Nefazodone Sertraline Venlafaxine Some tricyclics Anticonvulsants Carbamazepine	Antiarrhythmics Quinidine Lidocaine Calcium channel blockers Diltiazem Felodipine Nifedipine Verapamil Nonsedating antihistamines Astemizole Terfenadine Miscellaneous Cortisol Cyclosporine Dexamethasone Erythromycin Tamoxifen	Less genetic variability (i.e., all patients possess CyP450-3A4).	◆ SSRIs (weak effect) ◆ Ketoconazole ◆ Itraconazole ◆ Erythromycin (and other macrolide antibiotics) ◆ Cimetidine ◆ Nefazodone

Note. MAOIs = monoamine oxidase inhibitors; TCAs = tricyclic antidepressants. *Source.* Adapted from Stoudemire and Fogel[289a] and Gelenberg.[114a]

◆ A 53-year-old man lost consciousness for several minutes and was hospitalized 2 weeks after fluoxetine (20 mg/day) was added to his regimen of lorazepam (4 mg/day) and propranolol (80 mg/day), which he had taken for several years to manage anxiety.[77] His ECG showed *complete heart block* with an escape rhythm of 30 beats/minute, requiring pacemaker insertion. Fluoxetine interaction with propranolol was implicated because sinus rhythm returned 2 days after fluoxetine was withdrawn.

Note that fluoxetine can potentially inhibit the elimination of any drug that is oxidatively metabolized by the liver,[63] thus raising the drug's serum level (Table 1–2). Drugs so affected by fluoxetine include the following:[111,196]

◆ Most other psychotropic agents
◆ Cyclosporine
◆ Beta-blockers
◆ Some anticonvulsants
◆ Several antiarrhythmics

In addition, fluoxetine is highly protein bound (94%) and can displace other highly bound drugs such as digoxin or warfarin (Coumadin).[196]

Also, beware of heightened TCA cardiotoxicity when placing patients on fluoxetine-TCA combination therapy.

Finally, the psychopharmacologist Gelenberg feels that *atrial fibrillation and sinus bradycardia should be considered risks of fluoxetine treatment in the elderly and the cardiovascular population.*[114] However, note that these reports are rare and anecdotal. Remain vigilant about using fluoxetine in cardiovascular patients, but do not sacrifice clinical efficacy to overly cautious practice.

Sertraline. Sertraline (Zoloft) was first marketed in the United States in 1992; consequently, clinical experience with it in cardiovascular populations is limited. It is an even more selective reuptake inhibitor of serotonin than fluoxetine. It appears to be safe, without demonstrable effects on intraventricular conduction or electrocardiographic time intervals in healthy individuals.[125] One small study compared 50-, 100-, and 200-mg daily doses of sertraline with placebo:[10]

◆ One patient in the 100-mg group (*n* = 8) suffered a ventricular arrhythmia and was withdrawn from the study.
◆ One patient in the 200-mg group (*n* = 8) exhibited T-wave flattening and another showed a lengthened QT interval.

Larger premarketing studies do not appear to support early concern about sertraline's cardiovascular side effects,[144] but additional testing is necessary in cardiovascular patients.

Paroxetine. Paroxetine (Paxil) has been shown to be of similar efficacy to the TCAs, but has lower cardiovascular toxicity in animal models.[308] It has no effects on heart rate, blood pressure, or ECG in healthy men receiving single 20- to 40-mg doses.[308] One study showed mild but clinically significant increases in bleeding time in volunteers who took paroxetine and warfarin together, suggesting the need for caution when it is coadministered with oral anticoagulants.[302]

Miscellaneous Agents

Bupropion. Bupropion (Wellbutrin) is an aminoketone structurally unrelated to the TCAs that is relatively free of cardiac effects in healthy depressed individuals.[84,313] The clinical trial program in over 700 depressed patients found no significant change in heart rate, PR interval, QRS duration, and supine and standing blood pressure.[313]

◆ In a single-blind study of 12 patients with clinically significant postural hypotension on TCAs, bupropion (300–600 mg/day) was tolerated without statistically significant changes in heart rate or blood pressure.[84] Three patients had greater-than-placebo orthostatic drops in systolic pressure; bupropion may occasionally produce orthostatic effects in highly sensitive patients.
◆ Bupropion has fewer adverse cardiovascular effects than nortriptyline.[173a]

Two studies[252,255] specifically addressed the use of bupropion in patients with cardiovascular disease and confirmed a favorable side-effect profile.

Most recently, 36 inpatients with major depression and coexisting cardiovascular disease (left-ventricular impairment, *n* = 15; ventricular arrhythmias, *n* = 15; and/ or conduction disease, *n* = 21) were studied.[252] Cardiac drug regimens were continued and patients received bupropion for 3 weeks, with a mean dose of 442 mg/day. Cardiovascular functioning was measured by pulse, blood pressure, high-speed ECG, 24-hour portable ECG, and radionuclide angiography.

◆ Bupropion caused a statistically significant *increase* in supine systolic and diastolic blood pressure, with significant (but asymptomatic) orthostatic changes.

◆ Only one patient developed dizziness and fell in conjunction with an orthostatic drop of 40 points, necessitating discontinuation of bupropion.

◆ Bupropion had no effect on pulse rate, nor did it cause significant conduction complications or exacerbate arrhythmias.

◆ It did have to be discontinued in 14% of the patients because of adverse effects including exacerbation of baseline hypertension ($n = 2$), orthostatic hypotension ($n = 1$), rash ($n = 2$), and changing anginal pattern ($n = 1$).

Bupropion appears to be cardiovascularly safe in overdose.[281] Seizures—not CNS depression—have been described with bupropion overdose.[65,281,286] There are also anecdotal reports of delirium[9,292] and catatonia[140] appearing with bupropion.

Psychostimulants. Psychostimulants are increasingly used in treating depressed medically ill patients when anorexia, apathy, and profound hopelessness interfere with medical management.[177a,266,306] Sometimes the 2- to 3-week wait required for conventional antidepressants to take effect is too long; the depressed medical patient who is languishing—refusing to eat, drink, or cooperate with tests or rehabilitation—needs an antidepressant effect, stat! Often, such patients and their families will not consent to ECT, viewing it as one more "horrible ordeal." Moreover, many general hospitals do not have available ECT facilities. In situations like these, psychostimulants are invaluable. They are safe, relatively well tolerated, short acting, and quick to work in medical and surgical inpatients,[163–165,225,318] stroke patients,[148,199,209] rehabilitation patients,[13,56] the terminally ill,[41,134] the elderly,[238] and those in chronic care facilities.[156] There is also an increasing literature on the use of psychostimulants in depressed HIV-infected patients.[38,87,89,90,135,197,256]

Masand et al.[210] conducted a chart review of 198 patients with acute medical or surgical illnesses who had been treated with either dextroamphetamine (Dexedrine) or methylphenidate (Ritalin) for secondary depression. The medical diagnoses for these patients were as follows (most patients had more than one diagnosis):

◆ Cardiovascular ($n = 192$), including arrhythmias, CHF, coronary artery bypass graft, CAD, hypertension, peripheral vascular disease, and valvular disease

◆ Pulmonary ($n = 65$), including chronic obstructive lung disease, pneumonia, respiratory failure, lung cancer, and laryngeal/tracheal cancer

◆ Neurological ($n = 34$), including cerebrovascular accident, normal-pressure hydrocephalus, parkinsonism, and seizures

◆ Endocrinological ($n = 45$), including diabetes mellitus and thyroid disease

◆ Urological ($n = 35$), including renal failure and prostate and renal cancer

◆ Gastrointestinal ($n = 29$), including peptic ulcer disease, liver disease, and pancreatic disease

◆ Orthopedic ($n = 7$), including degenerative joint disease and fractures

The average daily doses were 9 mg/day of dextroamphetamine and 11 mg/day of methylphenidate. The results: 82% showed improvement after psychostimulant treatment, including 70% who demonstrated marked or moderate depressive improvement, usually within the first 2 days of treatment.

◆ The two medications did not significantly differ in efficacy.

◆ There were no significant differences across depressive diagnostic categories (*major depression* versus *adjustment disorder with depressed mood*).

◆ Only 3 out of 198 patients (2%) had relapses, which occurred between days 6 and 14 of treatment.

◆ No instances of medication-induced anorexia were observed; in fact, appetite actually improved in many patients undergoing psychostimulant trials.

◆ Adverse reactions occurred in 29 patients (15%), but side effects requiring psychostimulant discontinuation occurred in only 10% of trials (see below).

Methylphenidate and dextroamphetamine have been shown to also reduce sedation and opioid analgesic requirements in the pain management of cancer patients.[39,285]

Side effects. Psychostimulant side effects in the chart review study by Masand et al.[210] included (in descending order) the following:

◆ 4 cases each: confusion, agitation, anxiety

◆ 3 cases each: hypomania,[210a] paranoid delusions, sinus tachycardia

◆ 2 cases each: elevated blood pressure

◆ 1 case each: insomnia, dizziness, atrial fibrillation, spasticity, nausea, and visual hallucinations

Adverse effects on heart rate, blood pressure, or appetite were rare, and neither tolerance nor abuse have been regularly demonstrated with stimulants. In Masand et al.'s study, the referring internists, surgeons, and original consultants confirmed that they had encountered no psychostimulant abuse among these patients, corroborating the findings of others.[285]

However, there are several important psychostimulant drug interactions:[145]

◆ **Anticonvulsants** ⇒ Increased levels of phenobarbital, phenytoin, primidone
◆ **Guanethidine** ⇒ Decreased antihypertensive effect
◆ **MAOIs** ⇒ Hypertensive crisis
◆ **Oral anticoagulants** ⇒ Increased prothrombin time (methylphenidate)
◆ **TCAs** ⇒ Increased TCA blood levels
◆ **Vasopressors** ⇒ Increased pressor effect

Guidelines. Warneke[306] has suggested several guidelines for psychostimulant therapy; the following are pertinent to the medical population:

◆ The patient is depressed secondary to a medical illness or is elderly, a rapid response is required, and the side effects of conventional antidepressants must be avoided if possible.
◆ There is no history of substance abuse (relative contraindication).
◆ There is no previous history of an acute psychotic illness (relative contraindication).

The initial starting dose in fragile cardiovascular patients is 2.5 mg of either dextroamphetamine (given once before breakfast) or methylphenidate (given twice a day, usually before breakfast and after lunch), with careful monitoring of vital signs over the next 4 hours.[50] If the patient has tolerated the initial dose without incident but has failed to demonstrate any response to the medication, successively increase the medication over the next 2 or 3 days, monitoring vital signs.[50] Provided that vital signs are not adversely affected, Cassem[50] advises *pushing the medication to where there are demonstrable effects, such as improved mood or irritability.* He advises not abandoning the trial before at least some effect has been experienced by the patient. Persistent insomnia and only partial resolution of depressive symptoms on an adequate trial of psychostimulants are indications for trying another antidepressant.[50]

Alternatively, try pemoline (Cylert). Initial doses are 18.75 mg, raised slowly to 37.5 mg daily in the morning and at noon.[38] It has minimal sympathomimetic activity and can be given as tablets that can be sucked and absorbed directly through the buccal mucosa—bypassing the gastrointestinal tract. Pemoline has low abuse potential[52] and is not a controlled substance that requires special prescription forms. It may reversibly elevate liver enzymes, requiring regular monitoring of liver function tests.[229] There has been at least one case of pemoline-induced mania.[284]

There are no controlled studies of the safety or efficacy of long-term psychostimulants in medical patients.

Electroconvulsive Therapy

The autonomic changes associated with seizure activity, such as transient tachycardia and changes in blood pressure (which vary in type over the course of the seizure), pose the primary risks for patients with cardiovascular disease. A recent study found that the type of preexisting cardiac abnormality strongly predicted the type of cardiac complication that occurred during ECT.[72,167,322] However, most complications were transitory and did not interfere with the completion of ECT.[248] The greatest risk period for cardiac arrhythmias is during the seizure, when the sympathetic reaction predominates and tachycardia-related cardiac ischemia is most likely to occur, making beta-blocking agents particularly useful.[311] With adequate precautions, however, the adverse impact of an induced seizure on preexisting cardiac arrhythmias will likely be mild and transient, if not predictable. Guttmacher and Goldstein[124] have outlined the effect of ECT on the cardiovascular system in terms of the two physiological phases:

1. Marked initial and temporal parasympathetic discharge produces increased vagal tone, resulting in profound bradycardia in healthy subjects. Patients with cardiovascular disease are at risk for developing sinus arrest or conduction disturbances during this phase, although the routine use of anticholinergic agents has prevented cardiovascular complications caused by parasympathetic discharge.
2. The phase of parasympathetic discharge is followed by one dominated by sympathetic discharge. This is associated with hypertension, tachycardia, and, frequently, ventricular and other arrhythmias. Patients with all types of cardiovascular diseases are at risk during this period.

A history of MI is not a contraindication to ECT, but if the insult to the heart is recent or incompletely healed, the damaged myocardium is at risk for further injury as a result of the marked cardiovascular fluctuations that occur with each seizure.[310] An ideal waiting time has not been established, but some suggest that **6 weeks** is reasonable after uncomplicated MI without postinfarction angina, arrhythmia, or heart failure.[310] ECT has also been safely used in at least one depressed heart-transplant patient.[31] Patients with preexisting ventricular ectopy or bradycardia may be particularly prone to asystole or bradyarrhythmic-related ventricular contractions both during and after the seizure.[310]

Pre- and posttreatment pharmacological management greatly reduces the cardiovascular hazard in high-risk patients.[288] Although the prevalence of ECT-induced ECG abnormalities increases in patients with preexisting cardiac pathology, these effects are usually limited to the ictal and immediate postictal periods, even in patients with preexisting cardiovascular disease.[68,248]

Several factors predispose to prolonged asystole after ECT: cardiac history, failure to achieve a generalized seizure, and bilateral electrode placement.[68a,163a,198a,312a,319a]

- Atropine or glycopyrrolate are used to prevent vagal cardiovascular effects (bradycardia, ectopy) during and after the seizure.
- Acute blood pressure increases have been prevented by using agents such as trimethaphan (Arfonad), nitroprusside (Nipride), diazoxide (Hyperstat IV), hydralazine (Apresoline), and nitroglycerin.
- Lidocaine (Xylocaine) and propranolol (Inderal) are used in preventing and managing the sympathoadrenal cardiac arrhythmias associated with ECT.[1]
- Labetalol (Normodyne/Trandate; a mixed alpha- and beta-adrenergic blocker) was evaluated in a randomized, double-blind, placebo-controlled crossover study by Stoudemire and co-workers.[287,290] These researchers found that in 11 elderly depressed patients with cardiovascular disease, labetalol blunted the increase in mean arterial pressure and heart rate by up to 8% and 26%, respectively. Labetalol also decreased the frequency of atrial arrhythmias and premature ventricular contractions by 100% and 42%, respectively.
- Figiel and colleagues[91,92] supplemented the effect of labetalol by adding nifedipine (Procardia/Adalat), a calcium channel blocker. It was effective for 10 elderly patients whose blood pressures were not adequately controlled during ECT on labetalol alone. These authors noted no adverse effects, nor did nifedipine appear to shorten seizure duration.
- Beta-blockers are given to attenuate the postseizure adrenergic surge, which can lead to hypertension and arrhythmias. There is, however, a risk of asystole after beta-blockade. Premedication with anticholinergic drugs diminishes this risk.[198a]

Keep in mind that MAOIs may cause an intensified sympathetic response in ECT patients; Drop and Welch[78] recommend that MAOIs be discontinued at least 24–48 hours before ECT treatment. Concurrent administration of TCAs with ECT does not necessarily cause cardiovascular toxicity.[177]

Pacemakers and ECT

Mr. Doe should be reassured that his pacemaker can withstand the electrical current used in ECT and prevent it from reaching the heart. However, the pacemaker's endocardial electrode provides a low-resistance potential pathway to the myocardium if the patient is in contact with ground. It is essential to check grounding when using ECT in a pacemaker patient, and pacemaker wires should be checked for breaks or faulty insulation. Temporary pacemakers are external; they provide a ready pathway for current from improperly grounded monitoring equipment (even if equipment is turned off but a circuit is completed by an assistant who touches both patient and equipment simultaneously). Hence, temporary pacemakers are riskier than permanent (implanted) ones.

Demand pacemakers are inhibited by P or R waves; ECT-induced muscle potentials and contractions can also occasionally inhibit a demand pacemaker, resulting in severe bradycardia.[1] Analogously, synchronous pacemakers are triggered by P or R waves, and may produce tachycardia in response to ECT-induced muscle potentials. Converting the pacemaker to a *fixed*-mode operation avoids these possible side effects.

Comment. There seems to be consensus that for patients with conduction disease, the least risky and most effective treatment is not a drug, but rather ECT.[254] We await further studies of the newer antidepressants that compare their safety with that of ECT in the setting of cardiovascular disease (see Appendix O).

✦ SUMMARY

1. Untreated major depression predisposes to adverse medical outcomes.
2. Vegetative symptoms are not useful in diagnosing depression in the medically ill.
3. Rule out panic disorder in heart disease patients whose chest pain does not respond to usual antianginal medication, or in individuals complaining of chest pain without definable medical cause. The *pacemaker syndrome* is in the differential diagnosis of panic-like symptoms occurring in pacemaker patients.

4. Studies of the global type A behavior pattern have been replaced by those focusing on the specific components of hostility and anger. These affects have been shown to predispose to coronary artery disease (CAD), and serve as potential triggers for malignant arrhythmias and ischemia. They also predict cardiac mortality. Interventions aimed at modifying type A behaviors improve medical outcome.

5. Mental stress has a high association with myocardial ischemia and sudden cardiac death, individually. Unfortunately, it is not possible to rely on anginal pain to signal trouble; many episodes of myocardial ischemia are silent. Moreover, candidates for sudden cardiac death are not identifiable by the traditional risk factors for CAD, such as hypertension, smoking, and hypercholesterolemia.

6. Anxiolytics play an important role in reducing morbidity in coronary patients. Alprazolam (Xanax) has been the most widely studied, but is by no means unique in its effectiveness in the medical setting. Other reasonable alternatives include clonazepam (Klonopin), lorazepam (Ativan), and oxazepam (Serax). Preliminary evidence on buspirone (BuSpar) is promising.

7. The SSRIs have substantially different cardiac profiles than the tricyclics. Although they appear to be safe, they have not been systematically tested in patients with cardiovascular disease. Adverse cardiac side effects from fluoxetine (Prozac) have not been predicted by dose, age, or cardiac history. Be alert to adverse effects on the metabolism of other drugs.

8. Bupropion (Wellbutrin) appears to have a safe cardiac profile in this population. Problems are mainly limited to elevated blood pressure.

9. Psychostimulants are useful when an immediate antidepressant effect is needed. They have been shown to be safe in a variety of medical conditions, with few adverse side effects. Disadvantages include several drug interactions, restriction to patients without a psychotic or substance abuse history, and no controlled studies on their long-term use in medical patients.

10. Electroconvulsive therapy (ECT) is a safe and effective alternative to antidepressant medications in the cardiovascular patient.

☀ REFERENCES

1. Abrams R: Electroconvulsive Therapy, 2nd Edition. New York, Oxford University Press, 1992

2. Adsett C, Bruhn J: Short-term group psychotherapy for post-myocardial infarction patients and their wives. Can Med Assoc J 99:577–584, 1968

3. Ahmed I, Dagincourt P, Miller L, et al: Possible interaction between fluoxetine and pimozide causing sinus bradycardia. Can J Psychiatry 38:62–63, 1993

4. Alfredsson L, Karasek R, Theorell T: Myocardial infarction and psychosocial work environment: an analysis of the male Swedish working force. Soc Sci Med 16:463–467, 1982

5. Alfredsson L, Spetz C, Theorell T: Type of occupation and near-future hospitalization for myocardial infarction and some other diagnoses. Int J Epidemiol 14:375–388, 1985

5a. Allison T, Williams D, Miller T, et al: Medical and economic costs of psychologic distress in patients with coronary artery disease. Mayo Clin Proc 70:734–742, 1995

6. Almada S, Zonderman A, Shekelle R, et al: Neuroticism and cynicism and risk of death in middle-aged men: the Western Electric Study. Psychosom Med 53:165–175, 1991

7. American Psychiatric Association: Diagnostic and Statistical Manual of Mental Disorders, 3rd Edition, Revised. Washington, DC, American Psychiatric Association, 1987

8. American Psychiatric Association: Diagnostic and Statistical Manual of Mental Disorders, 4th Edition. Washington, DC, American Psychiatric Association, 1994

9. Ames D, Wirshing W, Szuba M: Organic mental disorders associated with bupropion. J Clin Psychiatry 52:53–55, 1992

10. Amin M, Lehmann H, Mirmiran J: A double-blind, placebo-controlled dose-finding study with sertraline. Psychopharmacol Bull 25:164–167, 1989

11. Anda R, Williamson D, Jones D, et al: Depressed affect, hopelessness, and the risk of ischemic heart disease in a cohort of U.S. adults. Epidemiology 4:285–942, 1993

12. Aromaa A, Raitasalo R, Reunanen A, et al: Depression and cardiovascular diseases. Acta Psychiatr Scand Suppl 377:77–82, 1994

13. Askinazi C, Weintraub R, Karamouz N: Elderly depressed females as a possible subgroup of patients responsive to methylphenidate. J Clin Psychiatry 47:467–469, 1986

14. Ausubel K, Furman S: The pacemaker syndrome. Ann Intern Med 103:420–429, 1983

15. Barefoot J, Dahlstrom W, Williams R, et al: Hostility, CHD incidence and total mortality: a 25-year follow-up study of 255 physicians. Psychosom Med 45:59–63, 1983

16. Barefoot J, Dodge K, Peterson B, et al: The Cook-Medley hostility scale: item content and ability to predict survival. Psychosom Med 51:46–57, 1989

17. Barefoot J, Patterson J, Haney T, et al: Hostility in asymptomatic men with angiographically confirmed coronary artery disease. Am J Cardiol 74:439–442, 1994

18. Barefoot J, Peterson B, Dahlstrom W, et al: Hostility patterns and health implications: correlates of Cook-Medley Hostility Scale scores in a national survey. Health Psychol 10:18–24, 1991

19. Barry J, Selwyn A, Nabel E: Frequency of ST segment depression produced by mental stress in stable angina pectoris from coronary artery disease. Am J Cardiol 61:989–993, 1988

20. Barsky A, Coles N, O'Donnell C, et al: Denial and silent ischemia: which comes first? (reply). JAMA 265:213, 1991

21. Barsky A, Hochstrasser B, Coles A, et al: Silent myocardial ischemia: is the person or the event silent? JAMA 264:1132–1135, 1990

22. Bass C: Chest pain and breathlessness: relationship to psychiatric illness. Am J Med 92:12S–17S, 1992

23. Bass C, Wade C: Chest pain with normal coronary arteries: a comparative study of psychiatric and social morbidity. Psychol Med 14:51–61, 1984

24. Beck A, Steer R, Garbin M: Psychometric properties of the Beck depression inventory: twenty-five years of evaluation. Clinical Psychology Review 8:77–100, 1988

25. Beitman B, Basha I, Flaker G, et al: Atypical or nonanginal chest pain: panic disorder or coronary artery disease? Arch Intern Med 147:1548–1552, 1987

26. Beitman B, Kushner M, Basha I, et al: Follow-up status of patients with angiographically normal coronary arteries and panic disorder. JAMA 265:1545–1549, 1991

26a. Benfield P, Ward A: Fluvoxamine: a review of its pharmacodynamic and pharmacokinetic properties, and therapeutic efficacy in depressive illness. Drugs 32:313–334, 1986

27. Bennett P, Carroll D: Cognitive-behavioural interventions in cardiac rehabilitation. J Psychosom Res 38:169–182, 1994

28. Bennett S: Perceived threats of individuals recovering from myocardial infarction. Heart Lung 21:322–326, 1992

29. Berkman L: The relationship of social networks and social support to morbidity and mortality, in Social Support and Health. Edited by Cohen S, Syme S. Orlando, FL, Academic Press, 1985, pp 241–262

30. Berkman L, Syme L: Social networks, host resistance, and mortality: a 9-year follow-up study of Alameda County residents. Am J Epidemiol 109:186–203, 1979

31. Bloch M, Admon D, Bonne O: Electroconvulsive therapy in a depressed heart transplant patient. Convulsive Therapy 8:290–293, 1992

32. Blumenthal J, Burg M, Barefoot J, et al: Social support, type A behavior, and coronary artery disease. Psychosom Med 49:331–340, 1987

33. Blumenthal J, McCubbin J: Physical exercise as stress management, in Handbook of Psychology and Health. Edited by Baum A, Singer J. Hillsdale, NJ, Lawrence Erlbaum, 1987, pp 303–331

34. Blumenthal J, Wei J: Psychobehavioral treatment in cardiac rehabilitation. Cardiol Clin 11:323–331, 1993

35. Blumenthal J, Williams R, Wallace A, et al: Physiological and psychological variables predict compliance to prescribed exercise therapy in patients recovering from myocardial infarction. Psychosom Med 44:519–527, 1982

36. Booth-Kewley S, Friedman H: Psychological predictors of heart disease: a quantitative review. Psychol Bull 101:343–362, 1987

37. Bradley L, Richter J, Scarinci I, et al: Psychosocial and psychophysical assessments of patients with unexplained chest pain. Am J Med 92(5A):65S–73S, 1992

38. Breitbart W, Mermelstein H: Pemoline: an alternative psychostimulant for management of depressive disorders in cancer patients. Psychosomatics 33:352–356, 1992

39. Bruera E, Chadwick S, Brennels C, et al: Methylphenidate associated with narcotics for the treatment of cancer pain. Cancer Treatment Reports 71:67–70, 1987

40. Buff D, Brenner R, Kirtane S, et al: Case report: dysrhythmia associated with fluoxetine. J Clin Psychiatry 52:174–176, 1991

41. Burns M, Eisendrath S: Dextroamphetamine treatment for depression in terminally ill patients. Psychosomatics 35:80–83, 1994

42. Cannon R, Quyyumi A, Mincemoyer R, et al: Imipramine in patients with chest pain despite normal coronary angiograms. N Engl J Med 330:1411–1417, 1994

43. Carney R, Freedland K, Rich M, et al: Ventricular tachycardia and psychiatric depression in patients with coronary artery disease. Am J Med 95:23–28, 1993

44. Carney R, Rich M, Freedland K, et al: Major depressive disorder predicts cardiac events in patients with coronary artery disease. Psychosom Med 50:627–633, 1988

45. Carney R, Rich M, Tevelde A, et al: Heart rate, heart rate variability and depression in patients with coronary artery disease. J Psychosom Res 32:159–164, 1988

46. Carney R, Rich M, Tevelde A, et al: Major depressive disorder in coronary artery disease. Am J Cardiol 60:1273–1275, 1987

47. Carter C, Maddock R, Amsterdam E, et al: Panic disorder and chest pain in the coronary care unit. Psychosomatics 33:302–309, 1992

48. Carter C, Maddock R, Zoglio M, et al: Panic disorder and chest pain: a study of cardiac stress scintigraphy patients. Am J Cardiol 74:296–298, 1994

49. Case R, Moss A, Case N, et al: Living alone after myocardial infarction. JAMA 267:515–519, 1992

50. Cassem N: Depression, in Massachusetts General Hospital Handbook of General Hospital Psychiatry, 3rd Edition. Edited by Cassem N. St. Louis, MO, Mosby Year Book, 1991, pp 237–268

51. Cavanaugh S: Depression in the medically ill: critical issues in diagnostic assessment. Psychosomatics 36:48–59, 1995

51a. Chernen L, Friedman S, Goldberg N, et al: Cardiac disease and nonorganic chest pain: factors leading to disability. Cardiology 86:15–21, 1995

52. Chiarello R, Cole J: The use of psychostimulants in general psychiatry: a reconsideration. Arch Gen Psychiatry 44:286–295, 1987

53. Chignon J-M, Lepine J-P, Ades J: Panic disorder in cardiac outpatients. Am J Psychiatry 150:780–785, 1993

54. Chochinov H, Wilson K, Enns M, et al: Prevalence of depression in the terminally ill: effects of diagnostic criteria and symptom threshold judgments. Am J Psychiatry 151:537–540, 1994

55. Claire R, Servis M, Gram D: Potential interaction between warfarin sodium and fluoxetine (letter). Am J Psychiatry 148:1604, 1991

56. Clark A, Mankikar G: d-Amphetamine in elderly patients refractory to rehabilitation procedures. J Am Geriatr Soc 27:174–177, 1979

57. Cobb L, Werner J: Predictors and prevention of sudden cardiac death, in The Heart. Edited by Hurst J. New York, McGraw-Hill, 1986, pp 538–546

58. Cohen S, Syme S (eds): Social Support and Health. New York, Academic Press, 1985

59. Cook W, Medley D: Proposed hostility and pharisaic-virtue scales for the MMPI. J Appl Psychol 238:414–418, 1954

60. Cooper D, Luceri R, Thurer R, et al: The impact of the automatic implantable cardioverter defibrillator on quality of life. PACE Pacing Clin Electrophysiol 4:306–309, 1986

61. Coplan J, Papp L, King D, et al: Amelioration of mitral valve prolapse after treatment for panic disorder. Am J Psychiatry 149:1587–1588, 1992

62. Cormier L, Katon W, Russo J, et al: Chest pain with negative cardiac diagnostic studies: relationship to psychiatric illness. J Nerv Ment Dis 176:351–358, 1988

63. Crewe H, Lennard M, Tucker G, et al: The effects of selective serotonin reuptake inhibitors on cytochrome P450-2D6 (CYP2D6) activity in human liver microsomes. Br J Clin Pharmacol 34:262–265, 1992

64. Dalack G, Roose S: Perspectives on the relationship between cardiovascular disease and affective disorder. J Clin Psychiatry 51 (7, suppl):4–9, 1990

65. Davidson J: Seizures and bupropion: a review. J Clin Psychiatry 50:256–261, 1989

66. Deanfield J, Kensett M, Wilson R, et al: Silent myocardial ischemia due to mental stress. Lancet 2:1001–1004, 1984

67. Deary IJ, Fowkes FG, Donnan PT, et al: Hostile personality and risks of peripheral arterial disease in the general population. Psychosom Med 56:197–202, 1994

68. Dec G, Stern T, Welch C: The effects of electroconvulsive therapy on serial electrocardiograms and serum cardiac enzyme values: a prospective study of depressed hospitalized inpatients. JAMA 253:2525–2529, 1985

68a. Decina P, Malitz S, Sackheim H, et al: Cardiac arrest during ECT modified by beta-adrenergic blockade. Am J Psychiatry 141:298–300, 1984

68b. Deedwania P: Mental stress, pain perception and risk of silent ischemia (editorial; comment). J Am Coll Cardiol 25:1504–1506, 1995

69. Dembroski T, MacDonald J, Herd J, et al: Effects of level of challenge on pressor and heart rate responses in type A and type B subjects. Journal of Applied Social Psychology 9:208–228, 1979

70. Dembroski T, MacDonald J, Williams R, et al: Components of type A, hostility, and anger in relationship to angiographic findings. Psychosom Med 47:219–233, 1985

71. Dembroski T, MacDougall J: Behavioral and psychophysiological perspectives on coronary-prone behavior, in Biobehavioral Bases of Coronary Heart Disease. Edited by Dembroski T, Schmidt T, Blumchen G. New York, Karger, 1983, pp 106–129

72. Devanand D, Roose S, Zielinski R, et al: Cardiovascular complication of ECT (reply). Am J Psychiatry 151:791, 1994

73. Doerfler L, Pbert L, DeCosimo D: Symptoms of posttraumatic stress disorder following myocardial infarction and coronary artery bypass surgery. Gen Hosp Psychiatry 16:193–199, 1994

74. Dorian B, Taylor C: Stress factors in the development of coronary artery disease. J Occup Med 26:747–756, 1984

75. Dougherty C: Longitudinal recovery following sudden cardiac arrest and internal cardioverter defibrillator implantation: survivors and their families. American Journal of Critical Care 3:145–154, 1994

76. Dracup K, Walden J, Stevenson L, et al: Quality of life in patients with advanced heart failure. J Heart Lung Transplant 11:273–279, 1992

77. Drake W, Gordon G: Heart block in a patient on propranolol and fluoxetine (letter). Lancet 343:425–426, 1994

78. Drop L, Welch C: Anesthesia for electroconvulsive treatment in patients with major cardiovascular risk factors. Convulsive Therapy 5:88–101, 1989

79. Ehlers A, Margraf J, Rother W, et al: Anxiety induced by false heart rate feedback in patients with panic disorder. Behav Res Ther 26:1–11, 1988

79a. Elliott S: Psychosocial stress, women and heart health: a critical review. Soc Sci Med 40:105–115, 1995

80. Ellison J, Milofsky J, Ely E: Bradycardia and syncope induced by fluoxetine in two patients. J Clin Psychiatry 51:385–386, 1990

81. Endicott J: Measurement of depression in patients with cancer. Cancer 53:2243–2247, 1984

82. Epstein S, Quyyumi A, Bonow R: Myocardial ischemia—silent or symptomatic. N Engl J Med 318:1038–1043, 1988

83. Esler M, Turbott J, Schwartz R, et al: The peripheral kinetics of norepinephrine in depressive illness. Arch Gen Psychiatry 39:285–300, 1982

84. Farid F, Wenger T, Tsai S, et al: Use of bupropion in patients who exhibit orthostatic hypotension on tricyclic antidepressants. J Clin Psychiatry 44:170–173, 1983

85. Feder R: Bradycardia and syncope induced by fluoxetine (letter). J Clin Psychiatry 52:139, 1991

86. Fernandez F: Depression and its treatment in cardiac patients. Tex Heart Inst J 20:188–197, 1993

87. Fernandez F, Adams F, Levy J: Cognitive impairment due to AIDS-related complex and its response to psychostimulants. Psychosomatics 29:38–46, 1988

88. Fernandez F, Levy J: Psychiatric diagnosis and pharmacotherapy of patients with HIV infection, in American Psychiatric Press Review of Psychiatry, Vol 9. Edited by Tasman A, Goldfinger SM, Kaufmann C. Washington, DC, American Psychiatric Press, 1990, pp 614–628

89. Fernandez F, Levy J, Galizzi H: Response of HIV-related depression to psychostimulants: case reports. Hosp Community Psychiatry 39:628–631, 1988

90. Fernandez F, Levy J: Psychopharmacology in HIV spectrum disorders. Psychiatr Clin North Am 17:135–148, 1994

91. Figiel G, DeLeo B, Zorumski C, et al: Combined use of labetalol and nifedipine in controlling the cardiovascular response from ECT. J Geriatr Psychiatry Neurol 6:20–24, 1993

92. Figiel G, McDonald L, Laplante R: Cardiovascular complication of ECT (letter). Am J Psychiatry 151:790–791, 1994

93. Finnegan D, Suler J: Psychological factors associated with maintenance of improved health behaviors in postcoronary patients. J Psychol 119:87–94, 1985

94. Fisch C: Effect of fluoxetine on the electrocardiogram. J Clin Psychiatry 46:42–44, 1985

95. Fleury J: An exploration of the role of social networks in cardiovascular risk reduction. Heart Lung 22:134–144, 1993

96. Follick M, Ahern D, Gorkin L, et al: Relation of psychosocial and stress reactivity variables to ventricular arrhythmias in the Cardiac Arrhythmia Pilot Study (CAPS). Am J Cardiol 66:63–67, 1990

97. Follick M, Gorkin L, Capone R, et al: Psychological distress as a predictor of ventricular arrhythmias in a post-myocardial infarction population. Am Heart J 116:32–36, 1988

98. Frank C, Smith S: Stress and the heart: biobehavioral aspects of sudden cardiac death. Psychosomatics 31:255–264, 1990

99. Frasure-Smith N: In-hospital symptoms of psychological stress as predictors of long-term outcome after acute myocardial infarction in men. Am J Cardiol 67:121–127, 1991

100. Frasure-Smith N, Lesprance F, Talajic M: Depression following myocardial infarction. JAMA 270:1819–1825, 1993

101. Frasure-Smith N, Prince R: The ischemic heart disease life stress monitoring program: impact on mortality. Psychosom Med 47:431–445, 1985

102. Freedland K, Carney R, Krone R, et al: Psychological factors in silent myocardial ischemia. Psychosom Med 53:13–24, 1991

103. Freedland K, Carney R, Rich M, et al: Depression in elderly patients with congestive heart failure. Journal of Geriatric Psychiatry 24:59–71, 1991

104. Freedland K, Lustman P, Carney R, et al: Underdiagnosis of depression in patients with coronary artery disease: the role of nonspecific symptoms. Int J Psychiatry Med 22:221–229, 1992

105. Fricchione G, Vlay L, Vlay S: Cardiac psychiatry and the management of malignant ventricular arrhythmias with the internal cardioverter-defibrillator (editorial). Am Heart J 128:1050–1059, 1994

106. Fricchione G, Vlay S: Psychiatric aspects of patients with malignant ventricular arrhythmias. Am J Psychiatry 143:1518–1526, 1986

107. Friedman M, Rosenman R: Type A Behavior and Your Heart. New York, Knopf, 1974

108. Friedman M, Thorensen C, Gill J, et al: Feasibility of altering type A behavior pattern after myocardial infarction. Circulation 66:83–92, 1982

109. Friedman M, Thorensen C, Gill J, et al: Alteration of type A behavior and reduction in cardiac recurrences in post myocardial infarction patients. Am Heart J 108:237–248, 1984

110. Friedman M, Thorensen C, Gill J, et al: Alteration of type A behavior and its effect on cardiac recurrence in post myocardial infarction patients: summary results of the recurrent coronary prevention project. Am Heart J 112:653–665, 1986

111. Fuller R, Rothbun R, Parli J: Inhibition of drug metabolism by fluoxetine. Res Commun Chem Pathol Pharmacol 13:353–356, 1976

112. Gardner S, Rutherford W, Munger M, et al: Drug induced supraventricular tachycardia: a case report of fluoxetine. Ann Emerg Med 20:194–197, 1991

113. Garrity T, Klein R: Emotional response and clinical severity as early determinants of six-month mortality after myocardial infarction. Heart Lung 4:730–737, 1975

114. Gelenberg A: Fluoxetine-induced arrhythmia. Biological Therapies in Psychiatry Newsletter 13:26, 1991

114a. Gelenberg A: The P450 family. Biological Therapies in Psychiatry Newsletter 18:29–31, 1995

115. Gerin W, Pieper C, Levy R, et al: Social support in social interaction: a moderator of cardiovascular reactivity. Psychosom Med 54:324–336, 1992

116. Giannuzzi P, Shabetai R, Imparato A, et al: Effects of mental exercise in patients with dilated cardiomyopathy and congestive heart failure: an echocardiographic Doppler study. Circulation 83 (4 suppl):II55–II65, 1991

117. Giubbini R, Galli M, Campini R, et al: Effects of mental stress on myocardial perfusion in patients with ischemic heart disease. Circulation 83 (4 suppl):II100–II107, 1991

118. Glass D, Lake C, Contrada R, et al: Stability of individual differences in physiological responses to stress. Health Psychol 2:317–341, 1983

119. Goldberg R, Morris P, Christian F, et al: Panic disorder in cardiac outpatients. Psychosomatics 31:168–173, 1990

120. Goldstein M, Niaura R: Psychological factors affecting physical condition: cardiovascular disease literature review. Psychosomatics 33:134–145, 1992

120a. Goldstein M, Niaura R: Cardiovascular disease, part I: coronary artery disease and sudden death, in Psychological Factors Affecting Medical Conditions. Edited by Stoudemire A. Washington, DC, American Psychiatric Press, 1995, pp 19–37

120b. Gottdiener J, Krantz D, Howell R, et al: Induction of silent myocardial ischemia with mental stress testing: relation to the triggers of ischemia during daily life activities and to ischemic functional severity. J Am Coll Cardiol 24:1645–1651, 1994

121. Grafing M, Lamberti J, Mostoufi-Moab E, et al: Treatment of panic disorder in coronary artery disease (letter). Am J Psychiatry 150:168, 1993

122. Greene W, Goldstein S, Moss A: Psychosocial aspects of sudden cardiac death. Arch Intern Med 129:725–731, 1972

123. Gruen W: Effects of brief psychotherapy during the hospitalization period on the recovery process in heart attacks. J Consult Clin Psychol 43:223–232, 1975

124. Guttmacher L, Goldstein M: Treatment of the cardiac-impaired depressed patient, II: lithium, carbamazepine, and electroconvulsive therapy. Psychiatr Med 6:34–51, 1988

125. Guy S, Silke B: The electrocardiogram as a tool for therapeutic monitoring: a critical analysis. J Clin Psychiatry 51 (12, suppl B):37–39, 1990

126. Hamilton M: A rating scale for depression. J Neurol Neurosurg Psychiatry 23:56–62, 1960

126a. Hanger H, Thomas F: Fluoxetine and warfarin interactions (letter). N Z Med J 108:157, 1995

127. Haynes S, Feinleib M, Kannel W: The relationship of psychosocial factors to coronary heart disease in the Framingham Study, III: eight-year incidence of coronary heart disease. Am J Epidemiol 111:37–58, 1980

128. Hecker M, Chesney M, Black G, et al: Coronary-prone behaviors in the Western Collaborative Group Study. Psychosom Med 50:153–164, 1988

129. Hedblad B, Ostergren P, Hanson B, et al: Influence of social support on cardiac event rate in men with ischaemic type ST segment depression during ambulatory 24-hour long-term ECG recording. Eur Heart J 13:433–439, 1992

130. Helmers K, Krantz D, Howell R, et al: Hostility and myocardial ischemia in coronary artery disease patients: evaluation by gender and ischemic index. Psychosom Med 55:29–36, 1993

131. Helsing K, Szklo M, Comstock G: Factors associated with mortality after widowhood. Am J Public Health 71:802–809, 1981

132. Hilbert G: Family satisfaction and affect of men and their wives after myocardial infarction. Heart Lung 22:200–205, 1993

132a. Hoffmann A, Pfiffner D, Hornung R, et al: Psychosocial factors predict medical outcome following a first myocardial infarction. Working Group on Cardiac Rehabilitation of the Swiss Society of Cardiology. Coron Artery Dis 6:147–152, 1995

133. Holland J, Morrow G, Schmale A, et al: A randomized clinical trial of alprazolam versus progressive muscle relaxation in cancer patients with anxiety and depressive symptoms. J Clin Oncol 9:1004–1011, 1991

134. Holmes T, Sabaawi M, Fragala M: Psychostimulant suppository treatment for depression in the gravely ill (letter). J Clin Psychiatry 55:265–266, 1994

135. Holmes V, Fernandez F, Levy J: Psychostimulant response in AIDS-related complex patients. J Clin Psychiatry 50:5–8, 1989

136. House J, Landis K, Umberson D: Social relationships and health. Science 241:540–545, 1988

137. Houston B, Chesney M, Black G, et al: Behavioral clusters and coronary heart disease risk. Psychosom Med 54:447–461, 1992

137a. Huyse F, Zwaan W, Kupka R: The applicability of antidepressants in the depressed medically ill: an open clinical trial with fluoxetine. J Psychsom Res 38:695–703, 1994

138. Ibrahim M, Feldman J, Sultz H, et al: Management after myocardial infarction: a controlled trial of the effect of group psychotherapy. Int J Psychiatry Med 5:253–268, 1974

139. Ironson G, Taylor C, Boltwood M, et al: Effects of anger on left ventricular ejection fraction in coronary artery disease. Am J Cardiol 70:281–285, 1992

140. Jackson C, Head L, Kellner C, et al: Catatonia associated with bupropion treatment (letter). J Clin Psychiatry 53:210, 1992

140a. Jain D, Burg M, Soufer R, et al: Prognostic implications of mental stress-induced silent left ventricular dysfunction in patients with stable angina pectoris. Am J Cardiol 76:31–35, 1995

141. Janne P, Reynaert C, Cassiers L, et al: Psychological determinants of silent myocardial ischaemia. Eur Heart J 8 (suppl G):125–129, 1987

142. Janne P, Reynaert C, Decoster P: Denial and silent ischemia: which comes first? (letter). JAMA 265:213, 1991

143. Janne P, Reynaert C, Decoster P, et al: The spouse as a possible anginal warning system in silent myocardial ischaemia. Eur Heart J 9 (suppl N):21–24, 1988

144. Jefferson J: Treatment of depressed patients who have become nontolerant to antidepressant medication because of cardiovascular side effects. J Clin Psychiatry Monogr 10:66–71, 1992

145. Jenike M: Handbook of Geriatric Psychopharmacology. Littleton, MA, PSG Publishing, 1985

146. Jenni M, Wollersheim J: Cognitive therapy, stress management training, and the type A behavior pattern. Cognitive Therapy 3:61–73, 1979

147. Johnson J, Hall E: Job strain, work place social support, and cardiovascular disease: a cross-sectional study of a random sample of the Swedish working population. Am J Public Health 78:1336–1342, 1988

148. Johnson M, Roberts M, Ross A, et al: Methylphenidate in stroke patients with depression. Am J Phys Med Rehabil 71:239–241, 1992

149. Jolley R, Lydiard R, Assey M, et al: Cardiovascular status of panic disorder patients with and without prominent cardiac symptoms. Psychosomatics 33:81–84, 1992

150. Jonas J, Cohon M: A comparison of the safety and efficacy of alprazolam versus other agents in the treatment of anxiety, panic, and depression: a review of the literature. J Clin Psychiatry 54 (suppl):25–45, 1993

151. Josephson M, Marchlinski F, Buxton A: The bradyarrhythmias: disorders of sinus node function and AV conduction disturbances, in Harrison's Principles of Internal Medicine, 12th Edition. Edited by Wilson J, Braunwald E, Isselbacher K, et al. New York, McGraw-Hill, Health Professions Division, 1991, pp 902–908

152. Julkunen J, Idanpaan-Heikkila U, Saarinen T: Components of type A behavior and the first-year prognosis of a myocardial infarction. J Psychosom Res 37:11–18, 1993

153. Kalbfleisch K, Lehmann M, Steinman R, et al: Reemployment following implantation of the automatic cardioverter defibrillator. Am J Cardiol 64:199–202, 1989

154. Kamarck T, Jennings J: Biobehavioral factors in sudden cardiac death. Psychol Bull 109:42–75, 1991

155. Kane FJ, Strohlein J, Harper R: Noncardiac chest pain in patients with heart disease. South Med J 84:847–852, 1991

156. Kaplitz S: Withdrawn, apathetic geriatric patients responsive to methylphenidate. J Am Geriatr Soc 23:271–276, 1975

157. Karasek R, Baker D, Marxer F, et al: Job decision latitude, job demands, and cardiovascular disease: a prospective study of Swedish men. Am J Public Health 71:694–705, 1981

158. Karasek R, Theorell T, Schwartz J, et al: Job, psychological factors, and coronary heart disease: Swedish prospective findings and U.S. prevalence findings using a new occupational inference method. Adv Cardiol 29:62–87, 1982

159. Kathol R, Noyes RJ, Williams J, et al: Diagnosing depression in patients with medical illness. Psychosomatics 31:434–440, 1990

160. Katon W: Panic disorder and somatization. Am J Med 77:101–106, 1984

161. Katon W: Chest pain, cardiac disease, and panic disorder. J Clin Psychiatry 51 (5 suppl):27–30, 1990

162. Katon W, Hall M, Russo J, et al: Chest pain: the relationship of psychiatric illness to coronary arteriography results. Am J Med 84:1–9, 1988

163. Katon W, Raskind M: Treatment of depression in the medically ill elderly with methylphenidate. Am J Psychiatry 137:963–965, 1980

163a. Kaufman K: Asystole with electroconvulsive therapy. J Intern Med 235:275–277, 1994

164. Kaufmann M, Murray G: The use of D-amphetamine in medically ill depressed patients. J Clin Psychiatry 43:463–464, 1982

165. Kaufmann M, Murray G, Cassem E: Use of psychostimulants in medically ill depressed patients. Psychosomatics 23:817–819, 1982

166. Kawachi I, Colditz G, Ascherio A, et al: Prospective study of phobic anxiety and risk of coronary heart disease in men. Circulation 89:1992–1997, 1994

166a. Kawachi I, Sparrow D, Vokonas P, et al: Symptoms of anxiety and risk of coronary heart disease: the Normative Aging Study. Circulation 90:2225–2229, 1994

167. Kellner C, Beale M: Cardiovascular complication of ECT (letter). Am J Psychiatry 151:789–790, 1994

168. Kennedy G, Hofer M, Cohen D, et al: Significance of depression and cognitive impairment in patients undergoing programmed stimulation of cardiac arrhythmias. Psychosom Med 49:410–421, 1987

169. Kenny R, Sutton R: Pacemaker syndrome. BMJ 293:902–903, 1986

170. Kenyon L, Ketterer M, Gheorghiade M, et al: Psychological factors related to prehospital delay during acute myocardial infarction. Circulation 84:1969–1976, 1991

171. Keren R, Aarons D, Veltri E: Anxiety and depression in patients with life-threatening ventricular arrhythmias: impact of the implantable cardioverter-defibrillator. PACE Pacing Clin Electrophysiol 14:181–187, 1991

172. Ketterer M: Secondary prevention of ischemic heart disease. The case for aggressive behavioral monitoring and intervention. Psychosomatics 34:478–484, 1993

173. Keys A, Taylor H, Blackburn H, et al: Mortality and coronary heart disease among men studied for 23 years. Arch Intern Med 128:201–214, 1971

173a. Kiev A, Masco H, Wenger T, et al: The cardiovascular effects of bupropion and nortriptyline in depressed outpatients. Ann Clin Psychiatry 6:107–115, 1994

174. Kimball C: Psychological responses to the experience of open heart surgery, I. Am J Psychiatry 126:348–359, 1969

175. King K, Reis H, Porter L, et al: Social support and long-term recovery from coronary artery surgery: effects on patients and spouses. Health Psychol 12:56–63, 1993

176. Kisely S, Creed F, Cotter L: The course of psychiatric disorder associated with non-specific chest pain. J Psychosom Res 36:329–335, 1992

177. Klapheke M: Potential drug-ECT interactions, I. Biological Therapies in Psychiatry Newsletter 14:33–36, 1991

177a. Klein R: The role of methylphenidate in psychiatry. Arch Gen Psychiatry 52:429–433, 1995

178. Kornecki E, Ehrlich Y, Lenox R: Platelet-activating factor–induced aggregation of human platelets specifically inhibited by triazolobenzodiazepines. Science 225:1454–1456, 1986

179. Koskenvuo M, Kaprio J, Rose R, et al: Hostility as a risk factor for mortality and ischemic heart disease in men. Psychosom Med 50:330–340, 1988

180. Kostis J, Rosen R, Cosgrove N, et al: Nonpharmacologic therapy improves functional and emotional status in congestive heart failure. Chest 106:996–1001, 1994

181. Kowey P, Marinchak R, Rials S: Things that go bang in the night (letter). N Engl J Med 327:1884, 1992

182. Krantz D, Durel L: Psychobiological substrates of the type A behavior pattern. Health Psychol 2:393–411, 1983

183. Krantz D, Hedges S, Gabbay F, et al: Triggers of angina and ST-segment depression in ambulatory patients with coronary artery disease: evidence for an uncoupling of angina and ischemia. Am Heart J 128:703–712, 1994

184. Krantz D, Helmers K, Bairey C, et al: Cardiovascular reactivity and mental stress-induced myocardial ischemia in patients with coronary artery disease. Psychosom Med 53:1–12, 1991

185. Krantz D, Manuck S: Acute psychophysiologic reactivity and risk of cardiovascular disease: a review and methodologic critique. Psychol Bull 96:435–464, 1984

186. Kravitz H, Fawcett J, Newman A: Alprazolam and depression: a review of risks and benefits. J Clin Psychiatry 54 (suppl):78–84, 1993

187. Kroenke K, Mangelsdorff A: Common symptoms in ambulatory care: incidence, evaluation, therapy and outcome. Am J Med 86:262–266, 1989

188. Kulik J, Mahler H: Emotional support as a moderator of adjustment and compliance after coronary artery bypass surgery: a longitudinal study. J Behav Med 16:45–63, 1993

189. Kuller L: Sudden death: definition and epidemiologic considerations. Prog Cardiovasc Dis 23:1–12, 1980

190. Kushner M, Thomas A, Bartels K, et al: Panic disorder history in the families of patients with angiographically normal coronary arteries. Am J Psychiatry 149:1563–1567, 1992

191. Lachar B: Coronary-prone behavior: type A behavior revisited. Tex Heart Inst J 20:143–151, 1993

192. Lacroix A, Haynes S: Gender differences in the stressfulness of workplace roles: a focus on work and health, in Gender and Stress. Edited by Barnett E, Baruch G, Biender L. New York, Free Press, 1987, pp 96–121

193. Ladwig K, Röll G, Breithardt G, et al: Post-infarction depression and incomplete recovery 6 months after acute myocardial infarction. Lancet 343:20–23, 1994

194. Langosch W, Seer P, Brodner G, et al: Behavior therapy with coronary heart disease patients: results of a comparative study. J Psychosom Res 26:475–484, 1982

195. Lantinger L, Sprafkin R, McCroskery J, et al: One-year psychosocial follow-up of patients with chest pain and angiographically normal coronary arteries. Am J Cardiol 62:209–213, 1988

195a. Legault S, Langer A, Armstrong P, et al: Usefulness of ischemic response to mental stress in predicting silent myocardial ischemia during ambulatory monitoring. Am J Cardiol 75:1007–1011, 1995

196. Lemberger L, Rowe H, Bosomworth J, et al: The effect of fluoxetine on the pharmacokinetics and psychomotor responses of diazepam. Clin Pharmacol Ther 43:412–419, 1988

197. Levenson J: Should psychostimulants be used to treat delirious patients with depressed mood? (letter). J Clin Psychiatry 53:69, 1992

198. Levenson J: Cardiovascular disease, in Psychiatric Care of the Medical Patient. Edited by Stoudemire A, Fogel B. New York, Oxford University Press, 1993, pp 539–555

198a. Liebowitz N, El-Mallakh R: Cardiac arrest during ECT: a cholinergic phenomenon? J Clin Psychiatry 54:279–280, 1993

199. Lingam V, Lazarus L, Groves L, et al: Methylphenidate in treating poststroke depression. J Clin Psychiatry 49:151–153, 1988

200. Littman A, Fava M, McKool K, et al: Buspirone therapy for type A behavior, hostility, and perceived stress in cardiac patients. Psychother Psychosom 59:107–110, 1993

201. Logue M, Thomas A, Barbee J, et al: Generalized anxiety disorder patients seek evaluation for cardiological symptoms at the same frequency as patients with panic disorder. J Psychiatr Res 27:55–59, 1993

202. Lown B: Sudden cardiac death: biobehavioral perspective. Circulation 76 (suppl I):I198–I201, 1987

203. Lown B, DeSilva R: Roles of psychologic stress and autonomic nervous system changes in provocation of ventricular premature complexes. Am J Cardiol 41:979–985, 1978

204. Luderitz B, Jung W, Deister A, et al: Patient acceptance of the implantable cardioverter defibrillator in ventricular tachyarrhythmias. PACE Pacing Clin Electrophysiol 16:1815–1821, 1993

205. Luderitz B, Jung W, Deister A, et al: Patient acceptance of implantable cardioverter defibrillator devices: changing attitudes. Am Heart J 127 (4 pt 2):1179–1184, 1994

206. MacDougall J, Dembroski T, Dimsdale J, et al: Components of type A, hostility, and anger-in: further relationships to angiographic findings. Health Psychol 4:137–152, 1985

207. Manuck S, Kaplan J, Adams M, et al: Behaviorally elicited heart rate reactivity and atherosclerosis in female Cynomologus monkeys (Macaca fascicularis). Psychosom Med 51:306–318, 1989

208. Manuck S, Kaplan J, Matthews K: Behavioral antecedents of coronary heart disease and atherosclerosis. Arteriosclerosis 6:2–14, 1986

209. Masand P, Murray G, Pickett P: Psychostimulants in poststroke depression. J Neuropsychiatry Clin Neurosci 3:23–27, 1991

210. Masand P, Pickett P, Murray G: Psychostimulants for secondary depression in medical illness. Psychosomatics 32:203–208, 1991

210a. Masand P, Pickett P, Murray G: Hypomania precipitated by psychostimulant use in depressed medically ill patients. Psychosomatics 36:145–147, 1995

211. Massie M, Holland J: The cancer patient with pain. Med Clin North Am 71:243–258, 1987

212. Matthews K, Glass D, Rosenman R, et al: Competitive drive, pattern A, and coronary heart disease: a further analysis of some data from the Western Collaborative Group Study. Journal of Chronic Disease 30:489–498, 1977

213. Matthews K, Haynes S: Type A behavior pattern and coronary disease risk: update and critical evaluation. Am J Epidemiol 123:923–960, 1986

213a. Mayou R, Bryant B, Forfar C, et al: Non-cardiac chest pain and benign palpitations in the cardiac clinic. Br Heart J 72:548–553, 1994

214. Mazzuero G, Temporelli P, Tavazzi L, et al: Influence of mental stress on ventricular pump function in postinfarction patients: an invasive hemodynamic investigation. Circulation 83 (4 suppl):II45–II54, 1991

215. McDaniel J, Musselman D, Porter M, et al: Depression in patients with cancer: diagnosis, biology, and treatment. Arch Gen Psychiatry 52:89–99, 1995

216. McLeod D, Hoehn S, Porges S, et al: Effects of alprazolam and imipramine on parasympathetic cardiac control in patients with generalized anxiety disorder. Psychopharmacology 107:535–540, 1992

217. Medalie J, Goldbourt U: Angina pectoris among 10,000 men, II: psychosocial and other risk factors as evidenced by a multivariate analysis of a five-year incidence study. Am J Med 60:910–921, 1976

217a. Meesters C, Smulders J: Hostility and myocardial infarction in men. J Psychosom Res 38:727–734, 1994

218. Mendels J, Chernoff R, Blatt M: Alprazolam as an adjunct to propranolol in anxious outpatients with stable angina pectoris. J Clin Psychiatry 47:8–11, 1986

219. Mendes de Leon C: Anger and impatience/irritability in patients of low socioeconomic status with acute coronary heart disease. J Behav Med 15:273–284, 1992

220. Mendes de Leon C, Powell L, Kaplan B: Change in coronary-prone behaviors in the Recurrent Coronary Preventions Project. Psychosom Med 53:407–419, 1991

221. Mitsibounas D, Tsouna-Hadjis E, Rotas V, et al: Effects of group psychosocial intervention on coronary risk factors. Psychother Psychosom 58:97–102, 1992

222. Mitsui T, Mizuno A, Hasegawa A, et al: Atrial rate as an indicator for optimal pacing rate and the pacemaking syndrome. Annales de Cardiologie et d'Angeiologie 20:371–379, 1971

223. Morse D, Martin J, Moshonov J: Stress induced sudden cardiac death: can it be prevented? Stress Medicine 8:35–46, 1992

224. Mukerji V, Beitman B, Alpert M, et al: Panic attack symptoms in patients with chest pain and angiographically normal coronary arteries. Journal of Anxiety Disorders 1:41–46, 1987

225. Murray G: Psychostimulants in general hospital psychiatry. Currents in Affective Illness 6:5–10, 1987

226. Musante L, Treiber F, Davis H, et al: Hostility: relationship to lifestyle behaviors and physical risk factors. Behav Med 18:21–26, 1992

227. Myers A, Dewar N: Circumstances attending 100 sudden deaths from coronary artery disease with coroner's necropsies. Br Heart J 37:1133–1143, 1975

228. Myrtek M, Fichtler A, Konig K, et al: Differences between patients with asymptomatic and symptomatic myocardial infarction: the relevance of psychological factors. Eur Heart J 15:311–317, 1994

229. Nehra A, Mullick F, Ishak K: Pemoline-associated hepatic injury. Gastroenterology 99:1517–1519, 1990

230. Niaura R, Goldstein M: Psychological factors affecting physical condition—cardiovascular disease literature review, II: coronary artery disease and sudden death and hypertension. Psychosomatics 33:146–155, 1992

230a. Niaura R, Goldstein M: Cardiovascular disease, part II: coronary artery disease and sudden death and hypertension, in Psychological Factors Affecting Medical Conditions. Edited by Stoudemire A. Washington, DC, American Psychiatric Press, 1995, pp 39–56

231. Nunes E, Frank K, Kornfeld D: Psychologic treatment for the type A behavior pattern and for coronary heart disease: a meta-analysis of the literature. Psychosom Med 48:159–173, 1987

232. Oldenburg B, Perkins R, Andrews G: Controlled trial of psychological intervention in myocardial infarction. J Consult Clin Psychol 53:852–859, 1985

233. Olsson G, Rehnquist N: Sudden death precipitated by psychological stress. Acta Medica Scandinavica 212:437–441, 1982

234. Orth-Gomr K, Unden A: Type A behavior, social support, and coronary risk: interaction and significance for mortality in cardiac patients. Psychosom Med 52:59–72, 1990

235. Pagani M, Mazzuero G, Ferrari A, et al: Sympathovagal interaction during mental stress: a study using spectral analysis of heart rate variability in healthy control subjects and patients with a prior myocardial infarction. Circulation 83 (4 suppl):II43–II51, 1991

235a. Pasternak R: Psychologic factors and course after myocardial infarction: maturing of a risk factor (editorial). Mayo Clin Proc 70:809–810, 1995

236. Patterson J: Alprazolam dependency: use of clonazepam for withdrawal. South Med J 81:830–836, 1988

237. Peters J, Alpert M, Beitman B, et al: Panic disorder associated with permanent pacemaker implantation. Psychosomatics 31:345–347, 1990

238. Pickett P, Masand P, Murray G: Psychostimulant treatment of geriatric depressive disorders secondary to medical illness. J Geriatr Psychiatry Neurol 3:146–151, 1990

238a. Potts S, Bass C: Psychological morbidity in patients with chest pain and normal or near-normal coronary arteries: a long-term follow-up study. Psychol Med 25:339–348, 1995

238b. Price V, Friedman M, Ghandour G, et al: Relation between insecurity and type A behavior. Am Heart J 129:488–491, 1995

239. Rabins P, Harvis K, Koven S: High fatality rates of late-life depression associated with cardiovascular disease. J Affect Disord 9:165–167, 1985

240. Rahe R: Anxiety and coronary heart disease in midlife. J Clin Psychiatry 50 (11 suppl):36–39, 1989

241. Rahe R, Romo M, Bennett L, et al: Recent life changes, myocardial infarction and abrupt coronary death. Arch Intern Med 133:221–228, 1974

242. Rahe R, Ward H, Hayes V: Brief group therapy in myocardial infarction rehabilitation: three- to four-year follow-up of a controlled trial. Psychosom Med 41:229–242, 1979

243. Rapp S, Vrana S: Substituting nonsomatic for somatic symptoms in the diagnosis of depression in elderly male medical patients. Am J Psychiatry 146:1197–1200, 1989

244. Razavi D, Delvaux N, Fravacques C, et al: Prevention of adjustment disorders and anticipatory nausea secondary to adjuvant chemotherapy: a double-blind, placebo-controlled study assessing the usefulness of alprazolam. J Clin Oncol 11:1384–1390, 1993

245. Razin A, Swencionis C, Zohman L: Reduction of physiological, behavioral, and self-report responses in type A behavior: a preliminary report. Int J Psychiatry Med 16:31–47, 1986

246. Reich P: Psychological predisposition to life-threatening arrhythmias. Annu Rev Med 36:397–405, 1985

247. Reich P, DeSilva R, Lown B, et al: Acute psychological disturbance preceding life-threatening ventricular arrhythmia. JAMA 246:233–235, 1981

248. Rice E, Sombrotto L, Markowitz J, et al: Cardiovascular morbidity in high-risk patients. Am J Psychiatry 151:1637–1641, 1994

249. Robinson K: Developing a scale to measure denial levels of clients with actual or potential myocardial infarctions. Heart Lung 23:36–44, 1994

250. Rockwood K, Dobbs A, Rule B, et al: The impact of pacemaker implantation on cognitive functioning in elderly patients. J Am Geriatr Soc 40:142–146, 1992

251. Roll M, Theorell T: Acute chest pain without obvious organic cause before age 40: personality and recent life events. J Psychosom Res 31:215–221, 1987

252. Roose S, Dalack G, Glassman A, et al: Cardiovascular effects of bupropion in depressed patients with heart disease. Am J Psychiatry 148:512–516, 1991

253. Roose S, Dalack G, Woodring S: Death, depression, and heart disease. J Clin Psychiatry 52 (6, suppl):34–39, 1991

254. Roose S, Glassman A: Cardiovascular effects of tricyclic antidepressants in depressed patients. J Clin Psychiatry Monograph 7:1–18, 1989

255. Roose S, Glassman A, Giardina E, et al: Cardiovascular effects of imipramine and bupropion in depressed patients with congestive heart failure. J Clin Psychopharmacol 7:247–251, 1987

255a. Rosal M, Downing J, Littman A, et al: Sexual functioning post-myocardial infarction: effects of beta-blockers, psychological status and safety information. J Psychosom Res 38:655–667, 1994

256. Rosenberg P, Ahmed I, Hurwitz S: Methylphenidate in depressed medically ill patients. J Clin Psychiatry 52:263–267, 1991

257. Rosenman R: The interview method of assessment of the coronary-prone behavior pattern, in Coronary-Prone Behavior. Edited by Dembroski T, Weiss S, Shields J, et al. New York, Springer-Verlag, 1978, pp 55–69

258. Rosenman R: Current and past history of type A behavior pattern, in Psychosomatic Risk Factors and Coronary Heart Disease: Indications for Predictive Therapy. Edited by Rosenman R. Bern, Germany, Hans Huber, 1981, pp 15–40

259. Roskies E: Stress Management for the Healthy Type A. New York, Guilford, 1987

260. Roskies E, Kearney H, Spevack M, et al: Generalizability and durability of treatment effects in an intervention program for coronary-prone (type A) managers. J Behav Med 2:195–207, 1979

261. Roskies E, Seraganian P, Oseasohn R, et al: The Montreal type A intervention project: major findings. Health Psychol 5:45–69, 1986

262. Rozanski A, Bairey C, Krantz D, et al: Mental stress and the induction of silent myocardial ischemia in patients with coronary artery disease. N Engl J Med 318:1005–1012, 1988

263. Rozanski A, Krantz D, Bairey C: Ventricular responses to mental stress testing in patients with coronary artery disease: pathophysiological implications. Circulation 83 (4 suppl):II137–II44, 1991

264. Ruberman W, Weinblatt E, Goldberg J, et al: Psychological influences on mortality after myocardial infarction. N Engl J Med 311:552–559, 1984

265. Russek L, King S, Russek S, et al: The Harvard Mastery of Stress Study 35-year follow-up: prognostic significance of patterns of psychophysiological arousal and adaptation. Psychosom Med 52:271–285, 1990

266. Satel S, Nelson J: Stimulants in the treatment of depression: a critical overview. J Clin Psychiatry 50:241–249, 1989

267. Scherck K: Coping with myocardial infarction. Heart Lung 21:327–334, 1992

268. Scherwitz L, Perkins L, Chesney M, et al: Cook-Medley Hostility Scale and subsets: relationship to demographic and psychosocial characteristics in young adults in the CARDIA study. Psychosom Med 53:36–49, 1991

269. Schleifer S, Macari-Hinson M, Coyle D, et al: The nature and course of depression following myocardial infarction. Arch Intern Med 149:1785–1789, 1989

270. Schwartz P: Stress and sudden cardiac death: the role of the autonomic nervous system. J Clin Psychiatry Monograph 2:7–13, 1984

271. Selwyn A, Braunwald E: Ischemic heart disease, in Harrison's Principles of Internal Medicine, 13th Edition. Edited by Isselbacher K, Braunwald E, Wilson J, et al. New York, McGraw-Hill, Health Professions Division, 1994, pp 1077–1085

272. Selwyn A, Ganz P: Myocardial ischemia in coronary disease. N Engl J Med 318:1058–1060, 1988

273. Shekelle R, Gale M, Ostfield A, et al: Hostility, risk of coronary heart disease, and mortality. Psychosom Med 45:109–114, 1983

274. Shell W, Swan H: Treatment of silent myocardial ischemia with transdermal nitroglycerin added to beta-blockers and alprazolam. Cardiol Clin 4:697–704, 1986

275. Shen W-K, Hammill S: Survivors of acute myocardial infarction: who is at risk for sudden cardiac death? Mayo Clin Proc 66:950–962, 1991

276. Shine K: Anxiety in patients with heart disease. Psychosomatics 25 (suppl):27–31, 1984

277. Siltanen P: Life changes and sudden coronary death. Adv Cardiol 25:47–60, 1978

278. Smith T, Allred K: Blood-pressure responses during social interaction in high- and low-cynically hostile males. J Behav Med 12:135–143, 1989

279. Smith T, Frohm K: What's so unhealthy about hostility? construct validity and psychosocial correlates of the Cook and Medley Ho scale. Health Psychol 4:503–520, 1985

280. Specchia G, Falcone C, Traversi E, et al: Mental stress as a provocative test in patients with various clinical syndromes of coronary heart disease. Circulation 83 (4 suppl):II108–II114, 1991

281. Spiller H, Ramoska E, Krenzelok E, et al: Bupropion overdose: a 3-year multi-center retrospective analysis. Am J Emerg Med 12:43–45, 1994

282. Steptoe A, Vogele C: Methodology of mental stress testing in cardiovascular research. Circulation 83 (4 suppl):II14–II24, 1991

283. Stern M, Pascale L, Ackerman A: Life adjustment postmyocardial infarction: determining predictive variables. Arch Intern Med 137:1680–1685, 1977

284. Sternbach H: Pemoline-induced mania. Biol Psychiatry 16:987–989, 1981

285. Stiebel V, Kemp K: Long-term methylphenidate use in the medically ill patient with organic mood syndrome. Psychosomatics 31:454–456, 1990

286. Storrow A: Bupropion overdose and seizure. Am J Emerg Med 12:183–184, 1994

287. Stoudemire A: Cardiovascular complication of ECT (letter). Am J Psychiatry 151:790, 1994

287a. Stoudemire A: Expanding psychopharmacologic treatment options for the depressed medical patient. Psychosomatics 36:S19–S26, 1995

287b. Stoudemire A (ed): Psychological Factors Affecting Medical Conditions. Washington, DC, American Psychiatric Press, 1995

288. Stoudemire A, Atkinson P: Use of cyclic antidepressants in patients with cardiac conduction disturbances. Gen Hosp Psychiatry 10:389–397, 1988

289. Stoudemire A, Fogel B (eds): Psychiatric Care of the Medical Patient. New York, Oxford University Press, 1993

289a. Stoudemire A, Fogel B: Psychopharmacology in medical patients: an update, in Medical-Psychiatric Practice, Vol 3. Edited by Stoudemire A, Fogel B. Washington, DC, American Psychiatric Press, 1995, pp 79–149

289b. Stoudemire A, Hales R: Psychological factors affecting medical conditions and DSM-IV: an overview, in Psychological Factors Affecting Medical Conditions. Edited by Stoudemire A. Washington, DC, American Psychiatric Press, 1995, pp 1–17

290. Stoudemire A, Knos G, Gladson M, et al: Labetalol in the control of cardiovascular responses to ECT in high risk depressed medical patients. J Clin Psychiatry 51:508–512, 1990

291. Stratton J, Halter J: Effect of a benzodiazepine (Alprazolam) on plasma epinephrine and norepinephrine levels during exercise stress. Am J Cardiol 56:136–139, 1985

292. Strouse T, Salehmoghaddam S, Spar J: Acute delirium and parkinsonism in a bupropion-treated liver transplant recipient (letter). J Clin Psychiatry 54:489–490, 1993

293. Suadicani P, Hein H, Gyntelberg F: Are social inequalities as associated with the risk of ischaemic heart disease a result of psychosocial working conditions? Atherosclerosis 101:165–175, 1993

294. Suarez E, Williams RJ: Situational determinants of cardiovascular and emotional reactivity in high and low hostile men. Psychosom Med 51:404–418, 1989

295. Suinn R: The cardiac stress management program for type A patients. Cardiovascular Rehabilitation 5:13–15, 1975

295a. Sundin O, Ohman A, Palm T, et al: Cardiovascular reactivity, type A behavior, and coronary heart disease: comparisons between myocardial infarction patients and controls during laboratory-induced stress. Psychophysiology 32:28–35, 1995

296. Tavazzi L, Zotti A, Rondanelli R: The role of psychologic stress in the genesis of lethal arrhythmias in patients with coronary artery disease. Eur Heart J 7 (suppl A):99–106, 1986

297. Theorell T, Lind E, Froberg J, et al: A longitudinal study of 21 subjects with coronary heart disease: life changes, catecholamine excretion and related biochemical reactions. Psychosom Med 34:505–516, 1972

298. Thockcloth R, Ho S, Wright W: Is cardiac rehabilitation necessary. Med J Aust 2:669–674, 1973

299. Thoits P: Conceptual, methodological, and theoretical problems in studying social support as a buffer against life stress. J Health Soc Behav 23:145–159, 1982

300. Trzcieniecka-Green A, Steptoe A: Stress management in cardiac patients: a preliminary study of the predictors of improvement in quality of life. J Psychosom Res 38:267–280, 1994

301. Tufo H, Ostfeld A, Shekelle R: Central nervous system dysfunction following open-heart surgery. JAMA 212:1333–1340, 1970

302. Tulloch I, Johnson A: The pharmacologic profile of paroxetine, a new selective serotonin reuptake inhibitor. J Clin Psychiatry 53 (2, suppl):7–12, 1992

302a. Turner L, Linden W, van der Wal R, et al: Stress management for patients with heart disease: a pilot study. Heart Lung 24:145–153, 1995

302b. van Driel R, Op den Velde W: Myocardial infarction and post-traumatic stress disorder. Journal of Traumatic Stress 8:151–159, 1995

303. Vlay S, Olson L, Fricchione G, et al: Anxiety and anger in patients with ventricular tachyarrhythmias: responses after automatic interval cardioverter defibrillator implantation. PACE Pacing Clin Electrophysiol 12:366–373, 1989

304. Vogel W, Miller J, DeTurck K, et al: Effects of psychoactive drugs on plasma catecholamines during stress in rats. Neuropharmacology 23:1105–1108, 1984

304a. Volkow N, Ding Y-S, Fowler J, et al: Is methylphenidate like cocaine? Arch Gen Psychiatry 52:456–463, 1995

304b. Wallace A, Kofoed L, West A: Double-blind, placebo-controlled trial of methylphenidate in older, depressed, medically ill patients. Am J Psychiatry 152:929–931, 1995

305. Walley T, Pirmohamed M, Proudlove C, et al: Interaction of fluoxetine and metoprolol (letter). Lancet 341:967–968, 1993

306. Warneke L: Psychostimulants in psychiatry. Can J Psychiatry 35:3–10, 1990

307. Warner M, Peabody C, Whiteford H, et al: Alprazolam as an antidepressant. J Clin Psychiatry 49:148–150, 1988

308. Warrington S, Lewis Y: Cardiovascular effects of antidepressants: studies of paroxetine in healthy men and depressed patients. Int Clin Psychopharmacol 6 (suppl 4):59–64, 1992

309. Weidner G, Friend R, Ficarrotto T, et al: Hostility and cardiovascular reactivity to stress in women and men. Psychosom Med 51:36–45, 1989

310. Weiner R, Coffey C: Electroconvulsive therapy in the medically ill, in Principles of Medical Psychiatry. Edited by Stoudemire A, Fogel B. Orlando, FL, Grune & Stratton, 1987, pp 113–134

311. Weiner R, Henschen G, Dellasega M, et al: Propranolol treatment of an ECT-related ventricular arrhythmia. Am J Psychiatry 136:1594–1595, 1979

312. Welin L, Tibblin G, Svardsudd K, et al: Prospective study of social influences on mortality. Lancet 1:915–918, 1985

312a. Wells D, Zelcer J, Treadrae C: ECT-induced asystole from a subconvulsive shock. Anaesth Intensive Care 16:368–373, 1988

313. Wenger T, Stern W: The cardiovascular profile of bupropion. J Clin Psychiatry 44:176–182, 1983

314. Wielgosz A, Nolan R: Understanding delay in response to symptoms of acute myocardial infarction: a compelling agenda. Circulation 84:2193–2195, 1991

315. Williams R, Anderson N: Hostility and Coronary Heart Disease. Edited by Elias J, Marshall P. Washington, DC, Hemisphere/Harper & Row, 1987, pp 17–37

316. Williams R, Chesney M: Psychosocial factors and prognosis in established coronary artery disease: the need for research on interventions. JAMA 270:1860–1861, 1993

317. Williams RJ: Do benzodiazepines have a role in the prevention or treatment of coronary heart disease and other major medical disorders? J Psychiatr Res 24 (suppl 2):51–56, 1990

317a. Wilner K, Lazar J, Apseloff G, et al: The effects of sertraline on the pharmacodynamics of warfarin in healthy volunteers (abstract). Biol Psychiatry (suppl) 29:354S–355S, 1991

318. Woods S, Tesar G, Murray G, et al: Psychostimulant treatment of depressive disorders secondary to medical illness. J Clin Psychiatry 47:12–15, 1986

319. Woolfrey S, et al: Fluoxetine-warfarin interaction (letter). BMJ 307:241, 1993

319a. Wulfson H, Askanazi J, Finck A: Propranolol prior to ECT associated with asystole. Anesthesiology 60:255–256, 1984

320. Yingling K, Wulsin L, Arnold L, et al: Estimated prevalences of panic disorder and depression among consecutive patients seen in an emergency department with acute chest pain. J Gen Intern Med 8:231–235, 1993

321. Zarzar M, Kingsley R: Use of fluoxetine in a person with cardiac arrhythmias (letter). Psychosomatics 31:235–236, 1990

322. Zielinski R, Roose S, Devanand D, et al: Cardiovascular complications of ECT in depressed patients with cardiac disease. Am J Psychiatry 150:904–909, 1993

323. Zotti A, Bettinardi O, Soffiantino F, et al: Psychophysiological stress testing in postinfarction patients: psychological correlates of cardiovascular arousal and abnormal cardiac responses. Circulation 83 (4 suppl):II25–II35, 1991

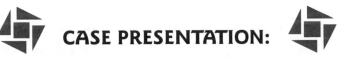

CASE PRESENTATION:

Mr. Smith: The Depressed, Post–Myocardial Infarction Patient

The cardiologist admits a 57-year-old man to the coronary care unit who has sustained an inferior-wall myocardial infarction (MI) 6 weeks ago with pneumococcal pneumonia. Mr. Smith had been maintained on trazodone (Desyrel) 350 mg per day prior to admission for depression and insomnia before his MI, with good therapeutic effect. Two weeks after admission, the cardiologist requests a psychiatric consultation to determine if trazodone should be started again.

The patient is stable clinically on quinidine for premature ventricular contractions, with no evidence at present of arrhythmias, congestive heart failure, or angina. The electrocardiogram (ECG) shows changes consistent with inferior-wall MI, and a rate-corrected QT interval (QTc) of 0.40 second (0.440 second is the upper limit of normal). Resting pulse is 80 and regular. Supine blood pressure is 140/90. Standing blood pressure is 120/88.

Past psychiatric history is notable for nonresponse to fluoxetine (Prozac), paroxetine (Paxil), and bupropion (Wellbutrin). He was unable to tolerate sertraline (Zoloft) even at small doses because of nausea and intractable headaches.

 QUESTIONS

Choose all that apply.

1. Mr. Smith has lost the will to live. He states that God is punishing him for all the wrongs he has committed in his life. He is self-deprecating, and admits to a pervasively dysphoric mood that does not lessen even when his daughter brings pictures of his new grandson. Although he expresses no active suicidal intent, he hopes that "nature will take its course" and states that it would "serve him right" to die from his illness. So far, Mr. Smith has been compliant with his medical regime. There is no psychotic symptomatology. He is cognitively intact except for diminished concentration. Although he has no appetite, his wife successfully encourages him to eat low-salt food that she brings from home. Assuming that Mr. Smith refuses ECT, what advice would you give the cardiologist about reinstituting trazodone?

    a. Warn the cardiologist that trazodone has antiarrhythmic effects requiring adjustments in class I antiarrhythmics like quinidine or procainamide.

    b. Discuss how trazodone has a high incidence of sinus tachycardia, even in the absence of orthostatic hypotension, and could potentially increase myocardial oxygen demand.

    c. Explain that trazodone may have negative inotropic effects on the heart.

    d. Caution that trazodone has been associated with aggravating preexisting ventricular irritability and heart block.

2. The decision is made to restart trazodone because of Mr. Smith's previous therapeutic response and his exacerbation when it was stopped. The cardiologist agrees to monitor the patient closely. Which of the following is/are *not* true regarding the orthostatic and anticholinergic side effects of antidepressant drugs?

    a. Trazodone has the advantage of producing few, if any, anticholinergic side effects.

    b. The less anticholinergic the drug, the less tachycardia it produces.

    c. Trazodone-digoxin interactions are rare.

    d. Trazodone has the advantage of producing a hypotensive effect less frequently than nortriptyline (Pamelor, Aventyl).

3. It is not uncommon to use intravenous lidocaine (Xylocaine) during the management of cardiac arrhythmias. All of the following would be typical of iv lidocaine *except . . .*

    a. Somnolence.

    b. Central nervous system (CNS) excitement.

    c. Psychosis.

    d. An anxious sense of doom.

4. Mr. Smith can no longer tolerate the orthostatic hypotension induced by trazodone. The cardiologist asks whether the tetracyclic antidepressant maprotiline (Ludiomil) is any different from medications with a tricyclic structure. You reply . . .

    a. The tetracyclic structure spares it from having the same spectrum of cardiovascular effects as the tricyclics.

    b. It induces significantly less orthostatic hypotension, resulting in fewer serious injuries from falls.

    c. Cardiovascular deaths have been reported in overdose.

    d. At normal therapeutic doses it slows conduction, like the standard tricyclics.

5. Mr. Smith and his family continue to refuse ECT. He has already failed trials of the newer generation antidepressants. It seems you have to decide whether to treat him with tricyclics or not. Periodic monitoring for postural hypotension is always important, but is especially crucial in patients like Mr. Smith, after MI. Imipramine (Tofranil) has been the most widely studied tricyclic antidepressant (TCA) in terms of this side effect. Which of the following is/are true?

    a. The orthostatic blood pressure changes secondary to imipramine generally disappear over a 4-week period for patients who develop this side effect.

    b. Many patients have postural hypotension on no medication. Those who are clinically asymptomatic are *less* likely to experience further orthostatic changes on TCAs than their symptomatic counterparts.

    c. Mr. Smith would be likely to sustain a systolic orthostatic drop on imipramine that is twice his baseline orthostatic change without imipramine.

    d. Significant orthostatic hypotension serves as a marker for plasma imipramine levels that are within the therapeutic range or above.

6. What is the most clinically relevant impact of congestive heart failure (CHF) on the use of TCAs?

    a. CHF exacerbates conduction defects.

    b. CHF lowers serum levels by increasing the apparent volume of distribution.

    c. CHF worsens on TCAs.

    d. CHF exacerbates orthostatic blood pressure changes.

7. Recent findings on the effects of quinidine-type antiarrhythmics in post-MI patients . . .

    a. Have shown increased mortality compared with placebo.

    b. Have supported using TCAs because of their quinidine-like effects.

    c. Have shown improved outcome compared with placebo-treated groups.

    d. Have led to recommendations of selective serotonin reuptake inhibitors (SSRIs) (despite their short track record in cardiovascular patients) or ECT over TCAs.

8. The mechanism of TCA-induced conduction disturbance is via . . .

    a. Alpha-adrenergic blockade

    b. Anticholinergic effects

    c. Blockade of inward sodium current

    d. Inhibition of calcium channels

9. All of the following are true regarding tricyclics *except* . . .

    a. Patients with prolonged QTc intervals after MI should not be given TCAs.

    b. Patients with medication-induced prolonged QTc intervals should not be given TCAs.

    c. In patients with second- or third-degree heart block, tricyclics are contraindicated even with a pacemaker.

    d. In patients with first-degree heart block, tricyclics may be used without a pacemaker.

10. The effect of adding a tricyclic to a quinidine regimen would be to . . .

    a. Decrease the likelihood of further arrhythmias via membrane stabilization.

    b. Dangerously increase the risk of heart block.

    c. Enhance inotropy (contractility).

    d. None of the above.

11. The term *conduction disease* covers a number of conditions, depending on the pathophysiology of the disorder. Which of the following is true about tricyclics and the specific types of conduction disturbance?

    a. *First*-degree heart block leads to higher degrees of atrioventricular (AV) block, especially on TCAs.

    b. The presence or absence of a pacemaker has little effect on whether a TCA can be used.

    c. Patients with *left* bundle branch block tend to be at lower risk for tricyclic-induced disturbances than patients with *right* bundle disease.

d. With a pacemaker in place, TCAs can be used in patients with bifascicular block, trifascicular block, or alternating bundle branch block.

12. What is true regarding TCAs in patients with conduction disease?
    a. Doxepin (Sinequan) is the tricyclic that alters conduction the least.
    b. Monitoring for medication-induced ECG changes must take into account that steady state is reached after three half-lives of the antidepressant.
    c. Compared with tricyclics, ECT is a less risky treatment for patients with bundle branch block.
    d. Adverse cardiac events become less likely with time for patients suffering conduction disease who have been successfully stabilized on long-term tricyclic therapy.

13. What are valid strategies for managing tricyclic-induced side effects?
    a. If a patient with preexisting bundle branch block shows an increase in QTc interval on amitriptyline (Elavil), switching to a less anticholinergic medication is likely to produce fewer effects on conduction.
    b. If a patient with preexisting orthostatic hypotension shows greater postural changes on a given dose of a tricyclic, lowering the medication dose is likely to bring some relief.
    c. If a patient with preexisting orthostatic hypotension shows more postural changes on a given tricyclic, changing to a different tricyclic is likely to bring some relief.
    d. None of the above.

14. You finally agree to try a tricyclic. Which of the following are true about Mr. Smith's psychopharmacological management?
    a. It would be important for Q waves in leads II, III, and aVF to resolve before instituting a tricyclic drug.
    b. A QTc interval of > 0.440 second poses particular risk.
    c. A pretreatment QRS complex of 0.08 second flags an increased risk for developing conduction abnormalities.
    d. The probability of producing significant tricyclic-induced ECG changes is dose related.

15. Treatments that might induce the "acquired" prolonged QT syndrome include:

a. ECT
b. Alprazolam (Xanax)
c. Nortriptyline (Pamelor, Aventyl)
d. Thioridazine (Mellaril)

16. If this were a healthy patient with a normal pretreatment ECG, which would be the most commonly observed ECG changes at therapeutic tricyclic levels?
    a. Increased heart rate
    b. ST-segment changes
    c. T-wave abnormalities
    d. QTc intervals ≥ 0.440 second

17. How does impaired myocardial contractility influence the psychopharmacology of depression?
    a. Tricyclics further impair left ventricular function.
    b. Impaired myocardial contractility predisposes to tricyclic-induced postural hypotension.
    c. When used in the setting of impaired myocardial contractility and CHF, nortriptyline (Pamelor, Aventyl) loses its advantage over other TCAs in producing the least postural hypotension.
    d. TCAs would be unlikely to contribute to decreased cardiac output.

18. Which are true regarding the use of psychotropics in the setting of atrial fibrillation?
    a. The potential for a tricyclic to convert atrial fibrillation to normal sinus rhythm would be a desirable therapeutic effect.
    b. New evidence supports avoiding tricyclics in the setting of chronic atrial fibrillation.
    c. Tricyclics often interact adversely with digoxin.
    d. Digoxin-tricyclic interactions have not been definitively documented.

19. The cardiologist has read that many psychiatrists feel that the dangers of monoamine oxidase inhibitors (MAOIs) have been overstated, as long as patients comply with diet and drug precautions. She has asked you to consider tranylcypromine (Parnate) for treating Mr. Smith. Which of the following are true regarding the relative advantages and disadvantages of MAOIs versus TCAs in treating this patient?
    a. Failure to develop postural hypotension within the critical first 2–3 weeks of MAOI therapy predicts that this side effect is unlikely to occur.
    b. MAOIs rarely cause cardiac rhythm disturbances.
    c. Patients without pretreatment baseline postural hypotension are unlikely to suffer MAOI treatment-emergent postural hypotension.

d. There is little cholinergic blockade with the MAOIs, so less likelihood of sinus tachycardia.

20. Which of the following psychiatric symptoms occur at *therapeutic* digoxin levels?
    a. Delirium
    b. Hallucinations
    c. Depression
    d. All of the above
    e. None of the above

21. Which of the following is/are *most* characteristic of digoxin toxicity?
    a. Mania
    b. Auditory disturbances
    c. Visual distortions
    d. Paranoid delusions

22. Before the tricyclic is added, Mr. Smith develops persecutory ideation and psychomotor agitation. He is medically stable and has had no changes in his medication regimen. Serum electrolytes and thyroid function tests are normal. His neurological exam and brain magnetic resonance imaging (MRI) are normal. The medical staff inquires about transfer to psychiatry for recurrent depression, since he is medically cleared. Which of the following considerations are true?
    a. A psychiatric syndrome due to medications has been sufficiently ruled out.
    b. The mental status changes could be entirely attributable to quinidine.
    c. Partial complex status epilepticus is high on the differential.
    d. None of the above is true.

Answers

1. Answer: d (p. 44)
2. Answer: d (pp. 41, 44)
3. Answer: a (p. 45)
4. Answer: c, d (p. 44)
5. Answer: c (p. 41)
6. Answer: d (p. 43)
7. Answer: a, d (pp. 39–40)
8. Answer: c (p. 39)
9. Answer: c (pp. 42–43)
10. Answer: b (p. 42)
11. Answer: d (pp. 42–43)
12. Answer: c (pp. 39–40)
13. Answer: c (pp. 39–41)
14. Answer: b, d (pp. 40–41)
15. Answer: c, d (p. 43)
16. Answer: a (p. 40)
17. Answer: b, d (pp. 41, 43)
18. Answer: b, d (p. 44)
19. Answer: b, d (pp. 44–45)
20. Answer: d (p. 45)
21. Answer: c (pp. 45–46)
22. Answer: b (p. 45)

The new-generation antidepressants, such as the SSRIs, appear to have safe cardiovascular profiles, which may make our discussion of heterocyclic antidepressants (tricyclics, tetracyclics, trazodone, amoxapine) and mono-amine oxidase inhibitors (MAOIs) seem extraneous—or worse, passé. But the psychiatrist who regularly consults on medically fragile patients knows that there is no such thing as a "routine" case, and that bad things happen with good medication. Of the newer antidepressants, only bupropion (Wellbutrin) has been systematically tested in the cardiovascularly ill. *Moreover, clinicians regularly encounter those patients who are nonresponders or who cannot tolerate the side effects of these medications.* Patient and family resistance to ECT still runs high, and may prove unworkable for individuals already overwhelmed by recent life-threatening medical events.

In short, one may find oneself mired in the old dilemma of choosing a TCA or an MAOI or doing nothing because it seems safer.[20] As previously reviewed, the growing literature on the relationship between major depressive disorder and cardiovascular morbidity, however, unambiguously demonstrates that untreated depression may be even more hazardous than medications that potentially affect the heart. We will review next the "old standbys"—tricyclics, heterocyclics, and MAOIs.

◈ TRICYCLIC ANTIDEPRESSANTS

Adverse Cardiovascular Effects

Adding a tricyclic may destabilize an antiarrhythmic drug regimen.[44] In addition, many patients have transitory conduction disturbances after an MI, making it sometimes difficult to accurately assess the conduction system. *Keep in mind when monitoring ECG parameters or serum levels that it requires approximately* **5 half-lives** *of the medication to achieve steady state.*[93]

At present there are no data available to guide the frequency of outpatient monitoring, but changes in the patient's medication regimen, symptoms, or medical status should serve as landmarks for checking ECGs and drug levels. Remember that *cardiovascular disease advances with time;* it is easy to be lulled into forgetting that your "stable" cardiovascular patients on long-term TCA maintenance are at progressive risk for conduction abnormali-

ties due to the advance of their underlying disease.[97] Check ECGs and serum antidepressant levels periodically.

Conduction and Rhythm

Tricyclics influence *conduction* by inhibiting the initial inward sodium ion (Na^+) current mediated by fast sodium channels, which in turn mediates phase 0 of the cardiac action potential, the initial rapid depolarization. They also prolong repolarization.[7] It is their anticholinergic properties that account for their effect on *heart rate*. Until recently, it was assumed that a patient with premature ventricular contractions who needed an antidepressant would benefit from TCAs, which have actions similar to "quinidine-like" class I antiarrhythmics.[106,110] It had been thought that TCAs would serve to both suppress the arrhythmia and treat the depression.

The main risk was thought to be the additive effects of combining TCAs with other class I antiarrhythmics. However, the disturbing results of a 1991 study showed that rather than reducing mortality, antiarrhythmic therapy with quinidine and other class I antiarrhythmics (e.g., moricizine [Ethmozine], flecainide) after MI actually *increased* mortality.[68,102]

◆ During the initial 2 weeks of moricizine treatment in the Cardiac Arrhythmia Suppression Trial (CAST) II, 17 of 665 patients receiving post-MI moricizine died or had a cardiac arrest, compared with only 3 of 660 who received placebo (2.6% versus 0.45%, respectively; $P < .001$).

There was also evidence of heightened mortality when these compounds were used for suppressing atrial fibrillation.[18,31] The psychopharmacologist Gelenberg[36] has offered the following perspective:

> For their first two decades, imipramine (Tofranil and others) and other TCAs were believed to be capable of causing or aggravating cardiac arrhythmias. This impression, however, came mainly from overdose cases, rather than from patients taking therapeutic doses. The assumption that TCAs cause arrhythmias was turned on its head in 1977 when Bigger et al.[8]

at Columbia reported that imipramine was an *antiarrhythmic* agent, capable of decreasing atrial and ventricular premature cardiac contractions. The investigators discovered that imipramine shared cardiac effects with quinidine [and others], . . . which classified it as a I-A type antiarrhythmic agent. From that time until recently, doctors assumed that a patient with premature ventricular contractions who needed an antidepressant would benefit from a TCA, which would decrease the extra beats and treat the depression simultaneously . . . A recent editorial from the same group,[41] who pioneered this field, casts these teachings in a different light. (p. 33)

In their 1993 *JAMA* editorial,[41] Glassman, Roose, and Bigger warned that until more specific information is available, it is safest to assume that TCAs have risks similar to those newly discovered for the class I antiarrhythmics. A. Stoudemire (personal communication, September 1993) has noted, however, that this issue constitutes an emerging controversy in the field of consultation-liaison psychiatry, as there are years of data supporting the *safe* use of tricyclics in post-MI patients without cardiac conduction disease. What, then, is the psychiatrist to use? In 1994, Roose and Glassman[84] proposed the following guidelines:

1. **Mild or moderate depression and ischemic heart disease:** Begin with an SSRI or perhaps bupropion (Wellbutrin). Consider a tricyclic only if the patient fails to respond.
2. **More severe melancholic depressions but with milder ischemic heart disease:** Begin with a tricyclic.

> This decision considers the increased morbidity and mortality associated with depression and balances the efficacy of the tricyclics in this population against the moderately increased risk of mortality that we infer to be associated with tricyclic use in these patients.[84] (p. 86)

3. **Severe ischemic heart disease:** Avoid tricyclics. As the severity of ischemic heart disease increases, the risk/benefit ratio begins to weigh against tricyclic use, even in the severely depressed melancholic patient.

Roose and Glassman[84] have written,

> In the final analysis, the treatment of the depressed patient with ischemic heart disease remains a complex problem for the informed clinician. At present we lack sufficient information on either the cardiovascular safety or the relative efficacy of available antidepressants to establish the risk/benefit ratio of these various treatments . . . The problem is that we lack the data to define [when the risk/benefit ratio begins to weigh against tricyclic use], and consequently, even within our own group, we cannot always reach consensus on how to treat the seriously depressed patient with symptomatic ischemic heart disease. (p. 86)

ECT is probably still the standard in terms of safety and effectiveness in these patients.[83] We await further developments.

Doxepin. The reader may occasionally hear that doxepin (Sinequan) has a superior cardiovascular profile. It does not. Early studies of patients who overdosed on tricyclics initially indicated that doxepin overdose resulted in less atrioventricular (AV) prolongation than other heterocyclic antidepressants.[1,13] Later studies showed methodological flaws in these data, and demonstrated that doxepin has no advantage over other tricyclics in affecting cardiac conduction.[67] For example, it was poorly tolerated in a recent prospective study of depressed patients with preexisting cardiac disease, who had a 41% dropout rate because of cardiovascular and other side effects.[81] Doxepin's alleged superior safety profile in the setting of cardiac conduction disease stands more as "persistent legend."[82] To repeat, "There is no evidence to suggest that one tricyclic is safer than another [in patients with conduction disease]" (p. 18).[44]

Electrocardiogram Changes

The effects of tricyclics on the ECG are *dose related* and reversible with discontinuation of the drug.[6] Tricyclics most commonly cause *increased heart rate.*

◆ True symptomatic tachycardia, with a heart rate of 130–140 beats/minute, is relatively rare.[83]
◆ Tricyclics increase the heart rate in inverse proportion to the drug-free baseline pulse[33,107]: the lower the baseline pulse, the greater the rise when the patient ingests the TCA.

◆ Mechanism: Although tricyclic antidepressants do slow HIS bundle conduction, this is not the mechanism for the tachycardia they produce. Their anticholinergic properties induce reflex sympathetic activity (and increased heart rate) via *vagal* ["-cholinergic"] blockade ["anti-"].[97]

Other less common ECG abnormalities include QRS widening, increased PR intervals, ST-segment and T-wave changes, QT-interval prolongation, and bradycardia.[48] New ST-segment changes and T-wave abnormalities should be investigated before they are attributed to the tricyclic.[85]

◆ A prolonged rate-corrected QT interval (QTc) (≤ 0.440 second) is a potentially malignant condition that heightens the risk for ventricular tachycardia,[32,92] especially in patients with pretreatment partial or incomplete heart block.[97] Life-threatening QT prolongation by tricyclics *alone* has been observed primarily in the setting of *overdose*.[34]

◆ A widened pretreatment QRS complex (≥ 0.11 second) identifies those patients at greater risk for subsequently developing conduction abnormalities on tricyclics.[97]

Persistent Q waves in leads II, III, and aVF are characteristic of an inferior-wall MI.[70] They persist after recovery and are not in themselves a contraindication to tricyclics.

Orthostatic Hypotension

Orthostatic hypotension is the most frequent side effect of TCA treatment and can produce significant post-MI morbidity (because of increased myocardial oxygen demand).[42,69] Orthostatic hypotension also predisposes to falls, especially in the elderly.[76,83] Tricyclic-induced hypotension is most likely secondary to relaxation of vascular smooth muscle (rather than via alpha-adrenergic blockade), resulting in peripheral vasodilation.[6,57,80] Many patients have postural hypotension on no medication; those who are asymptomatic (and therefore less likely to be identified unless baseline blood pressure is checked) are *no less likely* to experience further orthostatic changes on TCAs than are their symptomatic counterparts. *Always check* **every** *patient for postural changes before starting TCAs.*

◆ A difference greater than 10–15 mm Hg between the pretreatment lying and standing systolic blood pressures identifies patients vulnerable to postural hypotension on TCAs.[15,42]

• A patient on no medication whose systolic blood pressure falls more than 15 mm Hg on rising from a lying to a standing position (like Mr. Smith) is likely to sustain a decrease of about *twice* that on imipramine.[16]

◆ Glassman et al.[42] observed that the orthostatic drop may occur at lower-than-therapeutic plasma drug levels, and *remains constant* even as the dose is increased.

Unfortunately, *orthostatic changes do not disappear within 4 weeks, even if the patient is asymptomatic and has clinically accommodated to them.*[42]

> Clinically, this means that whatever drop a patient will undergo is unlikely to change as the dose of [TCA] increases; and conversely, decreasing the dose moderately, once at a therapeutic level, to diminish severe postural hypotension will result only in inadequate treatment of depression.[44] (p. 18)

Unlike the situation with conduction disease, in which all the tricyclics are potentially harmful,[14] the risk of a postural systolic drop is significantly reduced with at least one of the TCAs, nortriptyline (Pamelor, Aventyl).[41]

◆ Nortriptyline produces the least orthostatic hypotension of all the heterocyclics, including trazodone.[33,88,101,107]

◆ It has also been safely used in depressed heart transplant patients, with careful monitoring of plasma cyclosporine levels.[94]

As discussed in the section on congestive heart failure, CHF magnifies the risk of tricyclic-induced postural hypotension,[43,87] but nortriptyline does not lose its advantage over other TCAs even in this setting. It is the tricyclic of choice in cardiac patients, for the elderly, and for others vulnerable to orthostatic hypotension.[44,83]

Cardiotoxicity and Drug Metabolism

Recently, attention has focused on genetic differences of the hepatic cytochrome P450 system, which metabolizes most psychotropics. For example, Bluhm et al.[9] described a patient who developed desipramine toxicity (plasma level 764 ng/ml) and myocardial ischemia on conventional desipramine doses (250 mg/day). (The average serum concentration of desipramine on 200 mg has been reported as only 173 ng/ml.[35]) Using pharmacological probes, the authors found a pattern of poor drug metabolism—an inherited predisposition found in the patient, his mother, and one son.

Rudorfer[89] has written,

> The pharmacokinetic parameters for many psychoactive drugs are markedly altered in special patient populations. Both age and intercurrent disease strongly influence drug distribution and elimination, which means that treating all patients with standard dosing regimens can result in either undermedication or toxicity for many. Much of the information required to avoid potentially serious problems will be available from the patient's history and physical examination. Information about age, race, ethnic background, and other medical conditions that may alter drug metabolism can be obtained with relatively little effort. Although this information can be used to guide initial dosing, careful monitoring of drug plasma levels is also important, especially for drugs like TCAs, which have a relatively narrow therapeutic index and the potential for serious toxic reactions. (p. 54)

A series of excellent papers further details the pharmacokinetics of psychiatric drugs.[46,55,72,73]

Specific Cardiac Conditions

The absolute contraindications for using TCAs are surprisingly few. Obviously, collaboration with the cardiologist is crucial. Ongoing inpatient cardiology consultation, serial ECGs on an alternate-day basis during upward titration of the medication (remember that it takes five half-lives to reach steady state),[93] and 24-hour ambulatory (Holter) monitoring are helpful.

◆ **WARNING!** Additive effects on conduction delay can occur if tricyclics are combined with other class I antiarrhythmics, and there is new evidence[41,68,102] that this class of medications *predisposes*, rather than suppresses, fatal arrhythmias in post-MI patients (see discussion above).

Myocardial Infarction

No controlled data are available on the optimal waiting time after an MI for starting antidepressants. Formerly,

TCA therapy after uncomplicated MI was not controversial after a **6-week** waiting period[98] (the approximate time for healing of myocardial tissue). It was even thought[98] that TCAs could be started sooner, as long as there were no complications such as heart block, unstable CHF, or orthostatic hypotension (factors that could exacerbate angina and increase the likelihood of further ischemic events). However, the 1991–1992 data showing increased mortality with class I antiarrhythmics like quinidine have called these recommendations into question (see pp. 39–40).[41]

◆ Surprising data emerged from a retrospective case-control study of fatal cardiovascular disease in the United Kingdom.[103] Thorogood and co-workers found that the relative risk of a fatal MI was 17 times greater for young women (aged 16–39 years) who were currently using psychotropic drugs (benzodiazepines and tricyclics) than for those who were not. It is unclear whether these findings were due to the inherent risks of psychiatric illness, to the hazards of psychotropic drugs, or to the misattribution of a complex physical symptom, such as chest pain, to a psychogenic origin.[27]

Be cautious about abruptly stopping stable TCA regimens in patients who develop an MI, as sudden discontinuation may predispose to arrhythmias.[77]

Heart Block

Therapeutic plasma levels of tricyclics frequently prolong the PR, QRS, and QTc intervals in healthy people, and can occasionally cause malignant conduction disturbance.[38] Older patients are at particular risk (e.g., a 63-year-old man who had been free of underlying conduction disorders developed left bundle branch block at subtherapeutic serum levels of nortriptyline[47]); new onset of atrial fibrillation has occurred in elderly patients taking nortriptyline.[14]

◆ The risks of cardiovascular complications at therapeutic plasma tricyclic levels were compared in 155 patients with normal ECGs and 41 patients with prolonged PR interval and/or bundle branch block.[85] The occurrence of 2:1 AV block was significantly greater in patients with preexisting bundle branch block than in those with normal ECGs (9% versus 0.7%, respectively). Tricyclics had to be discontinued in 10% of the patients with preexisting bundle branch block because the QRS interval was prolonged by more than 25%.

Although patients with cardiac conduction disturbance are at relatively high risk for complications, the risk-benefit ratio should be assessed for each patient individually.

◆ **Prolonged QTc intervals:** Prolonged QTc intervals after MI bring a higher risk for subsequent fatal ventricular fibrillation; tricyclics, which may further prolong the QTc interval, are contraindicated in this setting,[97] especially if the QTc interval is longer than 0.440 second. Use caution if tricyclics are added to other class I antiarrhythmics (quinidine, procainamide), as there may be an additive effect on conduction delay.

  • Drugs such as quinidine, procainamide, disopyramide, the *phenothiazines,* and the *tricyclics* are the most common causes of the acquired QT syndrome,[97] which occurs primarily in the setting of overdose.[34] A very rapid form of ventricular tachycardia may occur, which frequently degenerates into ventricular fibrillation (torsade de pointes—polymorphic ventricular tachycardia).

  • As we will discuss later in this chapter, thioridazine (Mellaril) is the most cardiotoxic of the neuroleptics,[3,24,53,61] with quinidine-like properties similar to those of the tricyclics. Thioridazine and tricyclics should not routinely be combined.[16]

  • Neither ECT nor benzodiazepines (such as alprazolam [Xanax]) induce changes in the QT interval.

◆ **First-degree block:** First-degree heart block (PR interval > 0.20 second) is among the mildest forms of pathology and should not impede TCA treatment.[16,23] Although first-degree block theoretically predisposes to developing higher degrees of AV block, a 1987 study[85] demonstrated that it did *not* evolve into higher grades of AV block after tricyclic treatment. This finding was corroborated in another study.[23]

◆ **Second- to third-degree block/right versus left block:** It has not been possible to differentiate the relative risks for developing complications secondary to right versus left bundle branch block;[85] both groups are at some risk for progression to complete heart block. In patients with preexisting bundle branch block, it has been said that there is no such thing as a safe tricyclic.[83] Bifascicular or trifascicular block, alternating bundle-branch block, and second- or third-degree heart block represent more extensive

disease of the conduction system; tricyclics can be used *only if a pacemaker is in place.*[97]

Cassem[16] has reported using tricyclics in patients with relatively uncomplicated isolated left bundle branch block or hemiblock without evidence of second- or third-degree heart block. Conservative management would avoid tricyclics in these patients, however, unless there is continuous and intensive monitoring. TCAs also should not be used if there are syncopal episodes suggestive of Stokes-Adams attacks.[97]

Congestive Heart Failure

Although there were early indications that TCAs impaired the myocardium,[11,57,74,100] these studies were methodologically flawed because they relied on an imprecise measure of left-ventricular function (i.e., systolic time interval). This measure is dependent, in part, on the QRS duration, and reflects conduction more than left-ventricular function.[83] Subsequent, more precise studies[39,43,86,87,104] have shown no deleterious tricyclic effect on left ventricular function, even in patients with severe preexisting left ventricular impairment.

There is a catch, however—CHF *and impaired myocardial contractility markedly increase the risk of TCA-induced postural hypotension.*

◆ It was found that the rate of symptomatic orthostatic hypotension in medically healthy, depressed patients treated with imipramine was only 8%, compared with a rate of 50% in depressed CHF patients.[43,86,87]

◆ Nortriptyline retains its advantage over other TCAs in causing the least orthostatic hypotension,[43,87] making it the safest of its class for treating depression in CHF. However, case reports continue to emphasize that nortriptyline, like the other tricyclics, should be used with caution in patients with heart disease.[82]

It might seem logical that the volume of distribution of drugs increases in congestive heart failure because of fluid retention. However, fluid is retained *interstitially* in CHF,[93] while the *central* volume of distribution is *reduced.* Therefore, higher drug concentrations result from a given drug loading dose, so that smaller loading doses should be used.[93] Also, because *hepatic* blood flow and enzymatic activity are more markedly reduced in CHF than is renal function, drug toxicity occurs more readily in CHF with hepatically metabolized drugs (i.e., most psychotropics) than with those eliminated mainly by the kidney (e.g., lithium).[93]

Sick Sinus Syndrome

The sick sinus (bradycardia-tachycardia) syndrome refers to sinus node dysfunction that produces symptomatic bradyarrhythmias (sinus bradycardia, sinoatrial block, sinus arrest) and atrial tachyarrhythmias (paroxysmal atrial fibrillation, paroxysmal atrial flutter, and paroxysmal atrial tachycardia). The tricyclics can exacerbate sick sinus syndrome and *should not be used without a pacemaker*, since drugs with class I-A antiarrhythmic effects may depress the sinoatrial node.[97]

Atrial Fibrillation

It had been thought that tricyclics could be used in patients with *chronic* atrial fibrillation,[83] but data are accumulating that quinidine-like drugs heighten mortality when used for suppressing atrial fibrillation.[18,31] Conversion of new atrial fibrillation to normal sinus rhythm by a TCA would pose the risk of embolism.

Always monitor digoxin levels after adding a tricyclic; while digoxin-tricyclic interactions have not been specifically documented,[83] the TCAs' pharmacological cousin quinidine is known to increase digoxin levels.

⚜ MISCELLANEOUS AGENTS

Trazodone

A triazolopyridine derivative, trazodone (Desyrel) is chemically unrelated to tricyclic or tetracyclic agents. Trazodone's cardiovascular profile is substantially different from that of the tricyclics. It has few, if any, anticholinergic effects and thus does not increase heart rate. There are no known effects on myocardial contractility (inotropy). Trazodone is not considered to be a class I-A antiarrhythmic drug, like quinidine and the tricyclics; it does not predictably affect conduction when used in recommended doses. Overdose data show no cardiac abnormalities, including conduction problems. There have been no reports of fatalities secondary to trazodone overdose.[12,45,49,50,64,66] Patients with cardiovascular disease often have problems with fragmented sleep,[10] and trazodone is particularly useful as a hypnotic.

- ◆ However, Stoudemire and Atkinson[97] caution that trazodone's cyclic structure gives it the potential for inducing heart block.
- ◆ Although trazodone has no quinidine-like effects in experimental or overdose conditions, it has caused complete and first-degree heart block idiosyncratically.[54,75] Trazodone has also induced ventricular ar-

rhythmias in the elderly[105] and in patients with preexisting ventricular irritability, such as after MI.[56,71]
- ◆ Note that trazodone produces orthostatic hypotension *more frequently* than does nortriptyline.[79]
- ◆ There are two reports of digoxin toxicity occurring after the addition of trazodone.[21,75a] This is not a frequent interaction, but be sure to monitor digoxin levels when trazodone is administered concurrently.[17]

It is safest in high-risk patients to carefully increase trazodone and to monitor for ECG changes as you would with tricyclics.[97] Priapism is a rare but serious side effect of trazodone.

Maprotiline

First marketed in 1981 and touted as the first nontricyclic in the United States, the tetracyclic maprotiline (Ludiomil) was subsequently found to have essentially the same cardiovascular effects as the tricyclics. Side effects include slowing of conduction,[28,37] significant orthostatic hypotension with serious associated injuries,[19] and cardiovascular deaths in overdose.[19] Maprotiline lowers the seizure threshold, even at therapeutic doses,[22] and should not be used in patients with convulsive disorders.[6]

Amoxapine

Amoxapine (Asendin) was the second nontricyclic, non-MAOI drug available in the United States. It is the demethylated derivative of the neuroleptic loxapine (Loxitane), and thus has noradrenergic, serotonergic, and some antidopaminergic activity.[40] Although there are fewer cardiovascular complications in overdose compared with the TCAs,[25,51] amoxapine is ultimately more toxic in overdose because of seizures and rhabdomyolysis leading to myoglobinuria and acute renal failure.[62] It is now used infrequently. There are no reports in the literature of testing specifically in cardiovascular patients.

⚜ MONOAMINE OXIDASE INHIBITORS

In the era before SSRIs and bupropion (Wellbutrin), there were few antidepressant options for patients with conduction disease. The MAOIs were one of them. Although their side effects make the MAOIs less useful than the newer antidepressants, there are still those patients who respond to MAOIs and nothing else. It is important to know the cardiovascular profile of this group of drugs, which is substantially different from the TCAs.

◆ MAOIs have rarely been associated with cardiac rhythm disturbances or conduction abnormalities.[97]

◆ They have negligible effects on the ECG.[97]

◆ They do not have significant anticholinergic effects (and so do not induce the vagal blockade that causes cardiac acceleration).[97]

◆ They enhance myocardial contractility.[97]

There are several drawbacks. The most infamous side effect of MAOIs is hypertensive crisis; however, a far more common complication is orthostatic *hypotension*.[60] This effect is *more* likely with MAOIs than with TCAs.[15] In addition, MAOI orthostasis may occur for the first time well into the course of treatment (sometimes as late as 3–4 weeks), and unlike the TCAs, *cannot be predicted* by blood pressure at baseline. MAOIs also potentially interact with many cardiac medications,[48] including several antihypertensives and sympathomimetics.

⬥ PSYCHIATRIC SIDE EFFECTS OF CARDIAC DRUGS

Compiling a comprehensive list of drug reactions is like trying to hit a moving target. In consultation-liaison psychiatry, especially, it is hard to keep abreast of the new medications that appear in the medical subspecialties; the list often is based on anecdotal case reports, becomes outdated as soon as it is published, and can be only dimly recalled at the bedside. We find it more useful to assume that a medication (especially a new one) produces psychiatric sequelae or interacts with psychotropics until proven otherwise, and look up what is unfamiliar or unremembered. The excellent chapters by Levenson,[65] Stoudemire et al.,[99] and the recently revised volume by Ciraulo et al.[17] are good places to start.

Three cardiac medications merit special mention because they are "infamous" in producing psychiatric sequelae, *even without serum toxicity*. They are quinidine, lidocaine, and digoxin. In DSM-IV terminology, these sequelae would be grouped under the *substance-induced disorders* (see Appendix A), and specified according to the most prominent psychiatric symptom (e.g., 292.12: digoxin-induced psychotic disorder with hallucinations).

Quinidine

Quinidine's low therapeutic ratio requires constant vigilance.[7] Mental status changes such as psychosis, psychomotor excitement, confusion, and delirium may signal quinidine neurotoxicity, despite normal serum levels.[30,58]

Unfortunately, a history of psychiatric illness often leads to assumptions that the preexisting psychiatric condition is causing the mental status changes. Mr. Smith's persecutory ideation and psychomotor agitation could be entirely attributable to quinidine, even with normal serum levels. If medically feasible, he should be switched to another antiarrhythmic and reassessed psychiatrically off quinidine.

(Note that quinidine may inhibit the metabolism of certain psychotropics, such as desipramine and imipramine.[10a,95a,96a])

Lidocaine

Lidocaine (Xylocaine), especially when administered parenterally, induces CNS excitement—psychosis, anxiety, restlessness, tremors, and increased likelihood of grand mal seizures.[6]

◆ A 27-year-old woman with well-stabilized bipolar disorder experienced a psychotic reaction followed by a manic episode after 50 cc of intrathecal lidocaine, administered for removal of a pilonidal cyst.[78] She became extremely fearful, had visual hallucinations, and felt she "had died and been reborn." Although these sensations subsided over 24 hours, a frank manic episode ensued that eventually responded to lithium, carbamazepine, and haloperidol.

Psychotic reactions and "doom anxiety" have been reported in patients receiving intravenous lidocaine for cardiac arrhythmias.[90]

Digoxin

Digoxin precipitates a number of neuropsychiatric side effects, *even at therapeutic serum concentrations*. It is one of the most commonly prescribed drugs, with a relatively low margin of safety.[52] In fact, psychiatric symptoms may be an early warning of digoxin toxicity.

◆ For example, altered mental status, consisting of confusion and progressive lethargy, was the primary sign of digoxin neurotoxicity in a 65-year-old man whose serum digoxin level was within the therapeutic range.[96]

Others have reported similar cases.[5,30,30a,95,108,109] Neuropsychiatric symptoms of digoxin toxicity include disorientation, confusion, delirium, and hallucinations ("digitalis delirium").[52] Weakness, depression, and apathy may also occur.[29] Visual disturbances include white borders or halos on dark objects ("white vision") and disturbances of color vision, commonly with yellow or green coloration of objects, and less frequently, red, brown, and blue vision.[52]

◆ Clinical lore has it that the painter Vincent Van Gogh chewed on digitalis leaves, prompting the colorful visual effects so characteristic of his painting. Although of dubious art history value, this anecdote is a good way to remember digoxin toxicity.

Digoxin also causes depression at therapeutic serum levels.[83] In fact, a study of post-MI patients ($N = 190$) showed that after controlling for medical and sociodemographic factors, treatment with digoxin significantly ($P < .05$) predicted depression at 3–4 months after MI.[91] Corresponding rates for patients discharged without digoxin were significantly lower. No other medications, including beta-blockers, predicted depression.

Drug Interactions

As mentioned, lists of drug interactions and potential psychiatric side effects become outdated with each new drug that enters the market. We suggest that you consult a current *Physicians' Desk Reference* (PDR) or Ciraulo et al.[17] and briefly scan the literature before adding new psychotropics to a cardiac regimen or assuming a primary psychiatric syndrome before ruling out a medication effect. Some examples follow:

◆ **Propafenone (Rythmol):** This antiarrhythmic agent has caused toxicity when combined with desipramine (Norpramin), spiking a previously well-tolerated dose of 150 mg/day to a serum level of 2,092 nmol/L (therapeutic range 500–1,000 nmol/L).[59]

◆ **Bepridil hydrochloride (Vascor):** This new calcium channel blocker prolongs the QT interval and could potentiate QT lengthening by tricyclics, neuroleptics such as thioridazine (Mellaril), and pimozide (Orap).[2] Bepridil is used for treatment-resistant angina and may induce agranulocytosis, making coadministration with clozapine (Clozaril) potentially hazardous.

◆ **Cholestyramine resin (Cholybar, Questran):** This agent is used as an adjunct to dietary control for decreasing low-density lipoprotein (LDL) cholesterol. It has been found to bind TCAs, and should not be taken simultaneously with them.[4] Instead, TCAs should be taken 1 hour before or 4 hours after cholestyramine.

◆ **Pravastatin (Pravachol):** Four women with primary hypercholesterolemia became depressed during 12 weeks of treatment with this lipid-lowering agent.[63] In three of them, depressive symptoms were mild and reversible when the drug was discontinued. The fourth became suicidal.

◆ **Simvastatin (Zocor):** This lipid-lowering medication is in the same class as pravastatin and was linked to a variety of psychopathologic symptoms in four middle-aged hypercholesterolemic women.[26] In two patients with prior psychiatric histories, one become delusional and obsessional and the other developed murderous obsessive thoughts about her baby. Both were treated with clomipramine (Anafranil) and cognitive therapy; the latter was able to restart simvastatin. Two other women with no psychiatric histories became depressed, suicidal, and required psychiatric admission. They improved after simvastatin was withdrawn.

◆ **Diltiazem (Cardizem)** and <u>verapamil (Calan)</u> may impair metabolism of psychotropics metabolized by the cytochrome P450-3A4 isoenzyme, resulting in elevated psychotropic levels.[17]

❧ SUMMARY

1. The selective serotonin reuptake inhibitors (SSRIs) are not therapeutic for everyone and are not tolerated by every patient. The tricyclic antidepressants (TCAs) and the monoamine oxidase inhibitors (MAOIs) remain potential alternatives.

2. Adding a tricyclic may destabilize an antiarrhythmic drug regimen. Moreover, recent evidence suggests increased morbidity and mortality in post–myocardial infarction (MI) patients placed on quinidine-like antiarrhythmics. Extrapolations to the TCAs have led to similar warnings, although not everyone agrees. Recommendations for treating post-MI depression with TCAs have become more controversial.

3. Although TCAs differ in their anticholinergic and blood pressure effects, one tricyclic is no safer than any other in patients with conduction disease.

4. Pretreatment postural blood pressure changes may be asymptomatic, yet predispose to problems on tricyclics. Although patients may clinically accommodate, the orthostatic changes do not disappear with time. Congestive heart failure (CHF) magnifies the risk. Nortriptyline (Pamelor, Aventyl) produces the least orthostatic hypotension among the TCAs and trazodone (Desyrel).

5. Pacemakers make it possible to use TCAs in the setting of heart block.

6. Trazodone has the advantage of good hypnotic effects and almost no anticholinergic properties (and thus minimal sinus tachycardia).

7. MAOIs negligibly change the electrocardiogram (ECG), have rarely been associated with conduction or rhythm abnormalities, and have no significant anticholinergicity. Their main disadvantages are unpredictable orthostatic hypotension and many drug interactions.

8. It is best to assume that a cardiac drug will cause psychiatric side effects or interact with psychotropics until proven otherwise. *When in doubt, look it up.* Quinidine, lidocaine, and digoxin are notorious for producing psychiatric syndromes, even at therapeutic serum levels. The DSM-IV term for such syndromes is *substance-induced disorders*, which are specified according to the most prominent psychiatric symptom.

9. The new lipid-lowering medications appear particularly prone to interacting with psychotropics.

❧ REFERENCES

1. Ahles S, Swirtsman H, Halaris A, et al: Comparative cardiac effects of maprotiline and doxepin in elderly depressed patients. J Clin Psychiatry 45:460–465, 1984

2. Anonymous: Bepridil for angina pectoris. Med Lett Drugs Ther 33:53–54, 1991

3. Axelsson R, Aspenstrom G: Electrocardiographic changes and serum concentrations in thioridazine-treated patients. J Clin Psychiatry 43:332–335, 1982

4. Bailey D, Coffee J, Anderson B, et al: Interaction of tricyclic antidepressants with cholestyramine in vitro. Ther Drug Monit 14:339–342, 1992

5. Beller G, Smith T, Abelman W, et al: Digitalis intoxication: a prospective clinical study with serum level concentrations. N Engl J Med 284:989–997, 1971

6. Bernstein J: Handbook of Drug Therapy in Psychiatry, 3rd Edition. St. Louis, MO, Mosby Year Book, 1995

7. Bigger J, Hoffmann B: Antiarrhythmic drugs, in Goodman and Gilman's The Pharmacological Basis of Therapeutics, 8th Edition. Edited by Gilman A, Rall T, Nies A, et al. New York, Pergamon, 1990, pp 840–873

8. Bigger JJ, Giardina E, Perel J, et al: Cardiac antiarrhythmic effect of imipramine hydrochloride. N Engl J Med 296:206–208, 1977

9. Bluhm R, Wilkinson G, Shelton R, et al: Genetically determined drug-metabolizing activity and desipramine-associated cardiotoxicity: a case report. Clin Pharmacol Ther 53:89–95, 1993

10. Bradley T: Sleep disturbances in respiratory and cardiovascular disease. J Psychosom Res 37 (suppl 1):13–17, 1993

10a. Brosen K, Gram L: Quinidine inhibits the 2-hydroxylation of imipramine and desipramine but not the demethylation of imipramine. Eur J Clin Pharmacol 37:155–160, 1989

11. Burckhardt D, Raeder E, Muller V, et al: Cardiovascular effects of tricyclic and tetracyclic antidepressants. JAMA 239:213–216, 1978

12. Burgess C, Hames T, George C: The electrocardiographic and anticholinergic effects of trazodone and imipramine in man. Eur J Clin Pharmacol 23:417–421, 1982

13. Burrows G, Vohra J, Dumovic P, et al: Tricyclic antidepressant drugs and cardiac conduction. Prog Neuropsychopharmacol Biol Psychiatry 1:329–334, 1977

14. Caracci G, Reggev A: Atrial fibrillation and nortriptyline in the elderly. International Journal of Geriatric Psychiatry 8:577–580, 1993

15. Cassem N: Cardiovascular effects of antidepressants. J Clin Psychiatry 43:22–28, 1982

16. Cassem N: Depression, in Massachusetts General Hospital Handbook of General Hospital Psychiatry, 3rd Edition. Edited by Cassem N. St. Louis, MO, Mosby Year Book, 1991, pp 237–268

17. Ciraulo D, Shader R, Greenblatt D, et al. (eds): Drug Interactions in Psychiatry, 2nd Edition. Baltimore, MD, Williams & Wilkins, 1995

18. Coplen S, Antman E, Berlin J, et al: Efficacy and safety of quinidine therapy for maintenance of sinus rhythm after cardioversion: a meta-analysis of randomized control trials. Circulation 82:1106–1116, 1990

19. Crome P, Newman B: Fatal tricyclic antidepressant poisoning. J R Soc Med 72:649–653, 1979

20. Cunningham L: Depression in the medically ill: choosing an antidepressant. J Clin Psychiatry 55 (9, suppl A):90–97, 1994

21. Dec G, Jenike M, Stern T: Trazodone-digoxin interaction in an animal model. J Clin Psychopharmacol 4:153–155, 1984

22. Dessain E, Schatzberg A, Woods B, et al: Maprotiline treatment in depression. Arch Gen Psychiatry 43:86–90, 1986

23. Dietch J, Fine M: The effect of nortriptyline in elderly patients with cardiac conduction disease. J Clin Psychiatry 51:65–67, 1990

24. Donatini B, Le Blaye I, Krupp P: Transient cardiac pacing is insufficiently used to treat arrhythmia associated with thioridazine. Clin Pharmacol 81:340–341, 1992

25. Dugas J, Weber S: Amoxapine (Asendin, Lederle Laboratories). Drug Intelligence and Clinical Pharmacy 16:199–204, 1982

26. Duits N, Bos F: Depressive symptoms and cholesterol-lowering drugs (letter). Lancet 341:114, 1993

27. Editorial: Psychotropic drugs and myocardial infarction: cause for or caused by panic? Lancet 340:1069–1070, 1992

28. Edwards J, Goldie A: Mianserin, maprotiline and intracardiac conduction. Br J Clin Pharmacol 15 (1 suppl):249S–254S, 1983

29. Eisendrath S, Sweeney M: Toxic neuropsychiatric effects of digoxin at therapeutic serum concentrations. Am J Psychiatry 144:506–507, 1987

30. Eisenman D, McKegney F: Delirium at therapeutic serum concentrations of digoxin and quinidine. Psychosomatics 35:91–93, 1994

30a. El-Mallakh R, Hedges S, Casey D: Digoxin encephalopathy presenting as mood disturbance (letter). J Clin Psychopharmacol 15:82–83, 1995

31. Falk R: Flecainide-induced ventricular tachycardia and fibrillation in patients treated for atrial fibrillation. Ann Intern Med 111:107–111, 1989

32. Flugelman M, Tal A, Pollack S, et al: Psychotropic drugs and long QT syndromes: case reports. J Clin Psychiatry 46:290–291, 1985

33. Freyschuss U, Sjoqvist F, Tuck D, et al: Circulatory effects in man of nortriptyline, a tricyclic antidepressant drug. Pharmacology Clinics 2:68–71, 1970

34. Fricchione G, Vlay S: Psychiatric aspects of patients with malignant ventricular arrhythmias. Am J Psychiatry 143:1518–1526, 1986

35. Friedel R, Veith R, Bloom V, et al: Desipramine plasma levels and clinical response in depressed outpatients. Communications in Psychopharmacology 3:81–87, 1979

36. Gelenberg A: Back to the future: TCAs and arrhythmias. Biological Therapies in Psychiatry Newsletter 16:33, 36, 1993

37. Ghosh A: Cardiovascular effects of maprotiline, in New Dimensions in Antidepressants: Ludiomil. New York, Excerpta Medica, 1981

38. Giardina E, Bigger JJ, Glassman A, et al: The electrocardiographic and antiarrhythmic effect of imipramine hydrochloride at therapeutic plasma concentrations. Circulation 60:1045–1052, 1979

39. Giardina E, Bigger JJ, Johnson L: The effect of imipramine and nortriptyline on ventricular premature depolarizations and left ventricular function (abstract). Circulation 64 (suppl):IV316, 1981

40. Glassman A: The newer antidepressant drugs and their cardiovascular effects. Psychopharmacol Bull 20:271–280, 1984

41. Glassman A, Roose A, Bigger JJ: The safety of tricyclic antidepressants in cardiac patients (commentary). JAMA 269:2673–2675, 1993

42. Glassman A, Bigger JJ, Giardina E, et al: Clinical characteristics of imipramine-induced orthostatic hypotension. Lancet 1:468–472, 1979

43. Glassman A, Johnson L, Giardina E-G, et al: The use of imipramine in depressed patients with congestive heart failure. JAMA 250:1997–2001, 1983

44. Glassman A, Preudhomme X: Review of the cardiovascular effects of heterocyclic antidepressants. J Clin Psychiatry 54 (2, suppl):16–22, 1993

45. Gomoll A, Byrne J: Trazodone and imipramine: comparative effects on canine cardiac conduction. Eur J Pharmacol 57:335–342, 1979

46. Greenblatt D: Basic pharmacokinetic principles and their application to psychotropic drugs. J Clin Psychiatry 54 (9, suppl):8–13, 1993

47. Gross J, Zwerin G: Left bundle branch block developing in a patient with sub-therapeutic nortriptyline levels: a case report. J Am Geriatr Soc 39:1006–1007, 1991

48. Hackett T, Rosenbaum J, Cassem N: Cardiovascular disorders, in Comprehensive Textbook of Psychiatry, 5th Edition. Edited by Kaplan H, Sadock B. Baltimore, MD, Williams & Wilkins, 1989, pp 1186–1197

49. Hayes R, Gerner R, Fairbanks L, et al: ECG findings in geriatric depressives given trazodone, placebo, or imipramine. J Clin Psychiatry 44:180–183, 1983

50. Henry J, Ali C: Trazodone overdosage: experience from a poisons information service. Human Toxicology 2:353–356, 1983

51. Hetzman M, Goins R: Amoxapine and heart disease. J Clin Psychopharmacol 1 (6, suppl):70S–75S, 1984

52. Hoffman B, Bigger JJ: Digitalis and allied cardiac glycosides, in Goodman and Gilman's The Pharmacological Basis of Therapeutics, 8th Edition. Edited by Gilman A, Rall T, Nies A, et al. New York, Pergamon, 1990, pp 814–839

53. Huston J, Bell G: The effect of thioridazine hydrochloride and chlorpromazine on the electrocardiogram. JAMA 198:16–20, 1966

54. Irwin M, Spar J: Reversible cardiac conduction abnormality associated with trazodone administration (letter). Am J Psychiatry 140:945–946, 1983

55. Janicak P: The relevance of clinical pharmacokinetics and therapeutic drug monitoring: anticonvulsant mood stabilizers and antipsychotics. J Clin Psychiatry 54 (9, suppl):35–41, 1993

56. Janowsky D, Curtis G, Zisook S, et al: Ventricular arrhythmias possibly aggravated by trazodone. Am J Psychiatry 140:796–797, 1983

57. Jefferson J: A review of the cardiovascular effects and toxicity of tricyclic antidepressants. Psychosom Med 37:160–179, 1975

58. Johnson A, Dax R, Seldon M: A functional psychosis precipitated by quinidine. Med J Aust 153:47–49, 1990

59. Katz R: Raised serum levels of desipramine with the antiarrhythmic propafenone (letter). J Clin Psychiatry 52:432–433, 1991

60. Keck P, Carter W, Nierenberg A, et al: Acute cardiovascular effects of tranylcypromine: correlation with plasma drug, metabolite, norepinephrine, and MHPG levels. J Clin Psychiatry 52:250–254, 1991

61. Kemper A, Dunlap R, Pietro D: Thioridazine-induced torsade de pointes. JAMA 249:2931–2934, 1983

62. Kulig K, Rumack B, Sullivan JJ, et al: Amoxapine overdose: coma and seizures without cardiotoxic effects. JAMA 248:1092–1094, 1982

63. Lechleitner M, Hoppichler F, Konwalinka G, et al: Depressive symptoms in hypercholesterolaemic patients treated with pravastatin (letter). Lancet 340:910, 1992

64. Lesar T, Kinston R, Dahms R, et al: Trazodone overdose. Ann Emerg Med 12:221–223, 1983

65. Levenson J: Cardiovascular disease, in Psychiatric Care of the Medical Patient. Edited by Stoudemire A, Fogel B. New York, Oxford University Press, 1993, pp 539–555

66. Lippmann S, Bunch S, Abuton J, et al: A trazodone overdose (letter). Am J Psychiatry 139:1373, 1982

67. Luchins D: Review of clinical and animal studies comparing the cardiovascular effect of doxepin and other tricyclic antidepressants. Am J Psychiatry 140:1006–1009, 1983

68. Morganroth J, Goin J: Quinidine-related mortality in the short- to medium-term treatment of ventricular arrhythmias: a meta-analysis. Circulation 84:1977–1983, 1991

69. Muller O, Goodman N, Bellet S: The hypotensive effect of imipramine hydrochloride in patients with cardiovascular disease. Clin Pharmacol Ther 2:300–307, 1961

70. Myerburg R: Electrocardiography, in Harrison's Principles of Internal Medicine, 12th Edition. Edited by Wilson J, Braunwald E, Isselbacher K, et al. New York, McGraw-Hill, Health Professions Division, 1991, pp 850–860

71. Pohl R, Bridges M, Rainey JJ, et al: Effects of trazodone and desipramine on cardiac rate and rhythm in a patient with preexisting cardiovascular disease. J Clin Psychopharmacol 6:380–381, 1986

72. Preskorn S: Pharmacokinetics of antidepressants: why and how they are relevant to treatment. J Clin Psychiatry 54 (9, suppl):14–34, 1993

73. Preskorn S: Pharmacokinetics of psychotropic agents: why and how they are relevant to treatment. J Clin Psychiatry 54 (9, suppl):3–7, 1993

74. Raeder E, Burckhardt D, Neubauer H, et al: Long-term tri- and tetracyclic antidepressants, myocardial contractility, and cardiac rhythm. BMJ 2:666–667, 1978

75. Rausch J, Pavlinac D, Newman P: Complete heart block following a single dose of trazodone. Am J Psychiatry 141:1472–1473, 1984

75a. Rauch P, Jenike M: Digoxin toxicity possibly precipitated by trazodone. Psychosomatics 25:334–335, 1984

76. Ray W, Griffin M, Schaffner W, et al: Psychotropic drug use and the risk of hip fracture. N Engl J Med 316:363–369, 1987

77. Regan W, Margolin R, Mathew R: Cardiac arrhythmia following rapid imipramine withdrawal. Biol Psychiatry 25:482–484, 1989

78. Remick R, Gimbarzevsky B: Manic reactions to lidocaine anesthesia (letter). J Clin Psychopharmacol 10:442–443, 1990

79. Richelson E: Pharmacology of antidepressants in use in the United States. J Clin Psychiatry 43:4–11, 1982

80. Risch S, Groom G, Janowsky D: Interfaces of psychopharmacology and cardiology, I. J Clin Psychiatry 42:23–34, 1981

81. Roose S, Dalack G, Glassman A, et al: Is doxepin a safer tricyclic for the heart? J Clin Psychiatry 52:338–341, 1991

82. Roose S, Dalack G, Woodring S: Death, depression, and heart disease. J Clin Psychiatry 52 (6, suppl):34–39, 1991

83. Roose S, Glassman A: Cardiovascular effects of tricyclic antidepressants in depressed patients. J Clin Psychiatry Monograph 7:1–18, 1989

84. Roose S, Glassman A: Antidepressant choice in the patient with cardiac disease: lessons from the Cardiac Arrhythmia Suppression Trial (CAST) studies. J Clin Psychiatry 55 (9, suppl A):83–87, 1994

85. Roose S, Glassman A, Giardina E: Tricyclic antidepressants in depressed patients with cardiac conduction disease. Arch Gen Psychiatry 44:273–275, 1987

86. Roose S, Glassman A, Giardina E, et al: Nortriptyline in depressed patients with left ventricular impairment. JAMA 256:3253–3257, 1986

87. Roose S, Glassman A, Giardina E, et al: Cardiovascular effects of imipramine and bupropion in depressed patients with congestive heart failure. J Clin Psychopharmacol 7:247–251, 1987

88. Roose S, Glassman A, Siris S, et al: Comparison of imipramine and nortriptyline-induced orthostatic hypotension: a meaningful difference. J Clin Psychopharmacol 1:316–319, 1981

89. Rudorfer M: Pharmacokinetics of psychotropic drugs in special populations. J Clin Psychiatry 54 (9, suppl):50–54, 1993

90. Saravay S, Marke J, Steinberg M, et al: "Doom anxiety" and delirium in lidocaine toxicity. Am J Psychiatry 144:159–163, 1987

91. Schleifer S, Slater W, Macari-Hinson M, et al: Digitalis and beta-blocking agents: effects on depression following myocardial infarction. Am Heart J 121:1397–1402, 1991

92. Schwartz P, Wolf S: QT interval prolongation as predictor of sudden death in patients with myocardial infarction. Circulation 57:1074–1077, 1978

93. Shammas F, Dickstein K: Clinical pharmacokinetics in heart failure: an updated review. Clin Pharmacokinet 15:94–113, 1988

94. Shapiro P: Nortriptyline treatment of depressed cardiac transplant patients. Am J Psychiatry 148:371–373, 1991

95. Shear M, Sacks M: Digitalis delirium: report of two cases. Am J Psychiatry 135:109–110, 1978

95a. Skjelbo E, Brosen K: Inhibitors of imipramine metabolism by human liver microsomes. Br J Clin Pharmacol 34:256–261, 1992

96. Smith H, Janz T, Erker M: Digoxin toxicity presenting as altered mental status in a patient with severe chronic obstructive lung disease. Heart Lung 21:78–80, 1992

96a. Steiner E, Dumont E, Spina E, et al: Inhibition of desipramine 2-hydroxylation by quinidine and quinine. Clin Pharmacol Ther 43:577–581, 1988

97. Stoudemire A, Atkinson P: Use of cyclic antidepressants in patients with cardiac conduction disturbances. Gen Hosp Psychiatry 10:389–397, 1988

98. Stoudemire A, Fogel B: Psychopharmacology in the medically ill, in Principles of Medical Psychiatry. Edited by Stoudemire A, Fogel B. Orlando, FL, Grune & Stratton, 1987, pp 79–112

99. Stoudemire A, Fogel B, Gulley L, et al: Psychopharmacology in the medical patient, in Psychiatric Care of the Medical Patient. Edited by Stoudemire A, Fogel B. New York, Oxford University Press, 1993, pp 155–206

100. Taylor D, Braithwaite R: Cardiac effects of tricyclic antidepressant medication: a preliminary study of nortriptyline. Br Heart J 40:1005–1009, 1978

101. Thayssen P, Bjerre M, Kragh-Sorensen P, et al: Cardiovascular effects of imipramine and nortriptyline in elderly patients. Psychopharmacology 74:360–364, 1981

102. The Cardiac Arrhythmia Suppression Trial II investigators: Effect of the anti-arrhythmic agent moricizine on survival after myocardial infarction. N Engl J Med 327:227–233, 1992

103. Thorogood M, Cowen P, Mann J, et al: Fatal myocardial infarction and use of psychotropic drugs in young women. Lancet 340:1067–1068, 1992

104. Veith R, Rasking M, Caldwell J, et al: Cardiovascular effects of tricyclic antidepressants. N Engl J Med 306:954–959, 1982

105. Vitullo R, Wharton J, Allen N, et al: Trazodone-related exercise-induced nonsustained ventricular tachycardia. Chest 98:247–248, 1990

106. Vohra J, Burrows G, Hunt D, et al: The effect of toxic and therapeutic doses of tricyclic antidepressants drugs on intracardiac conduction. Europeann Journal of Cardiology 3:219–227, 1975

107. Vohra J, Burrows G, Sloman G: Assessment of cardiovascular side effects of therapeutic doses of tricyclic and anti-depressant drugs. Aust N Z J Med 5:7–11, 1975

108. Von Arnim T, Krawietz W, Vogt W, et al: Is the determination of serum digoxin concentration useful for the diagnosis of digitalis toxicity? Int J Clin Pharmacol Ther Toxicol 18:261–268, 1980

109. Wamboldt F, Jefferson J, Wamboldt M: Digitalis intoxication diagnosed as depression by primary care physicians. Am J Psychiatry 143:219–221, 1986

110. Weld F, Bigger J: Electrophysiological effects of imipramine on bovine cardiac Purkinje and ventricular muscle fibers. Circ Res 46:167–175, 1980

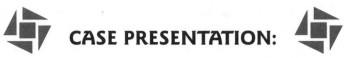

CASE PRESENTATION:

Ms. Anderson: The Manic Patient With Heart Disease and Hypertension

Ms. Anderson is a 45-year-old woman with a history of panic disorder and mitral valve prolapse who has been maintained for the past 6 months on imipramine (Tofranil) 125 mg per day with complete resolution of panic symptoms. (Clonazepam [Klonopin] was not effective.) She runs a successful retail business, but over the past month has begun to behave inappropriately with customers. She puns repeatedly in verbal interactions with them, making conversation impossible. At times Ms. Anderson has given merchandise away, much to the chagrin of her partner. Her bookkeeper notes large expenditures of cash. The patient feels little need for sleep, is distractible, and demonstrates euphoric mood. She has become convinced that she is Mary Magdalene and hears the voices of Jesus and Moses. She acknowledges feeling extremely anxious, and has been taking propranolol (Inderal) 10 mg bid prn for anxiety, as prescribed by her internist. Family history is notable for bipolar affective illness in her father and paternal uncle.

She is admitted to the psychiatry service. Mental status exam reveals an attractive but unkempt woman, heavily made up, with lipstick smeared haphazardly. Speech is pressured, with flight of ideas. Affect is silly. Mood is euphoric. She denies suicidal ideation. Thought content is notable for grandiose delusions of being the mother of God. She responds to voices telling her to sing hymns and praise the Lord. She denies hallucinations in other modalities. She is alert and fully oriented, and higher cognitive functions are intact except for difficulty concentrating.

Ms. Anderson's pulse is 80, and standing and supine blood pressure are 160/100. The physical exam is remarkable for mitral valve click. Holter monitoring shows frequent atrial premature beats. ECG reveals a QTc interval of 0.40 second (upper limit of normal is 0.44 second) and a QRS of 0.08 second (normal 0.04–0.10 second). Echocardiogram confirms the diagnosis of mitral valve prolapse. Thyroid function tests, serum B_{12}, sedimentation rate, antinuclear antibodies, and MRI of the brain are all normal. Serum imipramine and desipramine (Norpramin) levels are within the therapeutic range.

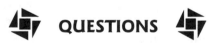

QUESTIONS

Choose all that apply.

1. The neuroleptic medication(s) that would be most cardiotoxic for Ms. Anderson are . . .
   a. Thioridazine (Mellaril).
   b. Perphenazine (Trilafon).
   c. Thiothixene (Navane).
   d. Molindone (Moban).

2. What are some relevant points about the effects of neuroleptics on the heart?
   a. ECG changes associated with thioridazine occur almost exclusively in the higher dose ranges (> 500 mg/day).
   b. Intramuscular phenothiazines may be safely used for patients who are bedridden or in four-point restraints, since these individuals are effectively incapable of postural changes.
   c. The ECG changes most frequently associated with phenothiazines are similar to those produced by quinidine.
   d. Haloperidol (Haldol) is the antipsychotic agent least likely to produce ECG change or cardiac abnormalities, except in patients with previous cardiovascular disease.

3. The cardiovascular effects of tricyclic antidepressants (TCAs) and antipsychotics . . .
   a. Are similar in the mechanisms by which they produce hypotension.

   b. Differ in that some neuroleptics affect conduction less than others, whereas all TCAs have an equal risk for this effect.
   c. Are additive when the two are prescribed together.
   d. All of the above.

4. Imipramine is discontinued. Ms. Anderson's ECG shows persistent runs of atrial premature contractions. Workup of her elevated blood pressure is consistent with essential hypertension. Her manic symptoms continue. The most common effect(s) of therapeutic lithium levels on the ECG of a healthy patient is/are:
   a. Tachycardia
   b. ST-segment changes
   c. Increased QT intervals
   d. T-wave flattening or inversion

5. Which of the following are true about lithium and the heart?
   a. Lithium most frequently inhibits conduction within the ventricles.
   b. Lithium causes sinus node dysfunction and first-degree atrioventricular (AV) block.
   c. Therapeutic lithium levels predispose to cardiac arrhythmias, even if congestive heart failure is stable.
   d. Alternatives to lithium should be used in CHF.
   e. Carbamazepine (Tegretol) is preferable to lithium when there is AV conduction delay.

6. Propranolol is also discontinued. What are significant factors in managing mania in the setting of heart disease?
   a. Synergistic interaction between lithium and propranolol may lead to sinus *bradycardia.*
   b. A history of myocardial infarction is a contraindication to lithium.
   c. The arrhythmogenic potential of hypokalemia and digitalis toxicity is exacerbated by lithium.
   d. All of the above.

7. Ms. Anderson does well but is lost to follow-up when she moves out of state. She returns to your office several years later, off all psychotropics. She is now 51 years old, hypertensive, with mild congestive heart failure (CHF) and angina. She is also quite depressed. Her local physician had placed her on a medication containing low-dose reserpine (Serpasil), and then methyldopa (Aldomet); when asked, she does not know why he selected those medications. All of the following are true *except . . .*

   a. Reserpine only rarely induces clinically significant depressive syndromes.
   b. Methyldopa-associated depressive syndromes occur at *standard* therapeutic doses.
   c. If reserpine or methyldopa were implicated in inducing depression, they should be discontinued before starting an antidepressant.
   d. Were Ms. Anderson to become psychotic again, she is at risk for toxic haloperidol-methyldopa interactions.

8. If furosemide (Lasix) were started, it could contribute to her depressive presentation through its effect on . . .
   a. Serotonin.
   b. Norepinephrine.
   c. Potassium.
   d. None of the above.

9. Which of the following are true about the potential role of psychological factors in hypertension?
   a. The interaction between psychological stressors and hypertension is thought to be mediated through the phenomenon of pressor reactivity.
   b. A positive relationship has been found between hypertension and suppressed—but not expressed—anger.
   c. The association between hypertension and suppressed hostility is not as substantial as other variables, such as obesity or social class.
   d. The majority of evidence confirms that behavioral treatments have a sustained effect in reducing hypertension.

10. Which of the following are true regarding the beta-blocking agents?
   a. The propranolol (Inderal)-induced psychotic syndrome is a *dose-related* phenomenon.
   b. The propranolol (Inderal)-induced depressive syndrome is a *dose-related* phenomenon.
   c. Propranolol's neuropsychiatric side effects are limited to the high dose ranges.
   d. The cardioselective beta-blockers (e.g., atenolol, metoprolol, nadolol) are as likely as propranolol to induce depression.

11. Ms. Anderson is taken off the methyldopa and her depression remits. Over the next year she does well psychiatrically, but develops crescendo angina and worsening CHF. She is not a candidate for angioplasty, and instead is advised to undergo coronary artery bypass graft (CABG) surgery. The surgery goes well, with minimal

time on cardiopulmonary bypass and adequate maintenance of blood pressure at all times. Upon awakening in the intensive care unit, however, she is paranoid and delusional. She fears that the insurance company is trying to rob her, and that the nurses want to cut her up into pieces. She responds to auditory hallucinations telling her to escape. When you arrive to interview her, she states, "You're too late. They've already killed my husband." She is agitated, alert, and oriented to person and place, but is wrong about the date. She refuses more detailed cognitive testing because she fears it can be used against her. Which are true regarding delirium following cardiotomy?

    a. Ms. Anderson's history of systemic hypertension probably placed her at higher risk for delirium.

    b. Abnormal postoperative electroencephalogram (EEG) results correlate with the occurrence of delirium following cardiotomy.

    c. The prevalence of postcardiotomy delirium has been declining with improvements in cardiopulmonary bypass technique.

    d. All of the above.

12. Ms. Anderson's paranoid symptoms respond rapidly to haloperidol 0.5 mg tid. By postoperative day 4, she is completely lucid and verbalizing appropriate concerns about recovery and prognosis. Which are valid statements?

    a. The duration of stay in the intensive care unit is a strong predictor of postcardiotomy delirium.

    b. Sleep deprivation often causes postcardiotomy delirium.

    c. A history of psychiatric illness is a risk factor for postcardiotomy delirium.

    d. The time on cardiopulmonary bypass is the strongest predictor of postcardiotomy delirium.

    e. None of the above.

Answers

1. Answer: a (p. 54)

2. Answer: c (p. 54)

3. Answer: b, c (p. 55)

4. Answer: d (p. 55)

5. Answer: b (p. 55)

6. Answer: a, c (pp. 55–56)

7. Answer: a (p. 57)

8. Answer: c (p. 57)

9. Answer: a (pp. 56–57)

10. Answer: b (p. 57)

11. Answer: b (p. 58)

12. Answer: e (p. 58)

⚐ NEUROLEPTICS AND THE HEART

Neuroleptics and the Electrocardiogram

Neuroleptic-induced ECG changes tend to be reversible after discontinuing the drug.[5,85] The *phenothiazines* are particular culprits, producing ECG effects similar to quinidine and myocardial ischemia:[7,28,85]

◆ T-wave depression, widening, notching, inversion, and flattening
◆ U waves
◆ Prolonged QT intervals

Other reported changes have included ST-segment flattening or depression,[6,7,56] first-degree atrioventricular (AV) block with conduction delay,[28,56] nonconducted premature atrial beats,[28,56] and atrial flutter with varying degrees of block,[28,56] particularly in patients receiving thioridazine (Mellaril) (see below).

Unlike tricyclic-induced hypotension, which occurs through vascular smooth muscle relaxation,[11,44,84] phenothiazine-induced hypotension occurs via alpha-adrenergic blockade.[11]

◆ The phenothiazines chlorpromazine (Thorazine), thioridazine (Mellaril), and mesoridazine (Serentil) can produce significant postural hypotension, and as well as systolic drops, *even while the patient is lying flat.*[10] The effect is enhanced when the medication is given intramuscularly or with other medications that lower blood pressure, such as antidepressants and antihypertensives.[9,82,85] This information is relevant for highly agitated, medically ill patients who may be confined to bed or in restraints; they may still "bottom out" their blood pressure on intramuscular phenothiazines even though they are incapable of changing position.
◆ Trifluoperazine (Stelazine), loxapine (Loxitane), and molindone (Moban) have less hypotensive action than do chlorpromazine (Thorazine) or thioridazine (Mellaril); haloperidol (Haldol) has the least hypotensive action of the antipsychotics.[10,102]
◆ *Haloperidol is the antipsychotic agent least likely to produce ECG changes or cardiac abnormalities,* and it retains this distinction even in patients with cardiovas-

cular disease.[29,102] However, as was discussed in the case of Mr. Davis (see Chapter 2), haloperidol has caused torsade de pointes (polymorphic ventricular tachycardia that frequently degenerates into ventricular fibrillation),[26,38,49,62,114,117] particularly when administered intravenously. Prolonged QT intervals, dilated cardiomyopathy, and a history of alcohol abuse predispose to this arrhythmia.[62]

Clozapine (Clozaril) has been only occasionally associated with cardiovascular events, although a recent case report[3] of new-onset ECG abnormalities (unifocal premature ventricular contractions [PVCs]) should remind clinicians of its structural similarity to the TCA imipramine (Tofranil). Bradycardia and somnolence have been described when fluoxetine was added to a pimozide regimen.[28a] (Pimozide can produce clinically significant cardiac depressant effects as a result of its calcium channel blocking action;[65b] it should not be coadministered with other calcium channel blockers.)

Thioridazine

As mentioned, *thioridazine* (Mellaril) is considered to be the most cardiotoxic of the neuroleptics.[15b]

◆ It possesses quinidine-like properties,[23] and thus should not be coprescribed with tricyclics or quinidine-like antiarrhythmics[17] without careful monitoring.
◆ Thioridazine can cause electrocardiogram abnormalities even at low doses.[5,7,11,42] One study reported that 90% of patients receiving less than 300 mg of thioridazine daily showed ECG changes.[7]
◆ It has been associated with sudden death[83] and also with torsade de pointes (polymorphic ventricular tachycardia). Ms. Anderson's prolonged QT intervals on imipramine would predispose to this arrhythmia if thioridazine were added.[48]
◆ Note that thioridazine is sometimes prescribed for patients with dementia who are agitated and need sedation, or who cannot tolerate the extrapyramidal side effects of the higher-potency neuroleptics. Be sure to monitor such patients, who are often elderly, for these often-overlooked cardiovascular side effects.

Neuroleptics, Antidepressants, and the Heart

Coadministering neuroleptics and TCAs exaggerates the potential conduction abnormalities of each, increasing the risk of cardiac toxicity.[112] If a patient requires both an antipsychotic and an antidepressant, choose a selective serotonin reuptake inhibitor (SSRI). If TCAs are unavoidable, use a secondary amine tricyclic (such as nortriptyline) combined with a high-potency neuroleptic (such as haloperidol), in order to minimize additive toxicity on pulse and blood pressure.[31] Keep in mind, however, that unlike neuroleptics, no one tricyclic has a cardiac *conduction* profile that is superior to any other.

✦ ANTIMANIC AGENTS AND THE HEART

Lithium

Unlike the tricyclics, which affect primarily ventricular conduction, lithium inhibits conduction within the *atrium*. Monitor for symptoms such as dyspnea, paroxysmal tachycardia, dizziness, and fainting, as well as abnormalities in resting pulse.

- The most common ECG effect of therapeutic levels of lithium in healthy patients is *T-wave flattening or inversion*, which is benign and reversible.[14a,15a,17,44a]
- Lithium *toxicity* has been associated with sinoatrial block, AV block, AV dissociation, bradyarrhythmias, ventricular tachycardia, and ventricular fibrillation.[20]
- Sinus node dysfunction and first-degree AV block, although uncommon, are the most common cardiac problems secondary to lithium,[64,100a,110,113] usually occurring when there is a vulnerable conduction system.[20,20a] As always, be especially careful with elderly patients and those with preexisting atrial conduction disturbances.[17,20a,86]

Congestive Heart Failure

There are contradictory data on using lithium in congestive heart failure (CHF); it has been reported both to induce and to ameliorate congestive failure.[20] Because there is little compelling evidence that it exacerbates congestive failure, DasGupta et al.[21] do not routinely recommend using alternatives to lithium.

- In moderate to severe CHF, diminished renal blood flow may produce *pre–renal azotemia* secondary to de-

creased cardiac output; this may cause lithium toxicity by decreasing lithium clearance.

Post–Myocardial Infarction

Some authors consider an acute myocardial infarction (MI) a temporary contraindication to lithium.[20] There is a case report, however, of a 59-year-old man with a 15-year history of bipolar illness whose lithium levels were safely maintained at 0.8–0.9 mEq/L throughout his MI and recovery.[91] It was also safely used in a patient undergoing coronary artery bypass graft (CABG) surgery.[114a] Obviously, use caution when prescribing any psychotropic after an MI.

Drug Interactions

As already advised, it is safest to assume that a medication (especially a new one) produces psychiatric sequelae or interacts with psychotropics until proven otherwise (refer to the volume by Ciraulo et al.[18a]). A brief survey of highlights follows. Note that lithium-vasodilator interactions (e.g., nitroglycerin, isosorbide [Isordil]) are absent; to our knowledge, they have not been described.

Increase Cardiac Toxicity

- Lithium and propranolol (Inderal) may have a synergistic effect on lowering heart rate.[8] This also could happen with other beta-blockers, which may be coprescribed for akathisia for lithium-induced tremor.[64,109]
- Hypokalemia and digitalis toxicity may enhance arrhythmogenic potential at even therapeutic serum lithium levels.[45,94]

Induce Manic States

- Clonidine (Catapres) withdrawal[17]
- Captopril (Capoten) administration[69]
- Rapid discontinuation of diltiazem (Cardizem) and atenolol (Tenormin) precipitated mania in a 44-year-old woman with hypomania and a family history of bipolar disorder.[96] It was thought that the diltiazem (which is a calcium channel blocker) may have protected against the expression of her bipolar illness.

Increase Lithium Toxicity

- Methyldopa (Aldomet)[16,66,67,107]
- Thiazide diuretics and furosemide (Lasix) ($\uparrow Na^+$ and K^+ excretion $\Rightarrow \uparrow$ lithium resorption[40a,45,45a])

Management: reduce lithium dose by 50% for a 50-mg dose of hydrochlorothiazide.[19]

◆ Angiotensin-converting enzyme (ACE) inhibitors, such as captopril (Capoten), lisinopril (Prinivil), and enalapril (Vasotec)[6a,18b,21,23a,25]

◆ The potassium-sparing diuretics amiloride (Midamor), spironolactone (Aldactone), and triamterene (Dyazide)[45]

◆ Indapamide (Lozol; an antihypertensive/diuretic of the indoline class of medications)[35]

◆ Calcium channel blockers, such as diltiazem (Cardizem) and verapamil (Calan), can cause symptoms of lithium toxicity (neurotoxicity, nausea, weakness, ataxia) even when serum lithium levels are within the therapeutic range.[73,74,106,115]

  • ⇒ verapamil + lithium: also associated with dysrhythmias[24]

  • ⇒ diltiazem + lithium: also associated with acute psychotic reactions[12]

Decrease Lithium Levels

◆ Acetazolamide (Diamox)[45,104]

◆ Sodium bicarbonate and sodium chloride[45]

Carbamazepine

Carbamazepine (Tegretol) has more cardiovascular toxicity than lithium.[14a,48a,50,101a] Kasarskis et al.[47] detailed a case history of carbamazepine-induced AV conduction disturbance and reviewed the literature on this agent's cardiovascular effects. Two patterns emerged from this review:

◆ At therapeutic or modestly elevated serum levels in the elderly: bradyarrhythmias and AV conduction delay[1]

◆ With massive carbamazepine overdose: sinus tachycardia

Although there is no distinct pattern of drug interactions with carbamazepine, beware of combining carbamazepine with medications known to affect AV nodal conduction, such as TCAs or antiarrhythmics. (Carbamazepine does interact with several cardiac medications, including diltiazem [Cardizem].[60]) Remember that this literature is not prospective, so it is not known whether carbamazepine induces dysfunction or worsens an already vulnerable conduction system.

Kasarskis and colleagues[47] have made the following recommendations for assessing carbamazepine cardiotoxicity:

◆ Obtain a baseline ECG in patients over the age of 50. Consider alternative therapy if there is evidence of heart block or AV conduction delay.

◆ ECGs should be repeated after reaching therapeutic serum carbamazepine levels. Reduce or discontinue drug if disturbances of AV conduction occur.

Valproic Acid

Valproic acid (Depakene) does not have adverse cardiac effects.[20a,55] Its most common side effects are transient gastrointestinal symptoms (anorexia, nausea, and vomiting), neurological symptoms (tremor, sedation, and ataxia), and asymptomatic serum hepatic transaminase elevations.[77] The most serious potential side effect of valproic acid is hepatotoxicity, which can lead to liver failure and death. This is a rare, idiosyncratic side effect, unrelated to dosage, and is more common in patients under age 10 who take multiple anticonvulsants.

⊕ PSYCHOLOGICAL FACTORS AFFECTING HYPERTENSION

The interaction between psychological factors and hypertension is thought to be mediated through the phenomenon of cardiovascular or "pressor" reactivity to stimuli.[25a,39,41,57,59,63,72,92,108] The hyperreactivity of heart rate and blood pressure to noxious stimuli may influence later vulnerability to hypertension, but no "hard" data in human models have yet proven this association. For example:

◆ Individuals with a family history of hypertension have greater cardiovascular reactivity than those without,[72] indicating a potential inherited diathesis for hypertension.

◆ In those who are already hypertensive, pressor reactivity may exacerbate and accelerate the disease process.[92]

Despite methodological problems, such as retrospective or cross-sectional design, the strength of the relationship between anger and hypertension is substantial, paralleling that of variables such as obesity and social class.[22] Studies have disclosed a positive relationship between hypertension and both expressed and unexpressed anger, indicating that the effects of stress on blood pressure may be influenced by coping styles for anger, interpersonal conflicts, and environmental stimuli.[41,57,92]

◆ For example, individuals who inappropriately use an assertive coping style may be predisposed to hypertension.[43]

Several studies have shown that psychological or behavioral treatments either reduced medication requirements or were more effective than medication alone.[32,100] Some studies have found sustained effects,[68] but unless **24-hour** ambulatory blood pressure monitoring offers confirmation, results must be interpreted with caution. Unfortunately, *sustained* effects are found to be minimal after treatment is terminated in studies using this methodology.[18,93] Psychotherapy, relaxation, and biofeedback improve quality of life in hypertensive subjects, but the impact of these interventions on the hypertension itself is modest, at best.[65]

Antihypertensive-Induced Depressive Disorder

Reserpine, Methyldopa, and Propranolol

In keeping with our antilist policy, only those antihypertensives that have been strongly associated with inducing depressive disorders are reviewed here. The most infamous are reserpine, methyldopa (Aldomet), and propranolol (Inderal). Antidepressant treatment should be deferred pending a trial off these medications.[11]

◆ **Reserpine (Serpasil)** is the antihypertensive most strongly correlated with producing secondary depressive states, even at low doses.[75] The affective changes have been attributed to depletion of catecholamine stores and occur even in the absence of a prior personal or family history of depression.[11] For those who think that reserpine is a medication of the past, note that a recent commentary[53] urged reserpine's resurgence because of its antihypertensive efficacy, tolerable side effects, and low cost (a 1-year supply is about as expensive as a 1-week supply of many newer agents).

◆ **Methyldopa (Aldomet)**—associated depression occurs even at standard therapeutic doses.[111] Vegetative symptoms seem to be more common than the psychological complaints of hopelessness, self-deprecation, and guilt.[54] Methyldopa may lead to confusional states when combined with haloperidol.[105] Some authors feel that methyldopa should be avoided in patients with psychiatric conditions.[54]

◆ **Propranolol (Inderal)** and the other beta-adrenergic blocking agents are used to treat cardiac arrhythmias,

angina, and hypertension. They are also gaining wider psychiatric application for aggression[33,78–80,99] and akathisia.[58,81] Of all the beta-blockers, it is propranolol that most often causes cognitive and behavioral side effects.[70,71] These appear to be twofold:

• Propranolol-induced *psychotic* disorder that is *dose independent:* Dissociation, hallucinations, and delusions may occur even at very small doses, especially in elderly patients.[11,27]

• Propranolol-induced *depressive* disorder that is *dose related:* This usually appears only at daily doses exceeding 120 mg.[11,34] The incidence of secondary depressive states with propranolol is controversial,[4,15,61,70,71,103] but has been estimated at between 0.5% and 20%.[34]

The more cardioselective beta-blockers, such as atenolol (Tenormin), metoprolol (Lopressor), and nadolol (Corgard), are less likely to cross the blood-brain barrier at ordinary therapeutic doses, and thus cause fewer psychiatric side effects compared with propranolol.[9,61,98] Patients with depressive symptoms on propranolol should be switched to an antihypertensive from another class or to a more selective beta-blocker, such as atenolol[30] or nadolol.[98]

◆ Beta-blockers are not contraindicated for patients with personal or family histories of mood disorders.[116] However, if a patient is already depressed or becomes depressed while taking a beta-blocker, consider alternatives.[116]

Miscellaneous Agents

◆ **Thiazide diuretics** and **furosemide (Lasix)** can produce hypokalemia ($\leq$ 3 mEq/liter) and hypovolemia. Patients may complain of symptoms that resemble depression, such as anergia, anorexia, constipation, dysphoria, lassitude, and weakness.[54] Check serum potassium before assuming that the patient requires antidepressant treatment.[11]

◆ **Clonidine (Catapres)** has a potentially sedating effect that can mimic the psychomotor retardation of depression, but without the pervasive dysphoria or hopelessness of a true depressive syndrome.[54] It can also induce a hypertensive crisis when combined with a monoamine oxidase inhibitor (MAOI).[11]

◆ **Nifedipine (Procardia)** has virtually no effect on mood, but may have subtle adverse effects on memory and visual-motor skills.[95]

Drug Interactions

As stated, assume that a medication will interact with one of the psychotropics until proven otherwise. A few more guidelines follow:

◆ It is safest to assume that most antihypertensives will interact adversely with MAOIs.

◆ Do not forget that diuretics and common vasodilators like nitroglycerin are likely to enhance the hypotensive properties of MAOIs and TCAs.[11]

◆ Diuretics may exaggerate the orthostatic effects of tricyclics by causing hypovolemia.[11] Conversely, the TCAs inhibit neuronal uptake—and thus the therapeutic effect—of several antihypertensive agents.[11,76]

◆ Serum TCA levels may be elevated by medications such as calcium channel blockers, causing conduction delays.[40] Check the particular drug pair before coprescribing them.

⚐ DELIRIUM AND THE CARDIAC PATIENT

After Cardiotomy

You will hear many theories about why cardiotomy ("open-heart surgery") leads a patient to become psychotic. Comments are offered about "ICU [intensive care unit] psychosis," enumerating the hours on bypass, days in the intensive care unit, noisiness of the unit, and the patient's hours without sleep. These theories confuse correlation with cause; although such factors often coincide with a distressed[13] postoperative patient, they do not *cause* psychosis, but *accompany* **delirium.**

Smith and Dimsdale[97] conducted a meta-analysis of 44 studies that examined the relationship between postcardiotomy delirium and 28 hypothesized risk variables. Many of their findings challenged prevailing clinical impressions:

◆ The prevalence of postcardiotomy delirium *has not declined* with improved technology, but has remained fairly constant over the years, hovering at an incidence of 32%.

◆ Gender, previous psychiatric illness, and intelligence failed to correlate with postcardiotomy delirium.

◆ Surprisingly, time on bypass did not robustly correlate with postcardiotomy delirium. Of 12 studies, 6 confirmed an effect; 5 found none, and 1 study reported a negative correlation between time on bypass and postoperative delirium.

◆ Correlation coefficients exceeding 0.30 were found only for noncongenital heart disease and the presence of postoperative EEG abnormality. (Note that EEG abnormalities in this context are indicative of the diffuse cerebral dysfunction of delirium rather than a seizure disorder. EEGs are often, but not universally, abnormal in delirium of any cause.)

◆ Strikingly, the most robust correlation was the inverse correlation between postcardiotomy delirium and preoperative psychiatric intervention ($r = -.60$). The psychiatric interviews in three studies[51,52,101] involved listening to the patient's fears, explaining the procedures, and cautioning the patient not to panic if postoperative confusion occurred. The reasons why preoperative psychological intervention would be associated with a lower incidence of delirium—a central nervous system (CNS) phenomenon—remain unclear. (The beneficial effects of psychiatric intervention on recovery after CABG surgery have been corroborated and reviewed in other papers.[90])

◆ No correlation was found between time in the intensive care unit and postcardiotomy delirium.[97]

◆ Sleep deprivation appeared modestly correlated with delirium, but sleep disturbance was a *consequence* of postcardiotomy delirium, not the *cause*,[36] which is true of other kinds of delirium.

Smith and Dimsdale[97] summarized their findings as follows:

> The high prevalence of postcardiotomy delirium and the fact that the prevalence is unchanged despite 25 years of ever more polished surgical and medical techniques suggest that we are not particularly close to understanding its etiology. The studies we have reviewed do not pinpoint any precise risk factor consistently . . . There are a number of tantalizing observations made by single studies; however, unfortunately, many of these observations have never been replicated. Where there was replication, one is struck by the relatively low order of magnitude of the estimated correlation with postcardiotomy delirium; the estimated correlation exceeded 0.30 for only two of the [statistically associated] risk factors: . . . postoperative EEG abnormality and noncongenital heart disease. This would appear to be an instance when clinical intuition is misleading. Postcardiotomy delir-

ium is as prevalent as ever, and the [physiological] risk factors are not understood. (p. 457)

As we will discuss in the case of Mr. Davis in Chapter 2, haloperidol (Haldol) is the treatment of choice for neuropsychiatric symptoms secondary to delirium. Unfortunately, subtle cerebral impairment may persist in up to one-third of postcardiotomy patients, even in those who have not been delirious.[2] The mechanism for this effect remains speculative.[37] Additional research is under way to quantify which biosocial factors might hasten and improve recovery from cardiac surgery.[14,46]

Intraaortic Balloon Pump

The intraaortic balloon pump (IABP) maintains hemodynamic stability during crescendo angina and cardiogenic shock, and provides perioperative support in the coronary care unit. It is associated with significant mental status changes; Sanders and colleagues[88,89] estimated in a retrospective chart review of 195 patients that approximately 34% of patients who underwent IABP placement developed delirium.

- Their sample was exposed to a significant number of medications, including narcotics (> 15 mg/day of morphine), benzodiazepines (> 15 mg/day of diazepam [Valium]), or neuroleptics (> 10 mg/day of intravenous haloperidol [Haldol]).
- The delirium associated with IABP treatment was rapid in onset (within the first 2 days after IABP insertion) and rapid in resolution (within hours after removing the IABP).
- The only risk factor for delirium was a history of seizures. Variables such as the medical indication for IABP placement, cardiac procedure, premorbid medical conditions, and duration of IABP did not differ significantly between delirious and nondelirious patients.
- Residual cognitive deficits and the need for psychiatric consultation upon hospital discharge were highly correlated with the diagnosis of IABP delirium.
- Sanders et al.[88] compared patients who received morphine infusions (> 200 mg/day) with those who received high doses of iv haloperidol (mean dose 135 mg/day) to control agitation. The morphine-treated patients had more complications while on IABP (e.g., pneumonia, lower limb ischemia, bleeding, stroke), a slightly higher mortality, longer hospital stays, and a higher incidence of residual organic brain syndrome.

The etiology of delirium associated with the IABP is unknown. Sanders and Cassem[87] speculate on several possibilities, including altered CNS perfusion caused by the counterpulsation hemodynamics; humoral factors related to the presence of a large, pulsating foreign body in the thoracic area (e.g., tumor necrosis factor or antihistamines); disinhibition secondary to benzodiazepine treatment; or akathisia secondary to neuroleptic therapy.[87]

SUMMARY

1. Unlike tricyclic antidepressants (TCAs), neuroleptics differ in their effect on cardiac conduction. Thioridazine (Mellaril) is the most cardiotoxic of the neuroleptics; haloperidol (Haldol) is the least.
2. Lithium is generally well tolerated in cardiovascular patients. The main effects of lithium are within the atrium (as opposed to the TCAs, which affect the ventricular conduction system). The most common benign electrocardiogram (ECG) effects of lithium are T-wave flattening or inversion. Be careful of the altered renal status that occurs in congestive heart failure. Also be alert to lithium-propranolol interactions, which may have a synergistic effect on lowering heart rate.
3. Carbamazepine (Tegretol) is more cardiotoxic than lithium.
4. Psychological and physiological factors interact to affect hypertension, but the effects of nonpharmacological interventions do not appear to be sustained once treatment stops.
5. As always, assume that antihypertensives produce psychiatric effects and interact with psychiatric medications. Prominent offenders in causing secondary depression are reserpine, methyldopa, and propranolol. Diuretics and vasodilators may exacerbate the hypotensive potential of monoamine oxidase inhibitors (MAOIs) and TCAs.
6. The etiology of delirium secondary to postcardiotomy or intraaortic balloon pump (IABP) therapy remains unclear. Management follows principles for any delirium, as discussed in the case of Mr. Davis (see Chapter 2).

REFERENCES

1. Ambrosi P, Faugre G, Poggi L, et al: Carbamazepine and pacing threshold (letter). Lancet 342:365, 1993
2. Anonymous: Brain damage and open-heart surgery. Lancet 2:364–366, 1989

3. Aronowitz J, Umbricht D, Safferman A, et al: Clozapine and new-onset ECG abnormalities (letter). Psychosomatics 36:82–83, 1995

4. Avorn J, Everitt D, Weiss S: Increased antidepressant use in patients prescribed beta-blockers. JAMA 255:357–360, 1986

5. Axelsson R, Aspenstrom G: Electrocardiographic changes and serum concentrations in thioridazine-treated patients. J Clin Psychiatry 43:332–335, 1982

6. Baldessarini R: Drugs and the treatment of psychiatric disorders, in Goodman and Gilman's The Pharmacological Basis of Therapeutics, 8th Edition. Edited by Gilman A, Rall T, Nies A, et al. New York, Pergamon, 1990, pp 383–435

6a. Baldwin C, Safferman A: A case of lisinopril-induced lithium toxicity. DICP Ann Pharmacother 24:946–947, 1990

7. Banchey M, Lee J, Amin R, et al: High and low potency neuroleptics in elderly psychiatric patients. JAMA 239:1860–1862, 1978

8. Becker D: Lithium and propranolol: possible synergism? (letter). J Clin Psychiatry 50:473, 1989

9. Bernstein J: Drug Interactions, in Massachusetts General Hospital Handbook of General Hospital Psychiatry, 3rd Edition. Edited by Cassem N. St. Louis, MO, Mosby Year Book, 1991, pp 571–610

10. Bernstein J: Psychotropic drug prescribing, in Massachusetts General Hospital Handbook of General Hospital Psychiatry, 3rd Edition. Edited by Cassem N. St. Louis, MO, Mosby Year Book, 1991, pp 527–569

11. Bernstein J: Handbook of Drug Therapy in Psychiatry, 3rd Edition. St Louis, MO, Mosby Year Book, 1995

12. Binder E, Cayabyab L, Ritchie D, et al: Diltiazem-induced psychosis and possible diltiazem-lithium interaction. Arch Intern Med 151:373–374, 1991

13. Blacher R (ed): Heart surgery: the patient's experience, in Psychological Experience of Surgery. Edited by Blacher R. New York, Wiley, 1987, pp 44–86

14. Blumenthal JA, Mank DB: Quality of life and recovery after cardiac surgery. Psychosom Med 56:213–215, 1994

14a. Boesen F, Andersen E, Jensen E: Cardiac conduction disturbances during carbamazepine therapy. Acta Neurol Scand 8:49–52, 1983

14b. Brady H, Horgan J: Lithium and the heart: unanswered questions. Chest 93:166–169, 1988

15. Bright R, Everitt D: β-blockers and depression: evidence against an association. JAMA 267:1783–1787, 1992

15a. Bucht G, Smigan L, Wahlin A, et al: ECG changes during lithium therapy: a prospective study. Acta Med Scand 216:101–104, 1984

15b. Buckley N, Whyte I, Dawson A: Cardiotoxicity more common in thioridazine overdose than with other neuroleptics. J Toxicol Clin Toxicol 33:199–204, 1995

16. Byrd G: Methyldopa and lithium carbonate: suspected interaction (letter). JAMA 233:320, 1975

17. Cassem N: Depression, in Massachusetts General Hospital Handbook of General Hospital Psychiatry, 3rd Edition. Edited by Cassem N. St. Louis, MO, Mosby Year Book, 1991, pp 237–268

18. Chesney M, Agras W, Benson H, et al: Nonpharmacologic approaches to the treatment of hypertension. Circulation 76 (suppl I):I104–I109, 1987

18a. Ciraulo D, Shader R, Greenblatt D, et al. (eds): Drug Interactions in Psychiatry, 2nd Edition. Baltimore, MD, Williams & Wilkins, 1995

18b. Correa F, Eiser A: Angiotensin-converting enzyme inhibitors and lithium toxicity (letter). Am J Med 93:108–109, 1992

19. Creelman W, Ciraulo D, Shader R: Lithium drug interactions, in Drug Interactions in Psychiatry. Edited by Ciraulo D, Shader R, Greenblatt D, et al. Baltimore, MD, Williams & Wilkins, 1989, pp 127–157

20. DasGupta K, Jefferson J: The use of lithium in the medically ill. Gen Hosp Psychiatry 12:83–97, 1990

20a. DasGupta K, Jefferson J: Treatment of mania in the medically ill, in Psychotropic Drug Use in the Medically Ill (Vol 21 of Advances in Psychosomatic Medicine). Edited by Silver P. New York, Karger, 1994, pp 138–162

21. DasGupta K, Jefferson J, Kobak K, et al: The effect of enalapril on serum lithium levels in healthy men. J Clin Psychiatry 53:398–400, 1992

22. Dimsdale J: Research links between psychiatry and cardiology: hypertension, type A behavior, sudden death, and the physiology of emotional arousal. Gen Hosp Psychiatry 10:328–338, 1988

23. Donatini B, Le Blaye I, Krupp P: Transient cardiac pacing is insufficiently used to treat arrhythmia associated with thioridazine. Clinical Pharmacology 81:340–341, 1992

23a. Drouet A, Bouvet O: Lithium and converting enzyme inhibitors. Encephale 16:51–52, 1990

24. Dubovsky S, Franks R, Allen S: Verapamil: a new antimanic drug with potential interactions with lithium. J Clin Psychiatry 48:371–372, 1987

25. Douste-Blazy P, Rostin M, Livarek B, et al: Angiotensin converting enzyme inhibitors and lithium treatment (letter). Lancet 1:1448, 1986

25a. Esler M, Lambert G, Ferrier C, et al: Central nervous system noradrenergic control of sympathetic outflow in normotensive and hypertensive humans. Clin Exp Hypertens 17:409–423, 1995

26. Fayer S: Torsade de pointes ventricular tachyarrhythmia associated with haloperidol (letter). J Clin Psychopharmacol 6:375–376, 1986

27. Finestone D, Manly D: Dissociation precipitated by propranolol. Psychosomatics 35:83–85, 1994

28. Fowler N, McCall D, Chou T, et al: Electrocardiographic changes and cardiac arrhythmias in patients receiving psychotropic drugs. Am J Cardiol 37:223–230, 1976

28a. Friedman E: Re: Bradycardia and somnolence after adding fluoxetine to pimozide regimen (letter). Can J Psychiatry 39:634, 1994

29. Fulop G, Phillips R, Shapiro A: ECG changes during haloperidol and pimozide treatment of Tourette's disorder. Am J Psychiatry 144:673–675, 1987

30. Gelenberg A: Depression, depressants, and antidepressants (editorial). Arch Intern Med 150:2245, 1990

31. Gelenberg A, Bassuk E, Schoonover S (eds): The Practitioner's Guide to Psychoactive Drugs, 3rd Edition. New York, Plenum Medical Book, 1991

32. Glasgow M, Engel B, D'Lugoff B: A controlled trial of a standardized behavioral stepped treatment for hypertension. Psychosom Med 51:10–26, 1989

33. Greendyke R, Schuster D, Wooten J: Propranolol in the treatment of assaultive patients with organic brain disease. J Clin Psychopharmacol 4:282–288, 1984

34. Griffen S, Friedman M: Depressive symptoms in propranolol users. J Clin Psychiatry 47:453–457, 1986

35. Hanna M, Lobao C, Stewart J: Severe lithium toxicity associated with indapamide therapy (letter). J Clin Psychopharmacol 10:379, 1990

36. Harrell R, Othmer E: Postcardiotomy confusion and sleep loss. J Clin Psychiatry 48:445–446, 1987

37. Harris D, Balley S, Smith P, et al: Brain swelling in the first hour after coronary artery bypass surgery. Lancet 342:586–587, 1993

38. Henderson R, Lane S, Henry J: Life-threatening ventricular arrhythmia (torsade de pointes) after haloperidol overdose. Hum Exp Toxicol 10:59–62, 1991

39. Herd J, Falkner O, Anderson D, et al: Psychophysiologic factors in hypertension. Circulation 76 (suppl I):189–194, 1987

40. Hermann D, Krol T, Dukes G, et al: Comparison of verapamil, diltiazem, and labetalol on the bioavailability and metabolism of imipramine. J Clin Pharmacol 32:176–183, 1992

40a. Himmelhoch J, Poust R, Mallinger A, et al: Adjustment of lithium dose during lithium-chlorothiazide therapy. Clin Pharmacol Ther 22:225–227, 1977

41. Houston B: Psychological variables and cardiovascular and neuroendocrine reactivity, in Handbook of Stress, Reactivity, and Cardiovascular Disease. Edited by Matthews K, Weiss S, Detre T, et al. New York, Wiley, 1986, pp 207–229

42. Huston J, Bell G: The effect of thioridazine hydrochloride and chlorpromazine on the electrocardiogram. JAMA 198:16–20, 1966

43. James S: Psychosocial precursors of hypertension: a review of the epidemiologic evidence. Circulation 76 (suppl I):160–166, 1987

44. Jefferson J: A review of the cardiovascular effects and toxicity of tricyclic antidepressants. Psychosom Med 37:160–179, 1975

44a. Jefferson J, Greist J: The cardiovascular effects and toxicity of lithium, in Psychopharmacology Update: New and Neglected Areas. Edited by Davis J, Greenblatt D. New York, Grune & Stratton, 1979, pp 65–79

45. Jefferson J, Greist J, Ackerman D, et al: Lithium Encyclopedia for Clinical Practice, 2nd Edition. Washington, DC, American Psychiatric Press, 1987

45a. Jefferson J, Kalin N: Serum lithium levels and long-term diuretic use. JAMA 241:1134–1136, 1979

46. Jenkins CD, Stanton BA, Jono RT: Quantifying and predicting recovery after heart surgery. Psychosom Med 56:203–212, 1994

47. Kasarskis E, Kuo C, Berger R, et al: Carbamazepine-induced cardiac dysfunction: characterization of two distinct clinical syndromes. Arch Intern Med 152:186–191, 1992

48. Kemper A, Dunlap R, Pietro D: Thioridazine-induced torsade de pointes. JAMA 249:2931–2934, 1983

48a. Kennebäck G, Bergfeldt L, Vallin H, et al: Electrophysiologic effects and clinical hazards of carbamazepine treatment for neurologic disorders in patients with abnormalities of the cardiac conduction system. Am Heart J 121:1421–1429, 1991

49. Kriwisky M, Perry G, Tarchitsky D, et al: Haloperidol-induced torsade de pointes. Chest 98:482–484, 1990

50. Labrecque J, Cote M, Vincent P: Carbamazepine-induced atrioventricular block. Am J Psychiatry 149:572–573, 1992

51. Layne O, Yudofsky S: Postoperative psychosis in cardiotomy patients. N Engl J Med 284:518–520, 1971

52. Lazarus H, Hagens J: Prevention of psychosis following open-heart surgery. Am J Psychiatry 124:1190–1195, 1968

53. Lederle F, Applegate W, Grimm R: Reserpine and the medical marketplace. Arch Intern Med 153:705–706, 1993

54. Levenson J: Cardiovascular disease, in Principles of Medical Psychiatry. Edited by Stoudemire A, Fogel B. Orlando, FL, Grune & Stratton, 1987, pp 477–494

55. Levenson J: Cardiovascular disease, in Psychiatric Care of the Medical Patient. Edited by Stoudemire A, Fogel B. New York, Oxford University Press, 1993, pp 539–555

56. Levinson D, Simpson G: Antipsychotic drug side effects, in Psychiatry Update: American Psychiatric Association Annual Review, Vol 6. Edited by Hales RE, Frances AJ. Washington, DC, American Psychiatric Press, 1987, pp 704–723

57. Light K: Psychological precursors of hypertension: experimental evidence. Circulation 76 (suppl I):167–176, 1987

58. Lipinski J, Zubenko G, Cochrane B, et al: Propranolol in the treatment of neuroleptic-induced akathisia. Am J Psychiatry 141:412–415, 1984

59. Manuck S, Krantz D: Psychophysiologic reactivity in coronary heart disease and essential hypertension, in Handbook of Stress, Reactivity, and Cardiovascular Disease. Edited by Matthews K, Weiss S, Detre T, et al. New York, Wiley, 1986, pp 11–34

60. Maoz E, Grossman E, Thaler M, et al: Carbamazepine neurotoxic reaction after administration of diltiazem. Arch Intern Med 152:2503–2504, 1992

61. McNeil G, Shaw P, Dock D: Substitution of atenolol for propranolol in a case of propranolol-related depression. Am J Psychiatry 139:1187–1188, 1982

62. Metzger E, Friedman R: Prolongation of the corrected QT and torsade de pointes cardiac arrhythmia associated with intravenous haloperidol in the medically ill. J Clin Psychopharmacol 13:128–132, 1993

63. Mills P, Dimsdale J, Nelesen R, et al: Patterns of adrenergic receptors and adrenergic agonists underlying cardiovascular responses to a psychological challenge. Psychosom Med 56:70–76, 1994

64. Mitchell J, MacKenzie T: Cardiac effects of lithium therapy in man. J Clin Psychiatry 43:47–51, 1982

65. Niaura R, Goldstein M: Psychological factors affecting physical condition: Cardiovascular disease literature review, II: coronary artery disease and sudden death and hypertension. Psychosomatics 33:146–155, 1992

65a. Niaura R, Goldstein M: Cardiovascular disease, part II: coronary artery disease and sudden death and hypertension, in Psychological Factors Affecting Medical Conditions. Edited by Stoudemire A. Washington, DC, American Psychiatric Press, 1995, pp 39–56

65b. Opler L, Feinberg S: The role of pimozide in clinical psychiatry: a review. J Clin Psychiatry 52:221–233, 1991

66. O'Regan J: Adverse interaction of lithium carbonate and methyldopa (letter). Can Med Assoc J 115:385, 1976

67. Osanloo E, Deglin J: Interaction of lithium and methyldopa (letter). Ann Intern Med 92:433–434, 1980

68. Patel C, Marmot M, Terry D, et al: Trial of relaxation in reducing coronary risk: four year follow-up. BMJ 290:1102–1106, 1985

69. Patten S, Brager N, Sanders S, et al: Manic symptoms associated with the use of captopril (letter). Can J Psychiatry 36:314–315, 1991

70. Paykel E, Fleminger R, Watson J: Psychiatric side effects of anti-hypertensive drugs other than reserpine. J Clin Psychopharmacol 2:14–39, 1982

71. Petrie W, Maffucci R, Woosley R: Propranolol and depression. Am J Psychiatry 139:92–93, 1982

72. Pickering T, Gerin W: Ambulatory blood pressure monitoring and cardiovascular reactivity for the evaluation of the role of psychosocial factors and prognosis in hypertensive patients. Am Heart J 116:665–672, 1988

73. Price W, Giannini A: Neurotoxicity caused by lithium-verapamil synergism. J Clin Pharmacol 26:717–719, 1986

74. Price W, Shalley J: Lithium-verapamil toxicity in the elderly. J Am Geriatr Soc 35:177–178, 1987

75. Quetsch R, Achor R, Litin E: Depressive reactions in hypertensive patients. Circulation 19:366–375, 1959

76. Ragheb M: Drug interactions in psychiatric practice. International Pharmacopsychiatry 16:92–118, 1981

77. Rall T, Schleifer L: Drugs effective in the therapy of the epilepsies, in Goodman and Gilman's The Pharmacological Basis of Therapeutics, 8th Edition. Edited by Gilman A, Rall T, Nies A, et al. New York, Pergamon, 1990, pp 439–443

78. Ratey J, Mikkelsen E, Bushell-Smith G, et al: β-blockers in the severely and profoundly mentally retarded. J Clin Psychopharmacol 2:103–107, 1986

79. Ratey J, Mikkelsen E, Sorgi P, et al: Autism: the treatment of aggressive behaviors. J Clin Psychopharmacol 7:35–41, 1987

80. Ratey J, Sorgi P, Lindem J, et al: Nadolol to treat aggression in psychiatric patients (NR182), in New Research Program and Abstracts: American Psychiatric Association 142nd Annual Meeting, San Francisco, CA, May 1989. Washington, DC, American Psychiatric Association, 1989, p 112

81. Ratey J, Sorgi P, Polakoff S: Nadolol as a treatment for akathisia. Am J Psychiatry 142:640–641, 1985

82. Ray W, Griffin M, Schaffner W, et al: Psychotropic drug use and the risk of hip fracture. N Engl J Med 316:363–369, 1987

83. Richardson H, Graupner K, Richardson M: Intramyocardial lesions in patients dying suddenly and unexpectedly. JAMA 195:254–260, 1966

84. Risch S, Groom G, Janowsky D: Interfaces of psychopharmacology and cardiology, I. J Clin Psychiatry 42:23–34, 1981

85. Risch S, Groom G, Janowsky D: The effects of psychotropic drugs on the cardiovascular system. J Clin Psychiatry 43:16–31, 1982

86. Roose S, Bone S, Haidorfer C, et al: Lithium treatment in older patients. Am J Psychiatry 136:843–844, 1979

87. Sanders K, Cassem E: Psychiatric complications in the critically ill cardiac patient. Tex Heart Inst J 20:180–187, 1993

88. Sanders K, Stern T, O'Gara P, et al: Delirium during intra-aortic balloon pump therapy: incidence and management. Psychosomatics 33:35–44, 1992

89. Sanders K, Stern T, O'Gara P, et al: Medical and neuropsychiatric complications associated with use of the intra-aortic balloon pump therapy. Journal of Intensive Care Medicine 7:154–164, 1992

90. Schindler B, Shook J, Schwartz G: Beneficial effects of psychiatric intervention on recovery after coronary artery bypass graft surgery. Gen Hosp Psychiatry 11:358–364, 1989

91. Schwarcz G, Lopez-Toca R: Continued lithium treatment after myocardial infarction (letter). Am J Psychiatry 139:255, 1982

92. Shapiro A: Psychological factors in hypertension: an overview. Am Heart J 116:632–637, 1988

93. Shapiro P: Nortriptyline treatment of depressed cardiac transplant patients. Am J Psychiatry 148:371–373, 1991

94. Shom M: Electrocardiographic changes during treatment with lithium and with drugs of the imipramine type. Acta Psychiatr Scand Suppl 169:258–259, 1963

95. Skinner M, Futterman A, Morrissette D, et al: Atenolol compared with nifedipine: effect on cognitive function and mood in elderly hypertensive patients. Ann Intern Med 116:615–623, 1992

96. Slagle D: The acute withdrawal of diltiazem and atenolol: a possible challenge to affective stability (letter). J Clin Psychopharmacol 9:381–382, 1989

97. Smith L, Dimsdale J: Postcardiotomy delirium: conclusions after 25 years? Am J Psychiatry 146:452–458, 1989

98. Sorgi P, Ratey J, Knoedler D, et al: Depression during treatment with beta-blockers: results from a double-blind placebo-controlled study. J Neuropsychiatry Clin Neurosci 4:187–189, 1992

99. Sorgi P, Ratey J, Polakoff S, et al: Adrenergic blockers for the control of aggressive behavior in patients with chronic schizophrenia. Am J Psychiatry 143:775–776, 1986

100. Southam M, Agras W, Taylor C, et al: Relaxation training: blood pressure reduction during the working day. Arch Gen Psychiatry 39:715–717, 1982

101. Surman O, Hackett T, Silverberg E, et al: Usefulness of psychiatric intervention in patients undergoing cardiac surgery. Arch Gen Psychiatry 30:830–835, 1974

102. Tesar G, Murray G, Cassem N: Use of high-dose intravenous haloperidol in the treatment of agitated cardiac patients. J Clin Psychopharmacol 5:344–347, 1985

103. Thiessen B, Wallace S, Blackburn J, et al: Increased prescribing of antidepressants subsequent to blocker therapy. Arch Intern Med 150:2286–2290, 1990

104. Thomsen K, Schou M: Renal lithium excretion in man. Am J Physiol 215:823–827, 1968

105. Thornton W: Dementia induced by methyldopa with haloperidol. N Engl J Med 294:1222, 1976

106. Valdiserri E: A possible interaction between lithium and diltiazem: case report. J Clin Psychiatry 46:540–541, 1985

107. Walker N, White K, Tornatore F, et al: Lithium-methyldopa interactions in normal subjects (abstract #34). Drug Intelligence and Clinical Pharmacy 14:638–639, 1980

108. Weder A, Julius S: Behavior, blood pressure variability, and hypertension. Psychosom Med 47:406–414, 1985

109. Weintraub M, Hes J, Rotmensh H, et al: Extreme sinus bradycardia associated with lithium therapy. Isr J Med Sci 19:353–355, 1983

110. Wellens H, Cats V, Durren D: Symptomatic sinus node abnormalities following lithium carbonate therapy. Am J Med 59:285–287, 1975

111. Whitlock F, Evans L: Drugs and depression. Drugs 15:53–71, 1978

112. Wilens T, Stern T, O'Gara P: Adverse cardiac effects of combined neuroleptic ingestion and tricyclic antidepressant overdose. J Clin Psychopharmacol 10:51–57, 1990

113. Wilson J, Kraus E, Bailas M, et al: Reversible sinus node abnormalities due to lithium carbonate therapy. N Engl J Med 294:1222–1224, 1976

114. Wilt J, Minnema A, Johnson R, et al: Torsade de pointes associates with the use of intravenous haloperidol. Ann Intern Med 119:391–394, 1993

115. Wright B, Jarrett D: Lithium and calcium channel blockers: possible neurotoxicity (letter). Biol Psychiatry 30:635–636, 1991

116. Yudofsky S: β-blockers and depression: the clinician's dilemma. JAMA 267:1826–1827, 1992

117. Zee-Cheng C, Mueller C, Seifert C, et al: Haloperidol and torsade de pointes (letter). Ann Intern Med 102:418, 1985

The Patient With Pulmonary Disease

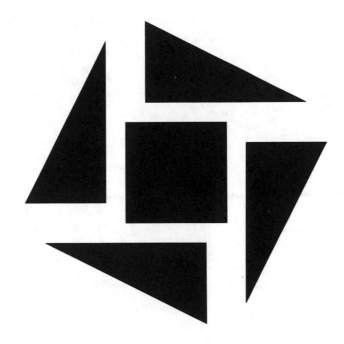

CHAPTER 2

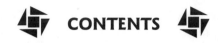

CONTENTS

■ Introduction to Chapter 2 67
■ Case Presentation: Mr. Davis: The Patient With
  Delirium and Lung Cancer 68
■ Questions 68
■ Answers 72
■ Discussion 73
  ◆ Psychotherapy With the Medically Ill 73
  ◆ Delirium 74
    Presenting Features 74
      Delirium or Dementia? 75
      Etiology 76
      Hypoxia 76
      "ICU Psychosis" 77
    Bedside Assessment of Delirium 77
      Mini-Mental State Examination 77
      Trail Making Tests 77
      Other Tests 77
    Management of Delirium 78
      Nonpharmacological Interventions 78
      Haloperidol in Delirium 79
      Haloperidol With Lorazepam 80
      Benzodiazepines 80
      Other Agents 80
          Droperidol 80
          Paralytic agents 81
          Miscellaneous agents 81
      Effects of Neuroleptics on Respiration . . 81
    Insomnia and Sundowning 81
    Ventilator Weaning 82
  ◆ Special Considerations in Lung Cancer 82
    Differential Diagnosis: Dyspnea, Anxiety,
      and Restlessness 82
      Adverse Neuropsychiatric Effects of Antiemetics 82
      Intracranial Metastases 82
      Paraneoplastic Syndromes 83
      Delirium in the Setting of Cancer 84
    Factors in Oncological Treatment 84
      Karnofsky Scale 84
      Benzodiazepines for Chemotherapy Patients . 84
      Doxorubicin 84
      Parenteral and Rectal Antidepressants . . . 85
      Lithium 85

◆ Summary 85
◆ References 86
■ Case Presentation: Mrs. Alberts: The Anxious,
  Depressed Asthmatic Patient 93
■ Questions 93
■ Answers 96
■ Discussion 97
  ◆ Coping With Chronic Lung Disease 97
    Psychological Precipitants 97
      Psychosocial Dysfunction 98
      Families 98
      Sexuality 99
    Medical and Psychological Factors 99
      Neuropsychiatric Effects of Chronic Hypoxia . 99
      *Mood, Subjective Dyspnea, and Objective
        Pulmonary Function* 100
      Physician-Related Assessment Factors . . . 101
    Psychotoxicity of Medications 101
      Steroids 101
      Theophylline and Bronchodilators 102
  ◆ Anxiety Disorders 102
    Somatization 102
  ◆ Major Depression 102
    Incidence 102
  ◆ Psychopharmacology 103
    Anxiolytics and Respiration 103
      Benzodiazepines 103
      Buspirone 104
      Other Anxiolytics 104
      Adverse Drug Interactions 105
    Neuroleptics 105
      Adverse Drug Interactions 105
    Antidepressants 105
      Efficacy 105
      Side Effects 105
      Tartrazine Dye 106
      Adverse Drug Interactions 106
    Electroconvulsive Therapy 106
    Psychotherapy 107
      Psychotherapy "Side Effects" 108
  ◆ Summary 108
  ◆ References 109

The two cases in this chapter have lung disease in common, but discuss very different issues. The lung cancer case explores delirium, the psychotherapy of the medically ill, and special considerations in cancer patients. The second case is more narrowly focused on asthma and chronic obstructive pulmonary disease (COPD). As mentioned, certain organizational decisions were arbitrary—some of these topics could have been just as appropriately included elsewhere.

Nonetheless, the cases and questions were designed to tap practically useful information. They are not intended to simulate an examination. As before, use the questions before, during, or after reading the text. There may be more than one correct answer.

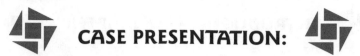
Mr. Davis is a 74-year-old man who recently retired as an editor at a publishing firm. He had been diagnosed with small-cell lung cancer 15 years ago. He had smoked for many years, but stopped at the time of his diagnosis. He was successfully treated with surgery and chemotherapy. His yearly checkups have revealed no evidence of disease. One month before the present referral, a new lesion was found on chest X ray. Workup was consistent with small-cell cancer of the lung, which was thought to be a new primary cancer rather than a recurrence. Although the patient was "confident" of a cure, he requested psychiatric referral for "support."

Mr. Davis had been in psychotherapy during his early 30s for help with his marriage. He had found it extremely useful in defining "how I was contributing to problems in the marriage." His first wife had died 20 years ago of a brain tumor. He had remarried 10 years ago and lived comfortably with his second wife, who was several years his junior.

He has never been on psychotropic medication or been hospitalized psychiatrically. Family history is negative for psychiatric illness. He denies any other pertinent medical history. He was on no medication at the time of referral. There is no history of substance abuse.

The patient is started on a regimen of vincristine (Oncovin), cyclophosphamide (Cytoxan), and doxorubicin (Adriamycin), with metoclopramide (Reglan) for nausea. He attends his twice-weekly psychotherapy visits in addition to regular visits to his oncologist.

Mr. Davis remains euthymic for the next 6 months, with appropriate concerns about recurrence. He talks a great deal about his love for adventurous sports, such as speedboat racing and mountain climbing. As a young man, he had participated in both. Free association to a dream about a boy who lost his baseball leads to memories of a serious illness when he was 6 years old, after he broke his leg while running after a trolley. He had never mentioned it to any of his doctors because "it happened over 60 years ago and there were no aftereffects." Since there were no antibiotics available at the time, the leg had become badly infected. He remembers the doctor whispering in the hall to his parents. Although he could not hear what was said, he remembered his father exclaiming, "No! I'd rather see him dead than grow up to be a man with only one leg. He'd be a cripple."

Despite an excellent working relationship with his psychiatrist, characterized by increasing insight and curiosity about himself, Mr. Davis begins to complain of "always feeling nervous for no reason." Several days after reporting the dream, he begins to experience persistent dread, restlessness, dry mouth, shortness of breath, and increasing fatigue. He becomes preoccupied with the effort to breathe, paces frequently, and develops difficulty sleeping. (He attributes his reaction to what was being discussed in psychotherapy.) When the psychiatrist queries him about the course of his treatments, he maintains that the doctors are pleased with his progress. He says that he is "going to lick this thing like I did 15 years ago."

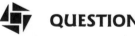 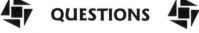 QUESTIONS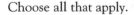

Choose all that apply.

1. Which of the following are *not* valid statements?
   a. Interpretation of Mr. Davis's implicit fear of burial should be the next psychodynamic intervention.
   b. The effects of the benzodiazepines on cognition make them useful in the setting of chemotherapy.
   c. A secondary psychiatric syndrome would be sufficiently ruled out if central nervous system (CNS) metastatic workup, a blood gas, and blood screen were negative.
   d. Among his medications, metoclopramide would be the most likely culprit for his anxiety-like symptoms.
   e. It is premature to start an anxiolytic.

2. Tricyclic antidepressants (TCAs) would be most likely to potentiate the cardiotoxic effects of which agent?
    a. Vincristine (Oncovin)
    b. Cyclophosphamide (Cytoxan)
    c. Doxorubicin ((Adriamycin)
    d. Metoclopramide (Reglan)
    e. None of the above

3. With the patient's consent, the psychiatrist confers with the oncologist, who reveals that the tumor is rapidly advancing and is inoperable. The oncologist confirms that Mr. Davis's recent blood gases have been slowly getting worse. Over the next few weeks, the patient deteriorates rapidly. He is hospitalized in the intensive care unit (ICU) with progressive respiratory failure, where he is intubated and you are called as the consultant. He manages to communicate that he is terrified that he will suffocate. Mr. Davis is tearful and sad, stating that he feels like dying. The nurses note that he seems to be talking to himself. He confided to one nurse in writing that an aide has poisoned his food in order to steal his insurance policy. The nurse says that he has conversations with his first wife, who has been dead for 20 years. They report that sometimes he appears oriented, but at other times he is "out of it." Mr. Davis has been briefly taken off all medications, but his mental status remains the same. Which of the following are true?
    a. Hypoxia should be expected to be accompanied by acute changes in mental status.
    b. The rate of change in level of oxygen saturation (Po_2) is the measure that most closely correlates with the occurrence of acute psychiatric symptoms.
    c. The severity of the neuropsychiatric symptoms secondary to hypercapnia has been found to correlate with the intensity of cerebrospinal fluid (CSF) acidosis.
    d. Carbon dioxide retention produces a maniclike psychosis resembling amphetamine intoxication.

4. You overhear the oncology staff discussing Mr. Davis's "Karnofsky." The Karnofsky Scale is a measure of . . .
    a. Chemotherapy toxicity.
    b. Performance status.
    c. Prognosis and survival.
    d. Metastatic disease.
    e. Mood in oncology patients.

5. Mr. Davis's blood gases improve while intubated, returning almost to baseline. Which of the following are true statements about the appropriateness of the Mini-Mental State Examination (MMSE) and the Trail Making Tests for evaluating Mr. Davis?

    a. The MMSE would be useful in assessing affective as well as cognitive changes.
    b. A disadvantage of the MMSE is that retesting would show significant practice effect, thereby limiting its usefulness in serially documenting Mr. Davis's cognitive change.
    c. Compared with the MMSE, the Trail Making Tests would be more likely to detect subtle cognitive dysfunction.
    d. Delirium is most sensitively assessed at the bedside using the MMSE.

6. Which of the following are true about other bedside tests of cognition?
    a. Writing functions are relatively resistant to the cognitive fluctuations of delirium, and impairments tend to occur late in the clinical course.
    b. Problems in reproducing a clock face specifically indicate right hemispheric dysfunction.
    c. The Isaacs Set Test asks the patient to sort cards by features such as shape, color, or number.
    d. None of the above.

7. Blood work is pending. Which of the following statements are true regarding Mr. Davis's neurological status?
    a. Psychiatric symptoms may occur *before* neurological findings in the setting of metastatic brain disease.
    b. Meningeal carcinomatosis rarely occurs without meningeal signs (e.g., fever, stiff neck).
    c. The three most common cancers that metastasize to the brain are those of the lung, breast, and prostate.
    d. The key clinical observation differentiating delirium from dementia is the level of psychomotor agitation.
    e. None of the above.

8. Which of the following are true about delirium in the cancer population?
    a. Cerebral metastases are the most common cause of delirium in this population.
    b. Delirium is particularly common in terminally ill cancer patients.
    c. Metabolic abnormalities are the most common cause of delirium in the cancer population.
    d. Delirium is relatively rare unless the patient is in the *terminal* phase of the cancer illness.

9. Which of the following are true regarding delirium in hospitalized patients?

a. Delirium presents as cognitive complaints in the majority of patients.
b. Psychoactive drugs are strongly associated with the risk of delirium in hospitalized elderly patients.
c. The occurrence of delirium identifies those elderly patients at risk for increased morbidity, but not mortality.
d. The most common behavioral marker for delirium in the elderly is disruptive behavior.
e. The goal of treatment is to calm agitation gradually, over the course of several days.

10. The medical intern requests advice on sedating Mr. Davis during the day, since he keeps pulling out his IV and is unable to cooperate with magnetic resonance imaging (MRI) scans of his brain and lungs. According to the current literature, which of the following would be *inappropriate* medications in this setting?
a. Intravenous diazepam (Valium)
b. Intravenous lorazepam (Ativan)
c. Oxazepam (Serax)
d. Intravenous haloperidol (Haldol)
e. Intramuscular haloperidol (Haldol)

11. Medications that have *not* been implicated in causing delirium include . . .
a. Antibiotics.
b. *Nonsteroidal* antiinflammatory agents (e.g., naproxen [Anaprox, Naprosyn]).
c. Propranolol in *low* doses.
d. H_2 antagonists used for peptic ulcer disease.
e. None of the above; they have all been implicated.

12. You learn that Mr. Davis's platelet count has dropped and that he has become severely thrombocytopenic. Regularly administered intramuscular injections are now inadvisable. Which of the following is *false* regarding the use of intravenous haloperidol for delirium?
a. Intravenous haloperidol produces quicker sedation than the intramuscular form.
b. Intravenous haloperidol has the disadvantage of producing more extrapyramidal side effects (EPS) compared with the oral form.
c. Hypotensive episodes are an *infrequent* complication following the administration of iv haloperidol.
d. Its mean half-life is shorter than those of the im or po forms.

13. Intravenous and/or intramuscular haloperidol are *contraindicated* in which of the following settings?

a. COPD
b. Head trauma
c. Meningeal carcinomatosis
d. Intraaortic balloon pump therapy
e. None of the above

14. In order to figure out a dosing schedule for Mr. Davis, it is important to know the equivalence dosages among different "types" of haloperidol. The equivalence dosage of 1 mg haloperidol iv has been empirically recommended to be . . .
a. 1 mg po.
b. 2 mg po.
c. 5 mg po.
d. 1 mg im.
e. 5 mg im.

15. Which of the following are true regarding the adverse effects of intravenous haloperidol?
a. It has been associated with progressive QT-interval widening.
b. Adverse effects have been described exclusively in the setting of preexisting electrolyte abnormalities.
c. At worst, the reported cardiovascular side effects have been limited to benign first-degree heart block (PR elongation).
d. The electrocardiogram (ECG) change that seems most likely to predispose to adverse cardiovascular events with iv haloperidol is sinus tachycardia.
e. The literature suggests that alcohol abuse may be a risk factor.

16. You have already given Mr. Davis 20 mg of iv haloperidol without side effects, but he is still psychotic and agitated. What is the maximum recommended 24-hour dosage?
a. 75 mg
b. 150 mg
c. 300 mg
d. No upper limit has been established

17. Mr. Davis continues to be quite agitated despite receiving 25 mg of intravenous haloperidol. He has become disruptive to the other ICU patients. Which of the following are true considerations about adding lorazepam (Ativan) at this point?
a. According to the literature, lorazepam should not be used in combination with haloperidol for elderly delirious patients.
b. Experts advise that single-agent therapy for agitated delirium is preferable to the haloperidol-lorazepam combination.

c. A ratio of 2 mg haloperidol to 1 mg lorazepam is recommended when the two are combined.

d. Treatments using the haloperidol-lorazepam combination have a lower incidence of EPS compared with those using haloperidol alone.

18. Which of the following are true regarding lorazepam (Ativan) for agitation?
    a. Active metabolites become a problem once the dose exceeds 10 mg.
    b. It has a wide therapeutic index.
    c. The maximum rate of iv administration is 0.5 mg/minute.
    d. The maximum single dose of lorazepam is 4 mg iv or im.
    e. The highest reported 24-hour dose of lorazepam for critically ill patients was no more than 85–90 mg.

19. Droperidol (Inapsine), a butyrophenone used as an adjunct to anesthesia, has advantages and disadvantages over haloperidol for delirious, agitated patients. Which of the following are false statements about droperidol compared with haloperidol?
    a. It has a slower onset of action.
    b. It has a shorter duration of action.
    c. It has a lower incidence of EPS.
    d. It has a higher incidence of hypotension.

20. Midazolam (Versed) is a benzodiazepine administered intravenously for sedation before certain medical procedures and as an adjunct to anesthesia. Some authors recommend it for treating delirium in the ICU. All of the following are true about midazolam except . . .
    a. It has a short half-life.
    b. There is the potential for respiratory depression.
    c. There is greater potential for iatrogenic overdose and toxicity with midazolam than with lorazepam (Ativan).
    d. Like lorazepam, midazolam's metabolism is relatively unaffected by liver dysfunction.

21. You and the oncologist confer and decide to start Mr. Davis on a neuroleptic. Which of the following are true regarding neuroleptics in psychotic patients with severe pulmonary disease?
    a. Neuroleptics usually have few adverse effects on respiration.
    b. The more sedating antipsychotic drugs are preferred because they lessen the need for benzodiazepines.

c. The single most serious neuroleptic side effect on respiratory function is the impact on secretions and the ability to clear them.

d. The potential risk of aspiration is increased by neuroleptics.

e. Most authors advise ordering the medications "as needed" (prn) to treat agitated, psychotic delirium.

22. Mr. Davis becomes more agitated and paranoid as evening approaches, and he experiences significant middle insomnia. What statements are accurate regarding insomnia in the delirious patient?
    a. Sodium amytal is a useful sleeping aid in this specific population.
    b. Antihistamines (e.g., diphenhydramine [Benadryl]) are innocuous alternatives to benzodiazepines for insomnia in the setting of delirium.
    c. The sedating phenothiazines are recommended to treat the insomnia of delirium, as long as effects on blood pressure are carefully monitored.
    d. Chloral hydrate in reduced doses is a practical hypnotic for delirium.
    e. Triazolam's (Halcion's) quick onset and short half-life make it widely recommended for the insomnia of delirium.

23. Which are *false* statements concerning benzodiazepines?
    a. Benzodiazepines should be avoided in treating the insomnia of delirium.
    b. Pharmacological interventions for insomnia should await the resolution of the delirium.
    c. Oxazepam (Serax) and temazepam (Restoril) have no active metabolites.
    d. Clonazepam (Klonopin) and lorazepam (Ativan) have no active metabolites.
    e. Adverse effects of benzodiazepines on delirium are attributable to the accumulation of metabolites.

24. If Mr. Davis were unable to tolerate oral medications, what parenteral medications would be deemed most appropriate for his insomnia while delirious?
    a. Perphenazine (Trilafon)
    b. Diazepam (Valium)
    c. Diphenhydramine (Benadryl)
    d. Lorazepam (Ativan)

25. Mr. Davis's delirium improves and the staff attempt to wean him off the ventilator. Repeated trials have been unsuccessful. He has become so anxious about the proce-

dure that your advice is again sought. Which of the following are recommended?

   a. Avoid all benzodiazepines.

   b. Avoid intravenous haloperidol.

   c. Classical behavioral techniques for inducing relaxation should be modified, because they paradoxically increase anxiety in this population.

   d. When using hypnosis for ventilator weaning of the anxious patient, *eliminate* the instruction to focus on deep breathing.

26. Mr. Davis's delirium clears. He is extubated and transferred to the regular ward for additional chemotherapy. A nasogastric tube has to be placed because of severe emesis, and he cannot take anything by mouth. Treatment options that have been investigated and found effective for depressed patients who cannot swallow oral antidepressants include which of the following?

   a. Dextroamphetamine (Dexedrine) suppositories

   b. Intramuscular imipramine (Tofranil)

   c. Intramuscular amitriptyline (Elavil)

   d. Intravenous amitriptyline (Elavil)

   e. Amitriptyline (Elavil) suppositories

   f. Doxepin (Sinequan) capsules per rectum

   g. Pemoline (Cylert)

   h. All of the above

⚕ Answers

1. Answer: a, c (pp. 73, 82–84)	14. Answer: b, d (p. 401)
2. Answer: b, c (p. 84)	15. Answer: a, e (p. 79)
3. Answer: c (pp. 76–77)	16. Answer: d (p. 401)
4. Answer: b (p. 84)	17. Answer: d (pp. 80, 401)
5. Answer: c (p. 77)	18. Answer: b, d (p. 401)
6. Answer: d (pp. 77–78)	19. Answer: a (p. 80)
7. Answer: a (pp. 75–76, 82–83)	20. Answer: d (p. 80)
8. Answer: b, c (p. 84)	21. Answer: a, d (pp. 80–81)
9. Answer: b (pp. 74–75, 78–79)	22. Answer: d (pp. 81, 402)
10. Answer: a (p. 81)	23. Answer: a, b (p. 80)
11. Answer: e (p. 76)	24. Answer: d (pp. 81, 402)
12. Answer: b (p. 79)	25. Answer: c, d (pp. 81–82)
13. Answer: e (p. 79)	26. Answer: h (pp. 84–85)

♨ PSYCHOTHERAPY WITH THE MEDICALLY ILL

Surgical patient to a consultant: "The tranquilizers can only do so much. I wish somebody would talk to me about this cancer thing . . . "[76]

The psychiatrist who consults on medical services regularly encounters some patients who require more than brief interventions; they are hungry to talk—to speak about their lives, to integrate their feelings about being ill, to try to make sense of the inevitable question, "Why me?" These issues arise with special urgency often, but not exclusively, in cancer patients, given the arduous, extended period of treatment, the close cultural association between cancer and death, and the manifold unconscious meanings of having a cancer diagnosis.

Bernhard and Ganz[24] have stated,

Good health has positive value and is associated with personal responsibility, whereas having a chronic or serious disease often is associated with a sense of personal failure. Even when an individual lung cancer patient has no known etiologic risk factors, the patient and significant others may still consider the patient responsible in some way for the disease . . . . (p. 219)

The multiple-choice format is ill suited to adequately review psychotherapy with the medically ill. A few resources follow for the interested reader:

♦ First coined by Viederman,[197] the "psychodynamic life narrative" is a psychotherapeutic technique geared specifically for the medically ill that explores the meaning of a particular illness within the context of a patient's entire life, rather than interpreting a single conflict or event.
♦ Werman's[202] 1981 paper stands as one of the most accessible technical comparisons of supportive psychotherapy and insight-oriented psychotherapy—concepts of particular relevance to working with people in crisis.

♦ Journals such as *Psychotherapy and Psychosomatics* (Karger) are less biologically oriented than many consultation-liaison journals, and regularly publish original articles about psychotherapy with medical patients.
♦ A useful series of papers on psychotherapy has appeared in the major consultation-liaison textbooks; topics addressed include principles of medical psychotherapy relative to coping with illness,[71,124,201] brief psychotherapy,[76,105] family therapy,[90] group therapy,[177] and caring for the dying patient.[42] These papers are informative and useful resources for approaching the current literature.

Interpreting Mr. Davis's implicit fear of burial would be premature on the basis of the presented material; it is not the most prominent theme. For example, there are indications that Mr. Davis's fears of bodily injury and helplessness predate his cancer and relate to feelings about himself as an intact, effective man. This trial inference would be based on observations about his early experience with illness and his associations to the dream. As Tavani[184] has pointed out, a patient's fantasies cannot be divined; if not elicited and addressed, they may interfere with the medical course and treatment. *Do not presume the meanings of an illness for a patient.* There will certainly be common elements among patients with the same illness; for example, fears of dying, burial, and suffocation are ubiquitous among lung cancer patients. However, remember that a seemingly obvious psychological or medical symptom can be overdetermined, having a plurality of meanings that are often unexpected, unpredicted, and highly individual to a particular patient. *Often there is unconscious overlap between preexisting conflicts and current reactions to the medical situation; the past merges with present reality into a "double whammy" of traumatic experience.* For Mr. Davis, interpretations that clarified his fears of becoming "unmanned" by the cancer and its treatment might help ease his anxiety. Try to avoid premature closure, as valuable opportunities for insight and relief may be missed.

♦ In addition, a patient's perception of the current medical status is colored by levels of defense, such as denial and displacement. The psychological dimension of lung cancer is particularly troubling because of the frequently self-introduced risk of cigarette smoking and the low survival rates.[78] For example, the conscious acknowledgment of the relationship between smoking and lung cancer is not simple;[20,68] some patients need to deny it.[102,139]

◆ Often, self-reports do not correlate with the objective disease course. For example, Mr. Davis was a veteran of psychotherapy, and was more willing to attribute his physical symptoms to anxiety about psychodynamics than he was to recognize that his disease was progressing. Be alert to patients who appear overly compliant in psychodynamic psychotherapy. How might their compliance serve as resistance to more painful realizations?

The psychotherapist's countertransference denial of the patient's medical deterioration is an occupational hazard, especially for patients who had been previously healthy, or "beat the odds" cancer survivors. It is painful for therapists, too, to acknowledge that the illness has recurred or that their patient is dying.

◆ Regular dialogue with the collaborating physicians— an unfamiliar strategy in the psychotherapy of medically healthy patients—helps the therapist stay realistic, minimizes collusion with the patient's denial, and reduces the likelihood of missing something medical.

Some of the more practical issues in psychiatric oncology (also known as psychooncology) are reviewed later in this chapter. Papers by Bernhard and Ganz[23,24,24a] and indispensable handbooks by Holland and colleagues at Memorial Sloan-Kettering Cancer Center[33,79] are particularly helpful.

⊕ DELIRIUM

Presenting Features

As detailed in several scholarly discussions of delirium,[109,116a,136,144c,172,192a,204] very little is known about its pathogenesis.[88,191] The discussion that follows is not comprehensive, but instead has abstracted the basics for clinical emphasis.

Table 2–1 presents the DSM-IV[10] diagnostic criteria for delirium due to a general medical condition.

Fluctuating consciousness is the hallmark of delirium. It occurs in approximately 10%–15%[21] of medical-surgical patients, with elderly patients at special risk.[111,161] Re-

Table 2–1.   DSM-IV criteria for delirium due to a general medical condition

A. Disturbance of consciousness (i.e., reduced clarity of awareness of the environment) with reduced ability to focus, sustain, or shift attention.

B. A change in cognition (such as memory deficit, disorientation, language disturbance) or the development of a perceptual disturbance that is not better accounted for by a preexisting, established, or evolving dementia.

C. The disturbance develops over a short period of time (usually hours to days) and tends to fluctuate during the course of the day.

D. There is evidence from the history, physical examination, or laboratory findings that the disturbance is caused by the direct physiological consequences of a general medical condition.

Coding note: If delirium is superimposed on a preexisting dementia of the Alzheimer's type or vascular dementia, indicate the delirium by coding the appropriate subtype of the dementia (e.g., 290.3, dementia of the Alzheimer's type, with late onset, with delirium).

Coding note: Include the name of the general medical condition on Axis I (e.g., delirium due to hepatic encephalopathy); also code the general medical condition on Axis III [DSM-IV provides the ICD-9-CM codes in its Appendix G].

Note.   Consult Appendix A for details on coding.
Source.   American Psychiatric Association 1994, p. 129.

covery is related inversely to age and duration of illness,[113] with mortality rates of elderly patients ranging from 15% to 30%.[112,155]

The prevalence, risk factors, and outcome of delirium were examined prospectively in one study of 229 elderly patients, in which 22% met criteria for delirium, and nondelirious patients constituted the control group.[60] Risk factors included the following:

◆ Abnormal sodium levels
◆ Greater illness severity
◆ Prior history of dementia
◆ Fever or hypothermia
◆ Psychoactive drug use
◆ Azotemia

The occurrence of delirium identified those elderly patients at greater risk for increased length of hospital stay, institutionalization, and mortality. (The latter appeared to be explained by greater severity of illness.) These results have been generally corroborated by other studies.[87,117]

Several points warrant clinical emphasis:

♦ "Hit and run" consultation is fraught with potential mistakes. Never rule out delirium based on one cross-sectional interview; if you see the patient during a period of relative lucidity, you may miss the disordered sensorium. Emphasize gathering longitudinal data from staff and family—your best sources of observational information—and assess the patient over time.

♦ The often-seen description of "unpredictable, fluctuating alertness and clouded sensory awareness" makes the diagnosis sound more obvious on paper than it often is at the bedside. *Delirium may be* **subtle** *and* **surreptitious** *in onset; you will be fooled if you suspect only blatant cognitive deficits.* In fact, a "classical" presentation of delirium with obvious cognitive problems occurs in only about 30% of consultations; other presentations are the rule—that is, 20% of delirium presents as anxiety or depression, 20% as hallucinations or delusions, and another 20% as inappropriate behavior (e.g., irascibility, uncooperativeness, attempts to leave against medical advice).[84,144a]

♦ *Delirium is a medical emergency.* Managing the psychosis and behavioral agitation is just the beginning; brain failure is in many ways analogous to acute congestive heart failure or acute renal failure. If not expeditiously treated, the underlying causes of delirium can produce permanent impairment. *An aggressive diagnostic investigation aimed at detecting metabolic or intracranial etiologies* is essential. Certain basic therapeutic interventions, such as correcting electrolyte abnormalities, constitute standard practice. Maintain diagnostic vigilance when there is no clear-cut etiology, even though the etiology seems "a little of this, a little of that"; for example, a urinary tract infection with slight hypercalcemia may not be dramatic, but it can devastate the brain functioning of a debilitated patient.

♦ *It is inappropriate to diagnose delirium and limit your involvement to an order for haloperidol.* Delirious patients need ongoing psychiatric follow-up and mental status assessment, as their agitation and cognitive impairment may significantly compromise their medical care.

♦ Because many requests for psychiatric consultation are for agitated patients who are later diagnosed as delirious, it is tempting to think of psychomotor agi-

tation as delirium's hallmark. It is not; the clinical emphasis on agitation is an artifact of who gets referred for consultation. Do not be diverted from a thorough workup because the patient appears placid; many delirious patients appear calm and in no obvious distress.[113] Our approach is to assume that a change in mental status is delirium until proven otherwise.

♦ It may come as a surprise that the most common behavioral marker for delirium in the elderly is *incontinence*, not disruptive behavior or agitation.[60] Delirium in these patients is often quiet, easily missed, and *may be mistaken for dementia.*

Delirium or Dementia?

The differential diagnosis of delirium "versus" dementia is often tricky; elderly patients are at highest risk for both, and algorithms detailing the distinction are fraught with exceptions. Moreover, the syndromes may coexist in the same patient.

♦ In general, the key clinical observation in differentiating delirium from dementia is the *state of consciousness;* the central problem in delirium is fluctuating alertness with distractible attention and clouded sensory awareness, interspersed with periods of lucidity. The demented patient generally has a relatively constant state of arousal. It is not feasible to diagnose dementia in a delirious patient unless there is a history of chronically progressive cognitive change antedating the delirious picture.

♦ Insomnia, nightmares, intermittent nighttime disorientation, and anxiety may be prominent features of both.[172]

Murray[140] has written,

> Attention, obviously, is linked to arousal, but there are different types of attention. A demented person may be sufficiently aroused, but he may be distracted by some persistent thought or sensory input and not attend to the matter at hand. The delirious patient can also be distracted, but it may have a different quality in that the "gain" of his arousal tends to vary, being either turned down or turned up. The delirious patient gives the impression of being oblivious to or, conversely, jumpy in response to environmental stimuli. The delirious person's arousal and correlative attention tends to vary more than that of the de-

mented person, who generally maintains a constant amount of arousal with a constant amount of attention or inattention. (p. 107)

When available, data about onset are helpful: the onset of delirium is typically rapid, developing within a few hours or days, often at night.[109] Dementia is usually gradual and progressive. Complete medical and neurological workup, integrated with clinical assessment and course, assists in making the distinction.

Etiology

The neuropathophysiology of delirium is not well understood, although anticholinergic mechanisms are under investigation.[101] The etiologies for delirium are multiple, ranging from toxic-metabolic causes to medication effects[44b] to structural neurological lesions. Rather than reproduce lists that are readily available in other sources, we will highlight several points on drug-induced delirium from the helpful paper by Slaby and Erle:[172]

◆ Propranolol (Inderal), even in low doses, may precipitate confusion and delirium, especially in the elderly.[63,147,158]

◆ Antibiotics are often overlooked in the etiology of delirium. High-dose intravenous penicillin, chloramphenicol, ofloxacin, norfloxacin, ciprofloxacin, gentamycin, tobramycin, and metronidazole have been associated with neuropsychiatric reactions.[128,173]

◆ Medications that act at H_2-histaminergic receptors (H_2 antagonists) inhibit gastric acid secretion and are used to treat peptic ulcers and reflux esophagitis.[37] They include cimetidine (Tagamet), ranitidine (Zantac), famotidine (Pepcid), and nizatidine (Axid). Cimetidine and ranitidine have been shown to produce neuropsychiatric side effects, including auditory and visual hallucinations, agitation, paranoia, disorientation, delirium, depression, and anxiety.[25,148] These problems are most common in the very young, in the elderly, and in patients with cirrhosis or uremia.[199] They also may interfere with the metabolism of drugs such as benzodiazepines, nifedipine (Procardia), metoprolol (Lopressor), and warfarin (Coumadin).[127,162]

◆ Antihypertensives can precipitate delirium either through direct CNS action (e.g., reserpine [Serpasil], methyldopa [Aldomet])[147] or via electrolyte disturbances.

◆ Nonsteroidal antiinflammatory agents can cause mental status changes. Psychotic reactions have occurred with sulindac (Clinoril), indomethacin (Indocin), tolmetin (Tolectin), and naproxen (Anaprox, Naprosyn).[100,176,179]

◆ Blood levels of theophylline (Theo-Dur), anticonvulsants, and digoxin (Lanoxin) should be regularly checked; these medications have been regularly implicated as offenders.

◆ Remain suspicious of antiarrhythmic agents until proven otherwise; as exhaustively reviewed by Levenson,[106] the majority of them induce neuropsychiatric side effects.

◆ Corticosteroids are notorious inducers of delirium (see Chapter 5).

◆ Psychotropic-induced delirium has occurred with anticholinergic medications, neuroleptic malignant syndrome, lithium toxicity, and the serotonin syndrome.[58] Benzodiazepine administration (e.g., of triazolam [Halcion]) and withdrawal (e.g., of alprazolam [Xanax]) may produce confusion and delirium, especially in elderly and brain-injured patients. Take care to fully evaluate psychotropic drug interactions in delirious patients.

◆ Just about every drug used to treat acquired immunodeficiency syndrome (AIDS) has been reported to produce neuropsychiatric side effects (see Chapter 6).

Finally, be aware of misleading stereotypes regarding narcotic-using patients. Most psychiatrists think of these medications in the context of the substance-abusing population, but the demographics of patients at risk for narcotic side effects are different in the general hospital. It is easy to overlook the role of narcotic analgesics since the typical medical patient often does not fit the "profile" of the substance abuser. Narcotic analgesic intoxication and withdrawal are widely documented to cause neuropsychiatric side effects, including those resembling delirium.[32,65,151]

Hypoxia

It is the *rate at which hypoxia develops* that determines the acute neuropsychiatric consequences of hypoxemia, not the absolute level of oxygen saturation.[14,74,92,109] As always, elderly patients are particularly vulnerable. In the setting of chronic hypoxia, for example, oxygen saturations as low as 60 mm Hg may produce few mental status changes, whereas abrupt declines from higher baselines usually result in delirium.[14,109] Similarly, acute increases of P_{CO_2} to 70 mm Hg will produce confusional states, whereas patients with chronic hypercapnia may have preserved alertness at levels as high as 90 mm Hg.[50]

- Hypercapnia produces a metabolic acidosis, and there is a correlation between the severity of the neuropsychiatric symptoms and the concomitant CSF acidosis.[150]
- Carbon dioxide retention produces anesthetic-like changes that resemble barbiturate intoxication,[92] not amphetamine psychosis.

Over half of even *mildly* hypoxemic patients show chronic impairments in concentration and recall, as well as difficulties in abstract reasoning, complex perceptual motor integration, and language function.[55,69,70,154] These deficits are often subtle. Neuropsychological evaluation may assist in making the diagnosis.

"ICU Psychosis"

The expression "ICU psychosis" implies that the environmental features of critical care settings can induce psychosis. Cassem and Hackett[43] have advised avoiding the term because it acts as a wastebasket distracter, invoked when the etiology of delirium is unknown. Attributing mental status changes to an environmental etiology may result in prematurely terminating a thorough differential diagnosis.[43] Of all causes of altered mental status in intensive care settings, *medications* are the most common offenders.[43]

Bedside Assessment of Delirium

Mini-Mental State Examination

The MMSE[59] is a quick bedside assessment instrument that can be administered repeatedly to track fluctuations in cognitive status. It taps orientation, registration, memory, attention, calculation, recall, visuospatial function, and language. A score of 20 or less out of 30 occurs with significant cognitive difficulties, such as dementia or delirium.[59] The scores identify changes in cognitive state over time, showing little practice effect. The MMSE does not assess mood or affect,[85] and may overlook thought disorder.[85] (Refer to Appendix B–1 for a copy of the MMSE.)

As recently reviewed by Nadler et al.,[141] the MMSE may produce both false-negative and false-positive results.[85,205,207] It may fail to detect subtle cognitive difficulties, especially in patients with mild diffuse cognitive dysfunction.[143,168] On the other hand, the MMSE may overestimate the deficits of patients who are neither demented nor delirious, but who have stable focal deficits such as aphasia, dyslexia, or dyscalculia. The MMSE should be interpreted as one component of the cognitive assessment rather than in isolation.

Trail Making Tests

The *Trail Making Tests* (Parts A and B)[157a] are more sensitive to detecting diffuse cognitive dysfunction. They tap attention, the ability to rapidly switch mental sets, and visuospatial ability. In Part A, the patient is asked to connect numbered circles in sequence by drawing a line as quickly as possible from one numbered circle to the next. In Part B, the circles contain either a number or a letter, and the patient is asked to draw a line in sequence from 1 to A, from A to 2, from 2 to B, from B to 3, and so forth. Both are timed tests, and age-corrected norms are available. Mildly confused patients may be able to perform Part A, but will have significant difficulty with Part B. See Appendix B–2 for norms.

Other Tests

Every clinician has his or her own array of bedside tests. It is useful to have strategies to supplement the MMSE or the Trail Making Tests. Some of the more easily administered tests in the critical care setting recommended by Wise and Cassem[205] include the following:

- **Constructional ability:** The degree of difficulty in drawing a clock face correlates with cognitive dysfunction and electroencephalogram (EEG) slowing. (It is not a specific test for right-hemispheric parietal dysfunction.)
- **Reitan–Indiana Aphasia Screening Test:**[76b] A very shortened version of a more extensive screening test consists of four tasks:
  1. Copy a square, Greek cross, and triangle *without lifting the pencil from the paper.*
  2. Name each copied figure.
  3. Spell each name.
  4. Repeat "He shouted the warning"; then explain and write it.

  This test may aid in discriminating between left- and right-hemisphere lesions; patients with the former can copy the designs but cannot write, whereas the patients with the latter can write but often cannot reproduce the designs.[108a]
- **Marie Three Paper Test:** The patient is given three different-sized pieces of paper and asked to take the biggest one and hand it to the examiner, take the smallest and throw it to the ground, and take the middle-sized one and place it in the patient's pocket.
- **Isaacs Set Test:**[89] A test of category-specific naming (cued naming, controlled word association) that assesses verbal fluency and screens for cognitive dysfunction. The patient is asked to name 10 items from

each of four categories: fruits, animals, colors, and towns. Scores below 15 out of a maximum of 40 indicate significant cognitive impairment. Patients with delirium or dementia often perseverate in this test.

◆ **Left-right tasks:** These not only assess left-right confusion but also tax the patient's ability to understand and manipulate information (e.g., "place your right hand on your left elbow; place your left hand on your right ear; place your right hand on your right elbow"). The unimpaired patient will realize that the last request is impossible, whereas confused patients will either attempt it or perseveratively repeat the first two tasks.[205]

◆ A new rapid bedside test of cognition has recently been developed.[93] Although targeted for patients with human immunodeficiency virus (HIV) infection who experience slowed mentation, poor concentration, and impaired psychomotor speed, the test may identify delirious patients as well. The test requires timed performance of a sequencing and category-switching task. Patients are asked to count to 20, to say the alphabet, and then to alternate between the numbers and letters: 1-A, 2-B, 3-C, and so forth. The number of correct alternation pairs produced in 30 seconds defines the score, with the maximum score being 52. The test takes less than 1 minute to conduct and correlates with deficits on the MMSE and the Trail Making B. A cutoff score of 15 correlates with an abnormal MMSE.

Impairment of writing (dysgraphia) is one of the most sensitive indicators of delirium.[1,198] For example, in 33 of 34 acutely confused patients, dysgraphia was manifested by clumsily drawn letters, reduplication of strokes (in letters like M and W), inability to align letters properly, problems with upward-downward letter orientation, and misspellings.[44] Clearing of the delirium was associated with resolution of the dysgraphia.

In the **Wisconsin Card Sorting Test,**[76a] the patient is asked to sort cards according to features such as shape, color, or number. The patient must empirically deduce the strategy used by the examiner, which periodically shifts during the test, requiring the patient to readjust his or her own sorting strategy. It is not a bedside test of cognitive dysfunction, but is used in assessing patients with frontal lobe damage.

Several authors[172a,192,193a] have recently reviewed various types of assessment instruments for delirium in greater detail, including nursing screening scales, symptom checklists, an analog scale, and interview schedule, and symptom rating scales.

Management of Delirium

Correcting the underlying pathophysiological problems is paramount in managing delirium. According to Tavani,[184] the goals of pharmacotherapy in the acutely agitated, medically ill patient are 1) to calm the patient sufficiently to aid in assessment; 2) to control behavior in order to facilitate the patient's medical treatment (e.g., prevent pulling out lines and tubes); 3) to minimize the effects of agitation and physical restraint on the cardiovascular, pulmonary, and other systems; and 4) to prevent self-harm or inadvertent harm to caretakers. It is important not to oversedate the patient, as this interferes with proper neuropsychiatric assessment and eventual rehabilitation.

Nonpharmacological Interventions

In their helpful review, Goldstein and Haltzman[66 (p. 249)] have detailed several nonpharmacological strategies for managing delirium in the intensive care setting:

◆ *Enhance cognitive function:* Reorient frequently; have clock, calendar, radio, and television in room; provide explanations and education

◆ *Enhance communication with family and staff:* Encourage writing if speaking is not possible; use letterboard, hand, or blink signals if patient is unable to write

◆ *Prevent self-harm and harm to staff:* Use mittens and restraints, employing the fewest restraints possible

◆ *Minimize environmental stresses:* Provide sensory stimulation but limit noise from alarms and equipment; maintain semblance of day-night cycle; transfer to general medical floor as soon as feasible; perform nonessential care during the day (to reduce nighttime disruptions)

◆ *Maximize patient's comfort:* Control pain adequately; try to mobilize from bed to chair; permit rest and limit unnecessary awakenings; invite family members to stay with patient to reduce suspiciousness and paranoia

◆ *Provide reassurance and support:* Show empathy; provide opportunities to ventilate

Haloperidol in Delirium

When agitation is accompanied by psychotic ideation, neuroleptics are the treatment of choice. (Note that neuroleptics were also found to be effective in reducing Delirium Rating Scale[193] scores in hypoactive delirium.[149]) High-potency neuroleptics (e.g., haloperidol [Haldol], thiothixene [Navane], fluphenazine [Prolixin]) have the fewest anticholinergic and orthostatic side effects. *The goal of treatment is to achieve complete calming of an agitated patient at the outset, not partial control or barely keeping up with agitation over several days.*[43] Haloperidol is the most commonly used high-potency neuroleptic agent in the medically ill. It has minimal effects on blood pressure, pulmonary artery wedge pressure, heart rate, and respiration.[15,41,107,175] The mechanism by which haloperidol ameliorates delirium is not clear; clinical improvement may be due to its sedative effects or antipsychotic properties, or to both.

Intramuscular haloperidol is used in most general consultation-liaison settings with good results,[109] but intravenous haloperidol is increasingly used in the intensive care setting. Many clinicians are not comfortable using iv haloperidol, since it has not been approved by the U.S. Food and Drug Administration (FDA). In some hospitals, physicians must administer it themselves, making it a potentially cumbersome treatment. However, many critical care experts discourage intramuscular injections,[43,184] citing erratic absorption, unnecessary discomfort, and elevation of muscle enzymes (creatine phosphokinase [CPK]). Moreover, in the oncology setting, thrombocytopenia and the risk of infection at injection sites often limits the number of intramuscular injections that can be safely given. The reader should at least be familiar with the data on intravenous haloperidol, and come to his or her own conclusions about its usefulness in practice.

There are several advantages of intravenous haloperidol over the intramuscular form:

◆ Quicker onset of action
◆ Fewer EPS[4,5,43,133,134]
◆ Shorter mean half-life (14 hours) compared with the intramuscular (21 hours) or oral (24 hours) forms

As with the intramuscular and oral forms of haloperidol, there is little, if any, effect on cardiovascular or pulmonary parameters except to normalize blood pressure when agitation has elevated it.[171] Hypotensive episodes are rare[43] and are almost invariably caused by hypovolemia.

Intramuscular and iv haloperidol are safe in treating patients with delirium on intraaortic balloon pump therapy, chronic obstructive pulmonary disease (COPD), head trauma, HIV infection, and epilepsy.[43,53,165] To date, haloperidol is contraindicated only in the setting of coma.

◆ Intravenous haloperidol may be used in patients receiving epinephrine drips, but a pressor other than epinephrine (e.g., norepinephrine) should be used after very large doses to avoid unopposed beta-adrenergic activity.[43]

◆ Cassem and Hackett[43] advocate obtaining permission to use intravenous haloperidol through a hospital's human studies committee, indicating that it is the drug of choice for the patient's welfare, is the safest drug, and is justifiable as innovative therapy.

Of concern, however, are a series of reports of torsade de pointes (polymorphic ventricular tachycardia that frequently degenerates into ventricular fibrillation) associated with iv haloperidol.[52,77,99,135,142,203,208] **Prolonged QT intervals** predispose to developing this arrhythmia. Two recent accounts described torsade de pointes with intravenous haloperidol:

◆ Wilt and colleagues[203] reported 4 cases of dysrhythmia on iv haloperidol and lorazepam (out of approximately 1,100 patients). All were in women, with the following diagnoses: two patients (ages 19 and 63) had status asthmaticus and prolonged baseline QTc intervals; one patient (age 74) had intermittent atrial fibrillation, hypothyroidism, and renal insufficiency, and developed congestive heart failure after respiratory arrest before being given haloperidol; and one patient (age 39) developed acute congestive heart failure as a complication of bacterial meningitis and was sedated with haloperidol. (Concurrently administered medications included a variety of antibiotics, steroids, bronchodilators, furosemide, digoxin, and nitroglycerin.) Doses ranged from 10 mg/4 hours to 580 mg/4 days. All patients had normal electrolytes, including calcium, magnesium, and potassium. *Progressive QT-interval widening was noted after haloperidol administration, and resolved after removal of the drug in 3 of the patients.*

◆ Metzger and Friedman[135] described three patients who developed torsade de pointes arrhythmia or QT lengthening with iv haloperidol (doses ranging from 115 to 825 mg). One patient (age 39) had preexisting dilated cardiomyopathy and right bundle branch block, and had suffered cardiac arrest prior to receiving haloperidol for agitated delirium. Another had COPD, alcohol abuse, a seizure disorder, and evidence of an older anterior myocardial infarction. The third had a history of multiple fractures, alcoholism, and cardiomyopathy.

These cases suggest that large doses of haloperidol require cardiac monitoring in seriously ill patients; risk factors for adverse side effects appear to be the following:

- Preexisting cardiac disease
- Prolonged baseline QT interval
- A history of alcohol abuse

Appendix C is a general guide to treating delirium using haloperidol and lorazepam, adapted from the cumulative recommendations and protocols of several authors.

Haloperidol With Lorazepam

Although controlled studies are lacking, many experts advise that combining haloperidol and lorazepam (Ativan) is synergistic and has *advantages over single-agent therapy* in managing agitation secondary to psychosis or delirium,[3,5,48,163,164] even in the elderly.[5] Lorazepam has no major active metabolites, possesses sedative properties, and has a wide therapeutic index that makes it safe. It is primarily eliminated through conjugation with glucuronic acid and does not rely on hepatic cytochrome P450 enzyme oxidation. Use the following ratio:

- **5 mg** po haloperidol to **1 mg** lorazepam[84]

The required dosage of each medication is *lower* in combination than when either is administered alone. No adverse cardiac or respiratory reactions have been reported. Fewer extrapyramidal side effects occur with this combination than when haloperidol is used alone.[134] See Appendix C for additional notes on administering lorazepam.

Benzodiazepines

It used to be taught that benzodiazepines were to be avoided in the setting of pulmonary disease or delirium. The slow, progressive accumulation of active metabolites occurring with long-acting agents like diazepam (Valium) or chlordiazepoxide (Librium) produced toxic effects in delirious patients, especially the elderly. The advent of the intermediate-duration benzodiazepines free of active metabolites, such as lorazepam (Ativan; po, im, or iv), oxazepam (Serax; po), and temazepam (Restoril; po), has changed this recommendation. These medications may be used for daytime sedation at dosages similar to or lower than those used for sleep.[113] The goal is to calm the restless or agitated patient while avoiding obtundation. If the patient requires repeated dosing, a small **standing dose** three to four times daily is more effective[43] than "as needed" dosing and may minimize the total amount of drug administered over a 24-hour period.[181]

Midazolam (Versed) is a benzodiazepine administered intravenously for sedation prior to medical procedures and as an adjunct to anesthesia.[130] It has several advantages for treating delirium in the ICU, such as rapid onset and short half-life (1–4 hours).[66] There are also several case reports demonstrating midazolam's efficacy for treating aggressivity, violence, and hyperarousal.[28,132] Shapiro and colleagues[170] recommend midazolam infusions of 0.1–2.0 μg/kg/minute for treatment of ICU agitation. Drawbacks, however, include the potential for respiratory depression, apnea, hypotension, and prolonged half-life in the setting of liver dysfunction and systemic illness. Goldstein and Haltzman[66] stress that the risk of iatrogenic overdose and toxicity is potentially greater with midazolam than with lorazepam. These limitations render lorazepam preferable to midazolam in managing delirium in the ICU, especially in nonintubated patients.

Although clonazepam (Klonopin) and triazolam (Halcion) also have no active metabolites, they are not currently used as first-line medications for delirium. (Low-dose triazolam [0.125–0.25 mg] is, however, gaining acceptance as a safe postoperative hypnotic when delirium is not present.[91])

Other Agents

Droperidol. Droperidol (Inapsine), a butyrophenone used as an adjunct to anesthesia, is already approved for intravenous administration by the FDA. It is not as commonly used as haloperidol for delirium,[60a] but some authors feel it is superior to haloperidol for delirious, agitated patients.[113] Compared with haloperidol, droperidol has a more rapid onset of action (within 5 minutes), a shorter duration of action (2–4 hours), and a lower incidence of EPS. Sedation is its main side effect. Dose ranges for acutely agitated patients are between 5 and 20 mg im (administered in unit doses of between 4 and 10 mg at separate injection sites) or iv (administered slowly when amounts > 10 mg are needed).[113] The medication may be repeated after 30 minutes if response to the first injection is inadequate.[83,159] Note that droperidol is a far more potent alpha-adrenergic antagonist than haloperidol, and is more likely to produce hypotension, particularly when it is combined with other agents.[43] However, more frequent adverse side effects have not been consistently confirmed.[187]

Paralytic agents. Some centers use paralytic agents to control agitation when other measures have failed and the agitation threatens critical procedures such as intraaortic balloon counterpulsation. Such medications include pancuronium bromide, metocurine, and *d*-tubocurarine.[160,186] These paralytic agents may have adverse psychological effects if patients are not adequately sedated with other medications. Medical complications include muscle atrophy, neuropathy, myopathic changes, and difficulty with ventilator weaning.[16] Goldstein and Haltzman[66] advise using paralytic agents *only* when all other measures to treat agitation and delirium have failed. They should be discontinued as quickly as possible.

Miscellaneous agents. Other medications that are currently being explored to manage ICU delirium and agitation include

- Flumazenil (Mazicon)[75,97]
- Etomidate (Amidate)[8]
- Propofol (Diprivan)[8,129,174]
- Isoflurane (Forane)[98]

Effects of Neuroleptics on Respiration

In general, neuroleptics are safe in moderate doses, usually with little effect on respiration.[18] However, neuroleptic-induced oversedation can worsen respiratory dysfunction in vulnerable patients, despite improvements in mental status.[81,206] The less-sedating antipsychotics, such as haloperidol, thiothixene (Navane), and fluphenazine (Prolixin),[49] are preferable but may cause bronchoconstriction.[180] *The most serious side effect of neuroleptics on respiratory function occurs when respiratory motility is impaired by dystonic effects on pharyngeal and laryngeal muscles.*[100a] Pure tardive respiratory dyskinesia is rare but may result from the long-term use of neuroleptics.[51,120,152,206] This syndrome can induce respiratory depression that significantly affects pulmonary function tests[200] and predisposes to aspiration. Laryngeal dystonia is an extremely rare form of acute dystonic reaction that presents as acute dyspnea. Like other dystonic reactions, it occurs within 24–48 hours after therapy is initiated or when dosage is increased.[189] It responds dramatically to intramuscular antihistaminic or antiparkinsonian agents. Monitoring the gag reflex during neuroleptic treatment may detect the development of laryngeal dystonia.[206]

Finally, neuroleptics with more pronounced anticholinergic and sedating effects, such as thioridazine (Mellaril) and chlorpromazine (Thorazine), can have untoward anticholinergic effects that are additive with atropine or other anticholinergic agents, and may potentiate the action of antihistamines.[188] They should be avoided.

Insomnia and Sundowning

Delirium usually is accompanied by disruptions in the sleep-wake cycle, often causing "sundowning"—the pa-

tient who was lethargic and sleeping by day becomes alert, agitated, and restless at night, often with no memory for the event.[26,84] *Normalizing sleep-wake cycle disturbances should be given high therapeutic priority.* Limiting noise if possible, maintaining some semblance of a day-night cycle (e.g., dim lights at night), providing all routine care during the day, and scheduling oral medications to minimize nighttime awakenings are useful nonpharmacological strategies.[66]

- Rapid eye movement (REM) suppression would be an undesirable side effect when treating insomnia secondary to delirium. Barbiturates cause both REM suppression and respiratory depression, and so should be avoided in delirium. These side effects can be minimized with judicious use of the shorter-acting benzodiazepines.[113]
- Liston[113] recommends chloral hydrate as an effective hypnotic in doses of 1–2 grams for middle or terminal insomnia, with a half-life of 4–12 hours, although it does depress REM.
- *Medications with **anticholinergic** properties, such as antihistamines (e.g., diphenhydramine [Benadryl]) and phenothiazines (e.g., chlorpromazine [Thorazine], perphenazine [Trilafon]), should be avoided*[115,185,194,195] in order to preserve cholinergic[101] functioning, which mediates attention, cognition, and memory.[84] Phenothiazines also lower the seizure threshold and may produce temperature dysregulation.[18,39,73]

Lorazepam (Ativan) in doses of 2–4 mg im at bedtime is effective for managing middle or terminal insomnia secondary to delirium.[113] Long-acting benzodiazepines with active metabolites (e.g., diazepam [Valium]) and highly anticholinergic medications (e.g., perphenazine [Trilafon], diphenhydramine [Benadryl])[185] should be avoided in the setting of delirium. Trazodone (Desyrel) in doses of 25–100 mg has also been effective.[66] Appendix D summarizes some of the recommendations for treating the insomnia and restlessness of delirium.

Ventilator Weaning

Anxiety interferes with ventilator weaning in a variety of ways. It can transiently increase metabolic demands and cardiac work, making further weaning impossible. It can induce fear and panic so that the patient becomes unable to comply with medical requests. The ventilator experience also can be psychologically traumatic, especially because of the inability to communicate.

Failure to wean may be due to hypoxia or hypercapnia, which may have recurred undetected. When anxiety interferes, administering low-dose lorazepam prior to weaning trials can be quite helpful,[43] but carefully monitor for respiratory depression if doses exceed 0.5–1.0 mg. Cassem and Hackett[43] use intravenous haloperidol when anxiety approaches near-panic. Psychostimulants may also be indirectly helpful for weaning apathetic or depressed patients.[92a,119]

Patients with respiratory problems are typically made anxious by the very thought or suggestion that they "breathe easily." Behavioral exercises for relaxation may paradoxically induce more anxiety if the technique—which classically encourages the subject to take slow, deep breaths—is not modified. Biofeedback has been used successfully to promote weaning.[1a,80] Hypnosis may also assist in the weaning process, but the instruction to breathe easily should be omitted from the hypnotic suggestion; instead, patients should be encouraged to concentrate either on a tranquil scene or on a single concept.[30,116]

Ventilator weaning has been discussed in more detail by several authors.[22,61,64,66,100b,131,145] We found the discussion by Goldstein and Haltzman[66] to be the most helpful.

✦ SPECIAL CONSIDERATIONS IN LUNG CANCER

Differential Diagnosis: Dyspnea, Anxiety, and Restlessness

Chronic dyspnea is agonizing. Panic about breathing and suffocating make the dyspnea worse. It would be premature, however, to start Mr. Davis on an anxiolytic at the onset of his symptoms.

The most appropriate interventions initially would be to consult with the oncologist about disease progression, to review medications for potential side effects, and to consider how psychodynamics and physiology are interacting.

Adverse Neuropsychiatric Effects of Antiemetics

Dopamine antagonist medications are widely used as antiemetics in the medical setting (e.g., prochlorperazine [Compazine], droperidol [Inapsine], promethazine [Phenergan]). *Early side effects are restlessness, pacing, and agitation—symptoms whose medication-induced etiology is often missed.*[18,54,56,103] Metoclopramide (Reglan) is a procainamide derivative and CNS dopamine antagonist that is highly effective in controlling chemotherapy-related emesis.[9] EPS such as akathisia often occur with high doses

of this agent.[167] When used chronically, such as in the treatment of diabetic gastroparesis and gastric atony, metoclopramide has also been associated with tardive dyskinesia.[62]

Mr. Davis's motor restlessness is most likely akathisia secondary to metoclopramide. Discontinuing the medication should improve this symptom, although it should be remembered that motor restlessness may also be a feature of impending delirium.

◆ Serotonin is thought to play an important role in chemotherapy-induced emesis. Ondansetron (Zofran) is a relatively new antiemetic with selective serotonin antagonist properties.[7,96] It has few adverse effects and appears to be well tolerated. There is, however, at least one case report each of dysphoria[144b] and a secondary anxiety disorder,[137] with symptoms of panic following the administration of ondansetron. Further research is needed to determine this agent's impact on mental status.

Intracranial Metastases

Intracranial metastases can involve the skull, the brain itself, and the craniospinal meninges (meningeal carcinomatosis). Cancer cells reach the brain by hematogenous spread. The most common primary cancer sites that metastasize to the brain (and that therefore are of special interest in mental status changes) are (in descending order of frequency) as follows:[6]

◆ Lung
◆ Breast
◆ Melanoma

(Colon, rectum, and kidney are the next most common primary sites; prostate cancer rarely metastasizes to the brain.[6]) The usual clinical picture consists of headache, focal weakness, *mental and behavioral abnormalities*, seizures, ataxia, aphasia, and signs of increased intracranial pressure.[6]

Mr. Davis's current presentation could be consistent with metastatic spread to the brain, which can present atypically as depressed mood, trembling, confusion, and forgetfulness *in the absence of other demonstrable neurological symptoms*.[6] Unfortunately, brain metastases are common in patients with lung cancer, occurring in at least 30%–40%.[78] When metastases to the brain present as headache and vomiting only, differential diagnosis becomes difficult and symptoms may be misattributed to a primary psychiatric etiology.[6]

For example, a 54-year-old man with a questionable history of nonspecific psychiatric illness presented with confusion, insomnia, and nausea over the course of 1 week.[190] On the day of admission, he could not recognize familiar faces. Negative computed tomography (CT) scan of the head, blood chemistries, toxicology screen, and neurological exam led the neurology consultant to erroneously conclude that the patient's presentation was probably due to "psychogenic" factors. The mental status examination, however, was consistent with delirium, showing reduced consciousness and severe cognitive difficulties. Further workup was pursued, with EEG revealing bitemporal abnormality with intermittent runs of rhythmic delta activity over the anterior temporal regions. Lumbar puncture confirmed the diagnosis of meningeal carcinomatosis.

The authors of this report[190] noted that the confounding variable in the initial evaluation was the prior history of psychiatric illness, which led the consultant to seize on a psychiatric explanation for "absent" neurological findings. Blustein and Seeman[27] have pointed out that psychogenic explanations may be sought, particularly in the absence of focal neurological signs, especially if the premorbid personality was regarded as "unstable" or "maladjusted."

Meningeal carcinomatosis is definitively documented on lumbar puncture. It usually presents with radiculopathies (particularly involving cauda equina), cranial nerve palsies, and dementia,[6] unlike bacterial meningitis, which presents with fever, stiff neck, and headache.

Paraneoplastic Syndromes

Even if there is no demonstrable evidence of metabolic or metastatic neurological disease or medication side effects, beware of prematurely rejecting the contribution of an oncological illness to the psychiatric picture. Nonendocrine, nonmetastatic neuropsychiatric syndromes occur as rare, remote effects of carcinoma. *They occur in the absence of metastatic spread or recurrence and can operate even after successful resection of the tumor.*[110] Lung cancer (particularly small [oat]–cell or undifferentiated bronchial carcinoma) can induce pathological changes in the brain even without CNS metastases (i.e., in the limbic gray matter). This type of paraneoplastic syndrome has been termed *limbic encephalitis* (also known as *paraneoplastic encephalopathy;* in DSM-IV nosology it would be classified as a psychiatric condition—e.g., delirium, psychosis, de-

mentia—"due to a general medical disorder.") Tumors of the ovary, breast, stomach, kidney, and colon have also been associated with limbic encephalitis.[146]

Patients present in a variety of ways: with dementia-like alterations of recent memory and other intellectual functions;[11,31,46,95,196] with severe anxiety or depression;[92] and/or with psychosis.[46,110,144] Amnesia may be the sole neuropsychological abnormality in some patients.[92] Catatonia has also been reported as the presenting symptom.[183] *Routine diagnostic tests, including CT scan and EEG, may be initially* **normal,**[45,47,94] *prompting the oft-heard, dreaded conclusion that the patient is "medically cleared" and should be transferred to psychiatry.* The following case example illustrates a situation in which a diagnosis of paraneoplastic syndrome should be considered:

We suspected a paraneoplastic syndrome in a 74-year-old woman with no prior psychiatric or medical history who had been admitted to the hospital septic from a urinary tract infection. As the infection resolved, the patient became less sedated and more blatantly psychotic. She had the delusion that there was a plot to kill her. Psychiatric consultation was requested several days later, after sepsis had resolved. The patient was thought by the medical staff to be suffering from "psychotic depression" and was medically cleared for transfer to psychiatry. Chest X ray, however, was notable for a midline mass. Bronchoscopy had been recommended but the patient had refused. Since she was afebrile, the house staff had decided to defer further workup until her "psychotic depression" cleared on antidepressants. MRI of the head and EEG were normal. Blood gases and blood work, including thyroid function tests and all serum electrolytes, were normal. Lumbar puncture was normal. The patient's family had noted personality changes over the previous 2 months, and reported that at times the patient had been paranoid and delusional during that period. She took no medications and had no substance abuse history. Family history was negative for psychiatric illness. There was no evidence of depressive content on mental status exam, but she was paranoid and delusional. There were no hallucinations. The patient performed within normal limits on the MMSE but could not do the Trail Making Test, Part B. She showed difficulty concentrating, a symptom that had been attributed to "pseudodementia." The diagnosis was made of psychotic disorder with delusions, probably due to a medical condition (DSM-III-R: *organic delusional syndrome*). Repeat lumbar puncture was normal. Repeat MRI of the head was negative, but a second EEG 1 week later showed diffuse slowing. The patient was medicated with haloperidol and consent was obtained for bronchoscopy. Biopsy results showed small-cell carcinoma.

Although not neuropathologically proven, the diagnosis of a paraneoplastic encephalopathy was suspected in this patient on the basis of mild encephalopathic signs (abnormal EEG, problems in sustained attention) with prominent delusions and no other etiology apparent in the extensive workup.

Paraneoplastic mental status phenomena should be considered in an oncological patient who presents with psychosis, personality changes, or cognitive deficits. *A preexisting psychiatric history may divert attention away from the diagnosis, especially when there are no focal neurological symptoms and imaging tests appear normal.* A paraneoplastic etiology is more apparent when a seizure disorder heralds or accompanies the psychiatric syndrome.[35,45,46,118,169]

Delirium in the Setting of Cancer

Delirium due to multiple etiologies is one of the most common psychiatric disorders among cancer patients, second only to depressive syndromes.[121] Its prevalence in cancer patients has been estimated at 15%.[57] Delirium is particularly common in terminally ill cancer patients, with an incidence of 50%–85% reported in two small studies.[36,122] The most common cause of delirium in cancer patients is probably metabolic derangement ("metabolic encephalopathy"),[109] with respiratory failure and hypercalcemia the major offenders. Delirium may be the initial presenting feature of cancer, occurring sometimes in the absence of cerebral metastases.[86] Interestingly, in a group of 100 cancer patients referred for psychiatric consultation, 40% had an "organic mental syndrome" but less than one-fifth had documentable evidence of cerebral metastases.[108] Forty percent of encephalopathic cancer patients referred for neurological consultation were found to suffer from metabolic disorders, most notably hepatic or uremic encephalopathy and hypercalcemia.[150] In addition, the narcotic analgesics used for cancer pain may exacerbate delirium.[32,104]

Factors in Oncological Treatment

Karnofsky Scale

You may hear oncologists and staff discuss "the patient's Karnofsky." The Karnofsky Scale assesses performance status or functional ability of cancer patients. It is an important independent predictor of prognosis and survival in lung cancer patients.[178] Briefly, criteria are as follows:[126]

- **Score of 80–100:** Able to carry on normal activity; no special care needed
- **Score of 50–70:** Unable to work; able to live at home and care for most personal needs; a varying amount of assistance is needed
- **Score of 0–40:** Unable to care for self; requires equivalent of institutional or hospital care; disease may be progressing rapidly

Benzodiazepines for Chemotherapy Patients

Benzodiazepines affect both short- and long-term memory,[19] but their most profound effects are on the consolidation processes whereby information is transferred from short- to long-term memory.[13] Interestingly, the amnestic side effects of benzodiazepines are uniquely useful for chemotherapy patients; they prevent the development of the conditioned response of anticipatory nausea and vomiting (e.g., nausea experienced when approaching the hospital for a medical appointment) by mitigating anxiety and producing an anterograde amnesia for the unpleasant experiences of chemotherapy.[103] This effect eliminates recall of adverse treatment-related experiences, such as vomiting, thus avoiding the conditioned response[29] of anticipatory nausea. Behavioral interventions, especially relaxation techniques (hypnosis, progressive muscle relaxation, systematic desensitization), also have been effectively used to control anxiety[17] and chemotherapy-related nausea.[12,67,157] Lorazepam (Ativan) is the most widely used anxiolytic in this setting, although alprazolam (Xanax)[156] and midazolam (Versed)[153] are also being studied.

Doxorubicin

Take care when prescribing psychotropics to patients who have received doxorubicin (Adriamycin). It is highly cardiotoxic and may potentiate the cardiotoxicity of TCAs and, anecdotally, lithium.[114]

Parenteral and Rectal Antidepressants

Depressed patients who are unable to take oral medications are frequently encountered on a consultation-liaison service. Alternative routes of administration that have been found to be effective include the following:

- Amitriptyline (Elavil) suppositories (50 mg in cocoa butter twice daily)[2]

- Doxepin (Sinequan) capsules per rectum (two 25-mg capsules at a time inserted directly without use of a suppository base; good blood levels resulted)[182]
- Intramuscular amitriptyline, doxepin, or imipramine (Tofranil)[123,125]
- Pemoline (Cylert) (the tablets can be dissolved in the mouth and absorbed through the oral mucosa, bypassing the gastrointestinal tract)[34,125]
- Dextroamphetamine (Dexedrine) suppositories[82]
- Intravenous amitriptyline (not approved for use in the United States, but shown effective and safe in European studies)[40,138]

(See also the cases of Mr. Doe [Chapter 1] and Mr. Lowe [Chapter 6] for discussion of the use of psychostimulants in the medically ill, and the recent paper by Burns and Eisendrath[38] on the use of these agents in terminally ill patients.) We have encountered no reports of using fluoxetine (Prozac) suppositories.

Santos et al.[166] have recently summarized additional details on the parenteral use of psychotropic agents.

Lithium

Lithium can be used in cancer patients, but should be withheld 1–2 days before chemotherapy because of the risk of dehydration and electrolyte imbalance.[72] Patients receiving cranial radiation for brain metastases are at risk for seizures and delirium; both conditions would complicate questions of lithium toxicity, which also lowers the seizure threshold.

❧ SUMMARY

1. A patient's perception of his or her illness is colored by levels of defense and previous life experience. Never presume the meanings of an illness for a particular patient. There will certainly be common themes among patients with the same illness, but with often unexpected, unpredicted meanings that are as individual as fingerprints. Often there is an unconscious overlap between preexisting psychological conflicts and reactions to the current medical events.

2. Akathisia is a side effect of many nonpsychiatric drugs, such as prochlorperazine (Compazine), droperidol (Inapsine), promethazine (Phenergan), and metoclopramide (Reglan).

3. Consider the possibility of brain metastases for mental status changes in cancer patients. The most common primary cancer sites that metastasize to the brain are (in descending order) lung > breast > melanoma. Behavioral and psychiatric abnormalities may be the harbingers of metastatic disease in the absence of other systemic signs.

4. Delirium is second only to depression in frequency of occurrence in psychiatrically symptomatic cancer patients, and is usually caused by metabolic factors. It should be suspected in cancer patients presenting with new psychiatric symptoms. Limbic encephalitis is a rare, fascinating variant of delirium. This paraneoplastic syndrome produces mental status changes in the absence of metastatic spread or cancer recurrence, and can occur even after successful resection of the tumor. Routine diagnostic tests, including computed tomography (CT) or magnetic resonance imaging (MRI) scans and electroencephalogram (EEG), may be initially normal. Limbic encephalitis is a diagnosis of exclusion, occurring most often in lung cancer.

5. "Hit and run" consultation is fraught with potential mistakes; delirium is most accurately diagnosed and managed based on longitudinal observations over time. Fluctuating consciousness is its hallmark. Delirium is often subtle in its symptoms and surreptitious in onset; you will be fooled if you seek only blatant cognitive deficits or agitation. It presents most often as anxiety, depression, psychosis, or inappropriate behavior, less often as obvious cognitive problems. The etiologies for delirium are multiple, ranging from toxic-metabolic causes to medication effects to structural neurological lesions. The underlying cause for delirium should be aggressively pursued; avoid attributing mental status changes to the environment—"ICU psychosis" is not a useful diagnostic category because it tends to abort differential diagnosis.

6. The goal of psychiatric management is to completely calm the agitated patient. Haloperidol (Haldol), in combination with lorazepam (Ativan), is the current preferred treatment for agitation. There are various algorithms for dosing, but most recommend neuroleptization on day 1 of delirium, liberally titrating to agitation, and then sequentially reducing the antipsychotic over the following few days as delirium resolves (see Appendix C, "Guide to Treating Delirium With Haloperidol and Lorazepam").

7. Some centers rely on intravenous haloperidol, citing its quicker onset of action, fewer extrapyramidal side effects (EPS), and shorter mean half-life over intramuscular forms. Others prefer more traditional ad-

ministration routes. Although haloperidol has minimal cardiac effects, prolonged QT intervals predispose to malignant arrhythmias when haloperidol is given intravenously. The most serious side effect of neuroleptics on respiratory function is laryngeal dystonia.

8. Delirium is usually accompanied by disruptions in the sleep-wake cycle, often causing the *sundowning* phenomenon. Normalizing sleep-wake cycle disturbances should be given high therapeutic priority (see Appendix D, "Managing Insomnia and Restlessness in Delirium").

REFERENCES

1. Aakerlund L, Rosenberg J: Writing disturbances: an indicator for postoperative delirium. Int J Psychiatry Med 24:245–257, 1994

1a. Acosta F: Biofeedback and progressive relaxation in weaning the anxious patient from the ventilator: a brief report. Heart Lung 17:299–301, 1988

2. Adams S: Amitriptyline suppositories (letter). N Engl J Med 306:996, 1982

3. Adams F: Neuropsychiatric evaluation and treatment of delirium in the critically ill cancer patient. Cancer Bulletin 36:156–160, 1984

4. Adams F: Emergency intravenous sedation of the delirious, medically ill patient. J Clin Psychiatry 49 (suppl 12):22–26, 1988

5. Adams F, Fernandez F, Andersson B: Emergency pharmacotherapy of delirium in the critically ill cancer patient: intravenous combination drug approach. Psychosomatics 27 (suppl 1):33–37, 1986

6. Adams R, Victor M: Principles of Neurology, 4th Edition. New York, McGraw-Hill Information Services, 1989

7. Ahn M, Lee J, Lee K, et al: A randomized double-blind trial of ondansetron alone versus in combination with dexamethasone versus in combination with dexamethasone and lorazepam in the prevention of emesis due to cisplatin-based chemotherapy. Am J Clin Oncol 17:150–156, 1994

8. Aitkenhead A, Pepperman M, Willatts S, et al: Comparison of propofol and midazolam for sedation in critically ill patients. Lancet 2:704–709, 1989

9. Albibi R, McCallum R: Metoclopramide: pharmacology and clinical application. Ann Intern Med 98:86–95, 1983

10. American Psychiatric Association: Diagnostic and Statistical Manual of Mental Disorders, 4th Edition. Washington, DC, American Psychiatric Association, 1994

11. Amir J, Galbraith R: Paraneoplastic limbic encephalopathy as a nonmetastatic complication of small cell lung cancer. South Med J 85:1013–1014, 1992

12. Andrykowski M, Jacobsen P: Anticipatory nausea and vomiting with cancer chemotherapy, in Psychiatric Aspects of Symptom Management in Cancer Patients. Edited by Breitbart W, Holland J. Washington, DC, American Psychiatric Press, 1993, pp 107–128

13. Angus W, Romney D: The effect of diazepam on patients' memory. J Clin Psychopharmacol 4:203–206, 1984

14. Austen F, Charmichael M, Adams R: Neurologic manifestations of chronic pulmonary insufficiency. N Engl J Med 257:579–590, 1957

15. Ayd F: Intravenous haloperidol therapy. International Drug Therapy Newsletter 13:20–23, 1978

16. Bachenberg K: Disuse atrophy. Crit Care Med 16:649–650, 1988

17. Baider L, Uziely B, De-Nour A: Progressive muscle relaxation and guided imagery in cancer patients. Gen Hosp Psychiatry 16:340–347, 1994

18. Baldessarini R: Drugs and the treatment of psychiatric disorders, in Goodman and Gilman's The Pharmacological Basis of Therapeutics, 8th Edition. Edited by Gilman A, Rall T, Nies A, et al. New York, Pergamon, 1990, pp 383–435

19. Barbee J: Memory, benzodiazepines, and anxiety: integration of theoretical and clinical perspectives. J Clin Psychiatry 54 (suppl):86–97, 1993

20. Berckman K, Austin J: Causal attribution, perceived control, and adjustment in patients with lung cancer. Oncol Nurs Forum 20:23–30, 1993

21. Beresin E: Delirium, in Inpatient Psychiatry: Diagnosis and Treatment. Edited by Sederer L. Baltimore, MD, Williams & Wilkins, 1983

22. Bergbom-Engberg I, Haljamae H: Assessment of patients' experience of discomforts during respirator therapy. Crit Care Med 17:1068–1072, 1989

23. Bernhard J, Ganz P: Psychosocial issues in lung cancer patients, I. Chest 99:216–223, 1991

24. Bernhard J, Ganz P: Psychosocial issues in lung cancer patients, II. Chest 99:480–485, 1991

24a. Bernhard J, Ganz P: Psychosocial issues in lung cancer patients. Cancer Treat Res 72:363–390, 1995

25. Billings R, Stein M: Depression associated with ranitidine. Am J Psychiatry 143:915–916, 1986

26. Bliwise D: What is sundowning? J Am Geriatr Soc 42:1009–1011, 1994

27. Blustein J, Seeman M: Brain tumors presenting as functional psychiatric disturbances. Canadian Psychiatric Association Journal 17:59–63, 1972

28. Bond W, Mandos L, Kurtz M: Midazolam for aggressivity and violence in three mentally retarded patients. Am J Psychiatry 156:925–926, 1989

29. Bovjerg D, Redd W, Jacobsen P, et al: An experimental analysis of classically conditioned nausea during cancer chemotherapy. Psychosom Med 54:623–637, 1992

30. Bowen D: Ventilator weaning through hypnosis. Psychosomatics 4:449–450, 1989

31. Brain W, Henson R: Neurological syndromes associated with carcinoma. Lancet 2:971–975, 1958

32. Breitbart W: Psychotropic adjuvant analgesics for cancer pain. Psycho-Oncology 1:133–145, 1992

33. Breitbart W, Holland J (eds): Psychiatric Aspects of Symptom Management in Cancer Patients. Washington, DC, American Psychiatric Press, 1993

34. Breitbart W, Mermelstein H: Pemoline: an alternative psychostimulant for management of depressive disorders in cancer patients. Psychosomatics 33:352–356, 1992

35. Brennan L, Craddock P: Limbic encephalopathy as a non-metastatic complication of oatcell lung cancer. Am J Med 75:518–520, 1983

36. Bruera E, Chadwick S, Weinlick A, et al: Delirium and severe sedation in patients with terminal cancer. Cancer Treatment Reports 71:787–788, 1987

37. Brunton L: Agents for control of gastric acidity and treatment of peptic ulcers, in Goodman and Gilman's The Pharmacological Basis of Therapeutics, 8th Edition. Edited by Gilman A, Rall T, Nies A, et al. New York, Pergamon, 1990, pp 897–913

38. Burns M, Eisendrath S: Dextroamphetamine treatment for depression in terminally ill patients. Psychosomatics 35:80–83, 1994

39. Byerley B, Gillin J: Diagnosis and management of insomnia. Psychiatr Clin North Am 7:773–789, 1984

40. Carton M, Cabarrot E, Lafforgue C: Interet de l'amitriptyline utilise comme antalgigue en cancerologie [The value of amitriptyline as an analgesic in cancer]. Gazette Medicale de France 83:2375–2378, 1976

41. Cassem N: Critical care psychiatry, in Textbook of Critical Care. Edited by Shoemaker W, Thompson W, Holbrook P. Philadelphia, PA, WB Saunders, 1984, pp 981–989

42. Cassem N: The dying patient, in Massachusetts General Hospital Handbook of General Hospital Psychiatry, 3rd Edition. Edited by Cassem N. St. Louis, MO, Mosby Year Book, 1991, pp 343–371

43. Cassem N, Hackett T: The setting of intensive care, in Massachusetts General Hospital Handbook of General Hospital Psychiatry, 3rd Edition. Edited by Cassem N. St. Louis, MO, Mosby Year Book, 1991, pp 373–399

44. Chedru F, Geschwind N: Writing disturbances in acute confusional states. Neuropsychologia 10:343–353, 1972

44a. Ciraulo D, Shader R, Ciraulo A, et al: The treatment the alcohol withdrawal, in Manual of Psychiatric Therapeutics, 2nd Edition. Edited by Shader R. Boston, MA, Little, Brown, 1994, pp 193–210

44b. Ciraulo D, Shader R, Greenblatt D, et al. (eds): Drug Interactions in Psychiatry, 2nd Edition. Baltimore, MD, Williams & Wilkins, 1995

45. Cornelius J, Soloff P, Miewald B: Behavioral manifestations of paraneoplastic encephalopathy. Biol Psychiatry 21:686–690, 1986

46. Corsellis J, Goldberg G, Norton A: "Limbic encephalitis" and its associations with carcinoma. Brain 91:481–496, 1968

47. den Hollander A, van Hulst A, Meerwaldt J, et al: Limbic encephalitis: a rare presentation of small-cell lung carcinoma. Gen Hosp Psychiatry 11:388–392, 1989

48. Dubin W, Feld J: Rapid tranquilization of the violent patient. Am J Emerg Med 7:313–320, 1989

49. Dudley D, Sitzman J: Psychosocial and psychophysiologic approach to the patient. Seminars in Respiratory Medicine 1:59–83, 1979

50. Dulfano M, Ishikawa S: Hypercapnia: mental changes and extrapulmonary complications. Ann Intern Med 63:829–841, 1965

51. Faheem A, Brightwell D, Burton G, et al: Respiratory dyskinesia and dysarthria from prolonged neuroleptic use: tardive dyskinesia. Am J Psychiatry 139:517–518, 1982

52. Fayer S: Torsade de pointes ventricular tachyarrhythmia associated with haloperidol (letter). J Clin Psychopharmacol 6:375–376, 1986

53. Fernandez F, Levy J, Mansell P: Management of delirium in terminally ill AIDS patients. Int J Psychiatry Med 19:165–172, 1989

54. Ferrando S, Eisendrath S: Adverse neuropsychiatric effects of dopamine antagonist medications: misdiagnosis in the medical setting. Psychosomatics 32:426–432, 1991

55. Fix A, Golden C, Daughton D, et al: Neuropsychological deficits among patients with COPD. Int J Neurosci 16:99–105, 1982

56. Fleishman S, Lavin M, Sattler M, et al: Antiemetic-induced akathisia in cancer patients receiving chemotherapy. Am J Psychiatry 151:763–765, 1994

57. Fleishman S, Lesko L: Delirium and dementia, in Handbook of Psychooncology. Edited by Holland J, Rowland J. New York, Oxford University Press, 1990, pp 342–355

58. Fogel B: Organic mental disorders, in Inpatient Psychiatry. Edited by Sederer L. Baltimore, MD, Williams & Wilkins, 1991, pp 121–252

59. Folstein M, Folstein S, McHugh P: Mini-Mental State: a practical method for grading the cognitive state of patients for the clinician. J Psychiatr Res 12:189–198, 1975

60. Francis J, Martin D, Kapoor W: A prospective study of delirium in hospitalized elderly. JAMA 263:1097–1101, 1990

60a. Frye M, Coudreaut M, Hakeman S, et al: Continuous droperidol infusion for management of agitated delirium in an intensive care unit. Psychosomatics 36:301–305, 1995

61. Gale J, O'Shanick G: Psychiatric aspects of respirator treatment and pulmonary intensive care. Adv Psychosom Med 14:93–108, 1985

62. Ganzini L, Casey D, Hoffman W, et al: The prevalence of metoclopramide-induced tardive dyskinesia and acute extrapyramidal movement disorders. Arch Intern Med 153:1469–1475, 1993

63. Gershon E, Goldstein R, Moss A, et al: Psychosis with ordinary doses of propranolol. Ann Intern Med 90:938–939, 1979

64. Gipson W, Sivak E, Gulledge A: Psychological aspects of ventilator dependency. Psychiatr Med 5:245–255, 1987

65. Goldberg R: Acute pain management, in Psychiatric Care of the Medical Patient. Edited by Stoudemire A, Fogel B. New York, Oxford University Press, 1993, pp 323–339

66. Goldstein M, Haltzman S: Intensive care, in Psychiatric Care of the Medical Patient. Edited by Stoudemire A, Fogel B. New York, Oxford University Press, 1993, pp 241–265

67. Gorfinkle K, Redd W: Anticipatory nausea and vomiting with cancer chemotherapy, in Psychiatric Aspects of Symptom Management in Cancer Patients. Edited by Breitbart W, Holland J. Washington, DC, American Psychiatric Press, 1993, pp 129–146

68. Gotay C: Why me? attributions and adjustment by cancer patients and their mates at two stages in the disease process. Soc Sci Med 20:825–831, 1985

69. Grant I, Heaton R, McSweeney A, et al: Brain dysfunction in COPD. Chest 77:308–309, 1980

70. Grant I, Heaton R, McSweeney A, et al: Neuropsychologic findings in hypoxemic COPD. Arch Intern Med 142:1470–1476, 1982

71. Green S: Principles of medical psychotherapy, in Psychiatric Care of the Medical Patient. Edited by Stoudemire A, Fogel B. New York, Oxford University Press, 1993, pp 3–30

72. Greenberg D, Younger J, Kaufman S: Management of lithium in patients with cancer. Psychosomatics 34:388–394, 1993

73. Greenblatt D, Shader R: Treatment of the alcohol withdrawal syndrome, in Manual of Psychiatric Therapeutics. Edited by Shader R. Boston, MA, Little, Brown, 1975

74. Griggs R, Arieff A: Hypoxia and the central nervous system, in Metabolic Brain Dysfunction in Systemic Disorders. Edited by Arieff A, Griggs R. Boston, MA, Little, Brown, 1992, pp 39–54

75. Gross J, Weller R, Conrad P: Flumazenil antagonism of midazolam-induced ventilatory depression. Anesthesiology 75:179–185, 1991

76. Groves J, Kucharski A: Brief psychotherapy, in Massachusetts General Hospital Handbook of General Hospital Psychiatry, 3rd Edition. Edited by Cassem N. St. Louis, MO, Mosby Year Book, 1991, pp 321–341

76a. Heaton R: Wisconsin Card Sorting Test. Odessa, FL, Psychological Assessment Resources, 1985

76b. Heimburger R, Reitan R: Easily administered written test for lateralizing brain lesions. J Neurosurg 18:301–312, 1961

77. Henderson R, Lane S, Henry J: Life-threatening ventricular arrhythmia (torsade de pointes) after haloperidol overdose. Hum Exp Toxicol 10:59–62, 1991

78. Holland J: Lung cancer, in Handbook of Psychooncology. Edited by Holland J, Rowland J. New York, Oxford University Press, 1990, pp 180–187

79. Holland J, Rowland J (eds): Handbook of Psychooncology. New York, Oxford University Press, 1990

80. Holliday J, Hyers T: The reduction of weaning time from mechanical ventilation using tidal volume and relaxation biofeedback. Am Rev Respir Dis 141:1214–1220, 1990

81. Hollister L: Adverse reactions to phenothiazines. JAMA 189:143–145, 1974

82. Holmes T, Sabaawi M, Fragala M: Psychostimulant suppository treatment for depression in the gravely ill (letter). J Clin Psychiatry 55:265–266, 1994

83. Hooper J, Minter G: Droperidol in the management of psychiatric emergencies. J Clin Psychopharmacol 3:262–263, 1983

84. Horvath T, Siever L, Mohs R, et al: Organic mental syndromes and disorders, in Comprehensive Textbook of Psychiatry, 5th Edition. Edited by Kaplan H, Sadock B. Baltimore, MD, Williams & Wilkins, 1989, pp 599–641

85. House R, Trzepacz P, Thompson T: Psychiatric consultation to organ transplant services, in American Psychiatric Press Review of Psychiatry. Vol 9. Edited by Tasman A, Goldfinger SM, Kaufmann C. Washington, DC, American Psychiatric Press, 1990, pp 515–536

86. Hughes G, Turner R: Hypernephroma presenting as acute delirium. J Urol 130:539–540, 1983

87. Inouye S, Viscoli C, Horwitz R, et al: A predictive model for delirium in hospitalized elderly medical patients based on admission characteristics. Ann Intern Med 119:474–481, 1993

88. Inouye SK: The dilemma of delirium: clinical and research controversies regarding diagnosis and evaluation of delirium in hospitalized elderly medical patients. Am J Med 97:278–288, 1994

89. Isaacs B, Kenmi A: The set test as an aid to the detection of dementia in old people. Br J Psychiatry 123:467–470, 1973

90. Jacobs J: Family therapy in the context of chronic medical illness, in Psychiatric Care of the Medical Patient. Edited by Stoudemire A, Fogel B. New York, Oxford University Press, 1993, pp 19–30

91. Jacobsen P, Massie M, Kinne D, et al: Hypnotic efficacy and safety of triazolam administered during the postoperative period. Gen Hosp Psychiatry 16:419–425, 1994

92. Jenike M: The patient with lung disease, in Treatments of Psychiatric Disorders: A Task Force Report of the American Psychiatric Association, Vol 2. Washington, DC, American Psychiatric Association, 1989, pp 939–948

92a. Johnson C, Auger W, Fedullo P, et al: Methylphenidate in the "hard to wean" patient. J Psychosom Res 39:63–68, 1995

93. Jones B, Teng E, Folstein M, et al: A new bedside test of cognition for patients with HIV infection. Ann Intern Med 119:1001–1004, 1993

94. Kalkman P, Allan S, Birchall I: Magnetic resonance imaging of limbic encephalitis. Can Assoc Radiol J 44:121–124, 1993

95. Khan N, Wieser H: Limbic encephalitis: a case report. Epilepsy Res 17:175–181, 1994

96. Kidgell A, Butcher M, Brown B: antiemetic control: 5-HT$_3$ antagonists: review of clinical results, with particular emphasis on ondansetron. Cancer Treat Rev 17:311–317, 1990

97. Klotz U, Walker S: Flumazenil and hepatic encephalopathy (letter). Lancet 1:155–156, 1989

98. Kong K, Willatts S, Prys R: Isoflurane compared with midazolam for sedation in the intensive care unit. BMJ 298:1277–1280, 1989

99. Kriwisky M, Perry G, Tarchitsky D, et al: Haloperidol-induced torsade de pointes. Chest 98:482–484, 1990

100. Kruis R, Barger R: Paranoid psychosis with sulindac (letter). JAMA 243:1420, 1980

100a. Kruk J, Sachdev P, Singh S: Neuroleptic-induced respiratory dyskinesia. J Neuropsychiatry Clin Neurosci 7:223–229, 1995

100b. LaFond L, Horner J: Psychosocial issues related to long-term ventilatory support. Problems in Respiratory Care 1:241–256, 1988

101. Leavitt M, Trzepacz P, Ciongoli K: Rat model of delirium: atropine dose-response relationships. J Neuropsychiatry Clin Neurosci 6:279–284, 1994

102. Lebovits A, Chalinian A, Gorzynski J, et al: Psychological aspects of asbestos-related mesothelioma and knowledge of high risk for cancer. Cancer Detect Prev 4:181–184, 1981

103. Lesko L: Nausea and vomiting: physiology and pharmacological management, in Handbook of Psychooncology. Edited by Holland J, Rowland J. New York, Oxford University Press, 1990, pp 414–433

104. Lesko L, Fleishman S: Treatment and support in confusional states. Recent Results Cancer Res 121:378–392, 1991

105. Levenson H, Hales R: Brief psychodynamically informed therapy for medically ill patients, in Medical Psychiatric Practice. Vol 2. Edited by Stoudemire A, Fogel B. Washington, DC, American Psychiatric Press, 1993, pp 3–37

106. Levenson J: Cardiovascular disease, in Psychiatric Care of the Medical Patient. Edited by Stoudemire A, Fogel B. New York, Oxford University Press, 1993, pp 539–563

107. Levenson J: High-dose intravenous haloperidol for agitated delirium following lung transplantation. Psychosomatics 36:66–73, 1995

108. Levine P, Silberfarb P, Lipowski Z: Mental disorders in cancer patients: a study of 100 psychiatric referrals. Cancer 42:1385–1391, 1978

108a. Lezak M: Neuropsychological Assessment, 2nd Edition. New York, Oxford University Press, 1983

109. Lipowski Z: Delirium: Acute Confusional States. New York, Oxford University Press, 1990

110. Lishman W: Organic Psychiatry, 2nd Edition. London, Blackwell Scientific, 1987

111. Liston E: Delirium in the aged. Psychiatr Clin North Am 5:49–66, 1982

112. Liston E: Diagnosis and management of delirium in the elderly patient. Psychiatric Annals 14:109–118, 1984

113. Liston E: Delirium, in Treatments of Psychiatric Disorders: A Task Force Report of the American Psychiatric Association, Vol 2. Washington, DC, American Psychiatric Association, 1989, pp 804–815

114. Lyman G, Williams C, Dinwoodie W, et al: Sudden death in cancer patients receiving lithium. J Clin Oncol 2:1270–1274, 1984

115. Maas H, Wils V: "Cholinergic score" and delirium (letter). J Neuropsychiatry Clin Neurosci 5:208–210, 1994

116. Malatesta V, West B, Malcolm R: Application of behavioral principles in the management of suffocation phobia: a case study of chronic respiratory failure. Int J Psychiatry Med 19:281–289, 1989

116a. Manos P: Neuropathogenesis of delirium (letter). Psychosomatics 36:156, 1995

117. Marcantonio E, Goldman L, Mangione C, et al: A clinical prediction rule for delirium after elective noncardiac surgery. JAMA 271:134–139, 1994

118. Markham M, Abeloff M: Small-cell lung cancer and limbic encephalitis (letter). Ann Intern Med 96:785, 1982

119. Masand P, Pickett P, Murray G: Psychostimulants for secondary depression in medical illness. Psychosomatics 32:203–208, 1991

120. Masm A, Granacher R: Clinical Handbook of antipsychotic Drug Therapy. New York, Brunner/Mazel, 1980

121. Massie M, Holland J: Psychiatry and oncology, in Psychiatry Update: The American Psychiatric Association Annual Review, Vol 3. Edited by Grinspoon L. Washington, DC, American Psychiatric Press, 1984, pp 239–256

122. Massie M, Holland J, Glass E: Delirium in terminally ill cancer patients. Am J Psychiatry 140:1048–1050, 1983

123. Massie M, Lesko L: Psychopharmacological management, in Handbook of Psychooncology. Edited by Holland J, Rowland J. New York, Oxford University Press, 1990, pp 470–491

124. Massie M, Lesko L: Psychotherapeutic interventions [for cancer patients], in Handbook of Psychooncology. Edited by Holland J, Rowland J. New York, Oxford University Press, 1990, pp 455–469

125. Massie M, Shakin E: Management of depression and anxiety in cancer patients, in Psychiatric Aspects of Symptom Management in Cancer Patients. Edited by Breitbart W, Holland J. Washington, DC, American Psychiatric Press, 1993, pp 1–21

126. Mayer D, Davies R, Moossa A: Investigating the oncologic patient: diagnosis and staging, in Comprehensive Textbook of Oncology, 2nd Edition. Edited by Moossa A, Schimpff S, Robson M. Baltimore, MD, Williams & Wilkins, 1991, pp 201–206

127. McCarthy D: Ranitidine or cimetidine. Ann Intern Med 99:551–553, 1983

128. McCartney C, Hatley L, Kessler J, et al: Possible tobramycin delirium. JAMA 247:1319, 1982

128a. McCartney J, Boland R: Anxiety and delirium in the intensive care unit. Crit Care Clin 10:673–680, 1994

129. McMurray T, Collier P, Carson I, et al: Propofol sedation after open heart surgery: a clinical and pharmacokinetic study. Anaesthesia 45:22–26, 1990

130. Midazolam. Medical Letter on Drugs and Therapeutics 28:73–76, 1986

131. Mendel J, Khan F: Psychological aspects of weaning from mechanical ventilation. Psychosomatics 21:465–471, 1980

132. Mendoza R, Djenderedjian A, Adams J, et al: Midazolam in acute psychotic patients with hyperarousal. J Clin Psychiatry 48:291–292, 1987

133. Menza M, Murray G, Holmes V, et al: Decreased extrapyramidal symptoms with intravenous haloperidol. J Clin Psychiatry 48:278–280, 1987

134. Menza M, Murray G, Holmes V, et al: Controlled study of extrapyramidal reactions in the management of delirious medically ill patients: intravenous haloperidol plus benzodiazepines. Heart Lung 17:238–241, 1988

135. Metzger E, Friedman R: Prolongation of the corrected QT and torsade de pointes cardiac arrhythmia associated with intravenous haloperidol in the medically ill. J Clin Psychopharmacol 13:128–132, 1993

136. Miller N, Lipowski Z, Lebowitz B (eds): Delirium: Advances in Research and Clinical Practice. New York, Springer, 1991

137. Mitchell K, Popkin M, Trick W, et al: Psychiatric complications associated with ondansetron. Psychosomatics 35:161–163, 1994

138. Mucha H, Lange E, Bonitz G: Amitriptylin in der psychiatrischen Therapie [Amitriptyline in psychiatric therapy]. Psychiatrie, Neurologie und Medizinische Psychologie (Leipz) 22:116–120, 1970

139. Mumma C, McCorkle R: Causal attribution and life-threatening disease. Int J Psychiatry Med 12:311–319, 1982

140. Murray G: Confusion, delirium, and dementia, in Massachusetts General Hospital Handbook of General Hospital Psychiatry, 3rd Edition. Edited by Cassem N. St. Louis, MO, Mosby Year Book, 1991, pp 89–120

141. Nadler J, Richardson E, Malloy P: Detection of impairment with the Mini-Mental State Examination. Neuropsychiatry, Neuropsychology, and Behavioral Neurology 7:109–113, 1994

142. Napolitano C, Priori S, Schwartz P: Torsade de pointes: mechanisms and management. Drugs 47:51–65, 1994

143. Nelson A, Fogel B, Faust D: Bedside cognitive screening instruments: a critical assessment. J Nerv Ment Dis 174:73–83, 1986

144. Newman N, Bell I, McKee A: Paraneoplastic limbic encephalitis: neuropsychiatric presentation. Biol Psychiatry 27:529–542, 1990

144a. Nicholas L, Lindsey A: Delirium presenting with symptoms of depression. Psychosomatics 36:471–479, 1995

144b. Oren D: Dysphoria after treatment with ondansetron (letter). Am J Psychiatry 152:1101, 1995

144c. Ovsiew F: Neuropathogenesis of delirium (letter). Psychosomatics 36:156, 1995

145. Parker M, Schubert W, Shelhamer J, et al: Perceptions of a critically ill patient experiencing therapeutic paralysis in an ICU. Crit Care Med 12:69–71, 1984

146. Patel A, Davila D, Peters S: Paraneoplastic syndromes associated with lung cancer. Mayo Clin Proc 68:278–287, 1993

147. Paykel E, Fleminger R, Watson J: Psychiatric side effects of anti-hypertensive drugs other than reserpine. J Clin Psychopharmacol 2:14–39, 1982

148. Picotte-Prillmayer D, DiMaggio J, Baile W: H2 blocker delirium. Psychosomatics 36:74–77, 1995

149. Platt M, Breitbart W, Smith M, et al: Efficacy of neuroleptics for hypoactive delirium (letter). J Neuropsychiatry Clin Neurosci 6:66, 1994

150. Plum F, Posner J: Diagnosis of Stupor and Coma, 3rd Edition. Philadelphia, PA, FA Davis, 1980

151. Portenoy R: Chronic pain management, in Psychiatric Care of the Medical Patient. Edited by Stoudemire A, Fogel B. New York, Oxford University Press, 1993, pp 341–363

152. Portnoy R: Hyperkinetic dysarthria as an early indicator of impending tardive dyskinesia. Journal of Speech and Hearing Disorders 44:214–219, 1979

153. Potanovitch L, Pisters K, Kris M, et al: Midazolam in patients receiving anticancer chemotherapy and antiemetics. Journal of Pain and Symptom Management 8:519–524, 1993

154. Prigatano G, Parsons O, Wright E, et al: Neuropsychological test performance in mildly hypoxemic patients with COPD. J Consult Clin Psychol 51:108–116, 1983

155. Rabins P, Folstein M: Delirium and dementia: diagnostic criteria and fatality rates. Br J Psychiatry 140:149–153, 1982

156. Razavi D, Delvaux N, Fravacques C, et al: Prevention of adjustment disorders and anticipatory nausea secondary to adjuvant chemotherapy: a double-blind, placebo-controlled study assessing the usefulness of alprazolam. J Clin Oncol 11:1384–1390, 1993

157. Redd W: Management of anticipatory nausea and vomiting, in Handbook of Psychooncology. Edited by Holland J, Rowland J. New York, Oxford University Press, 1990, pp 423–433

157a. Reitan R: Validity of the Trail Making Test as an indicator of organic brain damage. Percept Mot Skills 8:271–276, 1958

158. Remick R, O'Kane J, Sparling T: A case report of toxic psychosis with low-dose propranolol therapy. Am J Psychiatry 138:850–851, 1981

159. Resnick M, Burton B: Droperidol vs. haloperidol in the initial management of acutely agitated patients. J Clin Psychiatry 45:298–299, 1984

160. Rie M, Wilson R: Acute respiratory failure, in Care of the Critically Ill Patient. Edited by Tinker J, Rapid M. Berlin, Springer-Verlag, 1983, pp 311–340

161. Rosen J, Sweet R, Mulsant B, et al: The Delirium Rating Scale in a psychogeriatric inpatient setting. J Neuropsychiatry Clin Neurosci 6:30–35, 1994

162. Rubin C: Cimetidine and ranitidine (letter). JAMA 251:2211–2212, 1984

163. Salzman C, Green A, Rodriguez-Villa F, et al: Benzodiazepines combined with neuroleptics for management of severe disruptive behavior. Psychosomatics 27 (suppl 1):17–21, 1986

164. Salzman C, Solomon D, Miyawaki E, et al: Parenteral lorazepam versus parenteral haloperidol for the control of psychotic disruptive behavior. J Clin Psychiatry 52:177–180, 1991

165. Sanders K, Murray G, Cassem: High-dose intravenous haloperidol for agitated delirium in a cardiac patient on intraaortic balloon pump. J Clin Psychopharmacol 11:146–147, 1991

166. Santos A, Beliles K, Arana G: Parenteral use of psychotropic agents, in Medical Psychiatric Practice. Vol 2. Edited by Stoudemire A, Fogel B. Washington, DC, American Psychiatric Press, 1993, pp 113–137

167. Schulze-Delrieu K: Metoclopramide. N Engl J Med 305:28–33, 1981

168. Schwamm L, Van Dyke C, Kiernan R, et al: The neurobehavioral cognitive status examination: comparison with the cognitive capacity screening examination and the Mini-Mental State Examination in a neurosurgical population. Ann Intern Med 107:486–491, 1987

169. Scully R, Mark E, McNeely B: Case 30—1985: weekly clinicopathological exercises. N Engl J Med 313:249–257, 1985

170. Shapiro J, Westphal L, White P, et al: Midazolam infusion for sedation in the intensive care unit: effect on adrenal function. Anesthesiology 64:394–398, 1986

171. Skinner J: Regulation of cardiac vulnerability by the cerebral defense system. J Am Coll Cardiol 5:88B–94B, 1985

172. Slaby A, Erle S: Dementia and delirium, in Psychiatric Care of the Medical Patient. Edited by Stoudemire A, Fogel B. New York, Oxford University Press, 1993, pp 415–453

172a. Smith M, Breitbart W, Platt M: A critique of instruments and methods to detect, diagnose, and rate delirium. J Pain Symptom Manage 10:35–77, 1995

173. Snavely S, Hodges G: The neurotoxicity of antibacterial agents. Ann Intern Med 101:92–104, 1984

174. Snellen F, Lauwers P, Demeyere R, et al: The use of midazolam versus propofol for short-term sedation following coronary artery bypass grafting. Intensive Care Med 16:312–316, 1990

175. Sos J, Cassem N: Managing postoperative agitation. Drug Therapeutics 10:103–106, 1980

176. Sotsky S, Tossell J: Tometin induction of mania. Psychosomatics 25:626–628, 1984

177. Spira J, Spiegel D: Group psychotherapy of the medically ill, in Psychiatric Care of the Medical Patient. Edited by Stoudemire A, Fogel B. New York, Oxford University Press, 1993, pp 31–50

178. Stanley K: Prognostic factors for survival in patients with inoperable lung cancer. J Natl Cancer Inst 65:25–32, 1980

179. Steele T, Morton W: Salicylate-induced delirium. Psychosomatics 27:455–456, 1986

180. Steen S: The effects of psychotropic drugs on respiration. Pharmacol Ther 2:717–741, 1976

181. Stern T, Caplan R, Cassem N: Use of benzodiazepines in a coronary care unit. Psychosomatics 28:19–26, 1987

182. Storey P, Trumble M: Rectal doxepin and carbamazepine therapy in patients with cancer (letter). N Engl J Med 327:1318–1319, 1992

183. Tandon R, Walden M, Falcon S: Catatonia as a manifestation of paraneoplastic encephalopathy. J Clin Psychiatry 49:121–122, 1988

184. Tavani C: Perioperative psychiatric considerations in the elderly. Clin Geriatr Med 6:543–556, 1990

185. Tejera C, Saravay S, Goldman E, et al: Diphenhydramine-induced delirium in elderly hospitalized patients with mild dementia. Psychosomatics 35:399–402, 1994

186. Tesar G, Stern T: Evaluation and treatment of agitation in the intensive care unit. Journal of Intensive Care Medicine 1:137–148, 1986

187. Thomas E, et al: Droperidol versus haloperidol for chemical restraint of agitated and combative patients. Ann Emerg Med 21:407–413, 1992

188. Thompson W, Thompson T: Use of medications in patients with chronic respiratory disease. Adv Psychosom Med 14:136–148, 1985

189. Thompson W, Thompson T: Pulmonary disease, in Principles of Medical Psychiatry. Edited by Stoudemire A, Fogel B. Orlando, FL, Grune & Stratton, 1987, pp 553–570

190. Trachman S, Begun D, Kirch D: Delirium in a patient with carcinomatosis. Psychosomatics 32:455–457, 1991

191. Trzepacz P: The neuropathogenesis of delirium. Psychosomatics 35:374–391, 1994

192. Trzepacz P: A review of delirium assessment instruments. Gen Hosp Psychiatry 16:397–405, 1994

192a. Trzepacz P: Neuropathogenesis of delirium (reply). Psychosomatics 36:157, 1995

193. Trzepacz P, Baker R, Greenhouse J: A symptom rating scale for delirium. Psychiatry Res 23:89–97, 1988

193a. Trzepacz P, Dew M: Further analyses of the Delirium Rating Scale. Gen Hosp Psychiatry 17:75–79, 1995

194. Tune L, Carr S, Cooper T, et al: Association of anticholinergic activity of prescribed medications with postoperative delirium. J Neuropsychiatry Clin Neurosci 5:208–210, 1993

195. Tune L, Holland A, Folstein M, et al: Association of postoperative delirium with raised serum levels of anticholinergic drugs. Lancet 2:650–653, 1981

196. Van Sweden B, Van Peteghem P: Psychopathology in paraneoplastic encephalopathy: an electroclinical observation. J Clin Psychiatry 47:267–268, 1986

197. Viederman M: Use of a psychodynamic life narrative in the treatment of depression in the physically ill. Gen Hosp Psychiatry 3:177–181, 1980

198. Wallesch C, Hundsalz A: Language function in delirium: a comparison of single word processing in acute confusional states and probable Alzheimer's disease. Brain Lang 46:592–606, 1994

199. Weddington W, Muelling A, Moosa H: Adverse neuropsychiatric reactions to cimetidine. Psychosomatics 23:49–53, 1982

200. Weiner W, Goetz C, Nausieda P, et al: Respiratory dyskinesia: extrapyramidal dysfunction and dyspnea. Ann Intern Med 88:327–331, 1978

201. Weisman A: Coping with illness, in Massachusetts General Hospital Handbook of General Hospital Psychiatry, 3rd Edition. Edited by Cassem N. St. Louis, MO, Mosby Year Book, 1991, pp 309–319

202. Werman D: Technical aspects of supportive psychotherapy. Psychiatric Journal of the University of Ottawa 6:153–160, 1981

203. Wilt J, Minnema A, Johnson R, et al: Torsade de pointes associated with the use of intravenous haloperidol. Ann Intern Med 119:391–394, 1993

204. Wise M, Brandt G: Delirium, in The American Psychiatric Press Textbook of Neuropsychiatry, 2nd Edition. Edited by Yudofsky S, Hales R. Washington, DC, American Psychiatric Press, 1992, pp 291–308

205. Wise M, Cassem N: Psychiatric consultation to critical-care units, in American Psychiatric Press Review of Psychiatry, Vol 9. Edited by Tasman A, Goldfinger SM, Kaufmann C. Washington, DC, American Psychiatric Press, 1990, pp 413–432

206. Young L, Patel M: Respiratory complication of antipsychotic drugs in medically ill patients. Resident and Staff Physician 30:73–80, 1984

207. Yue M, Fainsinger R, Bruera E: Cognitive impairment in a patient with a normal Mini-Mental State Examination (MMSE). Journal of Pain and Symptom Management 9:51–53, 1994

208. Zee-Cheng C, Mueller C, Seifert C, et al: Haloperidol and torsade de pointes (letter). Ann Intern Med 102:418, 1985

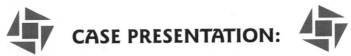
Mrs. Alberts is a 50-year-old woman with a 5-year history of asthma who is referred by her pulmonologist for evaluation. She feels that she is no longer coping as well as she used to. She lacks energy, is easily tearful, feels demoralized about her asthma, and "can't seem to snap out of it." She wakes up at 3 A.M. every morning, has diminished appetite (but no weight loss), and finds mornings "intolerable." She acknowledges transient suicidal ideation. Her boss suggested that she take some time off because she has become forgetful and has difficulty concentrating.

Mrs. Alberts has been experiencing repeated exacerbations of asthma requiring frequent adjustments in her medications, especially the steroids. A typical regimen for her is as follows: theophylline (Theo-Dur) 200 mg po od, albuterol (Proventil) inhaler 2–4 puffs/day, triamcinolone acetonide (Azmacort) inhaler 3 puffs tid, potassium (Slow K) (dosage variable), and Tums antacids. She has intermittently been on steroids in the past. She states that her theophylline dose is adjusted "according to how I feel": for example, when she experiences stomach upset, headache, and "not feeling like herself," her dose is halved. Most recently, her blood gases have been normal.

Mrs. Alberts has been hospitalized three times. The most serious of these occurred 2 years ago when she was rushed to the emergency room cyanotic and partially conscious. Her pulmonologist confirms that there were no medical or neurological sequelae. There are no other medical problems. She did not have asthma as a child.

The patient has been experiencing a very stressful time in the past 6 months. Her son has been having problems with cocaine addiction, but recently signed himself into a drug treatment center. Her husband, while quite supportive, is in danger of being laid off due to budget cuts. She works as an executive secretary. Although she enjoys her work, she finds it unpredictable and often stressful.

There is no past personal or family psychiatric history. There is no alcohol or substance abuse.

Mental status examination reveals an attractive middle-aged woman, well-groomed and fashionably dressed. Her speech is low in volume, slow in rate. Thought process is goal directed, coherent, and logical. Her affect is sad, and mood is depressed. She reports passive suicidal ideation. Thought content reveals no delusions or bizarre ideation. There are no hallucinations. She is alert and oriented for person, time, place, and situation. She scores 27 on the Mini-Mental State Examination (MMSE), with difficulty in concentration and recall.

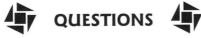

QUESTIONS

Choose all that apply.

1. During your initial interview with her, Mrs. Alberts briefly acknowledges that she nearly died from the acute exacerbation several years ago. What considerations would guide your psychological exploration of this event?

   a. Patients who respond to a "near miss" death from asthma with denial are more likely to develop secondary anxiety and psychiatric decompensation later on.

   b. Excessive independence in asthmatics is associated with a high hospitalization rate.

   c. Denial is less prominent in asthmatics who have experienced a "near miss" death from asthma than in those without this experience, partially because the realistic danger has been so compelling.

   d. Patients who decompensate psychiatrically following a "near miss" death from asthma are no more likely to have past personal or family psychiatric history than those who do not decompensate.

2. The psychosomatic literature on pulmonary disease has attempted to define the impact of anxiety on physical

illness by distinguishing "characterologic" symptomatology from illness-specific anxiety. Which of the following are true about the potential impact of anxiety on Mrs. Alberts's illness?

- a. Emotional factors are as potent as allergic factors in precipitating asthmatic attacks.
- b. High illness-specific anxiety and high characterological anxiety predict greater frequency of hospitalizations *independently* of illness severity.
- c. There is consensus among study results that show that patients with greater dyspnea have more impaired pulmonary function tests than those with fewer dyspneic complaints.
- d. All of the above.

3. Studies have shown that asthmatic patients with the best medical outcomes demonstrate . . .

- a. Low illness-specific anxiety and low characterological anxiety.
- b. High illness-specific anxiety and high characterological anxiety.
- c. High illness-specific anxiety and average characterological anxiety.
- d. Low illness-specific anxiety and average characterological anxiety.
- e. Average illness-specific anxiety and average characterological anxiety.

4. Mrs. Alberts and her pulmonologist have struggled for years to distinguish symptoms of anxiety from exacerbations of her respiratory disorder. For example, "asthma attacks" have been elicited in the doctor's office merely by suggesting that she will experience one. Her physician feels that sometimes her theophylline may have been inappropriately increased to medicate anxiety-related dyspnea rather than asthma, making the patient even more agitated and uncomfortable. Your help is requested in this dilemma. What are important factors?

- a. The rate of anxiety disorders in asthmatic patients is no higher than that in the general population.
- b. The induction of an "asthmatic attack" by suggestion points strongly to a component of conversion disorder, which has a higher incidence in asthmatic patients than in the general population.
- c. After correcting for medication side effects, the evidence argues against asthmatics having any greater biological diathesis for anxiety disorders than the general population.
- d. There is a predictable relationship between the perception of breathlessness and a given forced expiratory volume in 1 second (FEV_1).

- e. The medical assessment of asthma severity has been shown to be influenced by subjective, physician-dependent factors.

5. Which of the following variables are found to be significantly different in those asthmatics whose attacks are susceptible to suggestion?

- a. Age
- b. Gender
- c. Asthma severity
- d. Atopy
- e. None of the above

6. What statements are true about respiratory depression and benzodiazepines?

- a. Benzodiazepines reduce the ventilatory response to hypoxia.
- b. Benzodiazepines depress respiration primarily by causing muscle relaxation.
- c. Benzodiazepines cause respiratory depression mainly by reducing the ability to clear secretions.
- d. The respiratory-depressant effects of benzodiazepines can be partially bypassed by administering low-flow oxygen.
- e. Benzodiazepines reduce the ventilatory response to hypercapnia.

7. What are reasonable considerations in treating Mrs. Alberts's anxiety?

- a. Since benzodiazepines have respiratory-depressant effects even in healthy patients, consider using beta-blockers such as propranolol (Inderal).
- b. Hydroxyzine (Vistaril, Atarax) has become the anxiolytic of choice for highly anxious patients with severe lung disease.
- c. Consider using lorazepam (Ativan), which does not usually produce significant hypoxemia at low doses.
- d. Buspirone (BuSpar) does not depress respiration but tends to interact adversely with bronchodilators such as terbutaline (Bricanyl) and theophylline (Theo-Dur).
- e. Try to avoid all anxiolytics except diphenhydramine (Benadryl).

8. What statements may be true concerning cognitive difficulties in someone like Mrs. Alberts?

- a. Alertness is highly sensitive to even mild hypoxemia.
- b. Perceptual learning and problem solving tend to be preserved even in the setting of moderate hypoxemia (PaO_2 50–59 mm Hg).

c. The degree of hypoxemia closely parallels performance on pulmonary function tests.

d. Chronic obstructive lung disease (COLD) patients generally test within the average range of intelligence.

9. Mrs. Alberts's difficulties with concentration, recall, and dysphoria remain. She confides that she is upset that her sexual relationship with her husband, previously active and satisfying, has deteriorated since the onset of her asthma. All of the following are true except . . .

a. Asthmatic patients are at heightened risk for developing phobic avoidance of sexual situations compared with the general population.

b. A decrease in pulmonary function can produce deterioration in sexual function.

c. Depression associated with chronic illness accounts for most of the sexual dysfunction in patients with pulmonary disease.

d. Relationships between spouses have been shown to *improve* following a near-miss death from asthma.

10. The patient decides to take a leave of absence from her job because she is unable to concentrate on her work. She experiences transient suicidal ideation and awakens breathless in the middle of the night. She feels chronically fatigued and has lost interest in her usual activities. She is very afraid of becoming disabled and a burden to her family. Although her pulmonologist confirms an asthma exacerbation and has increased the bronchodilators, he feels her symptoms exceed what is attributable solely to her physical condition. The family is frightened by her deterioration. All of the following are true concerning depression in asthmatic patients except . . .

a. Asthmatic patients like Mrs. Alberts have a higher incidence of suicide than other medical patients, such as hypertensive patients.

b. Sleep apnea is likely to complicate evaluation of insomnia due to depression in this population.

c. Mrs. Alberts's level of disability would be expected to more closely correlate with her subjective *perception* of dyspnea than with her objective pulmonary function test results.

d. Mrs. Alberts's level of disability would be expected to more closely correlate with her *objective* pulmonary function test results than with her subjective perception of dyspnea.

e. Strong denial would pose a risk factor for asthma death.

11. The way you formulate the potential impact of Mrs. Alberts's mood disorder on her respiratory disease will have implications for your treatment strategy. Which of the following statements are *false?*

a. Anxiety, but not depression, influences dyspnea.

b. Both anxiety and depression influence dyspnea.

c. Depression could have an impact on Mrs. Alberts's respiratory disease even if she did not perceive herself as disabled.

d. Depression could have an impact on Mrs. Alberts's respiratory disease even if it did not affect her compliance with medical care.

e. *Objective* assessments of dyspnea are unlikely to be affected by depression.

12. Mrs. Alberts agrees to psychiatric hospitalization. On admission, her internist reports that her physical exam is unchanged. Thyroid function tests, routine blood work, and electrocardiogram (ECG) are normal. Neurological examination, electroencephalogram (EEG), and magnetic resonance imaging (MRI) of the brain are normal. Mrs. Alberts is relieved to be in the hospital, but continues to be extremely depressed. You consider that . . .

a. Tricyclic antidepressants (TCAs) do not depress respiratory drive, so would not require serial blood gas monitoring.

b. Antidepressants with anticholinergic effects would be preferred because they promote drying of bronchial secretions.

c. Psychiatric side effects are temporally related to ingesting theophylline and sympathomimetic bronchodilators, but are usually not dose related.

d. All of the above.

13. Caution should be used in administering certain antidepressants to the asthmatic patient with a history of allergy to . . .

a. Yellow or orange candy or soda

b. Chocolate

c. Fruit

d. Seafood

14. What are some of the important drug interactions to anticipate when treating a depressed patient with lung disease?

a. TCAs interfere with and diminish the effects of atropine.

b. The pressor effects of epinephrine are potentiated by TCAs.

c. It would be preferable to avoid TCAs in Mrs. Alberts because she is also on albuterol.

d. Physostigmine is the preferred treatment for anticholinergic side effects in asthmatic patients, as it also improves pulmonary function.

15. What treatments for depression should be avoided in patients like Mrs. Alberts?
   a. Selective serotonin reuptake inhibitors (SSRIs)
   b. Monoamine oxidase inhibitors (MAOIs)
   c. Nonsedating TCAs
   d. Electroconvulsive therapy (ECT)

16. What are some true statements concerning the techniques of psychotherapy with lung disease patients?

   a. Therapy is often focused on lessening the social intrusiveness of chronic obstructive pulmonary disease (COPD) patients, which tends to be more common than social isolation.
   b. The usefulness of group therapy for this population is limited.
   c. Behavior therapy to reduce anxiety by relaxation training may paradoxically exacerbate anxiety.
   d. Patients should be advised to bring their as-needed medications to their psychotherapy sessions.

🔲 Answers

1. Answer: b (pp. 97–98)
2. Answer: a, b (pp. 97–98, 100)
3. Answer: c (p. 98)
4. Answer: e (pp. 100, 101, 102)
5. Answer: e (p. 97)
6. Answer: a (p. 103)
7. Answer: c (p. 104)
8. Answer: d (pp. 99–100)
9. Answer: c (p. 99)
10. Answer: d (pp. 98, 100–101, 103)
11. Answer: a, e (p. 100)
12. Answer: a (pp. 102, 105–106)
13. Answer: a (p. 106)
14. Answer: b (p. 106)
15. Answer: b, d (pp. 105, 106)
16. Answer: c, d (pp. 107–108)

⬧ COPING WITH CHRONIC LUNG DISEASE

Asthma is a common disorder that affects between 0.3% and 7.9% of the U.S. population.[77] It is defined as a disease of airways that is characterized by increased tracheobronchial responsivity to many stimuli, causing widespread narrowing of the air passages.[113] *Chronic obstructive pulmonary disease* (COPD, or chronic obstructive lung disease [COLD]) is a condition in which there is chronic obstruction of airflow, despite periods of improvement, due to chronic bronchitis and/or emphysema.[76] Both illnesses have important psychiatric consequences and create an ever-growing pool of chronically ill, distressed individuals as both prevalence and survival increase.[111,128] Because the psychiatric literature for asthma and COPD overlap, we will review both conditions together rather than segregate them conceptually or medically. The reader is referred to the excellent series of review articles by Thompson and Thompson[169] for additional details.

(Ventilator weaning was discussed in the previous case, Mr. Davis. Complications of tuberculosis and antituberculous drugs will be discussed in Chapter 6.)

Psychological Precipitants

Psychological and emotional issues strongly affect the course of life-threatening asthma, as has been reviewed by Creer[28] and by Lehrer and colleagues.[100] It has been found, for example, that emotional precipitants of asthmatic attacks rival allergic factors and infection.[175] One case-control study found that psychological risk factors, such as depressive symptoms and parent-staff conflicts, were prominent in severely asthmatic children who subsequently died of asthma upon discharge.[165] Asthmatic attacks may be induced by psychological stimuli, such as "suggestion," *independently* of age, gender, asthma severity, atopy, or method of pulmonary assessment[72,77,78,106,159]—a finding that demonstrates the powerful (but as yet unspecified) interactions between higher brain functions and the respiratory system. A destructive cycle results of anxiety precipitating dyspnea, and dyspnea inducing more anxiety, interfering with medical and psychiatric interventions.[79] For example, generalized anxiety increases the likelihood that as-needed asthma medications will be used inappropriately.[112] Yellowlees and Kalucy[192] have written,

If the patient misperceives the major cause of his dyspnea as being anxiety, and does not treat his asthma with bronchodilators, then he is at risk, and conversely, if he treats his anxiety as if the problem were mainly asthma, then the bronchodilators he takes are likely to exacerbate the anxiety. (p. 631)

Many asthmatic and COPD patients withdraw from interpersonal contact to minimize their stress and the associated respiratory symptoms, resulting in significant social isolation and withdrawal.[62,103,107,170] These patients may consign themselves to living in "emotional straitjackets," fearful that significant emotional expression will trigger fatal symptoms. Asthmatic individuals often choose constricted "living space," both literally and socially,[103] retreating into the home and avoiding interaction with others. It has been shown that patients with few psychosocial supports tend to fare worse medically than those with more assistance.[11]

A number of early studies have explored the relationships among course of chronic pulmonary disease, denial, and anxiety. These studies frame anxiety as the concept of *panic-fear*.[22,37,93,95] *Characterological panic-fear* refers to an enduring response pattern of anxiety, panic, helplessness, or dependency. Illness-specific panic-fear occurs in response to a medical condition.

◆ Increased morbidity and mortality occur at both ends of the spectrum. Individuals with high illness-specific and high characterological anxiety were hospitalized more frequently and needed higher doses of medications, *regardless of the severity of their illness*.[22,37,93,95] Asthmatics with very low illness-specific and characterological anxiety tended to ignore their symptoms, did not respond appropriately to changes in their medical status, and complied poorly with medication. They tended to be prematurely discharged and later rehospitalized.

Denial is a necessary ingredient for adapting to adversity. It allows the individual to maintain hope and sustain constructive action in the face of anxiety, danger, and pain. It is the fine art of titrating denial that makes the difference between comfortable adjustment to a chronic illness and life-threatening indifference. Not surprisingly, asthmatic patients with the best medical outcomes in the panic-fear studies were those with only average characterological anxiety—which perhaps prevented them from being chronically flooded by anxiety—but high illness-specific anxiety, which signaled the need for medical attention in response to physical symptoms.

◆ Whereas denial in response to a life-threatening attack of asthma may guard against psychiatric sequelae, very intense denial is a risk factor for death from asthma.[193]

◆ Three defensive styles have been described in asthmatic patients:[38] 1) an appropriate, adaptive response to asthma management; 2) "hopeless dependency" on the physician and hospital staff; and 3) "inappropriate excessive independence." The latter is associated with high use of denial and high hospitalization rates.[36]

Yellowlees and Ruffin[193] studied patients who almost died from an asthmatic attack, but survived. Twenty-five patients who suffered a near-miss death from asthma underwent comprehensive psychiatric evaluation 13 months after the episode. The researchers had hypothesized that denial would not be high in these patients because the near-death experience would mitigate their ability to deny the illness and its implications. They found, to the contrary, that *all patients had very high denial.* They responded to the near-death experience in one of two ways: 1) they increased denial even further, or 2) they developed anxiety symptoms (40% were given psychiatric diagnoses at the time of assessment). Those who became psychiatrically symptomatic were more likely to have had personal and family psychiatric illness. The authors concluded that whereas strong denial may be normal and adaptive in asthma,

> high denial and the presence of psychiatric disorder are probably the worst combination, and psychiatric referral would seem appropriate . . . Clinicians have to be aware of the need to compromise in these high risk patients between attempting to modify excessively high levels of denial . . . while trying to minimize the risk of psychiatric decompensation with its potential for increased anxiety and dependence.[193] (p. 1302, italics added)

This research has important implications for psychiatrists: carefully focused anxiety reduction may minimize

asthmatic morbidity and mortality. Similarly, therapy addressing denial in low–panic-fear patients may enhance alertness to medical symptoms, improve compliance with medical care, and thus favorably influence outcome. Factors such as patient comfort, compliance with medical treatment, and attention to the realities of daily life enter into the art of managing denial in the medical setting. When compliance is jeopardized, denial should be tactfully challenged; when it is maintaining realistic patient comfort, support it.

Psychosocial Dysfunction

Individual personality styles, previous personal and medical experiences, and sociocultural factors affect how the asthmatic patient copes with the threat of worsening airway symptoms. For example, an inability to work may trigger depressive reactions, since employment is a highly prized and valued role for many patients.[87]

Several studies have assessed quality of life and psychosocial functioning in these patients.[62,69,91,115,136] Ambulatory and hospitalized patients with respiratory disease have been impaired on *all dimensions* compared with age-matched control subjects, particularly in areas such as household management, physical mobility, sleep and rest, social interactions, and recreation.[115] This finding demonstrates the major disturbances in daily living produced by chronic obstructive airways disease.[62] Of note, however, is that patients with richer psychosocial supports were more successful in protecting themselves from attacks of dyspnea, carried out treatment programs more carefully and responsibly, and generally outlived their counterparts who lacked such skills.[40]

Williams[182] and Rabinowitz and Florian[138] have recently reviewed the psychosocial issues of COPD patients more extensively.

Families

Chronic respiratory disease inevitably affects lifestyle and families.[129,150] Patients who have become phobic, reclusive, and extremely dependent burden their families enormously; those who react to loss and illness with anger may alienate potential supporters.[99] Asthma's life-threatening, sudden exacerbations engender anxiety and anger in families, especially when patients cope by denying their illness. Family members witness and remember the terrifying exacerbations, in contrast to the patient, who may be amnestic for some of the worst.[193]

◆ Significant disruptions occur in families of patients suffering a near-miss death from asthma.[193] Whereas the families wanted to overprotect the patients, the patients preferred to minimize their illness; anger, anxiety, and resentment were experienced by all. Anger tended to be suppressed by family members for fear of upsetting the patient and exacerbating the asthma.

For those who consciously or unconsciously believe in the destructive power of angry or negative feelings, fact and fantasy collide here. Interpersonal communication may deteriorate, and the psychosocial morbidity of the illness mushrooms.

◆ On the other hand, Yellowlees and Ruffin[193] found that marital relationships improved following a near-miss asthma death, with both partners becoming more aware of their mortality and their positive feelings toward each other.

Sexuality

The causes of sexual dysfunction in patients with pulmonary disease are varied. Some patients experience a decline in sexual function that parallels worsening pulmonary function tests, at times without identifiable psychiatric factors such as depression.[2,50,88] Concurrent illnesses (e.g., diabetes, hypertension) as well as medications may also interfere with sexual performance. Older patients are at particular risk. Asthmatic patients are additionally vulnerable to developing phobic reactions to situations that affect their breathing, such as showering, shaving, going to the toilet, eating alone, riding in elevators, or being away from home without an inhaler or a companion.[192] The pattern of avoidance is reinforced by reduced contact with asthmatic triggers or allergens in their daily lives. The dyspnea of sexual excitement may also become a feared trigger, producing conditioned avoidance of sexual activities or performance and interacting with preexisting conflicts about sexuality. A complex tangle of psychodynamics, learning, and physiology can result, highlighted by the disruptions of established roles already endured by the patient. Issues such as self-esteem, physical sense of well-being, perceptions about attractiveness, fears of rejection, previous sexual functioning, and fantasies about illness add to the patient's misery.

We advocate an eclectic approach that incorporates principles of psychodynamically informed psychotherapy with behavioral and cognitive techniques. The reader interested in the specific techniques of treating sexual dysfunction in medically ill patients is referred to the excellent review by Fagan and Schmidt.[45]

Medical and Psychological Factors

Neuropsychiatric Effects of Chronic Hypoxia

We next briefly summarize the highlights of the literature on cognitive dysfunction in COPD patients, which occurs in over half of even mildly hypoxemic patients[48,63,64,137] in areas such as

◆ Concentration
◆ Recall
◆ Abstract reasoning
◆ Complex perceptual motor integration
◆ Language function

Chronic hypoxia is associated with elevated hematocrit as well as with impaired memory.[15,184] Overall intelligence testing of patients with COPD places them in the average range, but with subtle cognitive changes that become most evident during times of stress.[66] It was thought that supplemental oxygen might reverse the difficulties,[12,70] but this has not been consistently corroborated.[75]

Remember that it is *the rate at which hypoxia develops* that determines the acute neuropsychiatric consequences of hypoxemia, not the absolute level of oxygen saturation.[4,68,83,105] In the setting of chronic hypoxia, for example, oxygen saturations as low as 60% may produce few changes, whereas abrupt changes usually result in delirium.[4,105] Similarly, acute increases of P_{CO_2} to 70 mm Hg will produce confusional states, while patients with chronic hypercapnia may preserve alertness at P_{CO_2} levels as high as 90 mm Hg.[44] Hypercapnia produces a metabolic acidosis, and there is a correlation between the severity of the patient's neuropsychiatric symptoms and the concomitant cerebrospinal fluid (CSF) acidosis.[135] Carbon dioxide retention produces anesthetic-like changes that resemble barbiturate intoxication,[83] not amphetamine psychosis.

One study combined data from two multicenter clinical trials to explore the nature and possible determinants of neuropsychological change in patients with COPD.[65] Patients were divided into three groups: mild hypoxemia ($P_{aO_2} > 59$ mm Hg; $n = 86$), moderate hypoxemia (P_{aO_2} 50–59 mm Hg; $n = 155$), or severe hypoxemia ($P_{aO_2} < 50$ mm Hg; $n = 61$). They were compared with age- and education-matched nonpatient controls. Although the rate of neuropsychological impairment in mildly hypoxemic patients was not substantially higher than in the control subjects, impairment was dramatically higher in those who were most severely hypoxemic.

◆ Clinical lore has flagged alertness as a sensitive indicator of oxygenation, but in this study *alertness was preserved even with moderate hypoxemia.* Alertness was affected only in *extreme* hypoxia.

This finding has implications for the consulting psychiatrist: estimating a patient's level of alertness at the bedside will have limited value in predicting cognitive functioning or level of hypoxemia; hypoxic, cognitively impaired patients may appear perfectly alert. Several other findings are notable:

◆ The effects of progressive hypoxemia became most apparent in *perceptual learning* and *problem solving,* the neuropsychological tests that are most sensitive to cerebral dysfunction.

◆ Surprisingly, other measures of disease severity, such as pulmonary function tests, did *not* predict the level of neuropsychological deficit.

◆ The degree of hypoxemia was *not* necessarily congruent with the extent of lung disease (as measured by pulmonary function tests). For example, some patients who were only mildly hypoxemic showed advanced lung disease.

These data suggest that neuropsychological abilities decline differentially in response to COPD. Factors beyond the objective degree of lung pathology influence brain dysfunction.[65] Nevertheless, hypoxemia seems to be a potent predictor of neuropsychological deficits. Elderly patients with chronic respiratory disease are particularly susceptible. Neuropsychological assessment may help shape a treatment program for them.

Mood, Subjective Dyspnea, and Objective Pulmonary Function

The assessment of dyspnea is controversial in the asthma literature; it is a complex symptom, with many elements that influence its perception and measurement.[130] Far from being a reliably measurable relationship, there is contradictory evidence regarding the subjective sense of dyspnea and corresponding measures of pulmonary function, with some studies reporting evidence of such a correlation[153,181] while others do not.[20,49,102,114,167,189]

◆ For example, there is wide variation among individuals in subjective dyspnea corresponding to any given forced expiratory volume in 1 second (FEV_1).[18]

Several explanations may account for this inconsistency:

◆ One is methodological: assessed dyspnea levels vary within a single patient and among different patients according to the method of assessment,[108,182] leading to proposals that more than one measure of dyspnea be used in research protocols.[90]

◆ Second, although emotional factors operate in all illnesses, such factors are particularly potent in respiratory disease—anxiety exacerbates and overlaps with the diseased lung's primary physical symptom, dyspnea. It often is impossible to tease apart the two.

Anxiety obviously affects breathing, but it is less apparent that ventilatory response to inhaled CO_2 is also affected by depression[3,151,152] and grief[80] in patients without lung disease. Mood also influences dyspnea in respiratory patients.[19,40,74] Several authors have investigated the effects of depression on objective and subjective measures of pulmonary function. Some of their findings follow:

◆ Depression is a significant predictor of self-rated dyspnea.[90]

◆ Dyspnea in patients with chronic pulmonary disease has been associated with hypoventilation in response to depressed mood.[42]

◆ Depression[29] and hypnosis-induced depressed mood[41] predispose to carbon dioxide retention.

◆ Depressed patients with chronic bronchitis have shown less exercise tolerance than their nondepressed counterparts.[126,126a]

◆ Psychosocial impairment significantly improved in depressed COPD patients on nortriptyline.[16]

Depression also correlates with self-rated *breathlessness.*[79]

◆ For example, Kellner and colleagues[90] examined the relationship of dyspnea to anxiety and depression in patients with chronic respiratory impairment. Anxiety and depression were measured with the Symptom Checklist–90[31a] and the Symptom Questionnaire.[89a,89b]

- They found that *self-rated breathlessness was significantly associated with self-rated depression,* and that *depression was predictive of breathlessness* in multiple regression analyses. When the sample was limited to patients with COPD, the results remained the same. These patients were significantly more depressed and anxious than matched family-practice patients.

- Moreover, results varied with the method of assessing dyspnea—a finding that highlights the lack of reliability in dyspnea assessment, which is influenced by emotional as well as physical factors.

These data have practical consequences for the psychiatrist working with asthmatic and COPD patients. *When complaints of dyspnea are disproportionate to the objective respiratory disease, they may signal treatable psychological distress.* The nature of the association between depression and pulmonary function remains speculative. What is unambiguous, however, is that disability more closely correlates with the *subjective* perception of dyspnea than with *objectively* measured pulmonary function,[69,84,183] and that affective state influences the *perception* of dyspnea.[178,179]

Physician-Related Assessment Factors

Despite the growing literature on the comorbidity of chronic medical conditions and mood disorders, a large percentage of affectively ill medical patients go unrecognized and untreated. As Zung and colleagues[194] have observed, many physicians do not consider the depressive symptoms to be adequate reason for further workup unless they are severe (e.g., suicidal ideation) or obvious (e.g., visible psychomotor retardation). Physicians may ignore depressive symptoms because the illness may be considered "reason enough" for patients to be depressed. In addition, the physical symptoms of medical disease often overlap with somatic symptoms of depression, making the two difficult to discriminate. This has important implications for patient management, since individuals with both a chronic illness and depression have been shown to be more disabled than those with either one.[161,180] Moreover, such comorbidity magnifies the costs of health care: depressed medical patients use more primary care services, especially emergency care, than do their chronically ill, nondepressed counterparts.[7,89]

Only a few studies have specifically examined the relationship between chronic respiratory patients and their physicians.[6,36] In one, the physician's personality was shown to influence medical assessments.[36] Physicians were rated for sensitivity to their patients' needs. The "low sensitivity" physicians related to their patients as specimens of "pulmonary pathology," whereas the high-sensitivity ones treated their patients as "whole human beings." The three physician groups (low, moderate, and high sensitivity) did not differ regarding medical decisions (e.g., length of hospitalization, amount of medication prescribed). However, *judgments of illness severity were found to be biased by physician sensitivity:*

◆ **Low-sensitivity physicians** were influenced more by the patient's personality than by objective indices of

pulmonary function, interpreting personality characteristics as reflecting illness severity, and confusing psychological and physical distress.
◆ **High-sensitivity physicians** distinguished between psychological and physical distress and were able to accurately interpret the severity of their patients' illness based on pulmonary function tests. However, certain medical decisions (such as the recommendation for oral steroids) were inappropriately influenced by patient personality variables. The authors[36] commented that these physicians tended to treat psychological problems as though they were medical.
◆ **Moderate-sensitivity physicians** were most objective and appropriate. They were best able to distinguish between psychological and physical distress, basing judgments of illness severity on pulmonary function results rather than personality.

Studies like these *are reminders than transference and countertransference reactions are not limited to the psychotherapy hour.* Psychiatrists are often asked to help negotiate the overlap of personality and psychodynamics occurring with "difficult patients" and "difficult physicians." This is one more arena in which psychological factors have an impact on treatment decisions and disease outcome.

Psychotoxicity of Medications

Steroids

Steroids are the pulmonary medications most often implicated in producing psychiatric side effects, which span the full spectrum of symptoms (refer to the extensive review in Chapter 5). A few brief points for emphasis follow:

◆ *Even low-dose steroids* may produce subclinical impairments in a patient's ability to process new information, filter out distracting information, and respond appropriately to environmental cues. For patients with chronic hypoxia, low-dose steroid therapy may exacerbate preexisting cognitive problems.
◆ Many patients are reluctant to comply with steroid treatment because of adverse side effects, leading to "steroid phobia"[30,131,187] and exacerbations of their pulmonary disease.
◆ Consider steroid administration and/or withdrawal in the differential diagnosis of new psychiatric symptoms ranging from anxiety through affective illness and psychotic disturbances.

Theophylline and Bronchodilators

Theophylline and sympathomimetic bronchodilators may induce anxiety, jitteriness, restlessness, irritability, and insomnia. These side effects are both dose- and temporally related to the medication. They are managed by tapering to the minimum therapeutic dose and by changing the specific type of theophylline preparation or the dosage timing. Theophylline toxicity produces marked anxiety, severe nausea, and sometimes delirium with psychotic features.

When theophylline exacerbates essential tremor, barbiturates or benzodiazepines may improve it;[170] remember, however, that beta-blockers are relatively contraindicated because of the potential for bronchospasm.

⚙ ANXIETY DISORDERS

There is a well-documented relationship between respiratory disease and anxiety disorders. The prevalence of anxiety disorders in asthmatic patients has been estimated at 34%,[191,193] a considerably higher rate than the 2%–5% prevalence estimated in the general population.[171] The reported prevalence of panic disorder among asthmatic[10,23,192] and COPD patients is also high—as much as 8%[85] to 24%.[190] Moreover, the hyperventilation that occurs with anxiety may in turn precipitate an asthmatic attack in susceptible patients.[71]

Theophylline, sympathomimetic bronchodilators, and steroid administration or withdrawal may also induce anxiety symptoms that are often difficult to distinguish from a primary anxiety disorder.

At a pathophysiological level, a number of factors suggest that asthmatic patients may have a biological diathesis for anxiety disorders:[22,192]

◆ Hyperventilation and hypersensitivity to carbon dioxide have been described in respiratory disease patients and those with panic disorder.[60]

◆ Panic attacks can be induced by CO_2 rebreathing, lactate acid infusion, or hyperventilation.[59] Could a similar mechanism also operate in patients with chronic airways obstruction,[190] in which hyperventilation occurs in response to a chronically elevated P_{CO_2} level? Might there be a subset of vulnerable asthmatic patients with a neurophysiological or neuroanatomical diathesis to panic attacks?

◆ Some preliminary evidence suggests a neurophysiological and/or a neuropathological basis for panic in patients with asthma. The respiratory centers in the brain stem are connected via the hippocampal formation to the parahippocampal region,[157] a major reception area for all sensory modalities that seems to be anatomically different in patients with panic disorder.[144,145] Positron-emission tomography (PET) has shown that patients susceptible to lactate-induced panic have abnormal hemispheric asymmetry of parahippocampal blood flow, blood volume, and oxygen metabolism.[145] These patients were abnormally susceptible to hyperventilation-induced panic, prompting speculation that hyperventilation may lead to parahippocampal abnormalities and continued panic attacks in asthmatic individuals via a feedback loop.[192] Hypothetically, a preexisting—possibly inherited—parahippocampal abnormality could make asthmatic patients more vulnerable to panic attacks.[192]

◆ Yellowlees and Kalucy[192] have speculated that imipramine's effectiveness in asthma may be due not only to imipramine's intrinsic bronchodilatory effect but also to a reregulation of the same autonomic hyperactivity thought to occur in panic patients. Hypothetically, there may be an inherited hypersensitivity of medullary chemoreceptors in panic disorder,[21] with administration of antipanic drugs (e.g., imipramine) reducing the response threshold of these neurons and thereby blocking the panic attack.[61]

Somatization

Although asthmatic patients do not have a higher incidence of conversion disorder, hypochondriasis, or malingering, some patients may somatize their anxiety,[19,37,90,168] presenting with chest discomfort, pain, or tightness accompanied by overt hyperventilation and dyspnea. This may represent a learned response to illness:

> The production of somatic symptoms related to the chest is as good an expression of anxiety as if the [asthmatic] patient were to tell his physician that he felt anxious.[192] (p. 631)

Consult the literature review on somatization in pulmonary patients by Thompson and Thompson[168] for additional details and several case examples.

⚙ MAJOR DEPRESSION

Incidence

Mrs. Albert's symptoms are consistent with major depression. Certainly, depression is common among lung disease patients.[2,40,62,115] Borson and colleagues'[16] review of the literature estimated the comorbidity of COPD and depression as exceeding 20%. In one report, COPD patients on long-term oxygen therapy showed a high degree of anxiety, depression, and low self-esteem and did not believe in the efficacy of their medical therapy.[14] A chart review study found that many asthmatic patients experienced at least fleeting suicidal ideation, with a significantly higher incidence of suicide and suicide attempts than in a group of hypertensive patients.[104]

- McSweeney and colleagues[116] have speculated that hypoxemia affects emotions by causing inadequate oxygenation of the limbic system and other brain areas that mediate emotional behavior. This hypothesis awaits confirmatory data.

The symptoms of chronic respiratory disease overlap with those of depression, such as fatigue, lethargy, and loss of interest in activities.[170] Vegetative symptoms are less useful than the quality of mood and the thought content in assessing depression.

- Sleep disruption is common in respiratory patients, complicating insomnia as an indicator of depression. It can be caused by nocturnal asthma attacks, coughing, or sleep apnea. Structural or functional impairment anywhere along the respiratory tract makes disturbed breathing during sleep more likely.[143]

⚕ PSYCHOPHARMACOLOGY

Anxiolytics and Respiration

Benzodiazepines

Normally, increased carbon dioxide is the physiological stimulus that drives breathing. Patients who have chronic lung disease and are hypercapnic lose their sensitivity to increased carbon dioxide (P_{CO_2}).

- As a result, they become more dependent on dips in oxygen saturation (i.e., hypoxia) to stimulate breathing.
- Thus, administering oxygen to chronically hypercapnic patients may cause them to stop breathing; it lessens their drive to breathe.[98]
- Benzodiazepines may further exacerbate the chronically hypercapnic patient's problem because they further reduce the ventilatory response to hypoxia.[98]
- In addition, this blunted sensitivity to hypoxia may induce more hypercapnia, initiating a vicious cycle: chronically increased P_{CO_2} leads to further *dependence* on hypoxia to drive breathing, but in the setting

of benzodiazepine-induced diminished *sensitivity* to hypoxia, there is further carbon dioxide retention.

- If this process occurs in a patient with marginal respiratory reserve, respiratory failure can rapidly follow.

The respiratory-depressant effects of the long-acting benzodiazepines, such as diazepam (Valium) and chlordiazepoxide (Librium), are well established.[24,26,73,82,97,139,172]

- Patients with moderate to severe COPD are at risk for carbon dioxide retention with long-acting oral benzodiazepines even at relatively low doses.[170]
- Respiratory depression gradually worsens as active metabolites accumulate, with the potential for significant benzodiazepine-induced carbon dioxide retention.[125]
- One study found that "pink puffers" (who do not retain carbon dioxide) *improved* their exercise tolerance with benzodiazepines,[124] but subsequent randomized, double-blind, placebo-controlled studies failed to substantiate this finding.[110,188] However, anxiety was not an inclusion criterion;[67] for example, the investigators in one of the studies[110] found no significant difference in anxiety scores of subjects receiving placebo and subjects receiving diazepam therapy, making a diagnosis of anxiety in their study population unlikely.
- Keep in mind that many patients with chronic respiratory disease suffer sleep apnea,[143] and that benzodiazepines are contraindicated in this condition.[119]

Studies on the respiratory effects of anxiolytics have used COPD subjects. Although all benzodiazepines cause some respiratory depression, intermediate-acting agents are the anxiolytics of choice,[83] since they have fewer respiratory-depressant effects than do sedative-hypnotics or barbiturates.[26,82] Several small studies have examined the intermediate-acting benzodiazepines:

- Subjects breathing elevated levels of carbon dioxide showed no respiratory change when they received intravenous oxazepam (Serax).[160] However, the sample was small (N = 4), and oxazepam has been approved by the FDA for oral use only.
- Oral temazepam (Restoril) has been associated with respiratory depression in healthy volunteers at 40 mg but not at 20 mg.[134]
- Both lorazepam (Ativan) and diazepam (Valium) induced respiratory depression with slight respiratory acidosis in COPD patients, but *lorazepam caused no significant hypoxemia.*[31]

◆ Surprisingly, another investigation reported *respiratory stimulation* after oral lorazepam.[39]

◆ In a case report of one patient, Greene and colleagues[67] found that a single 0.5-mg test dose of alprazolam (Xanax) produced significant improvement in objective and subjective assessments of dyspnea, anxiety, alertness, and other measures. Alprazolam produced no inhibition of the drive to breathe. Note, however, that withdrawal symptoms limit alprazolam's usefulness in the medically ill.

Based on these data, benzodiazepines should not be automatically rejected for patients with lung disease; when anxiety worsens respiratory function, their judicious use may actually improve respiratory status. Baseline blood gases and pulmonary consultation are necessary, of course, in deciding on the appropriateness of benzodiazepines. Blood gases should be rechecked following dose increments after steady state is reached. As discussed, lorazepam (Ativan) and oxazepam (Serax) have no active metabolites and are generally well tolerated in the medically ill. They are considered the benzodiazepines of choice in patients with lung disease.[83]

Buspirone

The nonsedating, nonaddictive azapirone anxiolytic buspirone (BuSpar) may be an alternative to benzodiazepines in pulmonary patients. Unlike diazepam, buspirone does not depress respiration in healthy volunteers, potentially making it a safer anxiolytic.[56,140,141] Although based on small studies, several trends reported in the literature are notable:

◆ Buspirone does not adversely interact with bronchodilators such as theophylline (Theo-Dur) and terbutaline (Bricanyl).[92]

◆ It has increased respiratory rate both in animal experiments and in preliminary studies with humans.[55,121]

◆ Buspirone has been used effectively in sleep apnea.[120] The patients in this study ($N = 5$) fell asleep sooner, slept longer, and slept more soundly on buspirone than on no medication. The number of episodes of apnea per hour decreased after buspirone, while the mean minimum arterial oxygen saturation remained unchanged. Because benzodiazepines should not be used in sleep apnea, buspirone may be a good alternative.

◆ Buspirone was prescribed in seven patients with anxiety disorders and obstructive lung disease at daily doses of 15–45 mg under open clinical conditions.[27] Six of the subjects were receiving continuous oxygen by nasal prongs, four had arterial carbon dioxide pressures of greater than 65 mm Hg, and five were awaiting lung transplantation. Two subjects discontinued the trial: one underwent transplantation, and the other developed delirium of unknown etiology. The mean anxiety ratings for the five subjects who completed the trial decreased by 44%; panic attacks fell from three per week to less than one per week. One patient was able to reduce his bronchodilators because of less panic anxiety. Several subjects reported less avoidance of anxiety-provoking situations and improved functional ability. None showed deterioration in respiratory function or increased carbon dioxide concentrations.

◆ Less promisingly, buspirone failed to improve anxiety or exercise tolerance in a double-blind, placebo-controlled randomized study of mildly anxious COPD patients ($N = 11$) given 30–60 mg/day for 6 weeks. There was no deterioration in respiratory function or exercise tolerance.[156]

The failure to improve anxiety in the last study is contrary to findings from several other studies, which have shown buspirone to be as effective as the benzodiazepines.[132] Moreover, an added advantage is that buspirone's pharmacokinetics do not always change in elderly patients.[54,132,146] More double-blind, placebo-controlled studies of buspirone are needed in moderately to severely anxious pulmonary patients to test its efficacy in this population. One potential drawback of buspirone, however, is that it often requires several days to weeks before a therapeutic effect is felt. Most medically ill patients require more immediate relief, especially in the hospital setting. For them, the benzodiazepines remain without peer.

Other Anxiolytics

The antihistamines, such as hydroxyzine (Vistaril, Atarax) and diphenhydramine (Benadryl), afford mild to moderate anxiolytic relief without respiratory depression[81] but may not be sufficiently effective for the severely anxious patient whose dyspnea and anxiety are mutually exacerbating.

Beta-blockers like propranolol are contraindicated for anxiolysis because they cause bronchoconstriction.[170]

Sedative-hypnotics and barbiturates (e.g., sodium amytal) have significant respiratory-depressant effects and should be avoided.

Adverse Drug Interactions

Anxiolytics generally do not adversely interact with common respiratory medications.

Neuroleptics

There are times when pulmonary patients are incapacitated by panic about suffocating, which worsens their dyspnea and psychological state. Although they need immediate relief, medical clearance for benzodiazepines may be withheld. In these situations, a brief course of low-dose, high-potency neuroleptics like haloperidol (Haldol)[163] can save the day, as long as dystonic effects on respiration do not occur.

◆ Alternatively, we have found that small doses of thioridazine (Mellaril) (10–25 mg po tid-qid prn anxiety) are safe and extremely effective for medically fragile patients. This agent does not depress respirations and, like the benzodiazepines, acts almost immediately. Because thioridazine's potential side effects are anticholinergic and cardiotoxic, it should not be used in the setting of delirium or conduction disease. Beware of additive anticholinergic effects with atropine, antihistamines, and some bronchodilators. We routinely check the ECG within the first week of thioridazine, as well as include blood pressure parameters before each as-needed dose (e.g., "hold for systolic blood pressure < 100, diastolic blood pressure < 60").

◆ Tardive dyskinesia is a risk of long-term treatment with all neuroleptics, so these agents should be used only as a brief intervention.

◆ An unexpected consequence of a neuroleptic order may be that the medical staff infers that the patient has been psychotic. Therefore, the rationale for starting a neuroleptic for anxiolysis should be documented clearly in the patient's chart.

Note that allergic asthma,[162] as well as respiratory arrest and depression,[47,51,53,147] has been associated with the novel antipsychotic clozapine (Clozaril). This medication should be used with careful respiratory monitoring.

Adverse Drug Interactions

The more sedating neuroleptics, such as thioridazine (Mellaril) and chlorpromazine (Thorazine), may produce additive anticholinergic effects with atropine, the atropine derivative ipratropium (Atrovent inhaler), and antihistamines.[170]

Antidepressants

Efficacy

Pulmonary disease poses few problems for antidepressant management.[83] The most experience has accumulated with tricyclics. Most TCAs have little or no effect on respiratory status as long as they are prescribed appropriately.[43,160,170] In fact, some (e.g., doxepin [Sinequan]) may act as mild bronchodilators[43] and may markedly improve the functional status of certain asthma patients.[192] Early studies established the efficacy and safety of the tricyclics in asthmatic patients.[57,118,166] Most recently, a double-blind, placebo-controlled study of depressed COPD patients showed that mood, certain respiratory symptoms, overall physical comfort, and day-to-day functioning significantly improved with nortriptyline (Pamelor, Aventyl).[16]

◆ MAOIs are more problematic because of the risk of interactions with epinephrine, which is used to treat acute asthmatic attacks.

◆ In an interesting anecdotal report,[58] a depressed patient suffering from severe asthma that required multiple trips to the emergency room for epinephrine injections was treated as an inpatient with MAOI therapy. Her suicidal depression had been refractory to standard tricyclic treatment. (SSRIs were not yet available.) The pulmonary consultant had carefully outlined a plan for managing the patient's asthma should an attack occur while receiving the MAOI. Her depression remitted after 4 weeks on the antidepressant, and to the surprise of all, she never had another asthma attack. Was the antidepressant acting specifically to relieve the respiratory pathology, perhaps by elevating endogenous catecholamine levels and therefore serving as a bronchodilator? Or was it the relief of her depression that contributed to the remission of asthmatic attacks? The answers to such questions await additional research.

There are no published controlled studies regarding the use of the newer antidepressants specifically in respiratory disease. These medications are usually well tolerated in medically ill patients, however, with rare cardiovascular effects. There are no known effects on respiration. We suggest cautiously trying them in this population, with careful monitoring, until more data become available.

Side Effects

Many pulmonary patients are elderly and have multisystem disease, so choose an antidepressant that minimizes side effects like hypotension, cardiotoxicity, and anticholinergic effects. Tricyclic anticholinergic effects may promote drying of bronchial secretions, making them more tenacious and promoting bronchial plugging.[83] Start with low doses and carefully titrate upward. Patients with compromised pulmonary status, especially COPD or sleep apnea, should generally receive the less-sedating tricyclic drugs,[170] like nortriptyline. Keep in mind that the synergistic effects of other sedating drugs, such as anxiolytics, may depress the respiratory drive.

◆ We know of only two reports describing a possible association of fluoxetine (Prozac) and pulmonary damage.[8,57a] These cases appear to involve idiosyncratic reactions.

Tartrazine Dye

Tartrazine (FD&C Yellow #5), a dye contained in several psychotropic drugs, can provoke severe bronchospasms for up to several hours after ingestion. Susceptible individuals may have a history of sensitivity to aspirin and bronchospasm from foods colored yellow or orange, such as soft drinks or candy.[148,149] Fortunately, only a small percentage of asthmatic patients respond with severe exacerbations,[155,174] and the pharmaceutical companies have been phasing out tartrazine.[170] It is best to avoid tartrazine-containing medications in patients with asthma or COPD, unless tartrazine sensitivity has been specifically excluded.[170]

Adverse Drug Interactions

The antidepressants have a number of adverse interactions with drugs prescribed for chronic respiratory disease. Refer to Ciraulo et al.[24a] for a more complete survey.

◆ Tricyclics potentiate the anticholinergic effects of the bronchodilator atropine[5] and its derivatives (e.g., ipratropium [Atrovent inhaler]).
◆ Tricyclics may also potentiate the pressor effects of epinephrine.[13]
◆ Progestational agents are sometimes given to patients with sleep apnea, and may elevate tricyclic levels by interfering with their hepatic metabolism.[170]
◆ It is usually safe to use TCAs with the more selective beta$_2$-agonists, such as terbutaline (Bricanyl), metaproterenol (Alupent), albuterol (Proventil), and isoetharine (Bronkometer).[170]
◆ MAOIs interact with a number of antiasthmatic medications (except the steroid inhalers). They intensify and prolong the effects of epinephrine, anti-

histamines, and anticholinergic agents.[5] MAOIs are contraindicated with sympathomimetic agents such as phenylephrine (Neo-Synephrine), pseudoephedrine (Novafed), ephedrine, and metaproterenol (Alupent).[170]

Physostigmine, which is used to reverse anticholinergic crisis, may precipitate bronchospasm in asthmatic patients and should be used with caution.[9]

We know of no reported interactions between the newer antidepressants and respiratory medications, except for several reports of the antiobsessional SSRI fluvoxamine (Luvox) causing toxic theophylline serum concentrations.[35a,141a,159a,170a,172a]

Electroconvulsive Therapy

Theophylline (Theo-Dur) produces one of the rare instances in consultation-liaison psychiatry in which ECT is relatively contraindicated.[1] Theophylline substantially increases the risk of inducing status epilepticus during ECT, with consequent brain damage or even death.[35,133] As reviewed by Rasmussen and Zorumski,[142] theophylline should be tapered in patients who must receive ECT.

Treatment of patients with COPD should focus on maximizing respiratory function prior to ECT; Welch[177] has pointed out that since the underlying problem is not a diffusion gradient, using 100% oxygen will not help. He suggests using aggressive pulmonary physical therapy in combination with bronchodilators and steroids first. Patients should bring their inhaler to the ECT treatment room, where it can be used several minutes before their treatment. Patients with COPD or asthma may be at relatively higher risk for bronchial spasm following ECT,[46] although opinion varies, with some feeling that there is no greater risk provided that beta-blockers are avoided.[177]

Knos and Sung[96] recommend spirometry prior to ECT to test pulmonary reserve. Values that indicate an increased risk for morbidity and mortality are as follows:[96]

◆ Forced vital capacity (FVC) < 50% predicted value
◆ Forced expiratory volume at 1 second (FEV$_1$) < 50% predicted (or < 2 L)
◆ FEV$_1$/FVC < 50%
◆ Maximal voluntary ventilation (MVV) < 50% predicted (or < 50 L/minute)
◆ Forced expiratory flow at 25%–75% of the vital capacity (FEF$_{25-75}$) < 50% predicted

They recommend that patients who do not meet these minimal criteria have their treatment optimized first by an internist. More seriously impaired patients should be managed in collaboration with a pulmonologist. Additional practical details regarding ECT in the medically ill can be found in the reviews by Knos and Sung,[96] Weiner and Coffey,[176] and Zwil and Pelchat.[195]

Psychotherapy

Most of the literature on the psychotherapy of chronic respiratory disease patients focuses on the role of psychological interventions in minimizing asthmatic attacks. As thoroughly summarized by Lehrer and colleagues,[101] these methodologies include psychoeducational approaches to the self-management of asthma,[25] family therapy, and stress management approaches such as relaxation therapies and biofeedback.

One of the goals of all psychotherapies is to reinforce the fact that dyspnea does not necessarily mean imminent death or danger. The belief that emotional expression or confrontation will cause fatal shortness of breath poses an important resistance in psychotherapy. Psychoanalytically informed, cognitive, and behavioral therapies all lessen the morbidity of chronic respiratory disease when patients are appropriately selected and sensitively managed.[170]

The early psychoanalytic literature posited that specific conflicts were etiological in developing psychosomatic illness. Asthma was one of the seven "classic" psychosomatic disorders. Its cause was thought to be a specific psychological conflict—namely, strong unconscious dependency wishes toward the mother, coupled with fears of separation from her.[52] Such a unifocal hypothesis is obsolete in current psychoanalytic thinking, confusing cause and effect. Contemporary psychoanalytic case reports demonstrate that powerful psychodynamic issues operate for most respiratory patients. Mushatt and Werby[127] have written,

> The argument as to whether clinical phenomena are psychosomatic or somatopsychic tends to become irrelevant if one utilizes [F.] Deutsch's concept of the mind-body-environment relationship.[32] Loss or disharmony in human relationships (with depression) or anticipation of loss or disruption of relationships (with anxiety) may be expressed in physical terms. Disturbance of physical function may evoke a sense of loss or threat of it in relation to key figures in the environment. (p. 83)

Conflicts about dependency and self-esteem and fantasies about the "toxic" effects of feelings are particularly

relevant to the pulmonary patient. Intense psychological states can exacerbate asthmatic attacks, and psychological conflict is a potent asthmatic trigger.

◆ For example, patients suffering from repeated asthmatic attacks may symbolically elaborate the physiological traumatic experience and may become preoccupied with the symbolic meanings of air, choking, and infection.[122,123]

When symbolic conflicts can precipitate an asthmatic attack, they become etiologically meaningful.[33,34] A patient's associations to these conflicts contain fantasies and memories concerning significant people in the patient's childhood and adult life. Several recent analytic case reports illustrate this observation[86,154,185] and review psychoanalytic conceptualizations of asthma in greater detail.

Clearly, not all patients are suitable for psychodynamically informed psychotherapy. However, sometimes the best "support" for a medically ill patient is clarifying psychological conflict and working toward insight. An approach that integrates techniques from several therapeutic methodologies, incorporating conflict resolution, pharmacotherapy, and behavioral techniques, offers patients the best chance for relief.

◆ For example, teaching asthmatic patients to systematically control their respiration through cognitive and behavioral methods, thus minimizing hyperventilation at the first suggestion of worsening dyspnea, could abort those attacks with a psychogenic/cognitive trigger.[58]
◆ Meany et al.[117] reported on the multimodal psychological treatment of an asthmatic patient using dreams, biofeedback, and pain behavior modification.
◆ Snadden and Brown[158] published excerpts of interviews with asthmatic patients concerning their experiences. The approach was qualitative, naturalistic, and narrative, and offered insights missing from the prevalent quantitative psychosomatic research. The asthmatic patient's need for a "mentoring relationship" was a consistent finding. This was defined as a protected relationship—with a physician, a health worker, or another asthmatic patient—in which learning, experimentation, and acquisition of illness-management skills could be developed. Not surprisingly, asthma imposed physical limitations on all participants, irrespective of the illness severity.
◆ Wise et al.[186] described a depressed 65-year-old woman with COPD who was treated with psychotherapy and buspirone (BuSpar). (A history of ventricular

irritability had precluded the use of antidepressants.) The authors used the life trajectory method of psychotherapy,[173] which frames a context for reactions to illness within the patient's life history. Other treatment modalities, including creative arts therapy and environmental support, were incorporated into a successful treatment plan. This case is a model for integrating psychosocial and biological approaches to the patient with severe pulmonary disease.

Group therapy[136,170] and self-help support groups[158] can be quite helpful for chronic respiratory patients, who are often socially isolated as a result of conditioned avoidance and fear.

Psychotherapy "Side Effects"

Interestingly, psychotherapy is not free of respiratory side effects—the confrontation of difficult feelings and situations may lead to hyperventilation and provoke an asthmatic attack. Patients should be encouraged to bring their as-needed medications (e.g., bronchodilator inhalers) to therapy sessions.[170] When patients "forget" to bring their medications, resistance to treatment can be discussed. Successful therapy can potentially reduce emergency room visits and hospital admissions. Breathing retraining can improve ventilation and minimize fears of dyspnea.

◆ Paradoxically, relaxation training may sometimes exacerbate asthmatic attacks[94] because of diminished signal anxiety and lessened vigilance toward early-warning symptoms. Ongoing monitoring and reassessment are important.

◆ Patients with respiratory problems are made anxious by the very suggestion that they "breathe easily." Behavioral exercises for relaxation may paradoxically induce *more* anxiety if the technique, which classically encourages the subject to take slow, deep breaths, is not modified for this population. Hypnosis may also be helpful for lung disease patients, but the instruction to breathe easily should be omitted from the hypnotic suggestion. Instead, patients should be encouraged to concentrate either on a tranquil scene or on a single concept.[17,109]

⚘ SUMMARY

1. Emotions and mood states—including depression—have powerful effects on pulmonary function. Anxiety can interfere with pulmonary assessment, begin-

ning a destructive cycle of anxiety-dyspnea-anxiety. For patients who believe in the destructive power of angry or negative feelings, fact and fantasy collide here. Interpersonal communication may deteriorate, and the psychosocial morbidity of the illness mushrooms. Phobic avoidance of anxiety-provoking situations, such as sexual encounters, may supervene. Panic disorder and depression are more prevalent among patients with chronic lung disease than among the general population.

2. Although denial in response to a life-threatening illness may guard against psychiatric sequelae, simultaneous high denial and psychiatric disorder are a dangerous combination. Factors such as patient comfort, compliance with medical treatment, and attention to the realities of daily life enter into the art of managing denial in the medical setting. When compliance is jeopardized, it is most constructive to challenge denial; when denial is maintaining realistic patient comfort, however, it should be supported.

3. Hypoxemia is associated with cognitive dysfunction in areas such as concentration, recall, abstract reasoning, complex perceptual-motor integration, and language function. Alertness remains relatively resistant to even moderate hypoxemia, and thus is not a sensitive indicator of diminished oxygenation. Stress will exacerbate these difficulties. It is the *rate* at which hypoxia develops that determines the acute neuropsychiatric consequences of hypoxemia, not the absolute level of oxygen saturation. Surprisingly, hypoxemia, dyspnea, and pulmonary function measures do not strictly covary. Dyspnea is a complex symptom, with many elements (including depression) influencing its perception and measurement.

4. Steroids, theophylline (Theo-Dur), and sympathomimetic bronchodilators are the pulmonary medications most often implicated in producing psychiatric side effects.

5. Physiologically, benzodiazepines reduce the ventilatory response to hypoxia, causing the response to hypercapnia to predominate and resulting in chronic respiratory acidosis and respiratory failure. In chronically hypercapnic patients who have lost their hypercapnic respiratory drive, the administration of low-flow oxygen further reduces the hypoxic drive, magnifying the respiratory-depressant effects of benzodiazepines even more. Although the respiratory-depressant effects of the longer-acting benzodiazepines (e.g., diazepam [Valium], chlordiazepoxide [Librium]) are well established, the intermediate-acting agents (e.g., lorazepam [Ativan], oxazepam

[Serax]) have few respiratory-depressant effects when used judiciously. They have no active metabolites and are generally well tolerated in medically ill patients. For patients whose anxiety worsens respiratory function, these medications may actually improve respiratory status. Baseline blood gases help determine the appropriateness of benzodiazepines. They should be rechecked following dose increments after steady state is reached. Keep in mind that many patients with chronic respiratory disease suffer sleep apnea and that benzodiazepines are contraindicated in this condition.

6. Buspirone (BuSpar) and antihistamines like hydroxyzine (Vistaril, Atarax) and diphenhydramine (Benadryl) appear safe but are not always effective. Beta-blockers like propranolol (Inderal) are contraindicated for anxiolysis because they cause bronchoconstriction. Sedative-hypnotics and barbiturates have significant respiratory-depressant effects and should be avoided. Anxiolytics generally do not create adverse drug interactions with the usual pulmonary medications.

7. When medical clearance is withheld for low-dose lorazepam (Ativan) or oxazepam (Serax), a panicky patient may benefit from a brief course of low-dose, high-potency neuroleptics, with careful monitoring for dystonic effects on respiration. Alternatively, low-dose thioridazine (Mellaril; 10–25 mg po tid-qid prn anxiety) is a safe, extremely effective anxiolytic for medically fragile patients. It does not depress respirations and, like the benzodiazepines, acts almost immediately. The immediate side effects are anticholinergic and cardiotoxic, so that it should be avoided in the setting of delirium or conduction disease. Tardive dyskinesia is a risk of long-term treatment with any neuroleptic, so thioridazine can be used only as a brief intervention. The rationale for starting it should be documented clearly in the patient's chart. There may be additive anticholinergic effects with atropine, the atropine derivative ipratropium (Atrovent inhalator), and antihistamines, particularly with the more sedating neuroleptics (e.g., thioridazine [Mellaril] and chlorpromazine [Thorazine]).

8. Pulmonary disease poses few problems to antidepressant management. Most tricyclic antidepressants (TCAs) have little or no effect on respiratory status as long as they are prescribed appropriately, and they may even act as mild bronchodilators. On the downside, many pulmonary patients are elderly and have multisystem disease, so choose the antidepressant that minimizes side effects such as hypotension, cardiotoxicity, and anticholinergicity. Monoamine oxidase inhibitors (MAOIs) are more problematic because of the risk of interactions with epinephrine, which is used to treat acute asthmatic attacks. The TCAs have a number of adverse interactions with drugs prescribed for chronic respiratory disease. There are no published controlled studies on the use of the newer antidepressants specifically in respiratory disease patients. These medications are usually well tolerated in medically ill patients, with rare cardiovascular effects. There are no known effects on respiration.

9. One of the rare instances in consultation-liaison psychiatry in which electroconvulsive therapy (ECT) is relatively contraindicated is for patients on theophylline, which substantially increases the risk of inducing status epilepticus, with consequent brain damage, or even death.

10. Various psychotherapeutic approaches minimize the adverse effects of chronic respiratory disease, including psychodynamic psychotherapy, psychoeducational approaches to the self-management of asthma, family therapy, and stress management approaches such as relaxation therapies and biofeedback. One of the goals of psychotherapies of all theoretical perspectives is to reinforce the fact that dyspnea does not necessarily mean imminent death or danger. The belief that expressing feelings or confronting certain situations will cause fatal shortness of breath poses an important resistance to any psychotherapy. Psychoanalytically informed, cognitive, and behavioral therapies all appear helpful in lessening the psychological and/or physical morbidity of chronic respiratory disease when patients are appropriately selected and sensitively managed.

❧ REFERENCES

1. Abrams R: Electroconvulsive Therapy, 2nd Edition. New York, Oxford University Press, 1992

2. Agle D, Baum G: Psychological aspects of chronic obstructive pulmonary disease. Med Clin North Am 61:749–758, 1977

3. Allen G, Hickie I, Gandevia S, et al: Impaired voluntary drive to breathe: a possible link between depression and unexplained ventilatory failure in asthmatic patients. Thorax 49:881–884, 1994

4. Austen F, Charmichael M, Adams R: Neurologic manifestations of chronic pulmonary insufficiency. N Engl J Med 257:579–590, 1957

5. Baldessarini R: Drugs and the treatment of psychiatric disorders, in Goodman and Gilman's The Pharmacological Basis of Therapeutics, 8th Edition. Edited by Gilman A, Rall T, Nies A, et al. New York, Pergamon, 1990, pp 383–435

6. Baron C, Lamarre A, Veilleux P, et al: Psychomaintenance of childhood asthma: a study of 34 children. J Asthma 23:69–79, 1986

7. Barsky A, Wyshak G, Klerman G: Medical and psychiatric determinants of outpatient medical utilization. Med Care 24:548–563, 1986

8. Bass S, Colebatch H: Fluoxetine-induced lung damage (letter). Med J Aust 156:364–365, 1992

9. Bernstein J: Handbook of Drug Therapy in Psychiatry, 3rd Edition. St Louis, MO, Mosby Year Book, 1995

10. Bernstein J, Sheridan E, Patterson R: Asthmatic patients with panic disorders: report of three cases with management and outcome. Ann Allergy 66:311–314, 1991

11. Blake RJ: Social stressors, social supports, and self-esteem as predictors of morbidity in adults with chronic lung disease. Fam Pract Res J 11:65–74, 1991

12. Block A, Castle J, Keitt A: Chronic oxygen therapy: treatment of COPD at sea level. Chest 65:279–288, 1974

13. Boakes A, Laurence D, Teoh P, et al: Interactions between sympathomimetic amines and antidepressant agents in man. BMJ 1:311–315, 1973

14. Borak J, Sliwinski P, Piasecki Z, et al: Psychological status of COPD patients on long term oxygen therapy. Eur Respir J 4:59–62, 1991

15. Bornstein R, Menon D, York E, et al: Effects of venesection on cerebral function in chronic lung disease. Can J Neurol Sci 7:293–296, 1980

16. Borson S, McDonald G, Gayle T, et al: Improvement in mood, physical symptoms, and functions with nortriptyline for depression in patients with chronic obstructive pulmonary disease. Psychosomatics 33:190–201, 1992

17. Bowen D: Ventilator weaning through hypnosis. Psychosomatics 4:449–450, 1989

18. Burdon J, Juniper E, Killian K, et al: The perception of breathlessness in asthma. Am Rev Respir Dis 126:825–828, 1982

19. Burns B, Howell J: Disproportionately severe breathlessness in chronic bronchitis. Q J Med (new series, XXXVIII) 151:274–294, 1969

20. Burrows B, Niden A, Barclay W, et al: Chronic obstructive lung disease, II: relationship of clinical and physiologic findings to severity of airway obstruction. Am Rev Respir Dis 91:665–678, 1965

21. Carr D, Sheehan D: Panic anxiety: a new biological model. J Clin Psychiatry 45:323–330, 1984

22. Carr R, Lehrer P, Hochron S: Panic symptoms in asthma and panic disorder: a preliminary test of the dyspnea-fear theory. Behav Res Ther 30:251–261, 1992

23. Carr R, Lehrer P, Rausch L: Anxiety sensitivity and panic attacks in an asthmatic population. Behav Res Ther 2:411–418, 1994

24. Catchlove R, Kafer E: The effects of diazepam on respiration in patients with obstructive pulmonary disease. Anesthesiology 34:14–18, 1971

24a. Ciraulo D, Shader R, Greenblatt D, et al. (eds): Drug Interactions in Psychiatry, 2nd Edition. Baltimore, MD, Williams & Wilkins, 1995

25. Clark N, Starr-Schneidkraut N: Management of asthma by patients and families. American Journal of Respiratory and Critical Care Medicine 149 (2 pt 2):S54–66; discussion S67–68, 1994

26. Cohn M: Hypnotics and the control of breathing: a review. Br J Clin Pharmacol 16:2455–2505, 1983

27. Craven J, Sutherland A: Buspirone for anxiety disorders in patients with severe lung disease. Lancet 338:249, 1991

28. Creer T: Emotions and asthma (editorial). J Asthma 30:1–3, 1993

29. Damas-Mora J, Grant L, Kenyon P, et al: Respiratory ventilation and carbon dioxide levels in syndromes of depression. Br J Psychiatry 129:457–464, 1976

30. Della Bella L: Steroidphobia and the pulmonary patient. Am J Nurs 92:26–29, 1992

31. Denaut M, Yernault J, DeCoster A: A double-blind comparison of the respiratory effects of parenteral lorazepam and diazepam in patients with COLD. Curr Med Res Opin 2:611–615, 1975

31a. Derogatis L, Rickels K, Uhlenhuth E, et al: The SCL-90 (SCL): a self-report symptom inventory. Behav Sci 19:1–15, 1974

32. Deutsch F (ed): Symbolization as a Formative Stage in the Mysterious Leap from the Mind to the Body. New York, International Universities Press, 1959

33. Deutsch L: Psychosomatic medicine from a psychoanalytic viewpoint. J Am Psychoanal Assoc 28:653–702, 1980

34. Deutsch L: Reflections on the psychoanalytic treatment of patients with bronchial asthma, in Psychoanalytic Study of the Child, Vol 42. Edited by Solnit A, Neubauer P. New Haven, CT, Yale University Press, 1987, pp 245, 253–254

35. Devanand D, Decina P, Sackeim H, et al: Status epilepticus following ECT in a patient receiving theophylline (letter). J Clin Psychopharmacol 8:153, 1988

35a. Diot P, Jonville A, Gerard F, et al: Possible interaction entre theophylline et fluvoxamine (letter). Therapie 46:170–171, 1991

36. Dirks J, Horton D, Kinsman R, et al: Patient and physician characteristics influencing medical decisions in asthma. Journal of Asthma Research 15:171–178, 1978

37. Dirks J, Jones N, Kinsman R: Panic-fear: a personality dimension related to intractability in asthma. Psychosom Med 39:120–126, 1977

38. Dirks J, Shraa J, Brown E, et al: Psycho-maintenance in asthma: hospitalization rates and financial impact. Br J Med Psychol 53:349–354, 1980

39. Dodson M, Yousseff Y, Madison S, et al: Respiratory effects of lorazepam. Br J Anaesth 48:611–612, 1976

40. Dudley D, Glaser E, Jorgenson B, et al: Psychosocial concomitants to rehabilitation in chronic obstructive pulmonary disease, I: psychosocial and psychological considerations. Chest 77:413–420, 1980

41. Dudley D, Holmes T, Martin C, et al: Changes in respiration associated with hypnotically induced emotion, pain, and exercise. Psychosom Med 26:46–57, 1963

42. Dudley D, Martin C, Holmes T: Dyspnea: psychologic and physiologic observations. J Psychosom Res 11:325–339, 1968

43. Dudley D, Sitzman J: Psychobiological evaluation and treatment of chronic obstructive pulmonary disease, in Chronic Obstructive Pulmonary Disease: A Behavioural Perspective. Edited by McSweeney A, Grant I. New York, Marcel Dekker, 1988, pp 183–236

44. Dulfano M, Ishikawa S: Hypercapnia: mental changes and extrapulmonary complications. Ann Intern Med 63:829–841, 1965

45. Fagan P, Schmidt C: Sexual dysfunction in the medically ill, in Psychiatric Care of the Medical Patient. Edited by Stoudemire A, Fogel B. New York, Oxford University Press, 1993, pp 307–322

46. Fawver J, Milstein V: Asthma/emphysema complication of electroconvulsive therapy: a case study. Convulsive Therapy 1:61–64, 1985

47. Finkel M, Schwimmer J: Clozapine—a novel antipsychotic agent (letter). N Engl J Med 325:518–519, 1991

48. Fix A, Golden C, Daughton D, et al: Neuropsychological deficits among patients with COPD. Int J Neurosci 16:99–105, 1982

49. Fletcher C, Elmes P, Fairbairn A, et al: The significance of respiratory symptoms and the diagnosis of chronic bronchitis in a working population. BMJ 2:257–266, 1978

50. Fletcher E, Martin R: Sexual dysfunction and erectile impotence in chronic obstructive pulmonary disease. Chest 81:413–421, 1982

51. Frankenburg F, Baldessarini R: Clozapine—a novel antipsychotic agent (letter). N Engl J Med 325:518, 1991

52. French T, Alexander F: Psychogenic factors in bronchial asthma. Psychosom Med Monogr 4:1–96, 1939–1941

53. Friedman L, Tabb S, Worthington J, et al: Clozapine—a novel antipsychotic agent (letter). N Engl J Med 325:518, 1991

54. Gammans R, Westrick M, Shea J, et al: Pharmacokinetics of buspirone in elderly subjects. J Clin Pharmacol 29:72–78, 1989

55. Garner S, Eldridge F, Wagner P, et al: Buspirone: an anxiolytic drug that stimulates respiration. Am Rev Respir Dis 139:945–950, 1989

56. Gelenberg A: Buspirone: seven-year update. J Clin Psychiatry 55:222–229, 1994

57. Goldbarb A, Venutolol F: The use of an antidepressant drug in chronically allergic individuals: a double-blind study. Ann Allergy 21:667–676, 1963

57a. Gonzalez-Rothi R, Zander D, Ros P: Fluoxetine hydrochloride (Prozac)–induced pulmonary disease. Chest 107:1763–1765, 1995

58. Gorman J: Psychobiological aspects of asthma and the consequent research implications (editorial). Chest 97:514–515, 1990

59. Gorman J, Askanazi J, Liebowitz M, et al: Response to hyperventilation in a group of patients with panic disorder. Am J Psychiatry 141:857–861, 1984

60. Gorman J, Fyer M, Goetz R, et al: Ventilatory physiology of patients with panic disorder. Arch Gen Psychiatry 45:31–39, 1988

61. Gorman J, Liebowitz M, Fyer A, et al: A neuroanatomical hypothesis for panic disorder. Am J Psychiatry 146:148–161, 1989

62. Grant I, Heaton R: Neuropsychiatric abnormalities, in Chronic Obstructive Pulmonary Disease, 2nd Edition. Edited by Petty T. New York, Marcel Dekker, 1985, pp 355–373

63. Grant I, Heaton R, McSweeney A, et al: Brain dysfunction in COPD. Chest 77:308–309, 1980

64. Grant I, Heaton R, McSweeney A, et al: Neuropsychologic findings in hypoxemic COPD. Arch Intern Med 142:1470–1476, 1982

65. Grant I, Prigatano G, Heaton R, et al: Progressive neuropsychologic impairment and hypoxemia. Arch Gen Psychiatry 44:999–1006, 1987

66. Greenberg G, Ryan J, Bourlier P: Psychological and neuropsychological aspects of COPD. Psychosomatics 26:29–33, 1985

67. Greene J, Pucino F, Carlson J, et al: Effects of alprazolam on respiratory drive, anxiety, and dyspnea in chronic airflow obstruction: a case study. Pharmacotherapy 9:34–38, 1989

68. Griggs R, Arieff A: Hypoxia and the central nervous system, in Metabolic Brain Dysfunction in Systemic Disorders. Edited by Arieff A, Griggs R. Boston, MA, Little, Brown, 1992, pp 39–54

69. Guyatt G, Townsend M, Berman L, et al: Quality of life in patients with chronic airflow limitation. British Journal of Diseases of the Chest 81:45–54, 1987

70. Heaton R, Grant I, McSweeney A, et al: Psychologic effects of continuous and nocturnal oxygen therapy in hypoxemia COPD. Arch Intern Med 143:1941–1947, 1983

71. Hibbert G, Pilsbury D: Demonstration and treatment of hyperventilation causing asthma. Br J Psychiatry 153:687–688, 1988

72. Horton D, Suda W, Kinsman R: Bronchoconstrictive suggestion in asthma: a role for airways hyperreactivity and emotions. Am Rev Respir Dis 117:1029, 1978

73. Huch R, Huch A: Respiratory depression after tranquilizers. Lancet 1:1267, 1974

74. Hudgel D, Cooperson D, Kinsman R: Recognition of added resistive loads in asthma: the importance of behavioral styles. Am Rev Respir Dis 126:121–125, 1982

75. Incalzi R, Gemma A, Marra C, et al: Chronic obstructive pulmonary disease: an original model of cognitive decline. Am Rev Respir Dis 148:418–424, 1993

76. Ingram R: Chronic bronchitis, emphysema, and airways obstruction, in Harrison's Principles of Internal Medicine, 12th Edition. Edited by Wilson J, Braunwald E, Isselbacher K, et al. New York, McGraw-Hill, Health Professions Division, 1991, pp 1074–1082

77. Isenberg S, Lehrer P, Hochron S: The effects of suggestion and emotional arousal on pulmonary function in asthma: a review and a hypothesis regarding vagal mediation. Psychosom Med 54:192–216, 1992

78. Isenberg S, Lehrer P, Hochron S: The effects of suggestion on airways of asthmatic subjects breathing room air as a suggested bronchoconstrictor and bronchodilator. J Psychosom Res 36:769–776, 1992

79. Janson C, Bjornsson E, Hetta J, et al: Anxiety and depression in relation to respiratory symptoms and asthma. American Journal of Respiratory and Critical Care Medicine 149 (4 pt 1):930–934, 1994

80. Jellinek M, Goldenheim P, Jenike M: The impact of grief on ventilatory control. Am J Psychiatry 142:121–123, 1985

81. Jenike M: Treating anxiety in elderly patients. Geriatrics 38:115–119, 1983

82. Jenike M: Handbook of Geriatric Psychopharmacology. Littleton, MA, PSG Publishing, 1985

83. Jenike M: The patient with lung disease, in Treatments of Psychiatric Disorders: A Task Force Report of the American Psychiatric Association, Vol 2. Washington, DC, American Psychiatric Association, 1989, pp 939–948

84. Jones P, Baveystock C, Littlejohns P: Relationships between general health measured with the sickness impact profile and respiratory symptoms, physiological measures, and mood in patients with chronic airflow limitation. Am Rev Respir Dis 140:1538–1543, 1989

85. Karajgi B, Rifkin A, Doddi S, et al: The prevalence of anxiety disorders in patients with chronic obstructive pulmonary disease. Am J Psychiatry 147:200–201, 1990

86. Karol C: The role of primal scene and masochism, in Psychosomatic Symptoms: Psychodynamic Treatment of the Underlying Personality Disorder. Edited by Wilson C, Mintz I. Northvale, NJ, Jason Aronson, 1989, pp 309–326

87. Kass I, Dykerhuis J, Rubin H: Correlation of psycho-physiological variables with vocational rehabilitation outcome in chronic obstructive pulmonary disease patients. Chest 67:433–440, 1975

88. Kass I, Updegraff K, Muffly R: Sex in chronic obstructive pulmonary disease. Medical Aspects of Human Sexuality 7:33–38, 1972

89. Katon W: Depression: relationship to somatization and chronic medical illness. J Clin Psychiatry 45:4–11, 1984

89a. Kellner R: Abridged Manual of the Symptom Questionnaire. Albuquerque, NM, University of New Mexico, 1976

89b. Kellner R: A symptom questionnaire. J Clin Psychiatry 48:268–274, 1987

90. Kellner R, Samet J, Pathak D: Dyspnea, anxiety, and depression in chronic respiratory impairment. Gen Hosp Psychiatry 14:20–28, 1992

91. Kent D, Smith J: Psychological implications of pulmonary disease. Clinical Notes on Respiratory Diseases 15:3–11, 1977

92. Kiev A, Domantay A: A study of buspirone coprescribed with bronchodilators in 32 anxious ambulatory patients. J Asthma 25:281–284, 1988

93. Kinsman R, Dirks J, Dahlem N, et al: Anxiety in asthma: panic-fear symptomatology and personality in relation to manifest anxiety. Psychol Rep 46:196–198, 1980

94. Kinsman R, Dirks J, Jones N, et al: Anxiety reduction in asthma: four catches to general application. Psychosom Med 42:397–405, 1980

95. Kinsman R, Luparello T, O'Banion K, et al: Multidimensional analysis of the subjective symptomatology of asthma. Psychosom Med 35:250–267, 1973

96. Knos G, Sung Y-F: ECT anesthesia strategies in the high-risk medical patient, in Psychiatric Care of the Medical Patient. Edited by Stoudemire A, Fogel B. New York, Oxford University Press, 1993, pp 225–240

97. Kronenberg R, Cosio M, Stevenson J, et al: The use of oral diazepam in patients with obstructive lung disease and hypercapnia. Ann Intern Med 83:83–84, 1975

98. Lakshminarawan S, Sahn S, Hudson L: Effects of diazepam on ventilatory responses. Clin Pharmacol Ther 20:173–183, 1976

99. Lane C, Hobfoll S: How loss affects anger and alienates potential supporters. J Consult Clin Psychol 60:935–942, 1992

100. Lehrer P, Isenberg S, Hochron S: Asthma and emotion: a review. J Asthma 30:5–21, 1993

101. Lehrer P, Sargunaraj D, Hochron S: Psychological approaches to the treatment of asthma (special issue: Behavioral Medicine: An Update for the 1990s). J Consult Clin Psychol 60:639–643, 1992

102. Leiner G, Abramovitz S, Lewis W, et al: Dyspnoea and pulmonary function tests. Am Rev Respir Dis 92:822–823, 1965

103. Lester D: The psychological impact of COPD, in Pulmonary Care. Edited by Johnson R. New York, Grune & Stratton, 1973, pp 341–353

104. Levitan H: Suicidal trends in patients with asthma and hypertension: a chart study. Psychother Psychosom 39:165–170, 1983

105. Lipowski Z: Delirium: Acute Confusional States. New York, Oxford University Press, 1990

106. Luparello T, Lyons H, Bleeker E, et al: Influences of suggestion on airway reactivity in asthmatic subjects. Psychosom Med 30:819–825, 1968

107. Lustig F, Haas A, Castillo R: Clinical and rehabilitation regime in patients with COPD. Arch Phys Med Rehabil 53:315–322, 1972

108. Mahler D, Weinberg D, Wells C, et al: The measurement of dyspnoea. Chest 85:751–758, 1984

109. Malatesta V, West B, Malcolm R: Application of behavioral principles in the management of suffocation phobia: a case study of chronic respiratory failure. Int J Psychiatry Med 19:281–289, 1989

110. Man G, Hsu K, Sproule B: Effect of alprazolam on exercise and dyspnea in patients with chronic obstructive pulmonary disease. Chest 90:832–836, 1986

111. Manton K: Future patterns of chronic disease incidence, disability, and mortality among the elderly: implications for the demand for acute and long-term health care. N Y State J Med 85:623–633, 1985

112. Mawhinney H, Spector S, Heitjan D, et al: As-needed medication use in asthma usage patterns and patient characteristics. J Asthma 30:61–71, 1993

113. McFadden EJ: Asthma, in Harrison's Principles of Internal Medicine, 12th Edition. Edited by Wilson J, Braunwald E, Isselbacher K, et al. New York, McGraw-Hill, Health Professions Division, 1991, pp 1047–1056

114. McGavin C, Artvinli M, Naoe H, et al: Dyspnoea, disability and distance walked: a comparison of estimates of exercise performance and respiratory disease. BMJ 2:241–243, 1978

115. McSweeney A, Grant I, Heaton R, et al: Life quality of patients with chronic obstructive pulmonary disease. Arch Intern Med 142:473–478, 1982

116. McSweeney A, Heaton R, Grant I, et al: COPD: socioemotional adjustment and life quality. Chest 77:309–311, 1980

117. Meany J, McNamara M, Burks V, et al: Psychological treatment of an asthmatic patient in crisis: dreams, biofeedback, and pain behavior modification. J Asthma 25:141–151, 1988

118. Meares R, Mills J, Horvath T: Amitriptyline and asthma. Med J Aust 2:25–28, 1971

119. Mendelson W: Pharmacotherapy of insomnia. Psychiatr Clin North Am 10:555–563, 1987

120. Mendelson W, Maczaj M, Holt J: Buspirone administration to sleep apnea patients (letter). J Clin Psychopharmacol 11:71–72, 1991

121. Mendelson W, Martin J, Rapoport D: Effects of buspirone on sleep and respiration. Am Rev Respir Dis 141:1527–1530, 1990

122. Mintz I: Air symbolism in asthma, in Psychosomatic Symptoms: Psychodynamic Treatment of the Underlying Personality Disorder. Edited by Wilson C, Mintz I. Northvale, NJ, Jason Aronson, 1989, pp 211–250

123. Mintz I: Treatment of a case of anorexia and severe asthma, in Psychosomatic Symptoms: Psychodynamic Treatment of the Underlying Personality Disorder. Edited by Wilson C, Mintz I. Northvale, NJ, Jason Aronson, 1989, pp 251–308

124. Mitchell-Heggs P, Murphy K, Minte K: Diazepam in the treatment of dyspnea in the "pink puffer" syndrome. Q J Med 49:9–20, 1980

125. Modei D, Berry D: Effects of chlordiazepoxide in respiratory failure due to chronic bronchitis. Lancet 2:869–870, 1974

126. Morgan A, Peck D, Buchanan D, et al: Effects of attitudes and beliefs on exercise tolerance in chronic bronchitis. BMJ (Clin Res Ed) 286:171–173, 1983

126a. Morgan A, Peck D, Buchanan D, et al: Psychological factors contributing to disproportionate disability in chronic bronchitis. J Psychosom Res 27:259–263, 1983

127. Mushatt C, Werby I: Grief and anniversary reactions in a man of sixty-two. International Journal of Psychoanalytic Psychotherapy 8:83–106, 1972

128. National Center for Health Statistics: National Health Interview Survey. Washington, DC, National Center for Health Statistics, 1984

129. Nocon A, Booth T: The social impact of asthma. Fam Pract 8:37–41, 1990

130. Nouwen A, Freeston MH, Cournoyer I, et al: Perceived symptoms and discomfort during induced bronchospasm: the role of temporal adaptation and anxiety. Behav Res Ther 32:623–628, 1994

131. Patterson R, Walker C, Greenberger P, et al: Prednisonephobia. Allergy Proc 10:423–428, 1989

132. Pecknold J, Matas M, Howarth B, et al: Evaluation of buspirone as an antianxiety agent: buspirone and diazepam versus placebo. Can J Psychiatry 34:766–771, 1989

133. Peters S, Wochos D, Peterson G: Status epilepticus as a complication of concurrent electroconvulsive and theophylline therapy. Mayo Clin Proc 59:568–570, 1984

134. Pleuvry B, Madison S, Odeh R, et al: Respiratory and psychological effects of oral temazepam in volunteers. Br J Anaesth 52:901–905, 1980

135. Plum F, Posner J: Diagnosis of Stupor and Coma, 3rd Edition. Philadelphia, PA, FA Davis, 1980

136. Post L, Collins C: The poorly coping COPD patient: a psychotherapeutic perspective. Int J Psychiatry Med 11:173–182, 1981–1982

137. Prigatano G, Parsons O, Wright E, et al: Neuropsychological test performance in mildly hypoxemic patients with COPD. J Consult Clin Psychol 51:108–116, 1983

138. Rabinowitz B, Florian V: Chronic obstructive pulmonary disease—psychosocial issues and treatment goals. Soc Work Health Care 16:69–86, 1992

139. Rao S, Sherbaniuk R, Prosad K, et al: Cardiopulmonary effects of diazepam. Clin Pharmacol Ther 14:182–184, 1973

140. Rapoport D, Greenberg H, Goldring R: Comparison of the effects of buspirone and diazepam on control of breathing (abstract). FASEB J 2:A1507, 1988

141. Rapoport D, Greenberg H, Goldring R: Differing effects of the anxiolytic agents buspirone and diazepam on control of breathing. Clin Pharmacol Ther 49:394–401, 1991

141a. Rasmussen B, Maenpaa J, Pelkonen O, et al: Selective serotonin reuptake inhibitors and theophylline metabolism in human liver microsomes: potent inhibition by fluvoxamine. Br J Clin Pharmacol 39:151–159, 1995

142. Rasmussen K, Zorumski C: Electroconvulsive therapy in patients taking theophylline. J Clin Psychiatry 54:427–431, 1993

143. Regestein Q: Sleep disorders in the medically ill, in Psychiatric Care of the Medical Patient. Edited by Stoudemire A, Fogel B, Gulley L, et al. New York, Oxford University Press, 1993, pp 485–515

144. Reiman E, Raichle M, Butler F, et al: A focal brain abnormality in panic disorder: a severe form of anxiety. Nature 310:683–685, 1984

145. Reiman E, Raichle M, Robins E, et al: The application of positron emission tomography to the study of panic disorder. Am J Psychiatry 143:469–477, 1986

146. Robinson D, Napoliello M, Schenk J: The safety and usefulness of buspirone as an anxiolytic drug in elderly versus young patients. Clin Ther 10:740–746, 1988

147. Sassim N, Grohmann R: Adverse drug reactions with clozapine and simultaneous application of benzodiazepines. Pharmacopsychiatry 21:306–307, 1988

148. Settipane G: Aspirin and allergic diseases: a review. Am J Med 74:102–109, 1983

149. Settipane G: The restaurant syndromes. New England and Regional Allergy Proceedings 8:39–46, 1987

150. Sexton D, Munro B: Living with a chronic illness: the experience of women with COPD. West J Nurs Res 10:26–44, 1988

151. Shershow J, Kanarek D, Kazemi H: Ventilatory response to carbon dioxide in depression. Psychosom Med 38:282–287, 1976

152. Shershow J, King A, Robinson S: Carbon dioxide sensitivity and personality. Psychosom Med 35:155–160, 1973

153. Shim C, Williams M: Evaluation of the severity of asthma: patients versus physicians. Am J Med 68:11–13, 1980

154. Silverman M: Power, control, and the threat to die in a case of asthma and anorexia, in Psychosomatic Symptoms: Psychodynamic Treatment of the Underlying Personality Disorder. Edited by Wilson C, Mintz I. Northvale, NJ, Jason Aronson, 1989, pp 351–364

155. Simon R: Adverse reactions to food additives. New England and Regional Allergy Proceedings 7:533–542, 1986

156. Singh N, Despars J, Stansbury D, et al: Effects of buspirone on anxiety levels and exercise tolerance in patients with chronic airflow obstruction and mild anxiety. Chest 103:800–804, 1993

157. Smith O, Devito J: Central neural integration for the control of autonomic responses associated with emotion. Annu Rev Neurosci 7:43–65, 1984

158. Snadden D, Brown J: The experience of asthma. Soc Sci Med 34:1351–1361, 1992

159. Spector S, Luparello T: Response of asthmatics to methacholine and suggestion. Am Rev Respir Dis 113:43–50, 1976

159a. Sperber A: Toxic interaction between fluvoxamine and sustained release theophylline in an 11-year-old boy. Drug Safety 6:460–462, 1991

160. Steen S, Amaha K, Martinez L: Effect of oxazepam on respiratory response to carbon dioxide. Anesthesia and Analgesia Current Researchers 45:455–458, 1966

161. Stewart A, Greenfield S, Hays R, et al: Functional status and well-being of patients with chronic conditions: results from the medical outcomes study. JAMA 262:907–913, 1989

162. Stoppe G, Muller P, Fuchs T, et al: Life-threatening allergic reaction to clozapine. Br J Psychiatry 161:259–261, 1992

163. Stoudemire A, Fogel B: Psychopharmacology in the medically ill, in Principles of Medical Psychiatry. Edited by Stoudemire A, Fogel B. Orlando, FL, Grune & Stratton, 1987, pp 79–112

164. Stoudemire A, Fogel B: Psychopharmacology in the medical patient, in Psychiatric Care of the Medical Patient. Edited by Stoudemire A, Fogel B, Gulley L, et al. New York, Oxford University Press, 1993, pp 155–206

165. Strunk R, Mrazek D, Fuhrmann G, et al: Physiologic and psychological characteristics associated with deaths due to asthma in childhood: a case-control study. JAMA 254:1193–1198, 1985

166. Sugihara H, Ishihara K, Noguchi H: Clinical experience with amitriptyline (Tryptanol) in the treatment of bronchial asthma. Ann Allergy 23:422–429, 1965

167. Sukumalchantra Y, Dinakara P, Williams M: Prognosis of patients with COPD after hospitalizations for acute ventilatory failure: a three-year follow-up study. Am Rev Respir Dis 93:215–222, 1966

168. Thompson W, Thompson T: Somatization and pulmonary disease. Psychiatr Med 10:77–91, 1992

169. Thompson W, Thompson T: Psychiatric disorders complicating treatment of patients with pulmonary disease. New Dir Ment Health Serv 57:117–130, 1993

170. Thompson W, Thompson T: Pulmonary disease, in Psychiatric Care of the Medical Patient. Edited by Stoudemire A, Fogel B. New York, Oxford University Press, 1993, pp 591–610

170a. Thomson A, et al: Interaction between fluvoxamine and theophylline. Pharm J 249:137, 1992

171. Tyrer P: Major common symptoms in psychiatry: anxiety. Br J Hosp Med 27:109–112, 1982

172. Utting H, Pleuvry B: Benzoctamine: a study of the respiratory effects of oral doses in human volunteers and interactions with morphine in mice. Br J Anaesth 47:987–992, 1975

172a. van den Brekel A, Harrington L: Toxic effects of theophylline caused by fluvoxamine. Can Med Assoc J 151:1289–1290, 1994

173. Viederman M: Use of a psychodynamic life narrative in the treatment of depression in the physically ill. Gen Hosp Psychiatry 3:177–181, 1980

174. Virchow C, Szczeklik A, Bianco S, et al: Intolerance to tartrazine in aspirin-induced asthma: results of a multicenter study. Respiration 53:20–23, 1988

175. Weiner H: Psychobiology and Human Disease. New York, Elsevier, 1977

176. Weiner R, Coffey C: Electroconvulsive therapy in the medical and neurologic patient, in Psychiatric Care of the Medical Patient. Edited by Stoudemire A, Fogel B. New York, Oxford University Press, 1993, pp 207–224

177. Welch C: ECT in medically ill patients, in The Clinical Science of Electroconvulsive Therapy. Edited by Coffey C. Washington, DC, American Psychiatric Press, 1993, pp 167–182

178. Wells K, Golding J, Burnam M: Psychiatric disorder and limitations in physical functioning in a sample of the Los Angeles general population. Am J Psychiatry 145:712–717, 1988

179. Wells K, Golding J, Burnam M: Affective, substance use, and anxiety disorders in persons with arthritis, diabetes, heart disease, high blood pressure, or chronic lung conditions. Gen Hosp Psychiatry 11:320–327, 1989

180. Wells K, Stewart A, Hays R, et al: The functioning and well-being of depressed patients. JAMA 262:914–919, 1989

181. Williams I, McGavin C: Corticosteroids in chronic airway obstruction: can the patient's assessment be ignored? British Journal of Diseases of the Chest 71:142–147, 1980

182. Williams S: Chronic respiratory illness and disability: a critical review of the psychosocial literature. Soc Sci Med 28:791–803, 1989

183. Williams S, Bury M: Impairment, disability and handicap in chronic respiratory illness. Soc Sci Med 29:609–616, 1989

184. Willison J, Thomas D, duBoulay G, et al: Effect of high hematocrit on alertness. Lancet 1:846–848, 1980

185. Wilson C: Parental overstimulation in asthma, in Psychosomatic Symptoms: Psychodynamic Treatment of the Underlying Personality Disorder. Edited by Wilson C, Mintz I. Northvale, NJ, Jason Aronson, 1989, pp 327–350

186. Wise T, Schiavone A, Sitts T: The depressed patient with chronic obstructive pulmonary disease. Gen Hosp Psychiatry 10:142–147, 1988

187. Woller W, Kruse J, Winter P, et al: Cortisone image and emotional support by key figures in patients with bronchial asthma: an empirical study. Psychother Psychosom 59:190–196, 1993

188. Woodcock A, Gross E, Geddes D: Drug treatment of breathlessness: contrasting effects of diazepam and promethazine in pink puffers. BMJ 283:343–346, 1981

189. Woolcock A, Read J: Improvement in bronchial asthma not reflected in forced expiratory volume. Lancet 2:1323–1325, 1965

190. Yellowlees P, Alpers J, Bowden J, et al: Psychiatric morbidity in patients with chronic airflow obstruction. Med J Aust 146:305–307, 1987

191. Yellowlees P, Haynes S, Potts N, et al: Psychiatric morbidity in patients with life-threatening asthma: initial report of a controlled study. Med J Aust 149:246–249, 1988

192. Yellowlees P, Kalucy R: Psychobiological aspects of asthma and the consequent research implications. Chest 97:628–634, 1990

193. Yellowlees P, Ruffin R: Psychological defenses and coping styles in patients following a life-threatening attack of asthma. Chest 95:1298–1303, 1989

194. Zung W, George D, Woodruff W, et al: Symptom perception by nonpsychiatric physicians in evaluating for depression. J Clin Psychiatry 45:26–28, 1984

195. Zwil A, Pelchat R: ECT in the treatment of patients with neurological and somatic disease. Int J Psychiatry Med 24:1–29, 1994

The Delirious Alcoholic Patient With Cirrhosis

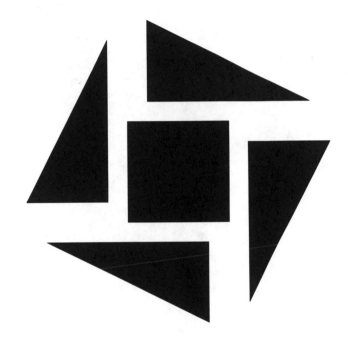

CHAPTER 3

CONTENTS

■ Introduction to Chapter 3 119
■ Case Presentation: Mr. Horton: The Delirious
   Alcoholic Patient With Cirrhosis 120
■ Questions 120
■ Answers 123
■ Discussion 124
   ◆ Alcoholic Hallucinosis 125
   ◆ Alcohol Withdrawal 125
      DSM-IV Criteria for Alcohol Withdrawal . . 126
      Treatment 126
   ◆ Alcohol Withdrawal Seizures 126
   ◆ Delirium Tremens 126
      DSM-IV Criteria for Alcohol Withdrawal
       Delirium 127
      Treatment 127
   ◆ Hepatic Encephalopathy 127
      Etiology 128
      Treatment 128

◆ Wernicke's Encephalopathy 130
   Etiology 130
   Treatment 130
◆ Korsakoff's Syndrome/Psychosis 131
   DSM-IV Criteria for Substance-Induced
     Persisting Amnestic Disorder 131
   Neuropsychology 131
◆ "Latent" Encephalopathy 132
◆ Diagnostic Workup 133
   Liver Function Tests 133
   Ammonia Levels 133
   Electroencephalogram 133
   Cerebrospinal Fluid 133
   Imaging Studies 133
◆ Liver Transplantation 134
◆ Psychopharmacology in Hepatic Failure 134
◆ Summary 136
◆ References 136

The patient with altered mental status, alcohol dependence, and chronic liver disease presents a diagnostic challenge. Alcohol intoxication, hepatic encephalopathy, Wernicke-Korsakoff syndrome, alcohol withdrawal, and alcohol withdrawal delirium (delirium tremens) have symptomatic overlap that can fool the unwary clinician. Moreover, they can coexist in the same patient. Quick differential diagnosis of such patients minimizes morbidity and mortality.

We decided to present one aspect of this conundrum. As in other chapters, the biological emphasis seeks to review often-forgotten basics; we in no way intend to minimize the importance of psychosocial issues. References are provided to supplement the psychosocial literature, which is covered only superficially.

As before, the questions are not intended to resemble a test, but are organized as an exercise in differential diagnosis. Therefore, the reader will derive maximal benefit from them by answering them in the arranged sequence. There may be more than one correct option.

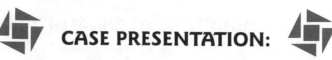

CASE PRESENTATION:
Mr. Horton: The Delirious Alcoholic Patient With Cirrhosis

Mr. Horton is a 33-year-old man with chronic alcoholism who is well known to the hospital staff: frequently in the past he has been brought to the emergency room acutely intoxicated after menacing passersby. He has had several admissions for hypothermia during the winter months and is marginally compliant with follow-up in the medical clinic for cirrhosis and hypertension. He has demonstrated the stigmata of liver disease for several years, including palmar erythema, spider nevi, and gynecomastia. Physical exam reveals that the liver is not enlarged. There is no psychiatric history other than several admissions for alcohol detoxification. He has never abused drugs.

You are asked to see him approximately 48 hours after admission to the emergency service for workup of hematemesis. Blood and urine on admission were negative for drugs or alcohol. He is awaiting transfer to the medical service, but there are no beds. He has been npo and has been receiving intravenous hydration. When you arrive, the patient is in Posey restraints because of agitation. He has already pulled out his lines twice.

On mental status exam, Mr. Horton appears frightened and his speech is slurred. He intermittently hallucinates, claiming he sees rats and spiders. He is convinced that the staff is trying to poison him. At times he breaks into inappropriate laughter. He is often alert then drowsy, and is oriented for person but not for date or place. Concentration is severely impaired, and he is distractible. Short-term recall is impaired. Remote memory seems grossly intact. He will not cooperate with other aspects of cognitive testing.

QUESTIONS

Choose all that apply.

1. The most frequent cause of psychosis in alcoholic patients is . . .
   a. Alcohol withdrawal delirium (delirium tremens [DTs])
   b. Hepatic encephalopathy
   c. Alcoholic hallucinosis
   d. Wernicke's encephalopathy
   e. Korsakoff's syndrome

2. As you listen to Mr. Horton's psychotic productions, you consider the differential diagnosis of his presentation. Which are true?
   a. The occurrence of vivid visual hallucinations in this setting is pathognomonic of DTs.
   b. DTs, alcoholic hallucinosis, and hepatic encephalopathy are all considered alcohol withdrawal syndromes.
   c. Paranoid delusions usually precede hallucinations in alcoholic hallucinosis and are related to them thematically.

   d. Had Mr. Horton presented with amusing or playful hallucinations, it would have argued against DTs.
   e. None of the above.

3. You present him with a blank piece of paper and ask him to read what it says; he confabulates that there are instructions to "leave this house of hell." He tries to jump out of bed. What finding(s) would be unique to Wernicke's encephalopathy, as opposed to hepatic encephalopathy, DTs, alcoholic hallucinosis, or the neurological effects of chronic alcohol abuse?
   a. Peripheral neuropathy
   b. Tremor
   c. Sixth-nerve palsy
   d. Confabulation

4. You carefully review the chart. Physical exam: as above. Vital signs: P:100, R:22, BP: 160/100, Temp: 99.0. Labs: hematocrit 32, hemoglobin 11. WBC 6,500 with normal differential. PT/PTT: mildly elevated. Arterial blood gas: pH 7.4, P_{CO_2} 40, P_{O_2} 90. Chemistries: BUN 35, creatinine 1.3, sodium 145, potassium 3.8; calcium, phos-

phorous, magnesium: normal. Blood alcohol level is zero. Blood and urine for toxicology are negative. SGOT, SGPT, GGTP are mildly elevated. Total bilirubin is minimally elevated. Serum ammonia is pending. Which are true?

  a. The minimally abnormal liver chemistries argue against Wernicke's encephalopathy.
  b. The minimally abnormal liver chemistries argue against hepatic encephalopathy.
  c. Normal brain-imaging studies, such as magnetic resonance imaging (MRI), would rule out a secondary psychiatric syndrome.
  d. A normal serum ammonia would definitively rule out hepatic encephalopathy.
  e. The minimal changes in liver function tests (LFTs) are probably a sign of severe liver failure.

5. Unfortunately, you do not know when Mr. Horton had his last drink. All of the following are true regarding the association between the cessation of drinking and alcohol-associated syndromes *except* . . .

  a. The risk of DTs is *highest* within the first 24 hours of the last drink.
  b. The risk of alcohol withdrawal seizures is *highest* within the first 24 hours of cessation of drinking.
  c. Alcoholic hallucinosis often follows a prolonged drinking bout.
  d. The onset of hepatic encephalopathy occurs independently of the last drink.
  e. The onset of Wernicke's encephalopathy occurs independently of the last drink.

6. Mr. Horton is disoriented for time and place and has visual hallucinations, sleep-wake cycle disturbance, and psychomotor agitation. Which of the following is the *least* likely diagnosis?

  a. DTs
  b. Hepatic encephalopathy
  c. Alcoholic hallucinosis
  d. Wernicke's encephalopathy

7. Which of the alcohol-related disorders resembles schizophrenia, especially when its association with drinking is not apparent?

  a. DTs
  b. Hepatic encephalopathy
  c. Alcoholic hallucinosis
  d. Wernicke's encephalopathy
  e. Korsakoff's syndrome

8. You consider starting Mr. Horton on a detoxification regimen. Which is an appropriate statement?

  a. Chlordiazepoxide (Librium) would be the detoxification agent of choice for Mr. Horton.
  b. Even without a detoxification regimen, Mr. Horton is probably past the peak time for alcohol withdrawal seizures but still at risk for the occurrence of DTs.
  c. Both DTs and mild withdrawal symptoms resolve within 3–4 days, with or without treatment.
  d. It is contraindicated to begin an alcohol detoxification regimen with chlordiazepoxide.

9. The medical student assigned to Mr. Horton asks you about whether "rum fits" are a form of epilepsy. You respond . . .

  a. They indicate an underlying seizure disorder that requires continued anticonvulsant prophylaxis.
  b. Patients with preexisting seizure disorders are at greater risk for alcohol withdrawal seizures.
  c. They present most typically as complex partial seizures.
  d. They are usually self-limited.

10. You learn that the patient is too agitated to cooperate with MRI scan of the head. The nursing staff is pressing you to medicate this patient, pronto! The medical intern awaits your instructions. You respond . . .

  a. Avoid all medication and use restraints instead.
  b. Since the patient may be in withdrawal and can take nothing by mouth, administer intravenous diazepam (Valium), carefully titrating according to symptoms.
  c. Since the patient may be in withdrawal and can take nothing by mouth, administer intravenous lorazepam (Ativan), carefully titrating according to symptoms.
  d. Agree with the intern's suggestion to sedate the patient with low-dose chlorpromazine (Thorazine) (because of its additional antiemetic properties).

11. Which of the following considerations are true regarding the pharmacokinetics in liver disease?

  a. Lithium metabolism and dosing remain unchanged in hepatic failure.
  b. Medications that primarily undergo glucuronidation, rather than oxidation, are more likely to have prolonged half-lives in hepatic failure.
  c. All benzodiazepines undergo Phase I metabolism.
  d. Intramuscular and intravenous administration of drugs bypass the first-pass metabolism.

12. The benzodiazepines that bypass oxidation by the cytochrome P450 system include the following:
    a. Lorazepam (Ativan)
    b. Halazepam (Paxipam)
    c. Triazolam (Halcion)
    d. Temazepam (Restoril)
    e. Oxazepam (Serax)
    f. Alprazolam (Xanax)
    g. Prazepam (Centrax)
    h. Clorazepate (Tranxene)
    i. Clonazepam (Klonopin)

13. Mr. Horton is given three intravenous doses of lorazepam 0.5 mg, which results in a mild reduction of his agitation. The MRI is still pending. Neurological examination shows diffuse hyperreflexia but no focal signs. He continues to actively hallucinate, talking to himself, fearful of taking anything by mouth because he believes it is "living poison of this satanic rite." Which of the following would be typical of a Wernicke's encephalopathic presentation?
    a. Apathetic, detached affect
    b. Psychomotor agitation
    c. History of a drinking binge
    d. Prominent paranoid delusions and auditory or visual hallucinations

14. The most important etiological factor in the development of Wernicke's encephalopathy is . . .
    a. Vitamin B_{12} deficiency.
    b. Thiamine deficiency.
    c. Folate deficiency.
    d. Alcohol intoxication.
    e. Ammonia load.

15. The medical student is confused about whether Mr. Horton's presentation is an example of "Korsakoff's psychosis." You respond that the term refers to the tendency of these patients to . . .
    a. Become delusional, with paranoid themes.
    b. Become delusional, with grandiose themes.
    c. Give false accounts of recent experiences.
    d. Resemble the very early visual hallucinatory stage of DTs.

16. All of the following would be true during the examination of a patient with Korsakoff's syndrome except . . .
    a. There are no concentration deficits evident on digit span.
    b. Alertness is preserved.
    c. Four items are not recalled after 2 minutes.

    d. A catastrophic reaction (e.g., crying) often occurs in response to the memory deficits.
    e. Social behavior is preserved.

17. What additional findings characterize patients with Korsakoff's syndrome?
    a. An inability to learn simple ward routines (procedural memory)
    b. A distortion of the temporal sequence of events
    c. Memory for emotionally charged information consistently better than for neutral material
    d. Blandness of affect and placidity
    e. Deficits similar to those of senile dementia of the Alzheimer type

18. Mr. Horton's cerebrospinal fluid (CSF) examination is normal. Serum ammonia level is still pending because the lab lost the tube. The electroencephalogram (EEG) is read as containing "5- to 7-cps (Hz) theta waves interspersed with alpha rhythm." Mr. Horton appears sedated but is rousable and able to talk. Which of the following is true about this patient's EEG?
    a. It is a normal variant.
    b. It indicates subdural hematoma.
    c. It is an artifact of the lorazepam.
    d. It could indicate impending coma.
    e. It is nonspecific as to etiology.

19. You are paged by a case worker at the men's shelter, who knows Mr. Horton well and reports that he has been too sick to drink for over 2 weeks. Mr. Horton has also been acting "peculiarly," with new onset of paranoid ideation. Given this information, the clinical picture, and the test results, which diagnosis is most likely?
    a. Hepatic encephalopathy
    b. DTs
    c. Subdural hematoma
    d. Alcoholic hallucinosis
    e. Wernicke's encephalopathy
    f. Korsakoff's psychosis

20. Precipitants of hepatic encephalopathy include . . .
    a. Benzodiazepines.
    b. Gastrointestinal bleeding.
    c. Chlorpromazine (Thorazine).
    d. Constipation.
    e. All of the above.

21. What is true concerning the neurological examination of patients with hepatic encephalopathy?
    a. Rigidity and hyperreflexia that fluctuate in parallel with the psychiatric symptoms are found.

b. Sensory abnormalities predominate over motor abnormalities.

c. Extrapyramidal features on motor exam are usually present.

d. Once neurological signs become evident, there tends to be unremitting progression to coma.

e. Psychiatric symptoms vary according to the etiology of the underlying liver pathology.

22. Which neurotransmitter has been implicated in the pathogenesis of hepatic encephalopathy?

a. Serotonin

b. Gamma-aminobutyric acid (GABA)

c. Dopamine

d. Acetylcholine

23. Several months later, you are asked to reevaluate Mr. Horton, who is being considered for liver transplantation. Which of the following are true regarding liver transplantation?

a. In the United States, alcohol dependence is an exclusion criterion.

b. Patient survival rates after transplantation are equivalent in alcoholic and nonalcoholic liver disease.

c. Graft survival rates are equivalent in alcoholic and nonalcoholic liver disease.

d. Preliminary figures show that relatively few patients are able to return to work and normal activity afterward.

24. It is quite common to be asked to consult on cirrhotic, alcoholic patients like Mr. Horton when they either are ready for discharge from the medical service or are already ambulatory outpatients. Although these patients have no overt evidence of encephalopathy, they are likely to have neuropsychological deficits that will impair their psychosocial adjustment. This condition has been termed "latent" encephalopathy or "subclinical delirium." What are true statements about latent encephalopathy?

a. Verbal and performance skills suffer approximately equal decrements.

b. The Trail Making Tests are not highly sensitive in identifying these patients.

c. There is close correlation between measurements of cerebral morphology on computed tomography (CT) or MRI scans and neuropsychological test performance of these patients.

d. EEG abnormalities often identify patients with latent encephalopathy.

Answers

1. Answer: a (p. 125)
2. Answer: e (pp. 124, 126–127)
3. Answer: c (p. 130)
4. Answer: e (pp. 128–129, 133)
5. Answer: a (pp. 126–127, 130)
6. Answer: c (p. 125)
7. Answer: c (p. 125)
8. Answer: b, d (pp. 124, 126–127)
9. Answer: b, d (p. 126)
10. Answer: c (pp. 127, 129)
11. Answer: d (pp. 134–135)
12. Answer: a, d, e, i (pp. 134–135)
13. Answer: a (p. 130)
14. Answer: b (p. 130)
15. Answer: c (pp. 131–132)
16. Answer: d (pp. 131–132)
17. Answer: b, d (pp. 131–132)
18. Answer: d, e (p. 133)
19. Answer: a (p. 124)
20. Answer: e (p. 129)
21. Answer: a, c (p. 128)
22. Answer: b (p. 129)
23. Answer: b, c (p. 134)
24. Answer: b (p. 132)

Why devote an entire case to hepatic encephalopathy rather than alcoholism? This decision was consistent with our aim to supplement the gaps in the consultation-liaison literature rather than to be comprehensive. Surprisingly, hepatic encephalopathy tends to be underemphasized and is only scantily reviewed in the major consultation-liaison texts. The care and treatment of the alcoholic patient is a subspecialty in itself, as detailed by other authors.[32] Our discussion highlights the medical issues of cirrhotic patients—many of whom are alcoholic—who often become psychiatrically symptomatic and present to the general psychiatrist.

The differential diagnosis of altered mental status, alcohol dependence, and chronic liver disease is complicated. Alcohol intoxication, hepatic encephalopathy, Wernicke-Korsakoff syndrome, alcohol withdrawal, and alcohol withdrawal delirium (delirium tremens) symptomatically overlap and may coexist in the same patient. Even the terminology can be confusing, since most of these syndromes are described in medical and neurological texts that do not use psychiatric nosology. Appendix E ("Differential Diagnosis of the Delirious Psychotic Patient With Cirrhosis") provides an overview of differential diagnosis. Also refer to Chapter 2, the case of Mr. Davis, for a review of delirium.

◆ In DSM-IV[1a] nosology, these syndromes would be termed as follows:
  - Alcohol hallucinosis ⇒ *alcohol withdrawal with perceptual disturbances* (if reality testing is intact) or *alcohol withdrawal psychotic disorder with hallucinations* (if reality testing is not preserved)
  - Delirium tremens (DTs) ⇒ *alcohol withdrawal delirium*
  - Hepatic encephalopathy ⇒ *delirium due to hepatic insufficiency*
  - Wernicke's encephalopathy ⇒ *delirium due to thiamine deficiency*
  - Korsakoff's syndrome ⇒ *alcohol-induced persisting amnestic disorder*

DTs and alcoholic hallucinosis occur during alcohol withdrawal; hepatic encephalopathy and the Wernicke-Korsakoff syndrome can occur *independently* of changes in alcohol consumption, but at times can resemble either DTs or alcohol intoxication. Subdural hematoma is a common complication of alcoholism, and because a clear history of head trauma is not always available, imaging studies such as the MRI are helpful. However, when brain imaging studies are normal, they often divert attention away from investigating a medical etiology. Mr. Horton's MRI of the brain is normal, and he is well past the critical period for the development of the alcohol withdrawal syndromes (2 weeks since his last drink). His presentation sounds initially consistent with DTs, and many clinicians would have reasonably treated him for this condition; it is only upon learning of the 2-week history of alcohol abstinence that it is possible to eliminate DTs and focus on the diagnosis of hepatic encephalopathy, also known as the *delirium of hepatic insufficiency*.

◆ *The psychiatrist may be the first to evaluate—and medicate—an agitated, psychotic cirrhotic patient who, unbeknownst to everyone, is in the very early stages of hepatic encephalopathy.*

It would have been an error, however, to have started Mr. Horton on long-acting benzodiazepines such as chlordiazepoxide (Librium) until hepatic encephalopathy had been ruled out. Lorazepam (Ativan) and oxazepam (Serax), which are intermediate-acting benzodiazepines that bypass the hepatic cytochrome P450 system and have no active metabolites, would have been more appropriate while the diagnosis remained ambiguous. All medications undergoing oxidative metabolism (Phase I) in the cytochrome P450 system of the liver should be avoided, with one exception: haloperidol may be used to treat the delirium of hepatic insufficiency.[110] Since it was highly likely that Mr. Horton was also in withdrawal, lorazepam was selected both to cover alcohol withdrawal and to sedate the patient. We discuss the hepatic metabolism of psychotropics later.

Most authors emphasize the variable nature of hepatic encephalopathy. Unlike DTs (which presents with agitated delirium, tremor, and unmistakable changes in vital signs) or Wernicke's encephalopathy (which has sudden onset and often distinct neurological features), the prodrome of hepatic encephalopathy may escape detection unless the clinician retains a high index of suspicion for its occurrence. The profile of at-risk patients easily allows them to present first to the psychiatric emergency room, where their symptoms may resemble primary psychiatric illness or be mistaken for alcohol intoxication or uncomplicated withdrawal. The diagnosis depends on clinical suspicion, confirmed by history, clinical features, and laboratory findings that exclude other etiologies. *Hepatic encephalopathy is usually a diagnosis of exclusion,*[79] *and may be misdiagnosed because it presents with psychiatric symptoms in the early stages that overlap with other syndromes.*

Lockwood[58] has written,

> While it may seem redundant to state that successful treatment [of hepatic encephalopathy] can only follow a correct diagnosis, this is worth emphasizing because of the high frequency with which relatively subtle alterations of mental capacity may be missed, unless thorough examinations are conducted . . . Decrements in mental capacity may be subtle and range from slight inattentiveness in a high-level executive to failure to eat usual meals at a shelter in a destitute alcoholic. (p. 177)

Clearly, there are many other causes of mental status changes in the setting of liver disease and alcohol abuse—for example, subdural hematoma, hypokalemia, hyponatremia, hypocalcemia, hypomagnesemia, hypoxia, hypoglycemia, and uremia. We shall limit our discussion to alcoholic hallucinosis, uncomplicated alcohol withdrawal, DTs, hepatic encephalopathy, Wernicke's encephalopathy, and the alcohol-induced (Korsakoff's) amnestic syndrome. The most frequent cause of psychotic symptoms in alcoholic individuals is DTs, occurring in about 15% of alcohol-dependent patients.[27] However, the occurrence and content of vivid visual hallucinations are not specifically diagnostic. A concise summary of diagnostic tests follows on page 133.

⚡ ALCOHOLIC HALLUCINOSIS

Alcoholic hallucinosis has auditory and/or visual hallucinations as its predominant symptom. Onset is classically within 48 hours of drinking cessation but can occur during drinking bouts.[28] Like DTs, the visual hallucinations may be of small animals, such as rodents and insects, characteristically moving rapidly on the walls, floor, or ceiling.[56] Visual disturbances such as blurring, flashes, and spots often accompany visual hallucinations.[88] Tinnitus is common, sometimes predating the appearance of auditory

hallucinations and persisting even after they clear.[88] The auditory hallucinations often begin as simple sounds (buzzing, roaring, bells) and gradually take on vocal form, usually the voices of friends or enemies that malign, threaten, or reproach the patient.[56]

- ◆ Sometimes the hallucinations are of a command nature, resembling those of paranoid schizophrenia. As mentioned, delusional elaborations typically *result from* the hallucinatory experiences, and usually do not precede them or arise in their absence.

Unlike DTs or the other deliria, alcoholic hallucinosis by definition occurs in a *clear sensorium* without confusion, psychomotor hyperactivity, or intense autonomic reactivity. These symptoms help to distinguish it from other syndromes. In the majority of cases, the symptoms remit within a few hours to days. Patients tend to preserve insight that the hallucinations are imaginary.[28]

- ◆ Preservation of insight affects the diagnostic coding in DSM-IV.[1a] When the patient shows intact reality testing (i.e., knows that his or her hallucinations are induced by the substance and do not represent external reality), the diagnosis for alcohol hallucinosis becomes *alcohol withdrawal with perceptual disturbances.* If hallucinations occur in the absence of intact reality testing, consider a diagnosis of *alcohol-induced psychotic disorder, with hallucinations.*

A small percentage of patients have been reported to evolve a chronic paranoid delusional state or frank schizophrenia,[95] although we could find no epidemiological studies verifying this. Antipsychotic drugs are the treatment of choice for the psychotic symptoms of alcoholic hallucinosis.[64]

⚡ ALCOHOL WITHDRAWAL

Symptoms of uncomplicated alcohol withdrawal include coarse tremors of the hands or tongue; nausea or vomiting; malaise; autonomic nervous system hyperactivity, manifested by tachycardia, sweating, and elevated blood pressure; anxiety; irritability; insomnia; and nightmares.[28] Peak symptoms occur 24–48 hours after the last drink and, in uncomplicated cases, subside within 5–7 days, even without treatment.[28] Uncomplicated alcohol withdrawal may progress to DTs or resolve spontaneously.

DSM-IV Criteria for Alcohol Withdrawal

The DSM-IV[1a, pp. 198–199] diagnostic criteria for alcohol withdrawal are as follows:

A. Cessation of (or reduction in) alcohol use that has been heavy and prolonged.

B. Two (or more) of the following, developing within several hours to a few days after criterion A:
    (1) autonomic hyperactivity (e.g., sweating or pulse rate > 100)
    (2) increased hand tremor
    (3) insomnia
    (4) nausea or vomiting
    (5) transient visual, tactile, or auditory hallucinations or illusions
    (6) psychomotor agitation
    (7) anxiety
    (8) grand mal seizures

C. The symptoms in criterion B cause clinically significant distress or impairment in social, occupational, or other important areas of functioning.

D. The symptoms are not due to a general medical condition and are not better accounted for by another mental disorder.

Specify if: **With Perceptual Disturbances**

Consult Appendix A for details on coding.

Treatment

A preset dosing schedule of benzodiazepines that is tapered over several days with hydration has long been the treatment of choice for alcohol withdrawal. A sample regimen for treating uncomplicated alcohol withdrawal symptoms with chlordiazepoxide (Librium) might be as follows:[18a,28,64]

◆ **Day 1:**
   • Chlordiazepoxide 25–100 mg po qid and
   • Chlordiazepoxide 25–50 mg po every 2 hours prn for agitation, tremors, and changes in vital signs
   • Thiamine 100 mg im stat and then 100 po daily
   • Folic acid 1 mg po daily
   • Multivitamin one per day
◆ **Then:**
   • Decrease day 1 dose by 20% in equally divided doses over the next 5–7 days.
◆ **Notes:**
   • Up to 400–600 mg of chlordiazepoxide may be given.
   • Vital signs must be carefully monitored.

• Chlordiazepoxide is poorly absorbed intramuscularly, so should not be given by this route.

Recently, however, modifications to this regimen have been explored:

◆ Bird and Makela[13] extensively reviewed the literature on the pros and cons of lorazepam (Ativan) as an alternative to drugs with longer half-lives.
◆ Saitz et al.[89] and Fuller and Gordis[31] had good results with symptom-triggered therapy, in which the benzodiazepine (chlordiazepoxide) was given only as needed to suppress withdrawal symptoms. This regimen used less medication and was quicker than the standard, fixed-dose approach, although the sample was not large enough to detect differences in rates of serious complications, such as seizures and DTs.

⚶ ALCOHOL WITHDRAWAL SEIZURES

Alcohol withdrawal seizures are also known in medical circles as "rum fits." They typically begin 7–48 hours after cessation of drinking, with over 60% of seizures occurring 17–24 hours after the last drink. Alcoholic patients presenting with their first seizure or focal seizures should have a workup for structural lesions (e.g., subdural hematoma). Seizures in alcoholic individuals usually do *not* indicate epilepsy and do not require prolonged anticonvulsant therapy,[7] although patients with preexisting seizure disorders are at greater risk for alcohol withdrawal seizures. Alcohol withdrawal seizures are frequently self-limited and require only supportive care.[28]

⚶ DELIRIUM TREMENS

DTs, also known as alcohol withdrawal delirium, usually begins 24–72 hours after the last drink, with 90% of patients showing symptoms within the first 7 days of abstinence.[64] Trzepacz[110] has noted that the onset of DTs may be delayed by the administration of anesthetic agents that cross-react with alcohol during surgery or other medical procedures, highlighting that *some patients may have delayed withdrawal or DTs in the postoperative period.* The prodrome, like any delirium, may begin with sleep cycle disturbances, restlessness, and fear. The patient easily startles, has vivid nightmares, and frequently awakens panicked from sleep.[56] Restlessness and anxiety increase as the illness progresses. The degree of impairment of consciousness varies widely among individuals and may shift from moment to moment in the same patient. The typical picture is of a hyperalert-hyperactive delirium with prominent psychotic features. Consciousness is rarely profoundly abnormal except in the terminal stages, but progressive disorientation and confusion may presage impending deterioration.[56]

Men develop DTs four to five times as often as women.[55] The syndrome usually occurs in alcoholic patients with a 5- to 15-year history of drinking who suddenly decrease their blood alcohol levels and also have major physical illness, such as trauma, infection, liver disease, or metabolic disorders.[28] Fortunately, only 1%–10% of alcoholic patients hospitalized for detoxification develop DTs.[40] Efforts are under way to find clinical predictors of DTs.[120a]

The visual hallucinations of DTs have been described as vivid, colorful, Lilliputian in size, and in constant movement.[56] Although apprehension and fear are typical, the hallucinations may also be amusing or playful in nature, resulting in affective states that are shifting and labile. Delusions are usually fragmented, transitory, and as changeable as the hallucinations. The patient is often markedly suggestible, enhancing the likelihood of illusions and confabulations. Unlike alcoholic hallucinosis, these psychotic symptoms occur with cognitive deficits and other symptoms of delirium.

DSM-IV Criteria for Alcohol Withdrawal Delirium

The DSM-IV[1a, pp. 131–132] diagnostic criteria for alcohol withdrawal delirium are as follows:

A. Disturbance of consciousness (i.e., reduced clarity of awareness of the environment) with reduced ability to focus, sustain, or shift attention.
B. A change in cognition (such as memory deficit, disorientation, language disturbance) or the development of a perceptual disturbance that is not better accounted for by a preexisting, established, or evolving dementia.
C. The disturbance develops over a short period of time (usually hours to days) and tends to fluctuate during the course of the day.
D. There is evidence from the history, physical examination, or laboratory findings that the symptoms in criteria A and B developed during, or shortly after, a withdrawal syndrome.

Note: This diagnosis should be made instead of a diagnosis of alcohol withdrawal only when the cognitive symptoms are in excess of those usually associated with the withdrawal syndrome and when the symptoms are sufficiently severe to warrant independent clinical attention. Consult Appendix A for details on coding.

Treatment

DTs is the most serious of the alcohol withdrawal syndromes.

♦ Deaths due to DTs may be from infections, fat emboli, or cardiac arrhythmia associated with hyperkalemia, hypokalemia, hyponatremia, hypophosphatemia, alcoholic ketoacidosis, hyperpyrexia, poor hydration, rhabdomyolysis, and hypertension.[28] Other complications include pancreatitis, gastritis, upper gastrointestinal (GI) bleeds, and hepatitis.

DTs constitutes a *medical emergency* and does *not* remit spontaneously, unlike uncomplicated alcohol withdrawal symptoms.[64] These patients are gravely ill and require intensive inpatient care, including intravenous hydration and benzodiazepines for sedation (e.g., diazepam 5–10 mg iv every 15–20 minutes until sedation is achieved).[64] Pharmacotherapy is designed to replace alcohol with a cross-tolerant sedative drug, which then can be tapered in a controlled manner.[7] Benzodiazepines are the drugs of choice because they are as effective as and less toxic than the alternatives—phenothiazines, barbiturates, or paraldehyde.[7] The long half-lives of benzodiazepines—such as diazepam (Valium) or chlordiazepoxide (Librium)—and their metabolites allow for drug levels to decline slowly over many days, creating a gradual withdrawal with relatively few abstinence symptoms.

♦ *However, benzodiazepines with active metabolites must be avoided until hepatic encephalopathy has been ruled out, because they can hasten the deterioration into coma.*[41]
♦ When in doubt, choose an agent like lorazepam (Ativan)—which has no active metabolites—over diazepam or chlordiazepoxide for treating the withdrawal symptoms in this context.
♦ Restraining paranoid patients may increase their agitation; a quiet environment will minimize agitation and allow the sedative medications to be more effective.[28]

⚕ HEPATIC ENCEPHALOPATHY

Hepatic encephalopathy may occur *independently* of alcohol intake, leaving the clinician without an obvious clue as to its etiology.

◆ DSM-IV[1a] lists hepatic encephalopathy as *delirium due to hepatic encephalopathy;* we prefer *delirium due to hepatic* **insufficiency,** because designating delirium as secondary to encephalopathy seems redundant.

Semantics aside, early prodromal signs of hypersomnia and sleep cycle inversion may progress to marked confusion, semicoma, and coma. Brain imaging studies are usually normal. The syndrome has been subdivided into clinical stages, which are defined by the progressive appearance of central nervous system (CNS) signs.[21]

◆ **Prodrome:** This stage presents as often subtle changes in personality, mood, psychomotor activity, and cognition.[33,70] Sleep cycle disturbances may result in nighttime wandering and confusion reminiscent of patients with dementia.[42,49] Symptoms may be more apparent to the patient's family and friends than to the physician.[34] The EEG is usually normal at this point,[41] and it is easy to overlook the underlying medical etiology. In their classic paper detailing the neuropsychiatric changes associated with hepatic disease, Summerskill et al.[100] described several patients who had been given psychiatric diagnoses (anxiety state, hysterical ataxia, depression) and were admitted to a psychiatric hospital. Liver disease was not immediately evident in these patients; neuropsychiatric symptoms were the *presenting* feature in 8 of the series of 17. Only 3 of the 17 were jaundiced, 7 had hepatomegaly, and 5 showed little evidence of hepatic dysfunction. Fetor hepaticus, splenomegaly, palmar erythema, spider nevi, finger clubbing, and loss of body hair were most useful in supporting the diagnosis. *It is now well established that* **personality changes,** *even without liver function test abnormalities, may be the initial presenting feature of hepatic failure, and that interepisode personality characteristics similar to those of frontal lobe syndromes may endure.*[56] Affective changes may show abrupt swings, ranging from depression to euphoria,[71] and at times paranoid reactions do occur.

◆ **Impending hepatic coma (precoma):** In this stage there is worsening of cognitive function and psychiatric symptoms, such as paranoid ideation, inappropriate behavior, mood disturbances (ranging from irritability to apathy or euphoria), and perceptual distortions.[21] *It is here that the differential diagnosis based on gross symptomatology most obviously overlaps with DTs.* There may be frank visual hallucinations. For example, one patient reported vivid, panoramic scenes of frightening bears and wolves.[100] The EEG is abnormal (often with 5- to 7–cycles per second [cps] theta waves) but nonspecific. Asterixis (liver flap)—a transient loss of wrist extensor postural tone when the hands are outstretched—often occurs at this point. It is best assessed by asking the patient to extend the hands or dorsiflex the wrists. Tremor is easy to miss when the patient's arms are restrained, as are Mr. Horton's. (Asterixis is not specific for a hepatic etiology, but also occurs in uremia, pulmonary disease, malnutrition, and polycythemia rubra vera.[86]) Aggressive intervention is crucial to prevent progression to the next phase.

◆ **Stupor and coma:** Without treatment, the patient's consciousness can rapidly deteriorate from alertness to drowsiness, and eventually to stupor and coma. Mortality and morbidity are high.

Fortunately, the onset of neurological symptoms does not always bode an inexorable downhill course; Lishman[56] has noted that the neurological abnormalities may worsen or remit from day to day, often in parallel with the variation in psychiatric symptoms. *Motor* symptoms predominate over sensory findings. There may be fluctuating rigidity of the trunk and limbs; grimacing and suck and grasp reflexes; exaggeration or asymmetry of tendon reflexes; Babinski signs; and focal or generalized seizures.[119] Pyramidal and extrapyramidal symptoms and signs can occur, such as dysarthria, ataxia, gross tremor, limb rigidity, hyperreflexia, and clonus. As mentioned, asterixis occurs at some point in almost every patient, but is nonspecific and may be seen in other encephalopathic conditions.[96] Other neurological abnormalities include constructional apraxia, dysphasia with perseverative speech disturbances, blurred vision, diplopia, and nystagmus.[56]

The most striking neuropathological finding in patients who die in hepatic coma is a diffuse increase in the number and size of protoplasmic astrocytes (Alzheimer type II astrocytes) in the deep layers of the cerebral cortex and in the lenticular nuclei, with little or no alteration in the nerve cells or other parenchymal elements.[119]

Etiology

The specific cause of hepatic encephalopathy is unknown. The most important factors in its pathogenesis are severe hepatocellular dysfunction and/or intrahepatic and extrahepatic shunting of portal venous blood into the systemic circulation, so that liver metabolism is largely bypassed.[79] As a result, toxic substances absorbed from the intestine are deprived of detoxification by the liver and produce metabolic abnormalities in the CNS. *Ammonia is the substance most often incriminated in the pathogenesis of hepatic encephalopathy, and recovery is often accompanied by declining blood ammonia levels.*[79] However, about 10% of encephalopathic patients have normal blood ammonia levels.[55] Other metabolites that may contribute to the delirium include mercaptans (derived from the intestinal metabolism of methionine), short-chain fatty acids, and phenol.

The neuropsychiatric disturbances are similar regardless of the underlying liver pathology (e.g., hepatocellular failure, portal hypertension, surgical portocaval anastomosis).[96] The shunt in primary hepatocellular failure, for example, is through the liver itself, because the cells are unable to completely metabolize the contents of the portal blood. In cirrhosis, the shunt occurs by way of the collateral vessels that develop during this disease.

Precipitants of hepatic encephalopathy are as follows:[79]

1. Increased nitrogen load: GI bleeding, excess dietary protein, azotemia, and constipation
2. Electrolyte imbalance: hypokalemia, alkalosis, hypoxia, and hypovolemia
3. Drugs: narcotics, tranquilizers, sedatives, and diuretics
4. Miscellaneous: infection, surgery, superimposed acute liver disease, and progressive liver disease

Several hypotheses have been proposed for the pathogenesis of hepatic encephalopathy, including the role of ammonia,[26] the synergistic actions of multiple toxins, the role of false neurotransmitters,[25] and the involvement of the gamma-aminobutyric acid$_A$ (GABA$_A$)–benzodiazepine neurotransmitter system.[69] Increased CNS GABA may reflect the failure of the liver to efficiently extract precursor amino acids[69] and may contribute to the potentially lethal impact of benzodiazepines, barbiturates, and chloral derivatives. As has been summarized by other authors,[33,43] strong evidence of a functional increase in GABA-ergic tone was found in an animal model of hepatic encephalopathy.[4,6,122] This hypothesis had led to investigations of the benzodiazepine receptor antagonist *flumazenil*.[3,93]

◆ Flumazenil may displace endogenous benzodiazepine-like substances from the GABA receptor.[69] Increased brain concentrations of substances inhibiting the binding of [³H]flumazenil to its receptors were found in some patients with hepatic encephalopathy due to fulminant hepatic failure.[5] In addition, there are reports of flumazenil-associated improvements in consciousness and reduced encephalopathic EEG changes in patients with different types of liver disease.[2,3,37,38,93]

Treatment

The treatment of hepatic encephalopathy, like that of any delirium, involves therapy of the underlying condition. Most psychotic symptoms and behavioral abnormalities will improve with medical treatment. In general, specific treatment is aimed at correcting the precipitating factors and eliminating nitrogenous products from the intestine.[79] In the setting of acute GI bleeding, blood in the bowel is evacuated with enemas and laxatives in order to reduce the nitrogen load.[79] Protein is excluded from the diet and constipation prevented. Ammonia absorption is decreased with lactulose (a nonabsorbable disaccharide) and intestinal ammonia production by bacteria reduced with the antibiotic neomycin.

Haloperidol is the neuroleptic of choice for the psychosis and agitation of hepatic encephalopathy.[113] Some authors feel that all benzodiazepines should be avoided in hepatic insufficiency, irrespective of their route of metabolism, unless an alcohol withdrawal regimen is necessary.[110] This recommendation is based on the benzodiazepines' potential to exacerbate the hypothesized increased GABA-ergic tone accompanying the hepatic delirium. Moreover, intramuscular and intravenous administration of haloperidol bypasses problems with absorption and first-pass metabolism, thereby increasing bioavailability.[113]

When benzodiazepines are necessary for coexisting withdrawal syndromes, administer only those avoiding oxidation in the cytochrome P450 system, such as lorazepam (Ativan) or oxazepam (Serax).[41,50,54,55,65,78,97] Unlike diazepam and chlordiazepoxide, these agents have no active metabolites, and their metabolism is virtually unaffected by liver disease.[46,50] Of the two, Jain and Shamoian[41] empirically prefer oxazepam for patients with parenchymal liver disease. If parenteral dosing becomes necessary, they use low-dose lorazepam.[41]

Unfortunately, we could locate no controlled studies comparing the efficacy and side effects of haloperidol versus lorazepam or oxazepam in the setting of hepatic encephalopathy. For now, treatment recommendations remain empirical. Certainly, the extensive experience with haloperidol on the liver transplant service at the University of Pittsburgh is reassuring.[113,114] Chlorpromazine (Thorazine), on the other hand, is unanimously to be avoided.

◆ WERNICKE'S ENCEPHALOPATHY

Like hepatic encephalopathy, Wernicke's encephalopathy may occur independently of alcohol intake. It is typically a global confusional state that has been termed a quiet, or "hypokinetic," delirium.[118] Patients demonstrate profound fatigue, apathy, impaired awareness and responsiveness, and derangements of perception and memory. These symptoms cause Wernicke's to resemble hepatic encephalopathy but render it easier to distinguish from DTs. Unlike DTs, which occurs in about 15% of alcohol-dependent patients, Wernicke-Korsakoff syndrome occurs in only about 3%–5%.[27]

Victor and colleagues[118] have described these patients in detail:

> [Patients were usually] inert and impassive, and they seemed detached and indifferent to everything and everybody in their environment and without any interest in their illness. Inattention was a conspicuous abnormality so that it was often difficult to engage the patient in a simple conversation. (p. 40)

Focal neurological findings are characteristic; ocular abnormalities were documented in more than 95% of patients with Wernicke's encephalopathy.[117] The most common findings are nystagmus and *ophthalmoplegia* (i.e., gaze paresis) such as sixth-nerve palsies producing lateral rectus weakness, or various forms of conjugate gaze paresis. (Sixth-nerve palsy does not characterize DTs, hepatic encephalopathy, or alcoholic hallucinosis.) Classically, Wernicke's encephalopathy has an abrupt onset of oculomotor disturbances, cerebellar ataxia, and mental confusion. Progression to frank stupor and coma may occur in as few as 10% and in as many as 80% of cases of Wernicke's encephalopathy.[72]

Confabulation is not unique to the Wernicke-Korsakoff syndrome. Peripheral neuropathy is common in alcoholic individuals but is not part of this syndrome.

Etiology

Thiamine deficiency plays a central role in the development of Wernicke's encephalopathy, which like any delirium, is considered a medical emergency. Although Wernicke's encephalopathy is not always related to alcohol withdrawal, some Wernicke's patients may coincidentally develop DTs, and some patients with DTs may develop Wernicke's. Thiamine deficiency causes a diffuse decrease in cerebral glucose utilization with resulting neurotoxicity. Wernicke's encephalopathy most often is associated with alcoholism, but can occur in any condition that causes thiamine deficiency (e.g., thyrotoxicosis, upper GI obstruction, severe anorexia, hyperemesis gravidarum, malabsorption syndrome, hemodialysis, prolonged intravenous feeding).[76,106]

Neuropathological findings in Wernicke's encephalopathy include punctate lesions in the periventricular, periaqueductal regions of the brain stem and diencephalon;[118] periventricular lesions of the dorsomedial nucleus of the thalamus, the hypothalamus, the mammillary bodies, the reticular activating system, the periaqueductal areas of the midbrain, and the floor of the fourth ventricle;[118] and loss of tissue[18] and edema[63] in the mammillary bodies.

Approximately 80% of patients who survive Wernicke's encephalopathy develop the Korsakoff amnestic syndrome.[82] However, many Korsakoff patients have no known history of prior Wernicke's encephalopathy.[15,16]

Treatment

Wernicke's encephalopathy is treated by medical management of the delirium and parenteral thiamine 100 mg initially, with upward titration until ophthalmoplegia resolves.[28] Oral thiamine is not always well absorbed:

◆ McNamara and colleagues[62] have described a 68-year-old woman admitted to a psychiatric hospital for a diagnosis of alcoholism. Her physical and mental status exams were normal except for some recent and remote memory deficits, and difficulty with tandem gait. She was begun on oral thiamine 100 mg daily and monitored for signs of alcohol withdrawal. Despite good inpatient nutrition and hydration by mouth (including large amounts of coffee) and no signs of alcohol withdrawal, the patient became increasingly confused, progressively disoriented, and amnestic. On day 3 she was switched to parenteral thiamine, with rapid resolution of the confusional state.

This case is a reminder that carbohydrate refeeding can precipitate acute thiamine deficiency, and the absorption of orally administered thiamine (already impaired in alcoholic patients) may be further blocked by both caffeinated and decaffeinated coffee[62] (often readily available on detox units). Psychiatrists who consult on such patients must be alert to the sometimes subtle presentations of this disease.

KORSAKOFF'S SYNDROME/ PSYCHOSIS

The original term *Korsakoff's psychosis*, which appears in the early literature, is in some ways a misnomer: psychotic symptoms such as delusions and hallucinations are not typical, although they can occur in the encephalopathic phase of the illness (i.e., the Wernicke delirium component).[118] A recent and more precise designation is DSM-IV's[1a] *alcohol-induced persisting amnestic disorder*, which emphasizes the memory deficits. Certainly the subsequent confabulation and evasiveness can seem like conviction about the unreal. Lishman[56] has written,

> Typically the patient gives a reasonably coherent but entirely false account of some recent event or experience, usually in relation to his own activities and often in response to suggestion by the examiner . . . The common "momentary type" [of confabulation] is brief in content, has reference to the recent past, and has to be provoked. The content can often be traced to a true memory which has become displaced in time or context. Much rarer is the "fantastic type" in which a sustained and grandiose theme is elaborated, usually describing farfetched adventures and experiences which clearly could not have taken place at any time. This form tends to occur spontaneously even without a provoking stimulus . . . . (p. 29)

Confabulation has been traditionally accepted as an integral feature of the syndrome, but is neither consistently present nor essential for the diagnosis.[118] Be sure to distinguish confabulation from delusions. Mr. Horton's delirious, agitated presentation is not characteristic of this syndrome.

DSM-IV Criteria for Substance-Induced Persisting Amnestic Disorder

The DSM-IV[1a, p. 162] diagnostic criteria for substance-induced persisting amnestic disorder are as follows:

A. The development of memory impairment as manifested by impairment in the ability to learn new information or the inability to recall previously learned information.

B. The memory disturbance causes significant impairment in social or occupational functioning and represents a significant decline from a previous level of functioning.

C. The memory disturbance does not occur exclusively during the course of a delirium or a dementia and persists beyond the usual duration of substance intoxication or withdrawal.

D. There is evidence from the history, physical examination, or laboratory findings that the memory disturbance is etiologically related to the persisting effects of substance use (e.g., a drug of abuse, a medication.)

Consult Appendix A for details on coding.

Neuropsychology

Several neuropsychological features characterize the Korsakoff amnestic syndrome.

♦ Both retrograde amnesia (impairing memory of material present before the onset) and anterograde amnesia (impairing new learning and memorization) are prominent,[75] although remote memories are better preserved than recent ones.

♦ Attention and perception of new material are intact, but retention is faulty. For example, patients are able to repeat three simple bits of information and understand what is wanted, but cannot retain the bits after distraction or learn them despite many repetitions. Memorization problems extend to all aspects of new learning: the names of persons and objects, nonsense syllables, a line of poetry, a card game, and all but the simplest motor tasks. "It seemed not to matter whether the information to be acquired was highly emotional or purely cognitive in nature, or by what sensory avenue the information was presented" (p. 43).[118]

♦ All types of memory are not equally affected. For example, patients can learn their way around the hospital ward and can acquire knowledge of simple ward routines. (This is called *procedural memory*.)

♦ Digit span is normal.

♦ In addition, the impairment of past memory is never complete. Patients may retain islets of information with varying degrees of accuracy but without their proper temporal sequence. A "telescoping" of events characteristically occurs (e.g., a patient who had been in a state mental hospital for 6 years reported that he had been there for only a few days).[118]

The descriptions of Victor and colleagues[118] remain among the most vivid in the literature:

We were quite unable to discern the factor(s) that governed what was forgotten and what was remembered. This aspect of the memory disorder seemed to follow no distinctive or consistent pattern. A patient might not recall seemingly important or emotionally charged events . . . but at the same time might be able to recall seemingly casual items or ones in which he or she was not personally involved . . . Similar inconsistencies were noted in regard to new memories. (p. 45)

The *catastrophic reaction* consists of hyperemotionality, restlessness, uncooperativeness, anxiety, tearfulness, and irritability, and occurs most characteristically with left-hemisphere lesions.[98] It is *not* typical of Korsakoff amnestic patients, who in the chronic stages of the illness are apathetic and placid, lack motivation, and show bland affect.[118] Korsakoff patients might admit to memory defects but without insight about the seriousness of their amnesia.

It was our impression that the patients were difficult to anger or to frighten, and although their emotional reactions were more or less appropriate, they were difficult to arouse.[118] (p. 45)

A progressive *global dementia*, such as senile dementia of the Alzheimer type, is *not* characteristic of Korsakoff amnestic disorder.[116,118] Although sensory, motivational, and visuospatial difficulties may occur, they are less prominent than the disordered memory and learning. Alertness is preserved with intact awareness of the patient's surroundings and without serious defects in social behavior. Also preserved are vocabulary, general language facility, long-standing motor skills and social habits, and the ability to recognize people known long before the illness. Apraxia and agnosia are not typical features, nor is aphasia; Korsakoff patients have normal speech and are able to write from dictation, copy figures, and draw simple objects like a clock from memory.

There is no effective treatment other than supportive management. Patients often require institutionalization or sheltered settings.[15] (See also the recent review by Kopelman.[48a])

❦ "LATENT" ENCEPHALOPATHY

Many cirrhotic patients without overt delirium suffer from subtle neuropsychological deficits that have been termed *latent* or *subclinical* encephalopathy.[24,36,85,91,92] Diagnostic

neuropsychological testing is more sensitive in identifying these individuals than is either the clinical neurological examination[35,81] or the EEG,[20,39] which may be normal.[80] Although useful in detecting delirium, the Trail Making Tests[81a] are of limited value in detecting latent hepatic encephalopathy, compared with other test batteries.[66]

◆ Performance skills are more often impaired than verbal skills, which may be normal;[36,92] such impairment interferes with a patient's ability to safely perform activities of daily living.[24,36,85,92]

◆ For example, patients with impaired short-term visual memory and delayed reaction times may be at risk when driving or operating machinery.

◆ The relationship between measurements of cerebral morphology (e.g., on CT scan) and neuropsychological test performance is controversial in these patients, with some studies emphasizing a close association between the two[12] while others find only a weak correlation.[66]

◆ Recently, regional cerebral blood flow in bilateral frontotemporal and right basal ganglia regions on single photo emission computed tomography (SPECT) brain scans was shown to be diminished in cirrhotic patients with visuopractic neuropsychological deficits characteristic of latent encephalopathy.[115] In summary, the clinical neurological exam, the EEG, brain imaging, and routine bedside tests of delirium do not identify those individuals at risk; instead, *formal neuropsychological testing appears to be the most sensitive and reliable.*[68] Batteries incorporating tests of intelligence, attention, learning, memory, psychomotor skills, language, and perceptual-spatial ability have been recommended for this specific patient population.[80] For screening purposes, tests of reaction time (e.g., the Vienna reaction time apparatus[45]) and short-term visual memory (e.g., the Benton visual retention test[8]) can detect the majority of compromised patients and are recommended for neuropsychiatric screening in the hepatology clinic.[66] These data should shape the psychiatric management of the ambulatory chronic alcoholic patient with cirrhosis, who may have cognitive deficits even in the absence of gross abnormalities on traditional mental status testing.

DSM-IV[1a] gives no specific instructions on how to code latent encephalopathy. Depending on the clinical findings, it may fit into *cognitive disorder not otherwise specified* (e.g., mild neurocognitive disorder), *amnestic disorder not otherwise specified*, or *dementia not otherwise specified*.

⚜ DIAGNOSTIC WORKUP

Liver Function Tests

Although liver function tests are indicators of hepatic disease, chronic, severe liver disease may cause "liver burnout," resulting in relatively *normal* serum enzyme levels and only modest hyperbilirubinemia.[57,58] All of the syndromes discussed in this chapter can coexist with liver function test results that fall within normal limits.[87]

Ammonia Levels

Although ammonia is widely believed to play a role in the pathogenesis of hepatic encephalopathy, the precise mechanism has yet to be clearly defined.[33] The value of serum ammonia levels is somewhat controversial. Several authors have reported significant correlations between elevations in arterial ammonia level and delirium,[29,59] and state that the blood ammonia level is helpful in establishing the diagnosis.[58] However, the magnitude of this value does not always correlate with the severity of the delirium.[86] In fact, there may be a stronger correlation between ammonia's CSF metabolites—glutamine and alpha-ketoglutaramate—and the clinical situation.[58]

Others have found that plasma levels of ammonia correlate poorly with hepatic encephalopathy[74] and may be abnormal in DTs as well.[42] Lockwood[58] advises that blood samples must be arterial, since venous ammonia levels may give spurious results due to unpredictable interactions between ammonia extraction and release by skeletal muscle. Hepatic encephalopathy is virtually always present when the blood ammonia concentration exceeds 3 mg/ml, but about 10% of patients with severe encephalopathy have levels within the normal range.[55] Moreover, patients with high ammonia levels may not be confused on mental status exam.[110]

The diagnosis of hepatic encephalopathy is usually one of exclusion; an elevated serum ammonia level in a delirious patient with hepatic insufficiency is highly suggestive of the diagnosis.[79]

Electroencephalogram

The EEG is of limited usefulness in the differential diagnosis of the delirious cirrhotic patient. It does have a role, however, in identifying those "psychiatric" presentations that may have a covert neurological underpinning. In the early stages of any delirium, for example, patients may have only ambiguous medical findings, and many authors advise using EEGs to assist diagnosis.

- The earliest change is slowing of the alpha rhythm and the appearance of 5- to 7-cps (*theta*) waves, most prominent in the frontal and temporal regions.[56]
- Although these changes are nonspecific for etiology, they flag an encephalopathic process in its early stages, often when other medical stigmata may be absent.
- These EEG changes may precede obvious changes in mental status[56] and may correlate with grades of neuropsychiatric abnormalities.[44,77]

Progressive impairments of consciousness show replacement of EEG alpha activity with theta waves. Eventually, *triphasic waves* make their appearance, portending a poor prognosis. Triphasic slow waves may also occur in patients with head injury, subdural hematomas, uremia, cerebral anoxia, infection, and electrolyte abnormalities.[86] Other metabolic derangements producing similar EEG changes include uremia, hypokalemia, anoxia, B_{12} deficiency, carbon dioxide retention, and the early stages of increased intracranial pressure.[56]

Although not specific for a hepatic source, these early EEG changes occurring in a conscious patient with the stigmata of liver disease, mental status changes, and no other findings are highly suggestive of delirium progressing to coma.[55]

During the height of delirium tremens, EEG rhythms show moderate increases in fast frequencies or may be in the normal range.[28]

Cerebrospinal Fluid

Lumbar puncture, including opening pressure, is usually normal in hepatic encephalopathy,[56] although increased protein may accompany evolution to coma.[96] There have also been reports of elevated CSF glutamine[29] and lactate levels,[121] although these levels are not routinely reported in CSF analysis.

There are no distinctive CSF findings in DTs, alcoholic hallucinosis, or Wernicke-Korsakoff syndrome.

Imaging Studies

CT or MRI scans of the brain are valuable in the differential diagnosis of mental status changes, but are of limited value in discriminating among metabolic causes of psychiatric symptoms. These tests exclude *structural* etiologies, such as subdural hematomas; chronic alcoholic patients are at high risk for head trauma. Unfortunately, often medical workup is prematurely abandoned and the patient is medically cleared if the MRI or CT scan was negative. *Think metabolic* until proven otherwise.

⬩ LIVER TRANSPLANTATION

Although we have not included a case example, the highlights of the liver transplantation literature follow, with references. This literature is covered more extensively by Trzepacz et al.[111,113,114] and others.[9,30,61,102]

Liver transplantation is increasingly being used for managing end-stage liver disease. Survival rates and quality of life have improved with advances in surgical techniques and immunosuppressive drugs. The 2-year survival rate is now 85%, with the highest mortality occurring within the first 6 months after transplant.[14]

Psychiatric assessment is routinely part of the screening process.[73a] To date, however, there is little research on what psychiatric criteria should be used to accept or reject a transplant candidate.[19,30] In Great Britain, for example, alcohol dependence has been considered a contraindication.[73] In the United States, however, alcoholism is not an absolute exclusion criterion for liver transplantation.[80a] Kumar et al.[51] found that only about 1 in 10 patients return to alcohol abuse after transplantation, but larger studies are required to support these data.[9,10] Moreover, patients with alcoholic liver disease have been shown to have graft survival rates equivalent to those of nonalcoholic control subjects, and have achieved equal levels of postoperative health.[40a,47] This favorable outcome has been shown in alcoholic patients despite significantly worse presurgical liver failure and morbidity.

Riether and Mahler,[83] in their review on suicide in liver transplant patients, emphasize that

> [t]he transplant team is responsible for rationing a scarce public commodity. This imposes a duty to place organs in those patients with the greatest chance for a successful outcome. (p. 576)

Organ transplantation may be successful even in individuals with significant psychopathology[101,104] For example, in a prospective study of 247 liver transplant candidates, Trzepacz and colleagues[111] found that half of them had a DSM-III[1] diagnosis, with 20% having adjustment disorders, 19% delirium, 9% alcohol dependence or abuse, 5% major depression, and 2% other substance abuse. They later retrospectively analyzed the transplantation and survival status for these patients[112] and found—optimistically—that survival status posttransplantation was *not* predicted by the presence of delirium or by pretransplantation differences in EEGs, cognitive tests, or serum albumin.

The severity of chronic neuropsychological deficits before liver transplantation has an impact on the quality of life after surgery.[109] Neuropsychological impairments of patients with severe liver disease improve after surgery but do not disappear.[108]

The quality of life after liver transplantation is good,[6a,19a,53,60,67,79a,84,103] with many patients able to return to work and normal activity after a single transplant.[107] Not surprisingly, patients requiring multiple transplants do more poorly, with organ rejection causing distress and often neuropsychiatric complications.[22,48,101,120] (See Singh et al.'s[99] exhaustive review of CNS lesions in liver transplant patients.) Medical noncompliance after transplantation may indicate an underlying psychiatric disorder that may respond to psychiatric intervention.[105]

The use of psychotropics in organ transplantation has been effectively reviewed elsewhere.[103,113,114] The following discussion highlights some of the major points regarding psychopharmacology in the setting of hepatic failure.

⬩ PSYCHOPHARMACOLOGY IN HEPATIC FAILURE

Pharmacokinetic changes may affect the mechanism and timing of a drug's absorption, distribution, metabolism, or excretion. Most psychotropic medications—other than lithium—are primarily metabolized by the liver. Hepatic insufficiency significantly affects medication clearance. The following are a few highlights:

◆ *Phase I metabolism:* Alters compounds by oxidation, reduction, or hydrolysis so as to prepare them for excretion or for further Phase II reactions.[94] Most Phase I oxidation reactions occur by the cytochrome P450 system. Phase I activity is decreased in liver disease. Clearance of drugs metabolized by Phase I reactions—for example, diazepam (Valium), chlordiazepoxide (Librium), alprazolam (Xanax), and triazolam (Halcion)—is reduced by 30%–66% in liver disease.[52] Other agents expected to have decreased clearance similar to that of diazepam in liver disease include clorazepate (Tranxene), prazepam (Centrax), halazepam (Paxipam), and flurazepam (Dalmane).[94] Cirrhosis decreases the activity and levels of enzymes, including the cytochrome P450 system.[94] Chlorpromazine (Thorazine)-induced hepatotoxicity and cholestasis occur when there is impaired sulfoxidation, another Phase I reaction.[52]

◆ *Phase II metabolism:* Consists of several conjugation pathways, usually resulting in the compound's inactivation.[94] The most common pathway is glucuronidation, which remains intact despite hepatic failure. This allows the clearance of Phase II–dependent medications, such as oxazepam (Serax), lorazepam (Ativan), and temazepam (Restoril), to be relatively preserved.[52]

The rate of hepatic metabolism is dependent on either 1) the rate of delivery of the drug to the hepatic metabolizing enzymes, in which liver blood flow is rate limiting; or 2) the intrinsic capacity of hepatic enzymes to metabolize the substrate, in which case the enzyme's saturation capacity is rate limiting.[52] Both may be impaired in cirrhosis; the former due to extrahepatic shunting, the latter by decreased enzyme activity.

◆ Classification as a *low-clearance drug* implies low affinity, slower metabolism, and enzyme saturation as rate limiting (e.g., diazepam, chlorpromazine).[114]

◆ *High-clearance drugs* are not enzyme dependent, but rather are flow dependent, and are metabolized as quickly as they can reach the liver (e.g., haloperidol [Haldol], tricyclic antidepressants, triazolam [Halcion]).[52] High-clearance drugs undergo significant *first-pass metabolism* (i.e., by the end of an orally administered drug's first pass through the liver, only a small fraction of the parent compound remains to enter the circulation).[52] For example, high-clearance drugs such as haloperidol are normally administered orally at 2–4 times the parenteral dose to compensate for extensive first-pass metabolism and to achieve equivalent blood levels and clinical response.[52] Moreover, intramuscular and intravenous administration of drugs avoids initial hepatic degradation, allowing direct entry into the systemic circulation.[52]

Some notes on sedating drugs:

◆ Patients with cirrhosis become more heavily sedated than healthy individuals when given benzodiazepines, with the greatest effects occurring in patients with severe liver dysfunction or a prior history of hepatic encephalopathy.[52]

◆ Haloperidol is the neuroleptic of choice for patients with hepatic disease, but very little has been written on its specific pharmacokinetics in liver failure. *Chlorpromazine's use in cirrhotic patients is unanimously advised against* because it can induce hepatotoxicity and cholestasis.[52]

Some notes on antidepressants and lithium in liver disease:

◆ The tricyclic antidepressants undergo extensive oxidative metabolism, often with active metabolites, and have long elimination half-lives.[52,94] Diminished hepatic delivery (e.g., shunting) and decreased functional liver tissue with diminished enzymatic activity will result in higher tricyclic blood levels in hepatic failure.[113] It is recommended that the initial dose be reduced by one-half to two-thirds, and that blood levels be monitored.[52] *Keep in mind that the constipation induced by tricyclic anticholinergic properties may exacerbate hepatic encephalopathy in susceptible individuals.*[94]

◆ Trazodone (Desyrel) has minimal hepatic excretion and little anticholinergic activity; it may be helpful in this population,[94] although we could find no specific studies.

◆ Fluoxetine (Prozac) ($t_{1/2}$ = 2–3 days) and its active metabolite norfluoxetine ($t_{1/2}$ = 7–9 days) are extensively hepatically metabolized. In cirrhosis, the mean elimination half-lives increase to 8 and 12 days, respectively.[23] Fluoxetine and norfluoxetine bind to hepatic cytochrome P450; they may interfere with the metabolism and clearance of other similarly metabolized drugs, potentially producing toxicity. In cirrhotic patients, dosages must be reduced or doses given less frequently,[17,90] since cirrhosis significantly reduces the clearance of fluoxetine and its metabolite.[11]

◆ Lithium is not protein bound; it is excreted by the kidney, and its metabolism is not directly affected by hepatic disease. It may be *indirectly* affected when ascites accompanies cirrhosis, increasing the water composition of the body. More lithium is required to produce the desired plasma levels, since the volume of distribution is increased.[52]

The interested reader should refer to two excellent papers by Leipzig[52] and Secor and Schenker[94] on the psychopharmacology of patients with hepatic and GI disease. Trzepacz et al.[113,114] provide an excellent general review of pharmacokinetics in organ failure. See also Appendix O ("Notes on the 'New' Antidepressants in the Medical Setting").

⟁ SUMMARY

1. The differential diagnosis of psychiatric symptoms in the cirrhotic patient must consider alcohol with-

drawal syndromes and the various etiologies of delirium associated with liver failure.

2. The psychotic *content* of cirrhotic patients has little value in differential diagnosis. Although the most common cause of psychosis for alcoholic cirrhotic patients is delirium tremens (DTs), there is a wide spectrum of conditions that also induces psychotic symptoms. Be wary of jumping to conclusions and abandoning a full medical and neurological workup because a patient's mental status "sounds like DTs" or "the MRI is normal." As the case of Mr. Horton demonstrates, the significant symptomatic overlap among syndromes mandates cautious and thorough medical evaluation.

3. Hepatic encephalopathy is often forgotten in the differential diagnosis of the psychotic alcoholic patient. It may present subtly as primary psychiatric symptoms, without its delirious character making itself obvious. Until hepatic encephalopathy has been definitively ruled out, benzodiazepines with long-acting metabolites (e.g., chlordiazepoxide [Librium], diazepam [Valium]) should be avoided. Lorazepam (Ativan) or oxazepam (Serax) are better choices for withdrawal symptoms—although, as mentioned, their potential to increase GABA-ergic tone in the central nervous system dictates vigilance in hepatic encephalopathy.

4. The psychopharmacology of hepatic failure requires cautious use of medications that undergo oxidative metabolism in the liver. This includes most psychotropics. Haloperidol (Haldol), although oxidized in the liver, has been safely used for the psychotic symptoms of hepatic encephalopathy.

⬥ REFERENCES

1. American Psychiatric Association: Diagnostic and Statistical Manual of Mental Disorders, 3rd Edition. Washington, DC, American Psychiatric Association, 1980

1a. American Psychiatric Association: Diagnostic and Statistical Manual of Mental Disorders, 4th Edition. Washington, DC, American Psychiatric Association, 1994

2. Bansky G, Meier P, Riederer E, et al: Effects of the benzodiazepine receptor antagonist flumazenil in hepatic encephalopathy in humans. Gastroenterology 97:744–750, 1989

3. Bansky G, Meier P, Ziegler W, et al: Reversal of hepatic coma by benzodiazepine antagonist (Ro 15-1788). Lancet 1:1324–1325, 1985

4. Basile A, Gammal S, Mullen K, et al: Differential responsiveness of cerebellar Purkinje neurons to GABA and benzodiazepine ligands in an animal model of hepatic encephalopathy. J Neurosci 8:2414–2421, 1988

5. Basile A, Hughes R, Harrison P, et al: Elevated brain concentrations of 1,4-benzodiazepines in fulminant hepatic failure. N Engl J Med 325:473–478, 1991

6. Bassett M, Mullen K, Skolnick P, et al: Amelioration of hepatic encephalopathy by pharmacologic antagonism of the GABA$_a$-benzodiazepine receptor complex in a rabbit model of fulminant hepatic failure. Gastroenterology 93:1069–1077, 1987

6a. Belle S, Porayko M: Improvement in quality of life after transplantation for recipients in the NIDDK Liver Transplantation Database. Transplant Proc 27:1230–1232, 1995

7. Benowitz N: Central nervous system manifestations of toxic disorders, in Metabolic Brain Dysfunction in Systemic Disorders. Edited by Arieff A, Griggs R. Boston, MA, Little, Brown, 1992, pp 409–436

8. Benton A: The Revised Visual Retention Test. New York, Psychological Corporation, 1974

9. Beresford T: Alcohol abuse and liver transplantation, in Psychiatric Aspects of Organ Transplantation. Edited by Craven J, Rodin G. Oxford, UK, Oxford University Press, 1992, pp 33–49

10. Beresford T, Schwartz J, Wilson D, et al: The short-term psychological health of alcoholic and non-alcoholic liver transplant recipients. Alcohol Clin Exp Res 16:996–1000, 1992

11. Bergstrom R, Beasley C, Levy N, et al: The effect of renal and hepatic disease on the pharmacokinetics, renal tolerance, and risk-benefit profile of fluoxetine. Int Clin Psychopharmacol 8:261–266, 1993

12. Bernthal P, Hays A, Tarter R, et al: Cerebral CT scan abnormalities in cholestatic and hepatocellular disease and their relationship to neuropsychological test performance. Hepatology 7:107–114, 1987

13. Bird R, Makela E: Alcohol withdrawal: what is the benzodiazepine of choice? Ann Pharmacother 28:67–71, 1994

14. Bismuth H: Liver transplantation: a subtle revolution. Br J Surg 74:339–340, 1987

15. Blansjaar B, Takens H, Zwinderman A: The course of alcohol amnestic disorder: a three-year follow-up study of clinical signs and social disabilities. Acta Psychiatr Scand 86:240–246, 1992

16. Blansjaar B, Van Dijk J: Korsakoff minus Wernicke syndrome. Alcohol Alcohol 27:435–437, 1992

17. Castiella A, Arenas J: Fluoxetine hepatotoxicity (letter). Am J Gastroenterol 89:458–459, 1994

18. Charness M, DeLaPaz R: Mammillary body atrophy in Wernicke's encephalopathy: antemortem identification using magnetic resonance imaging. Ann Neurol 22:595–600, 1987

18a. Ciraulo D, Shader R, Ciraulo A, et al: The treatment the alcohol withdrawal, in Manual of Psychiatric Therapeutics, 2nd Edition. Edited by Shader R. Boston, MA, Little, Brown, 1994, pp 193–210

19. Collis I, Lloyd G: Psychiatric aspects of liver disease. Br J Psychiatry 161:12–22, 1992

19a. Collis I, Burroughs A, Rolles K, et al: Psychiatric and social outcome of liver transplantation. Br J Psychiatry 166:521–524, 1995

20. Conn H, Leevy C, Vlahcevic Z, et al: Comparison of lactulose and neomycin in the treatment of chronic portal systemic encephalopathy. Gastroenterology 72:803–806, 1977

21. Davidson C, Gabuzda G: Hepatic coma, in Diseases of the Liver, 4th Edition. Edited by Schiff L, Schiff E. Philadelphia, PA, JB Lippincott, 1975, pp 466–499

22. Della Monica O, Alfani D, Berloco P, et al: Neuropsychiatric complications after liver transplantation: a single center experience. Transplant Proc 25:1771–1772, 1993

23. Dista Products Company: Prozac (fluoxetine hydrochloride). Indianapolis, IN, June 1992

24. Dunk A, Moore J, Symon A, et al: The effects of propranolol on hepatic encephalopathy in patients with cirrhosis and portal hypertension. Alimentary Pharmacology and Therapeutics 2:143–152, 1988

25. Editorial: Hepatic encephalopathy today. Lancet 1:489–491, 1984

26. Eichler M: Psychological changes associated with induced hyperammonemia. Science 144:886–888, 1964

27. Feuerlein W: Alkoholismus—Missbrauch und Abhaengigkeit, 3 Aufl. Stuttgart, Germany, Thieme, 1984

28. Franklin J, Frances R: Alcohol-induced organic mental disorders, in The American Psychiatric Press Textbook of Neuropsychiatry, 2nd Edition. Edited by Yudofsky S, Hales R. Washington, DC, American Psychiatric Press, 1992, pp 563–583

29. Fraser C, Arieff A: Hepatic encephalopathy. N Engl J Med 313:865–873, 1985

30. Freeman A, Davis L, Libb J, et al: Assessment of transplant candidates and prediction of outcome, in Psychiatric Aspects of Organ Transplantation. Edited by Craven J, Rodin G. Oxford, UK, Oxford University Press, 1992, pp 9–21

31. Fuller R, Gordis E: Refining the treatment of alcohol withdrawal. JAMA 272:557–558, 1994

32. Galanter M, Kleber H (eds): Textbook of Substance Abuse Treatment. Washington DC, American Psychiatric Press, 1994

33. Gammal S, Jones E: Hepatic encephalopathy. Med Clin North Am 73:793–813, 1989

34. Gazzard B, Price H, Dawson A: Detection of hepatic encephalopathy. Postgrad Med J 44:615–625, 1986

35. Gilberstadt S, Gilberstadt H, Zieve L, et al: Psychomotor performance defects in cirrhotic patients without overt encephalopathy. Ann Intern Med 140:519–521, 1980

36. Gitlin N, Lewis D, Hinkley L: The diagnosis and prevalence of subclinical hepatic encephalopathy in apparently healthy, ambulant, non-shunted patients with cirrhosis. J Hepatol 3:75–82, 1986

37. Grimm G, Katzenschlager R, Schneeweiss B, et al: Improvement of hepatic encephalopathy treated with flumazenil. Lancet 2:1392–1393, 1988

38. Grimm G, Lenz K, Kleinberger G, et al: Benzodiazepine antagonism improves hepatic encephalopathy due to fulminant hepatic failure: monitoring by multimodality evoked potentials, in Advances in Ammonia Metabolism and Hepatic Encephalopathy. Edited by Soeters P, Wilson J, Meijer A, et al. Amsterdam, Elsevier Sciences, 1988, pp 338–345

39. Hawkes C, Brunt P, Prescott R, et al: EEG-provocative tests in the diagnosis of hepatic encephalopathy. Electroencephalogr Clin Neurophysiol 34:163–169, 1973

40. Holloway H, Hales R, Wantanabe H, et al: Recognition and treatment of acute alcohol withdrawal syndrome. Psychiatr Clin North Am 7:729–743, 1984

40a. Howard L, Fahy T, Wong P, et al: Psychiatric outcome in alcoholic liver transplant patients. QJM 87:731–736, 1994

41. Jain H, Shamoian C: The patient with hepatic disease, in Treatments of Psychiatric Disorders: A Task Force Report of the American Psychiatric Association, Vol 2. Washington, DC, American Psychiatric Association, 1989, pp 930–939

42. Jefferson J, Marshall J (eds): Neuropsychiatric features of medical disorders. New York, Plenum, 1981

43. Jones E, Skolnick P, Gammal S, et al: The gamma-aminobutyric acid A ($GABA_A$) receptor complex and hepatic encephalopathy. Ann Intern Med 110:532–546, 1989

44. Kennedy J, Parbhoo S, MacGillivray B, et al: Effect of extracorporeal liver perfusion on the electroencephalogram of patients in coma due to acute liver failure. Q J Med 42:549–561, 1973

45. Klensch H: Die diagnostische Valenz der Reaktionszeitmesug bei vershiedenen Erkrankungen [The diagnostic significance of reaction time determination in various cerebral diseases]. Fortschr Neurol Psychiatr 41:575–581, 1973

46. Klotz U, Antonin K, Brugel H, et al: Disposition of diazepam and its major metabolite, desmethyldiazepam, in patients with liver disease. Clin Pharmacol Ther 21:430–436, 1977

47. Knechtle S, Fleming M, Barry K, et al: Liver transplantation for alcoholic liver disease. Surgery 112:694–701; discussion 701–703, 1992

48. Kober B, Kuchler T, Broelsch C, et al: A psychological support concept and quality of life research in a liver transplant program: an interdisciplinary multicentre study. Psychother Psychosom 54:117–131, 1990

48a. Kopelman M: The Korsakoff syndrome. Br J Psychiatry 166:154–173, 1995

49. Kornfeld D: Psychiatric aspects of liver disease, in Emotional Factors in Gastrointestinal Illness. Edited by Lindner A. Amsterdam, Excerpta Medica, 1973, pp 166–181

50. Kraus J, Desmond P, Marshall J, et al: Effects of aging and liver disease on disposition of lorazepam. Clin Pharmacol Ther 24:411–419, 1978

51. Kumar S, Basista M, Stauber R, et al: Orthotopic liver transplantation for alcoholic liver disease (abstract). Gastroenterology 96:A916, 1989

52. Leipzig R: Psychopharmacology in patients with hepatic and gastrointestinal disease. Int J Psychiatry Med 20:109–139, 1990

138

A CASE APPROACH TO MEDICAL-PSYCHIATRIC PRACTICE

53. Leyendecker B, Bartholomew U, Neuhaus R, et al: Quality of life of liver transplant recipients: a pilot study. Transplantation 56:561–567, 1993

54. Lichtigfeld F: Hepatic encephalopathy and delirium tremens—double jeopardy (letter). S Afr Med J 67:880, 1985

55. Lipowski Z: Delirium: Acute Confusional States. New York, Oxford University Press, 1990

56. Lishman W: Organic Psychiatry, 2nd Edition. London, Blackwell Scientific, 1987

57. Lockwood A: Hepatic Encephalopathy. Boston, MA, Butterworth-Heinemann, 1992

58. Lockwood A: Hepatic encephalopathy, in Metabolic Brain Dysfunction in Systemic Disorders. Edited by Arieff A, Griggs R. Boston, MA, Little, Brown, 1992, pp 167–182

59. Lockwood A, McDonald J, Reiman R, et al: The dynamics of ammonia metabolism in man: effects of liver disease and hyperammonemia. J Clin Invest 63:449–460, 1979

60. Lowe D, O'Grady J, McEwen J, et al: Quality of life following liver transplantation: a preliminary report. J R Coll Physicians Lond 24:43–46, 1990

61. Lucey M, Merion R, Beresford T (eds): Liver Transplantation and the Alcoholic Patient: Medical, Surgical, and Psychosocial Issues. New York, Cambridge University Press, 1994

62. McNamara M, Campbell J, Recupero P: Wernicke-Korsakoff syndrome (letter). J Neuropsychiatry Clin Neurosci 3:232, 1991

63. Mensing J, Hoogland P, Slooff J: Computed tomography in the diagnosis of Wernicke's encephalopathy: a radiological-neuropathological correlation. Ann Neurol 16:363–365, 1984

64. Mirin S, Weiss R, Greenfield S: Psychoactive substance use disorders, in The Practitioner's Guide to Psychoactive Drugs, 3rd Edition. Edited by Gelenberg A, Bassuk E, Schoonover S. New York, Plenum Medical Book, 1991, pp 243–279

65. Misra P: Hepatic encephalopathy. Med Clin North Am 65:209–226, 1981

66. Moore J, Dunk A, Crawford J, et al: Neuropsychological deficits and morphological MRI brain scan abnormalities in apparently healthy non-encephalopathic patients with cirrhosis. J Hepatol 9:319–325, 1989

67. Moore K, Jones R, Angus P, et al: Psychosocial adjustment to illness: quality of life following liver transplantation. Transplant Proc 24:2257–2258, 1992

68. Moss H, Tarter R, Yao J, et al: Subclinical hepatic encephalopathy: relationship between neuropsychological deficits and standard laboratory tests assessing hepatic status. Archives of Clinical Neuropsychology 7:419–429, 1992

69. Mullen K, Martin J, Mendelson W, et al: Could an endogenous benzodiazepine ligand contribute to hepatic encephalopathy? Lancet 1:457–459, 1988

70. Müller N, Klages U, Günther W: Hepatic encephalopathy presenting as delirium and mania: the possible role of bilirubin. Gen Hosp Psychiatry 16:138–140, 1994

71. Murphy T, Chalmers T, Eckhardt R, et al: Hepatic coma: clinical and laboratory observations on forty patients. N Engl J Med 239:605–612, 1948

72. Nakada T, Knight R: Alcohol and the central nervous system. Med Clin North Am 68:121–131, 1984

73. Neuberger J: Transplantation for alcoholic liver disease. BMJ 299:693–694, 1989

73a. Olbrisch M, Levenson J: Psychosocial assessment of organ transplant candidates: current status of methodological and philosophical issues. Psychosomatics 36:236–243, 1995

74. Pappas S, Ferenci P, Schafer D, et al: Visual evoked potentials in a rabbit model of hepatic encephalopathy, II: comparison of hyperammonemic encephalopathy, postictal coma and coma induced by synergic neurotoxins. Gastroenterology 86:546–551, 1984

75. Parkin A: The relationship between anterograde and retrograde amnesia in alcoholic Wernicke-Korsakoff syndrome. Psychol Med 21:11–14, 1991

76. Parkin A, Blunden J, Rees J, et al: Wernicke-Korsakoff syndrome of nonalcoholic origin. Brain Cogn 15:69–82, 1991

77. Parsons-Smith B, Summerskill W, Dawson A, et al: The encephalograph in liver disease. Lancet 2:867–871, 1957

78. Pillans P, Robins A, Straughan J: Drug therapy in patients with hepatic encephalopathy—suggested guidelines for sedation and treatment of delirium tremens—double jeopardy. S Afr Med J 66:711, 1984

79. Podolsky D, Isselbacher K: Cirrhosis of the liver, in Harrison's Principles of Internal Medicine, 12th Edition. Edited by Wilson J, Braunwald E, Isselbacher K, et al. New York, McGraw-Hill, Health Professions Division, 1991, pp 1340–1350

79a. Price C, Lowe D, Cohen A, et al: Prospective study of the quality of life in patients assessed for liver transplantation: outcome in transplanted and not transplanted groups. J R Soc Med 88:130–135, 1995

80. Puca F, Antonaci F, Panella C, et al: Psychomotor dysfunction in alcoholic and post-necrotic cirrhotic patients without overt encephalopathy. Acta Neurol Scand 79:280–287, 1989

80a. Raakow R, Langrehr J, Lohmann R, et al: Is orthotopic liver transplantation for end-stage alcoholic cirrhosis justified? Transplant Proc 27:1241–1242, 1995

81. Rehnstrom S, Simert G, Hansson J, et al: Chronic hepatic encephalopathy: a psychometrical study. Scand J Gastroenterol 12:305–311, 1977

81a. Reitan R: Validity of the Trail Making Test as an indicator of organic brain damage. Percept Mot Skills 8:271–276, 1958

82. Reuler J, Girard D, Cooney T: Wernicke's encephalopathy. N Engl J Med 312:1035–1039, 1985

83. Riether A, Mahler E: Suicide in liver transplant patients. Psychosomatics 35:574–578, 1994

84. Riether A, Smith S, Lewison B, et al: Quality-of-life changes and psychiatric and neurocognitive outcome after heart and liver transplantation. Transplantation 54:444–450, 1992

85. Rikkers L, Jenko P, Rudman D, et al: Subclinical hepatic encephalopathy: detection, prevalence and relationship to nitrogen metabolism. Gastroenterology 75:462–469, 1978

86. Rothstein J, McKhann G: Hepatic encephalopathy, in Current Therapy in Neurologic Disease—3. Edited by Johnson R. Philadelphia, PA, BC Decker, 1990, pp 352–356

87. Russell D, Keller F, Whitaker J: Episodic confusion and tremor associated with extrahepatic portacaval shunting in cirrhotic liver disease. Neurology 39:403–405, 1989

88. Sabot L, Gross M, Halpert E: A study of acute alcoholic psychoses in women. Br J Addict 63:29–49, 1968

89. Saitz R, Mayo-Smith M, Roberts M, et al: Individualized treatment for alcohol withdrawal: a randomized double-blind controlled trial. JAMA 272:519–523, 1994

90. Schenker S, Bergstrom R, Wolen R, et al: Fluoxetine disposition and elimination in cirrhosis. Pharmacol Ther 44:353–359, 1988

91. Schomerus H, Hamster W: Latent portasystemic encephalopathy. Digestion 14:5–6, 1976

92. Schomerus H, Hamster W, Blunck H, et al: Latent portasystemic encephalopathy, I: nature of cerebral functional defects and their effects on fitness to drive. Dig Dis Sci 26:622–630, 1981

93. Scollo-Lavizzari G, Steinmann E: Reversal of hepatic coma by benzodiazepine antagonist (Ro 15-1788). Lancet 1:1324–1325, 1985

94. Secor J, Schenker S: Drug metabolism in patients with liver disease. Adv Intern Med 32:379–406, 1987

95. Sellers E, Kalant H: Alcohol intoxication and withdrawal. N Engl J Med 294:757–762, 1976

96. Sherlock S: Diseases of the Liver and Biliary System, 6th Edition. Oxford, UK, Blackwell Scientific, 1981

97. Shull H, Wilkinson G, Johnson R, et al: Normal disposition of oxazepam in acute viral hepatitis and cirrhosis. Ann Intern Med 84:420–425, 1976

98. Silver J, Hales R, Yudofsky S, et al: Psychiatric consultation to neurology, in American Psychiatric Press Review of Psychiatry, Vol 9. Edited by Tasman A, Goldfinger SM, Kaufmann C. Washington, DC, American Psychiatric Press, 1990, pp 433–465

99. Singh N, Yu V, Gayowski T: Central nervous system lesions in adult liver transplant recipients: clinical review with implications for management. Medicine 73:110–118, 1994

100. Summerskill W, Davidson E, Sherlock S, et al: The neuropsychiatric syndrome associated with hepatic cirrhosis and an extensive portal collateral circulation. Q J Med 25:245–266, 1956

101. Surman O: Psychiatric aspects of organ transplantation. Am J Psychiatry 146:972–982, 1989

102. Surman O: Liver transplantation, in Psychiatric Aspects of Organ Transplantation. Edited by Craven J, Rodin G. Oxford, UK, Oxford University Press, 1992, pp 177–188

103. Surman O: Psychiatric aspects of liver transplantation. Psychosomatics 35:297–307, 1994

104. Surman O, Dienstag J, Cosimi A, et al: Liver transplantation: psychiatric considerations. Psychosomatics 28:615–621, 1987

105. Surman O, Dienstag J, Cosimi A, et al: Psychosomatic aspects of liver transplantation. Psychother Psychosom 48:26–31, 1987

106. Tan G, Farnell G, Hensrud D, et al: Acute Wernicke's encephalopathy attributable to pure dietary thiamine deficiency. Mayo Clin Proc 69:849–850, 1994

107. Tarter R, Erb S, Biller P, et al: Quality of life following liver transplantation: a preliminary report. Gastroenterol Clin North Am 17:207–217, 1988

108. Tarter R, Switala J, Arria A, et al: Subclinical hepatic encephalopathy: comparison before and after orthotopic liver transplantation. Transplantation 50:632–637, 1990

109. Tarter R, Switala J, Plail J, et al: Severity of hepatic encephalopathy before liver transplantation is associated with quality of life after transplantation. Arch Intern Med 152:2097–2101, 1992

110. Trzepacz P: Personal communication, November 1993

111. Trzepacz P, Brenner R, van Thiel D: A psychiatric study of 247 liver transplantation candidates. Psychosomatics 30:147–153, 1989

112. Trzepacz P, DiMartini A: Survival of 247 liver transplantation candidates. Gen Hosp Psychiatry 14:380–386, 1992

113. Trzepacz P, DiMartini A, Tringali R: Psychopharmacologic issues in organ transplantation, II: psychopharmacologic medications. Psychosomatics 34:290–298, 1993

114. Trzepacz P, DiMartini A, Tringali R: Psychopharmacologic issues in organ transplantation, I: pharmacokinetics in organ failure and psychiatric aspects of immunosuppressants and anti-infectious agents. Psychosomatics 34:199–207, 1993

115. Trzepacz P, Tarter R, Shah A, et al: SPECT scan and cognitive findings in subclinical hepatic encephalopathy. J Neuropsychiatry Clin Neurosci 6:170–175, 1994

116. Victor M: Alcoholic dementia. Can J Neurol Sci 21:88–99, 1994

117. Victor M, Adams R, Collins G: The Wernicke-Korsakoff Syndrome. Oxford, UK, Blackwell Scientific, 1971

118. Victor M, Adams R, Collins G: The Wernicke-Korsakoff Syndrome and Related Neurological Disease Due to Malnutrition (Contemporary Neurology Series, Vol 3). Philadelphia, PA, FA Davis, 1989

119. Victor M, Martin J: Nutritional and metabolic diseases of the nervous system, in Harrison's Principles of Internal Medicine, 12th Edition. Edited by Wilson J, Braunwald E, Isselbacher K, et al. New York, McGraw-Hill, Health Professions Division, 1991, pp 2045–2054

120. Vieta E, DePablo J, Cirera E, et al: Rapidly cycling bipolar II disorder following liver transplantation. Gen Hosp Psychiatry 15:129–131, 1993

121. Yao H, Sadoshima S, Fujii K, et al: Cerebrospinal fluid lactate in patients with hepatic encephalopathy. Eur Neurol 27:182–187, 1987

122. Yurdaydin C, Gu Z, Nowak G, et al: Benzodiazepine receptor ligands are elevated in an animal model of hepatic encephalopathy: relationship between brain concentration and severity of encephalopathy. J Pharmacol Exp Ther 265:565–571, 1993

The Patient With Kidney Disease

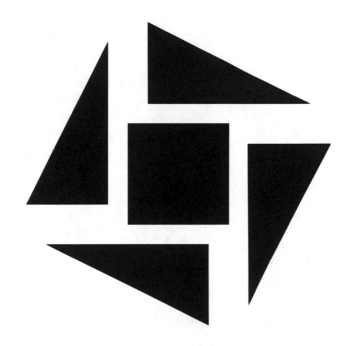

CHAPTER 4

CONTENTS

■ Introduction to Chapter 4 143
■ Case Presentation: Mrs. Freed: The Manic Patient
   in Renal Failure on Dialysis 144
■ Questions 144
■ Answers 147
■ Discussion 148
   ◆ Neuropsychiatric Presentations of Renal Failure 148
      Predictors of Neuropsychiatric Disturbance . 148
         Blood Urea Nitrogen 148
         Electroencephalogram 148
         Creatinine Clearance 148
      Dialysis-Related Neuropsychiatric Syndromes 149
         Disequilibrium Syndrome 149
         Dialysis Dementia 149
   ◆ Psychopharmacology in Renal Failure 149
      Nonrenal Factors 150
      Proteins and Protein Binding 150
      Unreliable Blood Levels 151
   ◆ Psychosis 151
      Neuroleptics 151
      Antiparkinsonian Medications 151
   ◆ Mania: Lithium and Kidney Physiology . . . 151
      The Controversy 151
         Effects on Tubular Functioning and
            Concentrating Ability 152
         Effects on Glomerular Function 153
         Proteinuria 153
         Histopathological Changes 153
      Using Lithium in the Setting of Renal Failure 153
         Maintenance Lithium 153
         Diuretics and Lithium 154
      Carbamazepine 154
      Valproate 154
   ◆ Summary 154
   ◆ References 156
■ Case Presentation: Mr. Barry: The Depressed
   Renal Patient and Transplantation 159
■ Questions 159
■ Answers 163
■ Discussion 164
   ◆ Coping With End-Stage Renal Disease 164
      A Digression About Disability Insurance . . . 164
      Illness Intrusiveness and Quality of Life . . . 165

Sexual Dysfunction 165
Hemodialysis Versus Continuous Abdominal
   Peritoneal Dialysis 166
Psychosocial Factors and Survival 166
◆ Depression and Anxiety 167
   Rational Treatment Withdrawal and Suicide . . 168
   Psychotherapy 168
      Compliance 169
      Behavioral and Cognitive Strategies 169
      Psychodynamics 170
   Medication 171
      Antidepressants 171
      Benzodiazepines 171
      Buspirone 172
      Chloral Hydrate 172
      Barbiturates 172
◆ Kidney Transplantation 172
   Candidates for Organ Transplantation 172
   Medical Risks of Transplantation 173
   Organ Donation 174
   Psychotherapeutic Issues 174
      Psychodynamic Concerns 174
      Psychological Preparation for Surgery 175
      Cadaver Versus Family Organ Recipients . . . 176
      Suicide 176
      Psychotherapy 177
   Neuropsychiatric Complications 177
      Infection 177
      Neurological Complications 177
      Corticosteroids 178
      Cyclosporine 178
      FK506 178
      OKT3 178
      Azathioprine 178
      Cimetidine 178
   Psychopharmacology 179
      Neuroleptics 179
      Anxiolytics 179
      Antidepressants 179
      Electroconvulsive Therapy 179
      Lithium 179
◆ Summary 180
◆ References 182

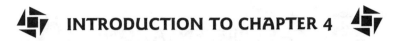

Every chronic medical illness is stressful, but the strain of end-stage renal disease (ESRD) is particularly exhausting—there is no physical or psychological respite. Work, family, meals, leisure, finances, sexuality, life expectancy—all are invaded by chronic renal failure. Perhaps more than any other chronic disease, ESRD imposes unremitting, multifaceted deprivation. In addition, tracing the fate of psychotropics in renal failure can lead to nightmarish flashbacks of renal physiology and organic chemistry; it is a labyrinth. Nonrenal factors confuse the issue. The easiest-to-trace blood protein, albumin, simply decreases in renal failure, but unfortunately is not the sole binder of psychotropics. As you will read, things get complicated.

This chapter reviews the practical consequences of these physiological changes for the renal patient. A concise guide to some of the legal issues, such as competency, living wills, and durable power of attorney, is provided in Appendix F. Use the questions following each vignette as you find most useful. There may be more than one correct option.

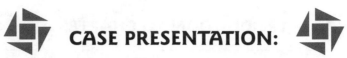

CASE PRESENTATION:

Mrs. Freed: The Manic Patient in Renal Failure on Dialysis

A colleague refers you Mrs. Freed, a 65-year-old woman with a 20-year history of bipolar affective illness treated with lithium. On three occasions in the past, Mrs. Freed had been noncompliant with lithium, become psychotic, and required hospitalization. On several occasions the patient refused lithium and attempts were made to substitute carbamazepine (Tegretol) or sodium valproate (Depakote). These medications had been unsuccessful and resulted in psychiatric hospitalization. Most recently, she responded to a brief course of haloperidol (Haldol) 3 mg twice daily for psychotic ideation.

Mrs. Freed had been stable for 2 years on lithium carbonate 1,200–1,500 mg/day, with blood levels ranging from 0.9 to 1.2 mEq/L. Several months ago, her internist noted progressively increasing creatinine. Lithium and diazepam (Valium; given for anxiety) were discontinued, her fluid was restricted, and the patient was placed on a 40-g low-protein diet. It was hoped that dialysis could be avoided. Mrs. Freed presents you with a printout of the most recent chemistries, remarkable for serum creatinine of 5.5 and a blood urea nitrogen (BUN) of 62. She has no other medical problems and is on no other medications.

Up to this time, the patient had been maintained on her usual doses of lithium. She has never been lithium toxic, clinically or by blood level, although polyuria has persisted for years. The family reports that in recent weeks she has begun wandering around the neighborhood, talking inappropriately to strangers, and unable to find her way back home. They say she is "giddy," unable to sleep, and has been making peculiar dietary indiscretions in her strictly kosher diet (such as bringing home a ham sandwich on one of her walks).

On mental status exam, Mrs. Freed reports feeling "great emotionally" but "tired all the time," and shows pressured speech. Her affect is silly and her mood euphoric. She occasionally breaks into song, singing "Oh, What a Beautiful Morning," ostensibly because she "feels happy." There is no suicidal ideation. Thought process is circumstantial. Thought content is notable for lack of bizarre or idiosyncratic ideation, but the patient insists, in an engaging, likable way, on trying to interview you about your personal life. There are no delusions or hallucinations. She is alert and oriented to person and place, but misreports the date by about 3 days. Recent memory, concentration, and recall are mildly impaired. Remote memory is intact. Proverbs and similarities are interpreted humorously but concretely. There is little insight, but she suspects "this visit has something to do with the lithium, which I haven't needed for years and will never take again."

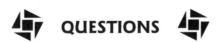

QUESTIONS

Choose all that apply.

1. You decide to request additional medical workup to evaluate possible etiologies for her mental status change. Assuming that magnetic resonance imaging (MRI) of the head, thyroid function tests, serum B_{12}, and folate are normal, what do you consider next?

   a. Mrs. Freed's mental status is fairly typical of the early changes of chronic renal failure.

   b. Characteristic electroencephalogram (EEG) changes for Mrs. Freed would include generalized synchronous paroxysmal spike and wave complexes.

   c. Mrs. Freed's BUN at the time of evaluation would more closely predict neuropsychiatric disturbance than would the rate of its change.

   d. Mrs. Freed's rate of change of BUN would more closely predict neuropsychiatric disturbance than would the BUN value itself.

   e. The EEG changes that occur in uremic encephalopathy are nonspecific with regard to etiology.

2. Mrs. Freed will probably require psychotropic medications. Which of the following most closely correlates with the development of neuropsychiatric symptoms?
    a. BUN
    b. Creatinine levels
    c. Creatinine clearance
    d. None of the above

3. What are true statements regarding medications in the setting of renal failure?
    a. The absorption of some medications by the small bowel changes in renal failure, even if hepatic metabolism remains intact.
    b. Hepatic metabolism of most psychotropic drugs is unchanged by renal failure.
    c. Ascites and edema require the use of lower doses of water-soluble or protein-bound medications.
    d. Aluminum-containing medications that are routinely administered in renal failure often precipitate psychotropic toxicity.

4. It is important to understand plasma protein binding in order to safely prescribe medications in renal failure. All of the following are true except . . .
    a. Most psychotropics have high protein-binding affinity.
    b. Lithium is not bound to protein.
    c. The bound component of the drug is responsible for the pharmacological activity.
    d. The protein binding of drugs by albumin decreases during renal failure.

5. Which of the following are true?
    a. The net result of the pharmacodynamic changes of advanced renal failure is that there is less free drug available compared with protein-bound drug.
    b. As a rule, the higher the protein-binding activity of a drug, the more dialyzable it is.
    c. Virtually all psychotropics are dialyzable.
    d. Albumin is the protein that is exclusively responsible for binding psychotropics and that is most affected by renal failure.
    e. None of the above.

6. Which of the following is true?
    a. Lipophilic psychotropics include tricyclic antidepressants (TCAs) and benzodiazepines, but not phenothiazines or lithium.
    b. Renal clearance of the hydrophilic psychotropics decreases during renal failure, resulting in potential toxicity.
    c. Renal clearance of the lipophilic psychotropics decreases during renal failure, resulting in potential toxicity.
    d. Blood levels are reliable indicators of active free drug during renal failure.

7. Most authors recommend that doses of psychotropics be empirically reduced in renal failure by a factor of approximately . . .
    a. One-fourth.
    b. One-third.
    c. One-half.
    d. Two-thirds.

8. Doses of lipophilic psychotropic medications should be reduced in renal failure because of . . .
    a. Diminished renal clearance.
    b. Heightened sensitivity to side effects.
    c. Impairments of cytochrome P450 metabolism.
    d. Increased likelihood of toxicity.

9. The family corroborates that Mrs. Freed has never been lithium toxic, but state that she did complain for many years of urinating a lot. Mr. Freed wants to know if the lithium had anything to do with his wife's developing kidney disease. To date, she has refused kidney biopsy. You formulate your response, taking into consideration that . . .
    a. Lithium-induced polyuria is initially reversible but may be associated with irreversible tubular damage.
    b. The lithium-induced impairments in concentrating capacity are most likely to be associated with lithium's effects on protein wasting, as opposed to tubular functioning.
    c. Recent studies have increasingly supported the safety of long-term lithium maintenance relative to the kidney.
    d. To date, no renal lesions specific to lithium-treated patients have been reported .
    e. To date, there has been no well-documented case of lithium-induced chronic renal failure progressing to chronic hemodialysis.

10. Which morphological and clinical changes of the kidney have been most commonly associated with lithium?
    a. Interstitial fibrosis
    b. Glomerular sclerosis
    c. Tubular atrophy
    d. Nephrotic syndrome

11. It is agreed that restarting lithium is the treatment of choice for Mrs. Freed, given the manic recurrence and his-

tory of nonresponse to carbamazepine (Tegretol). The family is unanimously in favor of this decision, because they fear another psychiatric hospitalization for Mrs. Freed without it. She agrees to comply. Which of the following are true?

    a. Lithium is contraindicated in acute renal failure, but not in chronic renal failure.

    b. The risk of significant lithium-induced glomerular damage compared with potential tubular damage is minimal.

    c. It is suggested in the literature that lithium levels be maintained no higher than 0.4 mEq/L in the setting of renal failure.

    d. Chronic renal failure has been proven to heighten the risk for lithium-induced renal impairment.

12. Mrs. Freed's nephrologist gives medical clearance to begin lithium and the family signs informed consent. If Mrs. Freed's usual lithium requirement has been 1,200 mg/day, how should her dosage be adjusted?

    a. If glomerular filtration rate (GFR) is greater than 50 ml/minute, her daily dosage should remain 1,200 mg/day.

    b. If GFR were 30 ml/minute, her daily dosage should be 600–900 mg/day.

    c. If GFR were approximately 20 ml/minute, her daily dosage should be 600–900 mg/day.

    d. All of the above.

13. As you are attempting to adjust lithium blood levels, Mrs. Freed's casual singing blossoms into the delusion that she is Ethel Merman. To the family's chagrin, she serenades the neighborhood nightly after the 11:00 news. The exhausted family and her nephrologist agree that an antipsychotic medication would be helpful. Her usual maintenance neuroleptic dose during a manic exacerbation has been 5 mg of haloperidol (Haldol). Which are true?

    a. Doses of haloperidol must be halved once GFR falls below 50 ml/minute.

    b. Haloperidol is not completely removed by dialysis.

    c. Phenothiazine neuroleptics are contraindicated because they hasten the progression of renal failure.

    d. Antiparkinsonian medications should not be used in the setting of renal failure.

14. Over the next 8 months, Mrs. Freed's psychosis resolves and she becomes euthymic. However, her creat-

inine clearance continues to decline and she becomes virtually anuric. The decision is made to begin hemodialysis, which Mrs. Freed accepts with surprising aplomb. She will be dialyzed three times a week. How should her psychiatric management proceed?

    a. Since lithium is completely dialyzed, it should be administered daily, except for weekends when she does not receive dialysis.

    b. She should receive a single oral dose after each dialysis treatment.

    c. Because she is virtually anuric, she is at risk for widely fluctuating lithium levels between dialysis sessions.

    d. Lithium could be administered in the dialysate.

15. In her second week of dialysis, Mrs. Freed is tapered off haloperidol and arrives to see you soon after her Monday dialysis. She appears disoriented and drowsy, and complains of headache. According to her husband, this also occurred last week. Her husband reports that her last dose of lithium was on Friday afternoon after dialysis. She has received no lithium today. Mrs. Freed is too sleepy to cooperate with your interview. Her lithium medication management has remained unchanged. What are the *most likely* diagnostic considerations at this point?

    a. Lithium toxicity

    b. Subdural hematoma

    c. Dialysis dementia

    d. Dialysis disequilibrium syndrome

16. The trace element that appears to be most consistently implicated in dialysis dementia is . . .

    a. Aluminum

    b. Cobalt

    c. Manganese

    d. Magnesium

    e. Iron

17. What factors would affect how diuretics interact with lithium?

    a. The diuretic's site of action on the nephron determines its effect on lithium.

    b. The tendency to deplete sodium would predispose to subtherapeutic lithium levels.

    c. Thiazide diuretics are likely to precipitate lithium toxicity.

    d. Most diuretics render lithium levels invalid.

✦ Answers

1. Answer: d, e (p. 148)
2. Answer: c (p. 148)
3. Answer: a, b (p. 150)
4. Answer: c (p. 150)
5. Answer: e (p. 150)
6. Answer: b (pp. 150–151)
7. Answer: b (pp. 149–150)
8. Answer: b (pp. 149–150)
9. Answer: a (pp. 151–153)
10. Answer: a, c, b (p. 153)
11. Answer: a, b (pp. 153–154)
12. Answer: d (p. 153)
13. Answer: b (p. 151)
14. Answer: b, d (p. 153)
15. Answer: b, d (pp. 149, 153)
16. Answer: a (p. 149)
17. Answer: a, c (p. 154)

◆ NEUROPSYCHIATRIC PRESENTATIONS OF RENAL FAILURE

Psychiatric consultation on a nephrology service can be confusing, given all the medical and psychological variables that potentially influence mental status. A clinical rule of thumb, however, is that the affective sequelae of renal failure are typically depressive syndromes.[71] There is also often symptomatic overlap between depression and early renal failure (i.e., malaise, apathy, fatigue, lethargy, memory disturbances).[71] Progression of renal insufficiency usually causes frank delirium, with alterations in consciousness, disorientation, disruption in memory function, and psychotic symptoms. The latter range from negativistic, combative behavior[57] to schizophreniform and paranoid symptoms.[44]

Only *rare* cases have appeared of secondary manic syndromes clearly and directly attributed to uremia.[22,61] Secondary mania may be a consequence of infection during dialysis,[15] and has been described as the initial presentation of progressive dialysis encephalopathy.[34] Benazzi[6] has recently corroborated the rarity of mania secondary to hemodialysis.

Mrs. Freed's symptoms represent a recurrence of her brittle bipolar illness, secondary to discontinuation of lithium prophylaxis, complicated by cognitive changes.

Predictors of Neuropsychiatric Disturbance

Blood Urea Nitrogen

Nephrology patients usually have a bewildering array of abnormal blood chemistries. It is often tempting to blame psychiatric symptoms on shockingly high BUN levels, wondering how a patient can have a mental status at all! Although BUN reflects the degree of renal impairment and loosely correlates with neuropsychiatric disturbance, the *absolute* urea level is *not* tightly related to the degree of neuropsychiatric impairment.[44]

◆ For example, patients dialyzed against solutions containing urea concentrations matching their own high baselines still demonstrate clinical improvement despite markedly abnormal BUNs.[43]

◆ In addition, infusion of large quantities of intravenous urea does not necessarily lead to central nervous system (CNS) toxicity.[35]

Rather than be distracted by BUN values that seem to be incompatible with mentation, pay attention to the *rate of BUN change*. This measure correlates more closely with mental status phenomena than does absolute BUN.[44] See Appendix G ("Neuropsychiatric Effects of Electrolyte and Acid-Base Imbalance").

Electroencephalogram

The EEG reflects elevations of blood urea:[63]

◆ BUN < 42 mg/100 ml: normal recordings
◆ BUN > 60 mg/100 ml: abnormal recordings

The EEG usually becomes abnormal within 48 hours of the onset of renal failure, and these abnormalities may persist for up to 3 weeks after starting dialysis.[24] *Loss of organized alpha activity* and *diffuse slowing* occur but are nonspecific and appear in other delirious states, such as delirium due to hepatic failure (hepatic encephalopathy).[24,40] Even triphasic waves may occur.

Generalized synchronous paroxysmal spike and wave complexes are characteristic of absence seizures, not delirium, and there would be no clinical reason to expect them in Mrs. Freed.

Creatinine Clearance

BUN does not always reliably measure kidney function, mostly because it depends on protein intake and catabolism. Although creatinine levels are better measures, they may also be misleading, since creatinine in its steady state depends on muscle mass as well as kidney function. Elderly or debilitated individuals may have relatively *low* BUNs, which falsely suggest "normal" renal function despite significant renal insufficiency.[37]

Creatinine clearance is the *most* useful, clinically available measure of renal function, and can be estimated from serum creatinine, without urine collection, by the following formula:[8]

Creatinine clearance =
Adult males: (140 − age) (body weight in kg) ÷
(72 × serum creatinine)
Adult females: (multiply above by factor of 0.85)

If oliguria is present in the setting of acute renal failure, creatinine clearance should be estimated as less than 10 ml/minute.[8]

Dialysis-Related Neuropsychiatric Syndromes

CNS abnormalities occur frequently among uremic patients.[24] Although no one etiological metabolic factor predominates, contributants include anemia, endocrinopathy, hypertension, and cardiovascular disease.[58] Acute changes in mental status require careful workup to rule out cerebral hemorrhage, seizure disorder, or dialysis disequilibrium. Anticoagulant therapy (to maintain patency of the shunts) and abnormal platelet function (secondary to chronic renal disease) predispose dialysis patients to subdural hematomas.[60] *Changes in mental status, when accompanied by symptoms of increased intracranial pressure or focal neurological signs, require emergency evaluation.*

Disequilibrium Syndrome

Dialysis disequilibrium is an acute delirious state that occurs during or soon after hemodialysis. It is caused by overly vigorous correction of azotemia, leading to osmotic imbalance and rapid shifts in pH. It is a transient disorder characterized by headaches, nausea, muscular cramps, irritability, agitation, drowsiness, and convulsions.[24,66] Psychosis may also occur.[58] Headache develops in approximately 70% of patients, whereas the other symptoms occur in 5%–10%, typically in individuals undergoing rapid dialysis or those in the early stages of a dialysis program.[66] The symptoms usually occur in the third to fourth hour of dialysis, but may also appear 8–48 hours after completing it.[66]

Dialysis Dementia

Dialysis dementia, also termed dialysis encephalopathy, is a progressive and fatal syndrome. It is fortunately a rare complication that occurs in chronic dialysis patients who have been dialyzed for a period *of at least 1 year,*[24] not a few days, like Mrs. Freed. Its incidence in 1987 was estimated at 0.2%, with a 29% fatality rate.[2] The syndrome usually begins with speech disturbance, such as stuttering, which progresses to dysarthria and dysphasia, at times with periods of muteness.[33] The dementia is global, with preservation of normal consciousness. The symptoms progress to focal and generalized myoclonus, focal and generalized seizures, personality changes, and psychotic episodes.[66] EEG abnormalities consist of bisynchronous, predominantly frontal or multifocal bursts of slow-wave discharges, associated with spikes and sharp waves.[66] The cerebrospinal fluid (CSF) is usually normal. Symptoms are initially intermittent, occurring during or immediately after dialysis and lasting for only a few hours.

Aluminum intoxication is most consistently implicated in the pathogenesis of dialysis dementia, with the aluminum content of brain gray matter in dialysis dementia patients reported to be 11 times the normal content.[24] The etiology remains somewhat controversial, however, because dialysate aluminum levels are not always elevated. In addition, affected patients were not always exposed to any more aluminum-containing antacids than were unaffected patients, nor were their brain aluminum levels consistently higher. Early cases may be reversible by instituting chelation therapy with deferoxamine; by reducing the dose of aluminum-containing phosphate-binding gels; and by using deionized water (which has no aluminum) to prepare dialysis solutions.[1,45] Altered psychomotor function has been described with even mildly elevated aluminum levels.[3] If left untreated, the symptoms gradually become more persistent and eventually permanent.[66] Once established, the syndrome is usually steadily progressive over a 1- to 15-month period.

Prevention of dialysis dementia centers on avoiding aluminum toxicity from the dialysis fluid and the aluminum salts used to regulate serum phosphate levels.[2] These preventive measures have been successful in decreasing the incidence of dialysis dementia.[18]

⚜ PSYCHOPHARMACOLOGY IN RENAL FAILURE

Fortunately, despite the physiological complexities of renal failure, a glance at the far right-hand column of Appendix H ("The Use of Psychotropics in Renal Failure") shows that few psychotropics require dose adjustments; of those that do, the most notable is lithium.

Although renal failure patients *theoretically* do not require dosage adjustments of most psychotropics, these patients are *clinically* quite vulnerable to adverse medication side effects at doses that healthy patients easily tolerate. The empirical ***"rule of two-thirds"*** advises lessening the side-effect risk by reducing usual medication doses by a factor of one-third—that is, by using two-thirds of a normal dose as an upper limit, even though renal failure does not necessarily lead to blood *levels* in the toxic range.[10,44]

◆   For example, a healthy patient might comfortably tolerate a nortriptyline blood level in the therapeutic range on 60 mg of medication; a patient in renal failure may mount the same blood level on the same dose of medication, but be more likely to have adverse side effects, such as sedation or dizziness. The rule of two-thirds advises using a maximum of only 40 mg of nortriptyline ($2/3 \times 60$ mg) to lessen the renal patient's risk of side effects.

A brief outline of some details of renal physiology is provided for the intrepid reader. Those wishing a more practical, easy-to-remember guide should refer to Appendix H, modified by the rule of two-thirds.

Nonrenal Factors

The nonrenal factors affecting drug metabolism include the following:

1. *Absorption:* Gastric absorption of psychotropic medication may be reduced by routinely administered aluminum-containing medication such as antacids, which form nonabsorbable complexes.[32] Even the absorption of some medications by the small bowel is decreased in renal failure, despite intact hepatic metabolism. The gastric alkalinizing effects of excess urea, which generates ammonia by the internal urea-ammonia cycle, may be responsible for this problem.[5]

2. *Hepatic metabolism:* Hepatic metabolism of psychotropic drugs is *not* reduced by renal failure; for example, glucuronidation by the liver *increases* during renal failure. Even more confusingly, other drugs (e.g., beta-blockers) may have their hepatic metabolism altered, causing increased amounts of active drug in the systemic circulation.[37]

3. *Volume of distribution:* Ascites and edema may increase the apparent volume of distribution of a drug, diluting out therapeutic blood levels and requiring *higher* doses of water-soluble or protein-bound medications. Volume of distribution shrinks in patients suffering from dehydration or muscle wasting, causing potential toxicity unless doses are reduced.

Proteins and Protein Binding

Most psychotropic medications (TCAs, benzodiazepines, phenothiazines, haloperidol) are lipophilic (lipid soluble) and strongly protein affinitive, and are not excreted by the kidneys. Lithium is hydrophilic (water soluble), is not protein bound, and is excreted unchanged by the kidneys.[42] There are several important consequences of these physiological facts:

1. *Free versus bound drug:* Renal failure profoundly alters the ratio of free (unbound) to bound drug. *It is the unbound or free component that is responsible for pharmacological activity.*
   - An example is the decrease in drug protein binding by *albumin* during renal failure.[37] Since there is diminished albumin concentration, it seems reasonable to expect higher concentrations of certain psychotropics because there is less protein available to bind them.[44] Wrong!
   - Generalizations like these are spurious because
     - *Volume of distribution* is also changed by decreased protein binding.
     - Many psychotropics bind to proteins *other than albumin* (which are less affected—or, maddeningly, actually *increase*—in renal failure).[37]

2. *Dialyzability:* In general, the higher the protein-binding activity of a drug, the less dialyzable it is. Lithium is almost completely removed by dialysis; in contrast, the majority of psychotropic medications are not.[37] Lithium toxicity is unlikely to be the cause of Mrs. Freed's Monday afternoon somnolence in your office because her lithium level can be assumed to be low (essentially zero) after dialysis, and her husband reports that she has had no lithium since Friday, 3 days before.

3. *Renal clearance:* Least complicated is the effect of renal failure on *hydrophilic* psychotropics like lithium: decreased renal function leads to decreased clearance, resulting in rising blood levels and potential toxicity. The metabolic effect on *lipophilic* agents is more complex and less predictable:
   - For some medications, an increase in free drug can lead to more rapid metabolism; for example, for benzodiazepines, hypoalbuminemia results in an increased free fraction of parent drug with compensatory rapid inactivation of drug and active metabolites through glucuronidation. Thus, counterintuitively, there is actually an *increase* in benzodiazepine clearance, with *lowered* plasma levels of active drug and shortened half-life.[44]
   - The situation for TCAs and phenothiazines is more ambiguous. Patients in renal failure on tricyclics have clearance rates[20,38] and steady-state plasma concentrations that are equivalent to[38] or even lower than[51] those of control subjects. Factors that may account for these findings include interindividual differences, intraindividual fluctuations, and competitive displacement of bound drug from protein by endogenous

uremic substances[46] (thereby freeing bound drug for inactivation by glucuronidation).

Unreliable Blood Levels

For those who imagine that drug blood levels might rescue them from this physiological conundrum, think again. *As long as glucuronidation by the liver remains intact during renal failure, the associated pharmacokinetic shifts render blood levels* **unreliable** *either as assays of free, therapeutically active drug or as guides for dosage adjustments.*[20,44,51] Blood levels may be easily misinterpreted; they may mislead about dose appropriateness because they do *not* reflect the alterations in protein binding and drug distribution that change the ratio of free to bound medication.[44]

Despite these problems, Levy[37] still feels that blood levels for medications like nortriptyline (Pamelor, Aventyl), which has a therapeutic window, may be better than dosing completely in the dark. The clinician who uses drug levels should be alert to their limitations in this setting, however, and not be lulled into a false sense of clinical security based on them.

✦ PSYCHOSIS

Neuroleptics

When psychotic reactions occur in ESRD, they often require neuroleptic management. According to Bennett et al.,[8] haloperidol does not require modifications based on GFR; dosages should be reduced empirically to minimize side effects, such as sedation. (Note that haloperidol is not completely removed by dialysis.[8]) Phenothiazines are not strictly contraindicated, but proceed cautiously because of potential sedation, anticholinergic toxicity, urinary retention, and orthostatic hypotension. They do *not* in themselves accelerate the progression of renal failure. Like haloperidol, phenothiazines are not dialyzable. They are generally not as well tolerated as haloperidol in medically fragile populations.

As mentioned, the rule of two-thirds advises lowering dosages by one-third to compensate for heightened sensitivity to side effects.

Antiparkinsonian Medications

Antiparkinsonian medications may be used in renal failure. However, we could locate no information on using benztropine mesylate (Cogentin) in patients with compromised renal function.

Although diphenhydramine (Benadryl) need not be reduced in renal failure,[8] note that its anticholinergic effects may predispose to urinary retention.

✦ MANIA: LITHIUM AND KIDNEY PHYSIOLOGY

The Controversy

The effects of prolonged lithium on the kidney have long been controversial. Controlling for confounding factors—such as the duration of affective illness and lithium treatment, the occurrence of transient episodes of toxicity in unmonitored patients, and the fact that many lithium-treated patients are on other psychotropics—has been difficult. Two critical reviews—one in 1988 by Schou[53] and one in 1989 by Waller and Edwards[70]—concluded that lithium does not lead to changes in GFR or predispose to renal failure, even when administered for many years. More recently, however, Gitlin[26] has reviewed the evidence for lithium-induced renal insufficiency and has cast a cautious eye on this optimistic view. He pointed out the following:

◆ The longitudinal studies examined by these reviews were of relatively short duration; the mean length of follow-up in the Waller and Edwards[70] review was less than 2 years.

◆ The longest follow-up study published at that time was by Løkkegaard and associates,[41] who examined renal function in lithium-treated patients for up to 17 years, with a mean follow-up interval of 10 years. Corrected for the normal age-related decline in GFR, creatinine clearance was not decreased after 7 years but was *significantly diminished* in the group treated for *17 years.* Moreover, two patients from the original cohort had discontinued lithium because of a decreased GFR and so were not examined. Gitlin[26] concluded that the effects of lithium treatment of greater than 10 years' duration remained unclear.

A brief scan of the studies since 1989 reveals the following:

◆ Conte et al.[14] studied 50 patients treated with lithium for a mean of over 6 years (range 1.5–14 years) who showed no change in renal function.

◆ Christensen and Aggernas[13] found no change in renal function in 14 patients treated with lithium for an average of 14 years (range 6–28 years).

◆ Stancer and Forbath[56] reported that renal insufficiency developed in 14 patients treated with lithium for more than 10 years (mean 15 years). One patient developed a serum creatinine level of 2.2 mg/100 ml and high parathormone levels.

◆ Hetmar et al.[31] reexamined 27 of the 46 patients they had studied 10 years previously.[29,30] Patients in the follow-up group were on lithium for a mean of more than 19 years (range 11.5–23.5 years). Although no decline in GFR was found, two patients had developed renal insufficiency. One patient showed a serum creatinine level of 2.26 mg/100 ml 3 years after lithium was discontinued and after recovering from acute drug-induced nephrotoxicity. Renal biopsy showed subacute tubulointerstitial nephritis. The other patient developed a serum creatinine of 3.2 mg/100 ml after 25 years of lithium treatment.

◆ Von Knorring et al.[67] described the first well-documented case of lithium-induced chronic renal failure that progressed to chronic hemodialysis. The patient's baseline serum creatinine had increased from 0.9 mg/100 ml to 2.1 mg/100 ml over 14 years of lithium treatment. Complete renal failure resulted from continued lithium treatment over the next 3.5 years. A renal biopsy showed chronic tubulointerstitial disease consistent with lithium-induced renal damage.

◆ In von Knorring and associates'[67] sample of patients who had been on lithium for more than 10 years, 11 of 66 (16.7%) had serum creatinine levels of more than 1.2 mg/100 ml.

◆ Most recently, Gitlin[26] found that 3 of 82 (3.7%) bipolar patients with normal baselines developed serum creatinine levels greater than 2.0 mg/100 ml. One patient progressed to chronic renal failure and hemodialysis, making him the second reported probable case of lithium-induced chronic renal failure. No common risk factor for renal disease among these patients was apparent.

◆ Additional reports continue to accumulate that advise caution.[7a]

Still unknown, however, is the rate of renal insufficiency in the general population or among bipolar patients who have never taken lithium. The absence of this information makes it difficult to distinguish lithium-induced renal failure from renal failure that might have occurred otherwise.[26] We agree that cautious optimism is necessary when prescribing lithium over the long term; our patient, Mrs. Freed, had no risk factors for renal disease other than 20 years of lithium maintenance. She had never been lithium toxic and had been compliant with careful pharmacological follow-up. Gitlin[26] has written,

[In conclusion,] among the recently published studies, there is evidence that between 0 and 5% of patients treated with lithium over a long period of time may develop signs of renal insufficiency. Additionally, the first two cases of renal failure progressing to dialysis probably as the result of lithium have now been reported . . . With increasing numbers of patients taking lithium for 15 years or more, we may need to be more cautious about describing the complete safety of lithium with very long-term use. Even if only 1% of the patients treated for a long time develop abnormalities in renal function (with the question of reversibility and progression still unknown), this might ultimately total a significant number of patients. (p. 278)

Gelenberg[25] advises caution for any patient whose creatinine level climbs gradually, and notes that the decision about how to proceed hinges on several questions:

◆ How stable has the patient been on lithium treatment, and what are likely repercussions of its discontinuation?

◆ If lithium is discontinued, what happens to the serum creatinine and creatinine clearance?

◆ Do other treatments, such as carbamazepine (Tegretol) and valproate (Depakote), protect the patient from mood episodes?

DasGupta et al.[19a] suggest that carbamazepine and valproate are preferred to lithium for manic patients with kidney disease. We next briefly summarize some of the other effects of lithium on the kidney.

Effects on Tubular Functioning and Concentrating Ability

Polyuria (24-hour urine volume > 3,000 ml) is a frequent side effect of lithium, occurring at any time during its administration, with estimated incidence between 2% and 35%.[7] It is related to reversible decreased tubular responsiveness to antidiuretic hormone, inducing a syndrome analogous to nephrogenic diabetes insipidus. Polyuria had been considered a benign condition, the reversible result of pharmacodynamic disturbance without histopathological changes.[52] However, case reports have appeared showing the following:

◆ Irreversible nephrogenic diabetes insipidus–like syndromes and morphological kidney changes have been found in lithium-treated patients who develop polyuria.[12,28]

◆ Impaired concentrating capacity up to 4 years after discontinuing lithium has also been demonstrated, an effect attributed to lesions of the cells lining the distal tubules and collecting ducts.[11,49,55] Concentrating ability was found to be inversely correlated with the proportion of atrophic tubules.[27]

◆ Two studies supported an association between the degree of lithium-induced nephrogenic diabetes insipidus and the extent of histopathological damage.[11,27]

◆ An association to renal tubular acidosis has appeared.[45a,45b]

Effects on Glomerular Function

Glomerular function is less affected by lithium than is tubular function.[7,9,53,54,64]

Proteinuria

A prospective 3-year study[4] of patients on lithium showed small but significant increases in urine protein excretion, but kidney function remained normal in the majority of subjects. These changes were not clinically meaningful. Routine urinalysis for protein is *not* usually advised because of the rarity of this side effect.[19]

Histopathological Changes

Specific distal-nephron lesions occurring in lithium-treated patients, but not in psychiatric control subjects,[67a,68,69] have included the following:

◆ Cytoplasmic swelling
◆ Accumulation of glycogen deposits
◆ Dilated tubules
◆ Microcyst formation

It is unclear whether these changes may lead to focal nephron atrophy after prolonged exposure to lithium, or if they are completely reversible.[12,53]

Interstitial fibrosis, glomerular sclerosis, and tubular atrophy were the most common pathological diagnoses in a review of seven studies of lithium-treated patients (N = 132).[7] It was estimated that less than 15% of patients showed morphological changes. Nephrotic syndrome is much rarer, with only 9 cases reported in association with lithium exposure.[72]

Using Lithium in the Setting of Renal Failure

Lithium is contraindicated in acute renal failure but not in chronic renal failure.[17,19,19a] It must be prescribed in conservative doses, with careful monitoring of serum levels and renal function. Creatinine clearance should be assessed at baseline and then every 3–6 months, with medical consultation sought for levels above 1.6 mg/ 100 ml.[26] Lithium levels should be maintained between 0.6 and 0.8 mEq/L.[19a] It is not yet known whether patients with chronic renal failure, preexisting glomerulonephritis, pyelonephritis, or tubulo-interstitial disease are at increased risk for lithium-induced renal impairment. Das-Gupta et al.[19a] feel it would be prudent to assume this to be the case. Although prolonged use of lithium sometimes reduces GFR,[21,65] the risk of significant glomerular damage is minimal.[50]

Maintenance Lithium

Lithium should be adjusted for undialyzed renal failure patients as follows[8] (see also Appendix H, "The Use of Psychotropics in Renal Failure"):

GFR (ml/minute)	Change in daily maintenance dose
> 50	Unchanged
10–50	Maintenance reduced to 50%–75% of usual
< 10	Maintenance reduced to 25%–50% of usual

Lithium is completely dialyzed;[62] one can assume that Mrs. Freed's serum lithium level, when she presents confused and somnolent in the consultant's office postdialysis, is zero and that lithium toxicity is unlikely.

Several authors have used lithium successfully in hemodialysis patients.[23,37,39,47,48,73] Because lithium given on nondialysis days can produce toxicity, it is usually synchronized with the dialysis schedule.

◆ *Lithium is either given in the dialysate during peritoneal dialysis[23] or administered as a single oral dose after each hemodialysis treatment.[19a]*

Predialysis blood work should include serum lithium levels—several times per week initially, and then monthly,[37] maintaining levels between 0.6 and 0.8 mEq/L.[19]

Anuria would result in interdialysis lithium levels that would be fairly consistent due to lack of kidney function, not widely fluctuating.

Diuretics and Lithium
A diuretic's site of action on the kidney determines whether it will cause lithium retention.

◆ For example, agents like furosemide (Lasix) and ethacrynic acid act at the Loop of Henle and do not acutely lead to decreased lithium excretion.[62]
◆ Potassium-sparing diuretics have a moderate effect on lithium retention.[36]
◆ Thiazide diuretics, which act at the proximal tubule, cause increased sodium and potassium excretion, and decrease lithium clearance by at least 40%.[36] *Reduce lithium by 50% when 50 mg of hydrochlorothiazide is added.*[16]

Remember to consult a reference source[13a] when lithium is coadministered with a diuretic in order to screen for potential side effects and toxicity.

Carbamazepine

Carbamazepine (Tegretol) can be used in renal failure, but it is not dialyzable.[58] It is preferred over phenobarbital and phenytoin for prospective transplant recipients with established seizure disorders. It is less likely than other anticonvulsants to accelerate prednisone metabolism by inducing liver microsomal enzyme systems and potentially precipitating graft rejection.[58] Complex partial seizures in the setting of renal failure and have been treated effectively with carbamazepine.[59] There is one report of acute renal failure in a carbamazepine-treated patient,[32a] which was thought to be an idiosyncratic hypersensitivity reaction. Nonetheless, significant effects on the kidney by carbamazepine are extremely rare.[19a] It is not yet known whether preexisting kidney disease predisposes to carbamazepine-induced renal dysfunction.[19a]

Valproate

DasGupta et al.[19a] suggest that valproate (Depakote) can probably be safely used in patients with preexisting renal disease, although data are lacking. Only 1%–3% of metabolized valproate is renally excreted.[36a]

⚘ SUMMARY

1. The mood changes of renal failure typically resemble depressive syndromes, often with symptomatic overlap between depression and early renal failure (i.e., malaise, apathy, fatigue, lethargy, memory disturbances). There are only *rare* cases of secondary manic syndromes directly attributed to uremia. Progression of renal insufficiency results in frank delirium, with alterations in consciousness, disorientation, disruption in memory function, and psychotic symptoms. The latter range from negativistic, combative behavior to schizophreniform and paranoid symptoms. Although blood urea nitrogen (BUN) reflects the degree of renal impairment and loosely correlates with neuropsychiatric disturbance, the absolute level of urea is not tightly correlated to the degree of neuropsychiatric impairment. Rather, monitor the *rate of change* in blood urea, a measure that more closely parallels mental status changes than does absolute BUN.

2. Central nervous system abnormalities occur frequently among uremic patients. While no one etiological metabolic factor predominates, contributing factors include anemia, endocrinopathy, hypertension, and cardiovascular disease. Acute changes in mental status require careful evaluation to rule out cerebral hemorrhage, seizure disorder, or dialysis disequilibrium. Anticoagulant therapy (to maintain patency of the shunts) and abnormal platelet function (secondary to chronic renal disease) predispose dialysis patients to subdural hematomas. *Changes in mental status, accompanied by symptoms of increased intracranial pressure or focal neurological signs, require emergency evaluation.* Dialysis disequilibrium is an acute brain syndrome that occurs during or soon after hemodialysis. It is caused by overly vigorous correction of azotemia, leading to osmotic imbalance and rapid shifts in pH. It is a transient disorder characterized by headache, nausea, muscular cramps, irritability, agitation, drowsiness, convulsions, and sometimes psychosis.

3. The fate of psychotropics in renal failure is variable because nonrenal factors (absorption, volume of distribution, hepatic metabolism) confuse the issue, and psychotropics are not exclusively bound by the easiest-to-trace blood protein, albumin, which simply decreases in renal failure. The far right-hand column of Appendix H ("The Use of Psychotropics in Renal Failure") shows that few psychotropics require dose adjustments; of those that do, the most notable is lithium. Although renal failure patients *theoretically* do not require dosage adjustments with most psychotropics, these patients are *clinically* quite vulnerable to adverse medication side affects at doses that

healthy patients easily tolerate. The empirical *rule of two-thirds* advises lessening the risk of side effects by reducing usual doses by a factor of one-third (i.e., using two-thirds of a normal dose as an upper limit).

4. Lithium is hydrophilic (water soluble), is not protein bound, and is excreted unchanged by the kidneys. In contrast, most psychotropic medications (tricyclic antidepressants [TCAs], benzodiazepines, phenothiazines, haloperidol [Haldol]) are lipophilic (lipid soluble) and strongly protein affinitive, and are not excreted primarily by the kidneys. In general, the higher the protein-binding activity of a drug, the less dialyzable it is. Lithium is almost completely removed by dialysis; in contrast, the majority of psychotropics are not.

5. Least complicated is the fate of hydrophilic psychotropics: decreased renal function leads to decreased clearance, resulting in mounting blood levels and potential toxicity. The metabolic effect on lipophilic agents is more complex and less predictable. For example, an increase in the free-drug component of some medications (e.g., benzodiazepines) can lead to more rapid metabolism, and thus to *increased* clearance, shortened half-life, and *lowered* plasma levels of active drug.

6. The situation for tricyclics and phenothiazines is more ambiguous. Patients in renal failure on TCAs have rates of clearance and steady-state plasma concentrations that are *equivalent* to or even *lower* than those of control subjects. Relevant factors include interindividual differences, intraindividual fluctuations, and competitive displacement of bound drug from protein by endogenous uremic substances.

7. As long as glucuronidation by the liver remains intact, the pharmacokinetic shifts of renal failure render blood levels unreliable either as assays of free, therapeutically active drug or as guides for dosage adjustments. Blood levels may be misleading because they do not reflect alterations in protein binding and drug distribution. Despite these problems, some feel that dosing according to blood levels for medications like nortriptyline (Pamelor, Aventyl), which has a therapeutic window, may be better than dosing completely in the dark. The clinician who uses blood levels should be alert to their limitations in renal failure.

8. Psychotic reactions often occur in end-stage renal disease and require neuroleptic management. Although it is not pharmacokinetically necessary to modify haloperidol based on glomerular filtration rate (GFR), doses should be reduced by two-thirds to minimize side effects such as sedation. Proceed cautiously when using phenothiazines, because of potential sedation, anticholinergic toxicity, urinary retention, and orthostatic hypotension. These agents generally are not as well tolerated as haloperidol in medically fragile patients.

9. The effects of prolonged lithium on the kidney have been controversial. Further, it has been difficult to control for confounding factors, such as the duration of affective illness and lithium treatment, the occurrence of transient episodes of toxicity in unmonitored patients, and the fact that many lithium-treated patients are on other psychotropics. Two critical reviews have concluded that lithium treatment does not lead to changes in GFR or to renal failure. A later review, however, cited evidence for lithium-induced renal insufficiency and was more circumspect. It is of concern that there are few data on patients followed for more than 10–15 years on lithium. In the existing data, there are indications that renal insufficiency developed in patients taking lithium for more than 10 years. Moreover, there are now at least two documented cases of lithium-induced chronic renal failure. Be sure to regularly monitor serum creatinine levels of lithium-treated patients every 6 months to 1 year, and to seek medical consultation for levels above 1.6 mg/100 ml.

10. Polyuria is a frequent lithium side effect, occurring at any time during the drug's administration. It has been considered a benign condition, the reversible result of pharmacodynamic disturbance without histopathological changes. However, case reports have appeared showing irreversible nephrogenic diabetes insipidus–like syndromes and morphological kidney changes in lithium-treated patients who develop polyuria.

11. Glomerular function is less affected by lithium than is tubular function. Proteinuria is rare. Cytoplasmic swelling, accumulation of glycogen deposits, dilated tubules, and microcyst formation have been described as specific distal nephron lesions occurring in lithium-treated patients but not in psychiatric control subjects. It is unclear whether these changes may lead to focal nephron atrophy after prolonged lithium exposure, or if they are completely reversible.

12. Lithium is contraindicated in acute—but not chronic—renal failure. It must be prescribed in conservative doses, with careful monitoring. Creatinine clearance should be assessed at baseline and then every 3–6 months. Lithium levels should be maintained between 0.6 and 0.8 mEq/L. Consult Appendix H ("The Use of Psychotropics in Renal Failure")

for advice on lithium adjustments in renal failure for patients who are not dialyzed. For dialyzed patients, lithium is usually synchronized with the dialysis schedule and given as a single oral dose after each hemodialysis treatment. Predialysis blood work should include serum lithium levels several times per week initially, and then monthly, maintaining levels between 0.6 and 0.8 mEq/L.

13. As mentioned in Chapter 1, our policy is to assume that a medication interacts with psychotropics until proven otherwise. Be sure to research the effects of medications such as diuretics and antihypertensives on lithium clearance, as many of these drugs will affect lithium levels.

14. Carbamazepine (Tegretol) and valproate (Depakote) are alternatives to lithium with less renal toxicity.

🔷 REFERENCES

1. Alfrey A: Dialysis encephalopathy. Kidney Int 29 (suppl):S53–S57, 1986

2. Alter M, Favero M, Miller J, et al: National surveillance of dialysis-associated diseases in the United States. Transactions—American Society for Artificial Internal Organs 35:820–831, 1989

3. Altmann P, Dhanesha U, Hamon C, et al: Disturbances of cerebral function by aluminum in haemodialysis patients without overt aluminum toxicity. Lancet 2:7–12, 1989

4. Amsterdam J, Jorkasky D, Potter L, et al: A prospective study of lithium-induced nephropathy: preliminary results. Psychopharmacol Bull 21:81–84, 1985

5. Anderson R, Gambertoglio J, Schrier R: Clinical Use of Drugs in Renal Failure. Springfield, IL, Charles C Thomas, 1976

6. Benazzi F: Mania during hemodialysis: causal or casual association? (letter). Am J Psychiatry 149:414, 1992

7. Bendz H: Kidney function in lithium-treated patients: a literature survey. Acta Psychiatr Scand 68:303–324, 1983

7a. Bendz H, Aurell M, Balldin J, et al: Kidney damage in long-term lithium patients: a cross-sectional study of patients with 15 years or more on lithium. Nephrology, Dialysis, Transplantation 9:1250–4125, 1994

8. Bennett W, Aronoff G, Golper T, et al: Drug Prescribing in Renal Failure: Dosing Guidelines for Adults, 3rd Edition. Philadelphia, PA, American College of Physicians, 1994

9. Boton R, Gaviria M, Batlle D: Prevalence, pathogenesis, and treatment of renal dysfunction associated with chronic lithium therapy. Am J Kidney Dis 10:329–345, 1987

10. Brater D: Drug Use in Renal Disease. Sydney, Australia, Aidis Health Science Press, 1985

11. Bucht G, Wahlin A: Renal concentrating capacity in long-term lithium treatment after withdrawal of lithium. Acta Medica Scandinavica 207:309–314, 1980

12. Burrows G, Davies B, Kincaid-Smith P: Unique tubular lesion after lithium (letter). Lancet 1:1310, 1978

13. Christensen E, Aggernas H: Prospective study of EDTA clearance among patients in long-term lithium treatment. Acta Psychiatr Scand 81:302–303, 1990

13a. Ciraulo D, Shader R, Greenblatt D, et al. (eds): Drug Interactions in Psychiatry, 2nd Edition. Baltimore, MD, Williams & Wilkins, 1995

14. Conte G, Vazzola A, Sacchetti E: Renal function in chronic lithium-treated patients. Acta Psychiatr Scand 79:503–504, 1989

15. Cooper A: Hypomanic psychosis precipitated by hemodialysis. Compr Psychiatry 8:168–174, 1967

16. Creelman W, Ciraulo D, Shader R: Lithium drug interactions, in Drug Interactions in Psychiatry. Edited by Ciraulo D, Shader R, Greenblatt D, et al. Baltimore, MD, Williams & Wilkins, 1989, pp 127–157

17. Csernansky J, Hollister L: Using lithium in patients with cardiac and renal disease. Hospital Formulary 20:726–735, 1985

18. Cummings J, Benson D: Dementia: A Clinical Approach, 2nd Edition. Boston, MA, Butterworth-Heinemann, 1992

19. DasGupta K, Jefferson J: The use of lithium in the medically ill. Gen Hosp Psychiatry 12:83–97, 1990

19a. DasGupta K, Jefferson J: Treatment of mania in the medically ill, in Psychotropic Drug Use in the Medically Ill (Vol 21 of Advances in Psychosomatic Medicine). Edited by Silver P. New York, Karger, 1994, pp 138–162

20. Dawling S, Lynn K, Rossner R, et al: The pharmacokinetics of nortriptyline in patients with chronic renal failure. Br J Clin Pharmacol 12:39–45, 1981

21. Depaulo JJ, Correa E, Sapir D: Renal glomerular function and long term lithium therapy. Am J Psychiatry 138:324–327, 1981

22. El-Mallakh R, Schrader S, Widger E: Mania as a manifestation of end-stage renal disease. J Nerv Ment Dis 175:243–245, 1987

23. Flynn C, Chandran P, Taylor M, et al: Intraperitoneal lithium administration for bipolar affective disorder in a patient on continuous ambulatory peritoneal dialysis. Int J Artif Organs 10:105–107, 1987

24. Fraser C: Neurologic manifestations of the uremic state, in Metabolic Brain Dysfunction in Systemic Disorders. Edited by Arieff A, Griggs R. Boston, MA, Little, Brown, 1992, pp 139–166

25. Gelenberg A: Lithium nephrotoxicity: new twists in an old story. Biological Therapies in Psychiatry 17:2–3, 1994

26. Gitlin M: Lithium-induced renal insufficiency. J Clin Psychopharmacol 13:276–279, 1993

27. Hansen H, Hestbech J, Sorenson J, et al: Chronic interstitial nephropathy in patients on long-term lithium treatment. Q J Med 48:577–591, 1979

28. Hestbach J, Hansen H, Amdisen A, et al: Chronic renal lesions following long-term treatment with lithium. Kidney 12:205–213, 1977

29. Hetmar O, Bolwig T, Brun C, et al: Lithium: long-term effects on the kidney. Acta Psychiatr Scand 73:574–581, 1986

30. Hetmar O, Brun C, Clemmesen L, et al: Lithium: long-term effects on the kidney, II: structural changes. J Psychiatr Res 21:279–288, 1987

31. Hetmar O, Povlsen U, Ladefoged J, et al: Lithium: long-term effects on the kidney—a prospective follow-up study 10 years after kidney biopsy. Br J Psychiatry 158:53–58, 1991

32. Hurwitz A: Antacid therapy and drug kinetics. Clin Pharmacokinet 2:269–280, 1977

32a. Imai H, Nakamoto Y, Kirokawa M, et al: Carbamazepine-induced granulomatous necrotizing angiitis with acute renal failure. Nephron 51:405–408, 1989

33. Jack R, Rabin P, McKinney T: Dialysis encephalopathy: a review. Int J Psychiatry Med 13:309–326, 1983/1984

34. Jack R, Rivers-Bulkeley N, Rabin P: Secondary mania as a presentation of progressive dialysis encephalopathy. J Nerv Ment Dis 171:193–195, 1983

35. Javid M, Settlage P: Effect of urea on cerebrospinal fluid pressure in human subjects. JAMA 160:943–949, 1956

36. Jefferson J, Greist J: Lithium and the kidney, in Psychopharmacology Update: New and Neglected Areas. Edited by Davis J, Greenblatt D. New York, Grune & Stratton, 1979, pp 81–104

36a. Kandrotas R, Love J, Gai P, et al: The effect of hemodialysis and hemoperfusion on serum valproic acid concentration. Neurology 40:1456–1458, 1990

37. Levy N: Psychopharmacology in patients with renal failure. Int J Psychiatry Med 20:325–334, 1990

38. Lieberman J, Cooper T, Suckow R: Tricyclic antidepressant and metabolite levels in chronic renal failure. Clin Pharmacol Ther 37:301–307, 1985

39. Lippman S, Manshadi M, Gultekin A: Lithium in a patient with renal failure on hemodialysis (letter). J Clin Psychiatry 45:444, 1984

40. Lockwood A: Hepatic encephalopathy, in Metabolic Brain Dysfunction in Systemic Disorders. Edited by Arieff A, Griggs R. Boston, MA, Little, Brown, 1992, pp 167–182

41. Løkkegaard H, Andersen N, Henriksen E, et al: Renal function in 153 manic-depressive patients treated with lithium for more than five years. Acta Psychiatr Scand 71:347–355, 1985

42. Mason R, McQueen E, Keary P, et al: Pharmacokinetics of lithium: elimination half-life, renal clearance, and apparent volume of distribution and schizophrenia. Clin Pharmacokinet 3:241–246, 1978

43. Merrill J, Legrain M, Hoigne R: Observations on the role of urea in uremia. Am J Med 14:519–520, 1953

44. Meyers B: The patient with renal disease, in Treatments of Psychiatric Disorders: A Task Force Report of the American Psychiatric Association, Vol 2. Washington, DC, American Psychiatric Association, 1989, pp 915–929

45. O'Hare J, Callaghan N, Murnaghan D: Dialysis encephalopathy. Medicine 62:129–141, 1983

45a. Ostrow D, Coe F, Wolpert E: A study of renal function in patients treated with a flexible dose lithium regimen. Journal of Psychiatric Treatment and Evaluation 4:269–278, 1982

45b. Perez G, Oster J, Vaamonde C: Incomplete syndrome of renal tubular acidosis induced by lithium carbonate. J Lab Clin Med 86:386–94, 1975

46. Piafsky K, Borga O, Odar-Cederlof I, et al: Increased plasma protein binding of propranolol and chlorpromazine mediated by disease-induced elevations of plasma alpha 1-acid glycoprotein. N Engl J Med 299:1435–1439, 1978

47. Port F, Kroll P, Rosenzweig J: Lithium therapy during maintenance hemodialysis. Psychosomatics 20:130–131, 1979

48. Procci W: Mania during maintenance hemodialysis successfully treated with oral lithium carbonate. J Nerv Ment Dis 164:355–358, 1977

49. Rabin E, Garston R, Weir R, et al: Persistent nephrogenic diabetes insipidus associated with long-term lithium carbonate treatment. Can Med Assoc J 121:194–198, 1979

50. Ramsey T, Cox M: Lithium and the kidney: a review. Am J Psychiatry 139:443–449, 1982

51. Sandoz M, Vandel S, Vande B: Metabolism of amitriptyline in patients with chronic renal failure. Eur J Clin Pharmacol 26:227–232, 1984

52. Schou M: Pharmacology and toxicology of lithium. Annu Rev Pharmacol Toxicol 16:231–243, 1976

53. Schou M: Effects of long-term lithium treatment on kidney function: an overview. J Psychiatr Res 22:287–296, 1988

54. Schou M, Vestergaard P: Prospective studies in a lithium cohort, II: renal function, water and electrolyte metabolism. Acta Psychiatr Scand 78:427–433, 1988

55. Simon N, Garber E, Arieff A: Persistent nephrogenic diabetes insipidus after lithium carbonate. Ann Intern Med 86:446–447, 1977

56. Stancer H, Forbath N: Hyperparathyroidism, hypothyroidism, and impaired renal function after 10 to 20 years of lithium treatment. Arch Intern Med 149:1042–1045, 1989

57. Stenback A, Haapanen E: Azotemia and psychosis. Acta Psychiatr Scand 43:30–38, 1967

58. Surman O: Hemodialysis and renal transplantation, in Massachusetts General Hospital Handbook of General Hospital Psychiatry, 3rd Edition. Edited by Cassem N. St. Louis, MO, Mosby Year Book, 1991, pp 401–430

59. Surman O, Parker S: Complex partial seizures and psychiatric disturbance in end-stage renal disease. Psychosomatics 22:134–137, 1981

60. Talalla A, Halbrook H, Barbour B, et al: Subdural hematoma associated with long-term hemodialysis for chronic renal disease. JAMA 212:1847–1849, 1970

61. Thomas C, Neale T: Organic manic syndrome associated with advanced uraemia due to polycystic kidney disease. Br J Psychiatry 158:119–121, 1991

62. Thomsen K, Schou M: The treatment of lithium poisoning, in Lithium Research and Therapy. Edited by Johnson F. New York, Academic Press, 1975, pp 227–236

63. Tyler R: Neurological complications of acute and chronic failure, in The Treatment of Renal Failure. Edited by Merrill J. New York, Grune & Stratton, 1965, pp 315–337

64. Vaamonde C, Milian N, Magrinat G: Longitudinal evaluation of glomerular filtration rate during long-term lithium therapy. Am J Kidney Dis 7:213–216, 1986

65. Vestergaard P, Amdisen A, Hansen H, et al: Lithium treatment and kidney function. Acta Psychiatr Scand 60:504–520, 1979

66. Victor M, Martin J: Nutritional and metabolic diseases of the nervous system, in Harrison's Principles of Internal Medicine, 12th Edition. Edited by Wilson J, Braunwald E, Isselbacher K, et al. New York, McGraw-Hill, Health Professions Division, 1991, pp 2045–2055

67. von Knorring L, Wahlin A, Nystrm K, et al: Uraemia induced by long-term lithium treatment. Lithium 1:251–253, 1990

67a. Walker R: Lithium nephrotoxicity. Kidney Int 44 (suppl 42):93–98, 1993

68. Walker R, Davies B, Holwill B, et al: A clinicopathological study of lithium nephrotoxicity. Journal of Chronic Diseases 35:685–695, 1982

69. Walker R, Dowling J, Alcorn D, et al: Renal pathology associated with lithium therapy. Pathology 15:403–411, 1983

70. Waller D, Edwards J: Lithium and the kidney: an update. Psychol Med 19:825–831, 1989

71. Wise T: The pitfalls of diagnosing depression in chronic renal disease. Psychosomatics 15:83–84, 1974

72. Wood I, Parmelee D, Foreman J: Lithium-induced nephrotic syndrome. Am J Psychiatry 146:84–87, 1989

73. Zetin M, Plon L, Vaziri N, et al: Lithium carbonate dose and serum level relationships in chronic hemodialysis patients. Am J Psychiatry 138:1387–1388, 1981

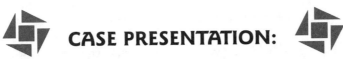
Mr. Barry is a 51-year-old man who has developed end-stage renal disease (ESRD) secondary to uncontrolled hypertension. He returns to psychotherapy for help in coping with his illness. The patient had been a highly decorated helicopter pilot in Vietnam who worked with the medical rescue team. After returning to the United States, he started a successful business in the garment industry. He had been married, but he divorced his first wife approximately 10 years previously when he learned that she was having an affair. Although it had been obvious that she was staying out "later and later," at times to 4:00 in the morning, ostensibly to "work late," Mr. Barry claims that he "never suspected" that she was involved with another man. Once he learned the truth, he refused to speak to her, nor would he answer her telephone calls or letters. He had no further communication with her other than to arrange to ship her belongings to her new address and work out terms of the divorce. He was steadfast in his position that she was "out," all the while maintaining that he was not angry, just "fed up."

Around this time, he sought psychiatric help because of panic disorder and major depression, both of which responded well to imipramine (Tofranil) 150 mg/day and clonazepam (Klonopin) 0.5 mg twice daily, with chloral hydrate 500 mg hs prn for insomnia. He remained in psychotherapy for a year. Mr. Barry acknowledged that he had always been an anxious person and a perfectionist. Although well liked and respected by colleagues and co-workers as fair, honest, and "a regular guy," he "suffered greatly" when confronted with what he perceived as others' incompetence on the job. He was unwilling to explore his denial about his wife's behavior or his subsequent refusal to have any contact with her. In therapy, he became quite dependent on his female psychiatrist. Although he was conscientious and punctual about psychotherapy appointments, he was not psychologically minded and could work in therapy only concretely. For example, he could not reflect on his own perfectionistic behavior and the meanings of others' incompetence; instead, supportive suggestions, such as the creation of an imaginary personal diary entitled "Barry's Believe It Or Not," brought humor and symptomatic relief.

He was lost to follow-up, except for occasional Christmas cards reporting that he had a girlfriend and was doing well. He returns to therapy soon after being told of progressive renal failure and the probability of needing dialysis. He feels constantly anxious, has been unable to fall asleep, and has been preoccupied with how "things were spinning out of control" because he could not attend to the details of his business. His appetite is poor, and he admits that he did not adhere to the diet prescribed by his physician because "there's nothing to eat on it." He is terrified about the possibility of renal transplantation, stating that he saw what happened to people in Vietnam and did not want to be "anyone's guinea pig." There is no drug or alcohol abuse. Family history is negative for psychiatric illness.

Mental status exam reveals an ill-appearing but meticulously groomed man with articulate, nonpressured speech. His affect is worried. Mood is anxious. His thought process is goal directed, coherent, and logical. Thought content concerns the specifics of the medical stressors he now faces. There are no delusions or hallucinations. He is alert and completely oriented, and higher cognitive functions are intact.

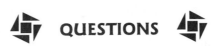

QUESTIONS

Choose all that apply.

1. The focus of Mr. Barry's worries centers on the practical—available treatment options, logistics, dietary restrictions, and fears of becoming unemployed. In order to distinguish realistic concerns from his characteristic denial and displacement, you must be familiar with some specifics of treatment. Which of the following are true?

a. Hemodialysis requires 4–6 hours per treatment, three times a week.
b. ESRD patients must learn to substitute a vegetarian type of diet that emphasizes fruits and vegetables, with fluid restrictions.
c. For most patients, full-time employment before dialysis predicts the return to full-time employment after settling into a regular dialysis schedule.
d. Different treatment modalities (hemodialysis, continuous ambulatory peritoneal dialysis, transplantation) tend to show fairly consistent outcomes on measures of quality of life.

2. It is recommended that Mr. Barry have a magnetic resonance imaging (MRI) for headaches of recent onset. However, he is very anxious and is not able to tolerate the test on the first try. Which of the following medications should be avoided in an ESRD patient?
a. Sodium amytal
b. Oxazepam (Serax)
c. Lorazepam (Ativan)
d. Buspirone (BuSpar)
e. Clonazepam (Klonopin)

3. Sleep in ESRD . . .
a. Tends to be restless.
b. Is associated with hypersomnia secondary to the central nervous system (CNS) depressant effects of uremia.
c. Is interrupted by sleep apnea syndrome.
d. Tends to be relatively preserved unless there is an intercurrent affective disorder.

4. Which of the following is true of lorazepam in the setting of renal failure?
a. Doses should be halved for every 10-point reduction of glomerular filtration rate (GFR).
b. It is preferred because of its short half-life.
c. It is preferred because of its lack of active metabolites.
d. It is dialyzable.

5. What is true about the half-life of lorazepam in ESRD?
a. It is unchanged as long as hepatic metabolism remains intact.
b. It is shortened.
c. It exceeds the half-life of clonazepam in healthy patients.
d. In ESRD, oxazepam and lorazepam have comparable half-lives.

6. All of the following are likely to be true of sexual functioning of ESRD patients such as Mr. Barry *except* . . .
a. There is usually only minimal change in libido.
b. There is high prevalence of physiologically based impotence.
c. There is decreased testosterone and spermatogenesis.
d. There is decreased orgasmic capacity for dialysands.

7. Mr. Barry begins to feel hopeless and constantly dysphoric, and develops transient suicidal ideation. He reveals that he has had difficulty performing sexually for a long time. Which of the following are true?
a. The medical severity of Mr. Barry's illness predicts the intensity of depression that he will experience.
b. Uremia produces depression-like symptoms.
c. ESRD patients in the early treatment stages are more vulnerable to depression than later on.
d. All of the above.

8. Which of the following study findings about decisions to terminate long-term dialysis are *false*?
a. The suicide and rational treatment withdrawal rates are roughly equivalent in ESRD patients.
b. Diabetes is a strong risk factor for rational elective treatment withdrawal.
c. The occurrence of new medical complications is not helpful in flagging patients at risk for suicide.
d. The majority of ESRD patients who elect to terminate dialysis do so because they are depressed.
e. The majority of patients terminally ill with diseases other than ESRD who commit suicide do so because they are depressed.

9. What has been found regarding the association between depression in ESRD and outcome studies of medical course?
a. ESRD morbidity varies independently of the occurrence of depression.
b. Depressive symptoms are associated with more frequent medical hospitalization.
c. Patients who describe their lives as happy overall have the longest survival times.
d. Age correlates more with decreased survival time in ESRD than does severity of depression.

10. The concept of *illness intrusiveness* refers to how an illness interferes with important facets of a person's life.

True statements about studies of ESRD illness intrusiveness are . . .

  a. The three life domains of physical well-being and diet, work and finances, and marital and family relations are just about equally adversely affected.
  b. The perception of illness intrusiveness is relatively independent of nonrenal stressors.
  c. Higher family income inversely correlates with the magnitude of perceived ESRD intrusiveness.
  d. ESRD patients with paid employment report better quality of life.

11. Illness intrusiveness has an impact on the following life domains. Which are arranged in correct descending order of impact?

  a. Religious expression > Finances > Marital and family relationships > Work
  b. Marital and family relationships > Religious expression > Finances
  c. Work and finances > Marital and family relationships > Religious expression
  d. None of the above are true, because they are affected fairly equivalently.

12. Mr. Barry feels hopeless, with guilty ruminations that he has "done this to myself." Pharmacological intervention becomes necessary. Which of the following are true?

  a. Antidepressants should be reserved for those ESRD patients whose depression jeopardizes their condition.
  b. The half-lives of tricyclic antidepressants (TCAs) do *not* increase in the setting of ESRD.
  c. The pharmacokinetics of TCAs dictate that the dosing interval be increased to compensate for ESRD.
  d. Drug plasma levels are the "gold standard" of pharmacological management in these patients.

13. You learn that the nephrologist has decided to add recombinant erythropoietin. Which of the following would you expect to see as a consequence?

  a. Anergia
  b. Decline in sexual functioning
  c. Worsened depression
  d. Enhanced psychological well-being

14. What potential side effect(s) of bupropion (Wellbutrin) is/are most likely to be exacerbated by ESRD?

  a. Seizures
  b. Hypotension
  c. Delirium
  d. Hypertension
  e. Restlessness

15. What potential side effect(s) of monoamine oxidase inhibitors (MAOIs) is/are most likely to be exacerbated by ESRD?

  a. Seizures
  b. Hypotension
  c. Delirium
  d. Hypertension
  e. Restlessness

16. Mr. Barry's depression begins to resolve with nortriptyline (Pamelor; Aventyl) 30 mg daily and lorazepam (Ativan) 0.25 mg bid. He adapts to the hemodialysis schedule with difficulty, but gradually befriends the dialysis staff and feels more comfortable. The nephrologist tells you, however, that despite being a model patient, Mr. Barry adamantly refuses to discuss the possibility of transplantation. When approached about it, he politely insists, "That option is out. I don't want to talk about it." He denies that he is anxious about the procedure, maintaining that it is "too experimental" and he'd "rather stick to what I know." He is also quite afraid of "catching cancer" from the donated organ, but refuses to explore these fears. This sounds quite familiar, as it is similar to the way Mr. Barry has coped with other stressful life events, like the divorce. Knowing that insight would be optimal but limited for this patient, and that he is most amenable to a supportive strategy, what might you tell Mr. Barry about renal transplantation?

  a. Successful transplantation offers hope for a life similar to what was experienced before the onset of renal failure.
  b. Kidney transplantation has been associated with improvement in sexual functioning.
  c. It is possible for patients to return to work in 4–6 months.
  d. Mr. Barry's fears that he can "catch cancer" if he undergoes transplantation are unfounded.
  e. The majority of patients return to work.

17. Mr. Barry becomes less resistant to discussing transplantation with the nephrologist, who feels he would be a good candidate. To help care for Mr. Barry, you want to become familiar with the techniques for controlling graft rejection, which include immunosuppressant drugs, graft radiation, and total lymphatic irradiation. The most important immunosuppressant drugs are prednisone, azothioprine, antithymocyte globulin, anti–T cell subtype mono-

clonal antibodies, and cyclosporine. Which of the following are atypical complications of renal transplantation?
  a. A high incidence of steroid psychosis
  b. Manic-type states secondary to viral encephalitis
  c. Worsened diabetic control for patients with diabetes mellitus
  d. Opportunistic infections

18. All of the following have been associated with cyclosporine except . . .
  a. More frequent adverse steroid side effects.
  b. Increased incidence of tremor.
  c. Greater propensity for seizures.
  d. Psychotic symptoms.
  e. Lithium toxicity.

19. What side effects do psychotropics and cyclosporine have in common?
  a. Neuroleptic malignant syndrome
  b. Tremor
  c. Conduction defects
  d. All of the above

20. The dialysis team wants you actively involved in planning for Mr. Barry's eventual transplantation. Which of the following are valid statements?
  a. Whereas quality of life is affected by depression, *graft* outcome tends to be independent of affective disorder.
  b. Organ donors are at high risk for postoperative morbidity and mortality.
  c. Transplantation outcome is affected by co-occurrence of personality disorders.
  d. The number of psychiatric exclusion criteria for transplantation has dwindled.

21. The transplant team asks you to help with Mr. Barry's preoperative teaching. So far, they have been unsuccessful, because he keeps saying "I don't want to know. Just do it." Each of the following findings on the value of preoperative teaching and psychological preparation for surgery has been reported except . . .
  a. Preoperative teaching decreases postoperative requests for analgesics.
  b. Anxiety before surgical procedures adversely influences postoperative coping skills.
  c. Preoperative preparation by a psychiatrist has been associated with less frequent postoperative delirium.
  d. Psychological preparation for elective surgery reduces length of hospital stays.

22. Which of the following is/are true about psychiatric syndromes in renal transplant recipients?
  a. The most common anxiety disorder in these patients is panic disorder.
  b. Mental status disturbances occur in the majority of patients postoperatively.
  c. The suicide risk in renal transplant patients is equivalent to that of the general population.
  d. None of the above.

23. Transplant patients receive organs from either biologically related live donors or unrelated cadaver donors. What has been found regarding the psychological adjustment of patients receiving these two types of transplants?
  a. Outcome studies show similar psychological adjustment for recipients, although the psychodynamics may be different.
  b. Related organ donors have a high rate of postoperative psychological disorders.
  c. Cadaver organ recipients have poorer psychological adaptation than related organ recipients.
  d. Related organ recipients have poorer psychological adaptation than cadaver organ recipients.

24. Several new immunosuppressants, antivirals, antifungals, and antibiotics are now available and being used in the transplantation setting. Which of the following are true statements about them?
  a. Only the antibiotics have *not* been associated with secondary hallucinosis and delusional states.
  b. Delirium has been described with all four classes of medications.
  c. Tremor occurs more with the immunosuppressant agents than with the other three classes of medications.
  d. The antiviral acyclovir (Zovirax) is generally not useful in this population, yet it is relatively free of neuropsychiatric side effects.
  e. None of the immunosuppressants match the low toxicity and high effectiveness of cyclosporine.

25. What is a potential side effect of adding antidepressants to regimens that include cyclosporine or other immunosuppressant agents?
  a. Increased graft rejection
  b. Frontal lobe symptoms
  c. Lowered seizure threshold
  d. Pseudobulbar symptoms

26. The literature has advised against using which of the following psychiatric treatments in transplant patients?
    a. MAOIs
    b. TCAs
    c. Electroconvulsive therapy (ECT)
    d. Selective serotonin reuptake inhibitors (SSRIs)
    e. Lithium
    f. Benzodiazepines
    g. Buspirone (BuSpar)
    h. Bupropion (Wellbutrin)
    i. Trazodone (Desyrel)

27. For kidney transplant patients with bipolar affective illness who require antimanic prophylaxis, which of the following are true?
    a. There is consensus that lithium should be avoided because of the possibility it could damage the new kidney.
    b. The best way to calculate lithium dosages for these patients is to use creatinine clearance and a pharmacokinetic model.
    c. Organ recipients who receive kidneys from living consanguineous donors can be expected to show near-*normal* renal functioning *within hours* after transplant.
    d. Compared with consanguineous allograft recipients, cadaver organ recipients must wait longer for their renal function to stabilize.

28. Which of the following are among the common psychotherapeutic issues of transplant patients?
    a. They tend to identify with some characteristic of the organ donor.
    b. Becoming healthy again is experienced as a blessing rather than something stressful.
    c. Their psychodynamic responses to surgery resemble those of general surgical patients.
    d. They fare more poorly psychologically when specific demographic information about their deceased organ donor is revealed.

Answers

1. Answer: a (pp. 164, 166)
2. Answer: a (p. 172)
3. Answer: a, c (p. 168)
4. Answer: c (p. 172)
5. Answer: c, d (p. 172)
6. Answer: a (pp. 165–166)
7. Answer: b, c (pp. 167–168)
8. Answer: a, e (p. 168)
9. Answer: b (pp. 166–167)
10. Answer: c, d (p. 165)
11. Answer: c (p. 165)
12. Answer: b (p. 171)
13. Answer: d (p. 166)
14. Answer: a (p. 171)
15. Answer: b (p. 171)
16. Answer: a, b, c (pp. 172–174)
17. Answer: a, b (pp. 177–178)
18. Answer: a (p. 178)
19. Answer: b (pp. 177–178)
20. Answer: c, d (pp. 173–174)
21. Answer: b (pp. 175–176)
22. Answer: d (pp. 176–177, 179)
23. Answer: a (p. 176)
24. Answer: b, c (pp. 177–178)
25. Answer: c (p. 178)
26. Answer: a (p. 179)
27. Answer: c, d (pp. 179–180)
28. Answer: a (pp. 174–175)

◈ COPING WITH END-STAGE RENAL DISEASE

Although Mr. Barry's premorbid personality, psychodynamics, and defensive style will undoubtedly influence how he copes with illness, many of his present fears are realistic. To comply with low-sodium, low-potassium, low-protein, and low-fluid diets, patients must eliminate almost all fruits and vegetables, ration only small amounts of meats and fish, and endure strict fluid restrictions. Family members often hover in disapproval when the patient's compliance wavers, creating misunderstandings and tension. Vacations must be planned around the availability of satellite dialysis units, with the attendant anxiety about relying on unknown doctors, unfamiliar staff, and the knowledge that even moderate dietary "cheating"— surely forgivable for any dieter on vacation—can lead to medical catastrophe.

Not all dialysis patients cope poorly.[109] Denial, for example, is an important defense that allows one to selectively titrate levels of awareness and is often adaptive in the medical setting. Personality variables, such as the need for independence and the ability to use denial effectively, will affect coping and comfort.

◆ For example, low denial scores in ESRD patients were associated with significantly greater mood and sleep dysfunction than were high denial scores.[104]
◆ Dialysis patients who rejected dependency and effectively handled anger more successfully adapted to their illness.[142]

The demands of thrice-weekly dialysis would intrude on most full-time occupations, however great the motivation to work. Sadly, many hemodialysis patients who were employed before their illness no longer work full-time.[120] Many choose to have "off the books" activity and retire disabled from full-time work.[167]

Unfortunately, return to work remains the Achilles' heel in the overall rehabilitation of the patient with ESRD . . . Studies have consistently shown that the longer patients have been unemployed, the less likely they are to return to work.[87] This is due to many factors, including economic disincentives associated with the availability of disability benefits and the potential loss of benefits through part-time employment. Second, experienced workers who have been chronically unemployed may not have positions available to them to which they can readily return.[89] (p. 829)

A Digression About Disability Insurance

While disability coverage is a godsend for patients incapacitated by illness, it can create economic quicksand that stymies psychological and occupational rehabilitation. It is important for consultation-liaison psychiatrists to know some facts about disability insurance:

◆ The best (and most expensive) disability policies are noncancellable, and have "own occupation" and partial disability riders.
  • The *own-occupation rider* states that a person will be considered "disabled" if unable to perform his or her *specific* occupation (e.g., a surgeon with a tremor who can no longer operate would be considered disabled with an own-occupation rider, even though he or she can still earn a living providing nonsurgical services).
  • A *partial-disability rider* permits part-time employment while still providing prorated disability income to supplement earnings.
  • A *noncancellable policy* prohibits the carrier from dropping the patient as long as the premiums are paid.

Unfortunately, most patients own the less expensive, cancelable policies without partial disability or own-occupation provisions. Attempting to earn an income again under these circumstances is a gamble with high stakes: patients risk zero reimbursement if they can perform *any* job for *any* income, however distant from their own occupation or below their standard of living. They may be *permanently* dropped by the carrier if they are judged to be "no longer disabled." Should there be a medical exacerbation, these patients are financially stranded, mired in an insurance no man's land, except for the meager allowance provided by social security.

These factors run counter to the psychological needs of recovering patients who seek to transform their "sick identity" back to health, normalcy, and productivity. The coup de grace is that chronically ill individuals (or their working spouses) often will *never* qualify for reinsurance by another insurance carrier provided by a new employer, and so may decline new job opportunities in order to stay insurable.

The secondary *psychological* disability of this insurance catch-22 enhances the psychological morbidity of an already formidable illness. A recent paper by Meyerson and Lawn[184] provides an extended discussion of some of these issues.

Illness Intrusiveness and Quality of Life

Illness intrusiveness refers to an illness's direct or indirect interference with important facets of an individual's life.[63,64,66–68] For example, direct interference refers to the physiological effects of irreversible renal failure itself, the consequences of the treatment regimen, and/or the presence of nonrenal complications, such as cardiovascular disease.[67] Examples of indirect interference are attitudinal shifts by family and friends that influence a patient's adjustment to his or her disease. Illness intrusiveness may be particularly potent in its effect on general psychosocial well-being.[63] Moreover, the psychosocial stressors resulting from the illness undoubtedly affect compliance with fluid and dietary restrictions, and therefore ultimately affect morbidity.[47,125,128,237,238,248]

The quality of life in ESRD also depends on several nonrenal variables. Devins et al.[67] studied illness intrusiveness in 200 ESRD patients receiving different treatments (hemodialysis, continuous abdominal peritoneal dialysis [CAPD], or renal transplantation). They found that interference in life domains greatly differed across treatments. Expectably, perceived illness intrusiveness correlated significantly with the following:

- Treatment time requirements
- Uremic symptoms
- Intercurrent nonrenal illnesses
- Fatigue
- Difficulties in daily activities

Moreover, increased psychosocial well-being and decreased distress were associated with fewer negative life events, richer social networks, involvement in paid employment, and higher annual family income. The occurrence of negative stressful, *nonrenal* life events signifi-

cantly increased perceived illness intrusiveness. The authors[67] proposed that

> the co-occurrence of independent stressful life events potentiates the intrusions imposed by ESRD, augmenting their impact on lifestyles, activities, and interests. Alternatively, such co-occurrences may simply compromise the individual's ability to cope with the demands of the illness situation—for example, either by competing for available attention, energies, and efforts or by amplifying the overall perception of the magnitude of intrusions to be negotiated. (p. 135)

Note that the burden of ESRD was not equivalent across all life domains.[67] The two domains that were especially affected, regardless of treatment modality, were physical well-being and diet, and then work and finances. Less adversely affected were marital and family relations, recreation, and social relationships outside the family. Life domains such as self-improvement/self-expression, religious expression, and community and civic activities were least affected.

ESRD, like many chronic illnesses, is a family affair.[97,254] Be sure to include family members in your interventions.

Sexual Dysfunction

Sexual dysfunction is common in dialysis patients, even in the absence of affective illness.[6,38,165,171] One nationwide questionnaire reported partial or complete impotence in 56% of dialysis patients and 43% of transplant patients.[164] It seems that sexual function does partially depend upon the degree of renal function.[167] Dialysis patients of both genders experience a marked decrease in libido and frequency of sexual intercourse once they become uremic,[167,169] with some showing abnormal hypothalamic-pituitary functioning.[76] For women dialysands, there may be diminished capacity for orgasm.[169] For men, there is a high prevalence of physiologically based impotence,[211] a reduction of testosterone, and decreased spermatogenesis.[268] Antihypertensive medications may further diminish libido in both sexes and cause impotence in males. Some men with persistent impotence become candidates for a penile prosthesis.[181,198,268]

Depression, disrupted family roles, and the psychological impact of losing urination exacerbate sexual difficulties.[45,62,92,166] Sexual performance may start as stable or normal predialysis,[70] but decline postdialysis and remain impaired. However, deteriorating sexual function that is markedly disproportional to the progression of renal disease suggests factors other than the strictly physiological.

◆ For example, one anecdotal report described restored erectile and ejaculatory ability in a diabetic patient only 3 days after renal transplantation, highlighting the powerful interaction of psychodynamics with physiology.[70]

Hemodialysis Versus Continuous Abdominal Peritoneal Dialysis

The demands of dialysis are sobering; this is no trivial procedure, however routine it may seem.

◆ Hemodialysis circulates the blood extracorporeally and may produce major complications, such as stroke and cardiac emergencies. It requires 4–6 hours daily three times a week.

◆ In CAPD, dialysis solution remains in the peritoneal cavity except for drainage periods, followed by reinstallation of fresh solution five times a day. After each exchange cycle, all tubing is disconnected, the chronic indwelling catheter capped, and the patient is free to go about daily activities.[209] Exchanges typically occur four to five times daily, requiring 30–60 minutes each, and are self-administered. The most common medical complication is peritonitis.

Quality-of-life comparisons between hemodialysis and CAPD have varied, with some studies showing improvements for CAPD patients over hemodialysis patients[176,187,194,300] and others showing no difference in psychosocial outcomes.[86,250] There are often body-image problems with CAPD due to the abdominal distention caused by the fluid in the abdominal cavity,[117] but CAPD has the advantage over hemodialysis of improved patient independence. Home hemodialysis and CAPD appear to be psychologically superior to hospital-based treatments, but the measurable magnitude of the difference has varied.[86,187,250] There are methodological problems with quality-of-life studies: ESRD patients are never randomized to receive a particular form of dialysis or transplantation,[161] and treatment-assignment bias is well known.[245]

◆ Quality-of-life differences were demonstrated across four modalities of treatment (in-center hemodialysis, CAPD, renal transplant, and cadaver transplant) in a study of 459 ESRD patients.[138] However, after ad-

justing for variables such as demographics, primary cause of ESRD, and comorbid illness, significant differences among the four modalities *declined.*

In general, however, most studies have shown *superior* quality of life after renal transplantation compared with all other treatments.[86,124,187,203,228,305]

Anemia is quite prevalent in ESRD and can severely limit rehabilitation. *Recombinant erythropoietin* for the anemia of chronic renal failure significantly improves the quality of life for dialysis patients.[77,195,299] Better energy level, improved psychological well-being, and enhanced sexual functioning have been reported with this medication.[89] Erythropoietin avoids the adverse effects of transfusion but has been associated with hypertension, thrombosis of vascular access, and hyperkalemia.[292]

Psychosocial Factors and Survival

As in the psychosocial literature on other illnesses, the relationship between psychosocial factors and ESRD survival is variable.[146] For example:

◆ Depression (as measured by the Basic Personality Inventory) was a better predictor of (shorter) survival than was age or even a composite physiological index that incorporated 19 chemical and clinical variables.[33]

◆ Depressive symptoms (on the Depression Adjective Check List) were associated with higher mortality and more frequent medical hospitalizations in 53 hemodialysis patients who had been on dialysis for durations ranging from zero to 150 months.[196]

◆ Another study demonstrated that in 47 hemodialysis patients, those who died within the first year of initiating dialysis were more likely to have been depressed (on the Minnesota Multiphasic Personality Inventory [MMPI][123a]) than those who survived longer.[304]

◆ Mortality at 10-year follow-up in center- and home-dialysis patients ($N = 64$) was better correlated with age and depressive symptomatology (on the Beck Depression Inventory[18a]) than with medical variables.[241]

Other studies have failed to corroborate the relationship between psychological variables and decreased survival time in ESRD:

◆ Depression did not predict survival in a group of 97 patients receiving hemodialysis, CAPD, or transplant.[68] Notably, those who described their lives as happy overall had the *shortest* survival times.

◆ No relationship between depressive symptoms (Likert Scale) and survival emerged in another study of 78 hemodialysis and CAPD patients over 70 years of age.[132]

Unfortunately, outcome studies of psychosocial intervention in ESRD have been uncontrolled or poorly controlled, and have tended to use a nonrandomized design.

◆ For example, one study showed that support-group participants on dialysis lived longer than nonparticipants, even after controlling for 13 psychosocial and physiological covariates.[106] However, the design was nonrandomized, and details of when patients joined the group and the duration of their participation were not reported.

The failure to control for disease severity[13] or to use assessment instruments specifically validated for ESRD[52] may confound these studies and account for the conflicting results.[160]

Quite apart from depression's potential impact on the immune system, depressed ESRD patients are more likely to show poor self-care, noncompliance (diet, medication, dialysis), and poor medical follow-up.[161] Smoking, alcoholism, drug abuse, and other medical problems such as myocardial infarction[28] and reduced aerobic capacity[40] may contribute to an adverse ESRD outcome. Moreover, depression is already associated with increased mortality even in the population at large.[190]

Large, prospective, long-term outcome studies on renal transplantation are under way.[295] Levenson and Glochieski have written,[161]

> Surprisingly, there do not appear to have been any psychiatric studies of chronic renal failure prior to the end stage when dialysis or transplantation are required, although there are large numbers of such patients medically followed for years. Such patients, in fact, have been the subject of a number of studies examining the progression of renal failure as a function of dietary protein intake and blood pressure control. Depression and noncompliance would be very interesting cofactors to examine in pre–end-stage renal disease patients. The interaction between depression-[related] noncompliance in all forms of treatment for ESRD remains an important area for

future research. Controlled intervention trials for treatment of depression, examining medical, psychiatric, and health services outcomes, would be valuable. (p. 387)

⚄ DEPRESSION AND ANXIETY

To say that dialysis patients experience anxiety and depression is to state the obvious. Worry and dysphoria may invade everything—self-esteem, prognosis, sexual performance, ability to cope with dialysis stressors, and the expectations of staff and family. As always, patients who have a premorbid history of psychiatric disorders have a particularly difficult time.

◆ An interesting side note: Masturbatory behavior has been anecdotally observed among dialyzed men and has been understood as a type of anxious discharge,[167] similar to reports of masturbation occurring in soldiers about to face combat situations.[213] Needless to say, this behavior is not popular with dialysis staff, and psychiatric consultation may be requested for help in dealing with it.

Prevalence rates for major and minor depression (by Research Diagnostic Criteria [RDC][250a]) were 6.5% and 18%, respectively, among 124 hemodialysis patients in a recent study.[127] Prevalence estimates of depression in ESRD patients have varied widely, however.[161a] Methodological problems have included sample heterogeneity (disease type, e.g., systemic lupus erythematosus [SLE], hypertension; duration of renal failure; and treatment type), variations in assessment instruments, and differences in diagnostic criteria. Uremia itself produces depressive-like symptoms (irritability, decreased appetite and libido, insomnia, apathy, fatigue, poor concentration) that may be misattributed to a primary psychiatric condition.[123,169,246] In addition, ESRD patients may be affected by other medical conditions that mimic depressive states or cause secondary mood disorders, such as anemia, electrolyte disturbances, or underlying systemic disease (e.g., SLE).[161] Medications such as antihypertensives and steroids may produce depressive side effects.

As in other medically ill populations, the nonsomatic symptoms (e.g., depressed mood, suicidal ideas, guilt, loss of interest, discouragement) best distinguish ESRD patients with and without affective illness.[54,127] Physical factors related to medical status (tiredness, sleep disturbance, cramps, pruritis, headache, nausea, dyspnea, joint pain) adversely affect mood and quality-of-life indices.[16]

◆ Note that restless sleep,[65] restless leg syndrome, and sleep apnea syndrome[145,182,289] occur frequently in ESRD. Fractured, nonrestorative sleep contributes to illness intrusiveness[65] and should be given therapeutic priority.

Adjustment disorders are the most common of the less-severe depressive states,[262] with patients most vulnerable during the early stages of treatment.[153,262] Even in a field as quantifiable as nephrology, psychodynamics are inescapable: *It has been found that the patient's perception of illness predicts the occurrence of depression better than the objective illness severity or the extent of role disruption.*[231] Appropriate psychiatric treatment may improve the perception of these physical complaints.[57]

Rational Treatment Withdrawal and Suicide

The psychiatrist may be asked to assist patients in making decisions about dialysis, transplantation, or treatment termination.[37,227] The true suicide rate in dialysis has not been systematically established and estimates have varied widely,[161] but it is thought to be much more common in dialysis patients than in the general population or in other chronic illnesses.[2,122] Certainly, dialysis patients can easily commit suicide; they may sever fistulas, exsanguinate, go on potassium binges, or skip a few dialysis runs.[169] On the other hand, assumptions that "most" dialysis patients "want to commit suicide" because of the stressors they endure can lead to therapeutic nihilism and are not supported by the statistical facts. Some of the data on suicide rates come from studies on decisions to stop treatment:

◆ "Treatment-withdrawal" samples are a heterogeneous group, including nondepressed individuals who wish to live but who have made a rational decision to terminate treatment as well as those who are depressed and who actively want to die (i.e., commit suicide).
◆ Rational treatment withdrawal accounts for approximately 20%–25% of all ESRD deaths.[193,223] Two factors were strongly associated with this decision: 1) the presence of diabetes and 2) increasing age (> age 60).[193]
◆ Suicide (i.e., motivated specifically by the wish to die) accounts for only 1%–2% of these deaths.[31,193,223] For these patients, there were no new medical complications before their death that might have predicted suicide. Little information has been reported about these patients.

Rational treatment withdrawal is not synonymous with the active desire to kill oneself by suicide.[126a] Never assume that a depressed ESRD patient who is expressing the wish to stop treatment is "justified"—some may be seeking reassurance or support, or may be suffering a treatable psychiatric illness such as psychosis, an anxiety disorder, or major depression.[105,113,126,189] Many patients feel more optimistic about continuing dialysis after their depression has been treated or certain of their fears explored in psychotherapy.

◆ Beware of therapeutic nihilism: most completed suicides among terminally ill patients occur in the setting of clinical depression or impaired judgment.[30,45a,238a,264]
◆ Depression affects decision making; for example, acceptability of life-sustaining interventions was significantly lower in clinically depressed patients, who showed a change of heart when depression was no longer present.[98]

The literature on rational treatment withdrawal has been explored in further detail in several papers.[14,27a,30,56,154,192,227,242,264]

Psychotherapy

Several factors make ESRD patients particularly challenging to work with in psychotherapy:[37]

◆ The effects of uremia and electrolyte imbalance often profoundly affect energy, mental alertness, and the ability to remember.
◆ The time-consuming regimens required of dialysis patients are of unparalleled complexity. When other medical problems, such as diabetes, also require attention, the cognitive demands would overload anyone. Psychotherapy may seem like one more burden.
◆ ESRD patients are often candidates for more than one type of treatment. Informed consent in these cases requires the processing of a large volume of material by a patient who may already be overwhelmed.

In her excellent paper on improving decision making in ESRD patients, Campbell[37] advises nephrologists to avoid several pitfalls when discussing dialysis options. Since consultation-liaison psychiatrists often assist patients in exploring complex decisions (e.g., whether to remain on dialysis or to pursue kidney transplantation), we found several of her warnings—which are really about maintaining neutrality—particularly relevant:

- *The "I'll compare both treatments" trap:* Although physicians may be tempted to use this approach because it seems so logical and time efficient, "patients may end up confused or glassy-eyed while nodding and agreeing that, of course, they understand" (p. 176).[37] To new dialysis patients, there is nothing more confusing that an approach that details comparisons. Explain treatments first individually, and then compare them sparingly to allow the patient to review.

- *The trap of complex explanations:* It is easier for health care professionals to speak the technical shorthand that they use with colleagues. It takes more work to distill complicated medical concepts into simple explanations for the patient, whose concentration is already burdened by illness and fear.

- *The trap of prejudging who would or would not do well:* It is hard not to prejudge who would or would not do well with particular treatments based on previous experiences with other patients. Every patient is unique and should not be judged on the basis of first impressions. Try to give each patient the chance to make an educated decision for him- or herself.

- *The trap of deciding what you think would be best:* Patients often ask their physicians, including their psychiatrists, "Yes, but what do *you* think I should do? What treatment is best?" Beware of offering a quick opinion, as there are pitfalls if you do so, such as the patient's continued dependency on "experts" and abdication of making responsible decisions. It is better for patients to work through the decision making for themselves with your help, if requested.

- Finally, be careful of making sweeping generalizations, creating bias with length of discussion time, or using biased wording that propels the patient down one decision path and not another.

Compliance

Consultation-liaison psychiatrists are often asked to help noncompliant patients whose medical care is in jeopardy.[94] Failure to comply with fluid and dietary restrictions, especially, can have dire consequences for health and survival.

- Plough and Salem[206] found that dietary indiscretion was the primary and immediate cause of death from congestive heart failure in ESRD.

- Excessive fluid overload is a widespread problem for more than one-third of ESRD patients,[55] and is a major cause of death.[298]

- Patients report being preoccupied with *thirst,* and in one study ranked *fluid compliance* as the most stressful of 30 physiological and psychological stressors.[15]

More favorable compliance occurs in patients who have an internal locus of control,[141,207] less-marked anger and hostility,[210] and a high degree of self-control and frustration tolerance.[226] Patients with more supportive families, characterized by greater cohesion, expressiveness, and less intrafamily conflict, have better adherence to fluid-intake restrictions.[47] Stress adversely affects dietary compliance, even when it is minor.[128]

Behavioral and Cognitive Strategies

Most of the reports on compliance strategies use a behavioral or cognitive model.

- ESRD patients provided with educational strategies specifically aimed at basic information concerning normal kidney function, kidney disease, dietary management of renal failure, dialysis, and transplantation survived an average of 4.6 months longer before requiring the initiation of renal replacement therapy (e.g., dialysis) compared with those who received their hospitals' standard education materials.[26]

- Two male hemodialysis patients were described in another study who had been noncompliant with fluid restrictions.[263] The authors proposed a treatment model that emphasized a biosocial approach, including a nonmoralistic attitude, flexibility in dialysis schedules, and psychological intervention early in the course of dialysis.

- Hegel and colleagues[125] compared a cognitive with a behavioral intervention to determine relative effectiveness in reducing interdialysis weight gain (a measure of fluid-restriction compliance) in 8 male hemodialysis patients. The behavioral model consisted of positive reinforcement (using incentives such as lottery tickets and a private television), shaping, and self-monitoring. The cognitive model offered counseling designed to modify health beliefs (i.e., problem solving to develop strategies to overcome barriers to treatment adherence; information about the potential negative/positive health consequences of poor/good adherence; information to correct misconceptions or lack of knowledge regarding dialysis or renal disease). Both interventions produced immediate reductions in weight gain, but the behavioral intervention was superior in maintaining these reductions. Combining the interventions resulted in no improvement over the behavioral intervention alone. Continuation of self-monitoring procedures maintained improvements up to 2 months posttreatment.

The **Health Belief Model** used in this study is worth further mention. It was originally devised by Becker and Maiman[19] as a way of defining how personal health beliefs interact to affect compliance with medical care. The model identifies five criteria that we have found clinically useful in guiding interventions with noncompliant patients:

1. Perceived **susceptibility** to negative health consequences caused by poor compliance with medical advice.
2. Perceived **seriousness** of these consequences.
3. Perceived **costs** versus benefits of performing the prescribed adherence behavior.
4. Perceived **barriers** (i.e., the degree of difficulty in incorporating the adherence behavior into the person's lifestyle).
5. Degree of **concern** about the disease itself and its consequences.

◆   For example, Mr. Barry (like many newly diagnosed ESRD patients) was initially noncompliant with the strict fluid restrictions prescribed by his nephrologist, although he followed other aspects of his diet with his usual precision. We learned that Mr. Barry thought that the extra fluid intake could be "taken off" by hemodialysis, and was willing to spend "an extra hour or two" on the dialysis machine in exchange for diminished thirst, which he found uncomfortable. He had little understanding of how he could be jeopardizing his health with this behavior, since he thought dialysis and the kidneys operated along a simplistic plumbing model of "fluid in, fluid out." An educational intervention was tailored for this patient, explaining basics of how fluid and electrolyte shifts affected blood pressure and the heart. Helping him devise his own logbook of fluid intake (with provisions for occasional "splurges") capitalized on his obsessional style and improved his adherence to the fluid restrictions.

Psychodynamics

Although we could locate no studies systematically applying insight-oriented techniques, there are several interesting anecdotal reports on the psychodynamics of dialysis patients. In one, a 38-year-old woman undergoing hemo-

dialysis was referred because of noncompliance.[150] It was learned that the patient had been repeatedly raped and sexually abused by her stepfather when she was 5–10 years old. Dialysis for this patient meant losing control over her body and a repetition of being physically intruded upon by caretakers.

Other interesting reports occur in the French literature. In one, the analysis of a 33-year-old woman on dialysis revealed fantasies connected with vampires.[202] Another report explored the use of conjoint medical and psychoanalytic perspectives in four patients undergoing long-term hemodialysis.[178] It demonstrated that significant differences often exist between the physician's and the patient's perceptions of the disease and its treatment. Other authors have speculated on the symbolic and mythological underpinnings of urine and the loss of micturition.[92]

Never assume that you know the meanings of an illness for a particular patient. For example, 80 patients on a renal unit were interviewed to assess their psychiatric status and social functioning, and then reinterviewed 1 year later. An incidental finding was that despite problems, 11 patients commented *positively* on some aspect of their experience.[129] House reported,[129]

> Typical comments were: "I feel as if I've grown up . . . as if I'm more aware of what life's all about." "Every day is a bonus now . . . I'm always hopeful." Several people commented that they worried less over unimportant things and "noticed life" more. These comments were often made by people who had at some time recovered from a medical crisis, and did not necessarily reflect current mental state . . . It is clear that individual statements about the value of life on treatment are not related, in a simple direct way, to current levels of social or physical function. (p. 449)

Because denial is high in these patients as a group,[167] a call for help should be responded to quickly. Renal patients tend to feel very much "overdoctored,"[169] and Freyberger[102] has suggested that psychotherapy will have a better chance of success if conducted in conjunction with clinic visits or dialysis runs. However, psychotherapy sessions conducted on a dialysis unit may forfeit privacy and may be necessarily brief, ego supportive, and pragmatic in focus.[268]

Itschaki[134] has further reviewed psychosocial issues pertaining specifically to the geriatric nephrology patient.

Medication

Antidepressants

By far, there is the most clinical experience with the tricyclic antidepressants (TCAs), which have been safely and widely used to medicate depression in renal failure. From the strictly pharmacological point of view, the half-lives of cyclic antidepressants do not change in ESRD, so it is not necessary to modify the dose or interval[21] (see Appendix H). Pharmacokinetics should not supersede clinical judgment, however; remember the **rule of two-thirds** cautions about the heightened sensitivity to side effects of standard medication doses.[268] Some guidelines follow:

- Surman[268] advises beginning TCA therapy empirically with the equivalent of 25 mg desipramine (Norpramin) and titrating upward in 25-mg increments on successive dialysis days, after carefully monitoring for anticholinergic effects, orthostatic hypotension, or other side effects.
- When sleep disorder is prominent, doxepin (Sinequan)[268] and trazodone (Desyrel)[43,73,214] are appropriate choices.
- Some authors feel that nortriptyline is particularly useful because of its therapeutic window,[168] while others caution that drug plasma levels in the setting of renal failure are inaccurate.[183] (See discussion on Mrs. Freed.)
- Elderly patients and those with other medical problems should be treated with special caution.
- Fluoxetine (Prozac) and its active metabolite norfluoxetine are extensively hepatically metabolized, with renal excretion only a minor elimination route. One study[12] found no correlations between the degree of renal dysfunction and rate of elimination, volume of distribution, or protein binding. Plasma concentrations of fluoxetine and norfluoxetine were not significantly changed by hemodialysis.[12] Another study[24] found that daily administration of 20 mg fluoxetine for more than 2 months to renally impaired, depressed hemodialysis patients produced steady-state fluoxetine and norfluoxetine plasma concentrations comparable to those in depressed patients with normal renal function.
    - Remember, however, that fluoxetine is highly protein bound (94%) and can displace other highly bound drugs, such as digoxin or warfarin (Coumadin).[159] Fluoxetine may also induce elevated plasma levels of cyclosporine, beta-blockers, some anticonvulsants, several antiarrhythmics, and other psychotropics.[110,159]
- Although dosage adjustments are pharmacokinetically unnecessary in renal failure,[23] fluoxetine's long half-life and ESRD patients' vulnerability to side effects makes it advisable to start at doses even lower than two-thirds (e.g., 10 mg every other day).[268]
- Be especially cautious about electrolyte monitoring. The electrolyte imbalances of ESRD may predispose to seizures, which could potentiate lowering of the seizure threshold by bupropion (Wellbutrin)[259] and other antidepressants.[137] (The risk of seizures increased with bupropion when doses exceeded the recommended maximum of 450 mg/day.[259]) Information concerning the dialyzability of bupropion or its metabolites is limited. Dialysis has not been associated with a change in its blood levels, although bupropion and its metabolites are almost completely excreted through the kidney, so may accumulate in renally impaired patients.[180] Initial treatment should be at reduced doses, and patients should be closely monitored for toxic effects. It may be wisest to choose antidepressants other than bupropion for nephrology patients until there is more definitive experience.
- To date, there has been no specific clinical trial experience of paroxetine (Paxil) in depressed renal patients, although increased plasma concentrations of paroxetine occur in the setting of renal impairment (personal communication, SmithKline Beecham Pharmaceuticals, July 1994). Increasing mean plasma concentrations have been demonstrated with decreasing renal function, although half-life was only significantly prolonged in patients with severe renal impairment.[74] The manufacturer's recommended initial dose for patients with severe renal impairment is 10 mg once daily. Daily doses should not exceed 40 mg.
- The total clearance of venlafaxine (Effexor) and O-desmethylvenlafaxine is markedly decreased in renal disease; dosage adjustment is necessary for patients with creatinine clearance below 30 ml/minute.[274]
- The MAOIs have been described as useful in ESRD patients[168] but can potentiate the orthostatic hypotension that commonly occurs immediately after dialysis runs.
- Standard ECT can be used in nephrology patients.[268]

Benzodiazepines

With the exception of barbiturates, almost all psychotropic medications can be used in renal failure.[22] (See discussion on Mrs. Freed.) As mentioned, hypoalbuminemia causes an increased free fraction of parent drug with compensatory rapid inactivation of drug and active metabolites through glucuronidation. Thus, counterintuitively, there may be actually an *increase* in the clearance of some benzodiazepines, with *lowered* plasma levels of active drug and shortened half-life.

Lorazepam (Ativan) and oxazepam (Serax) are preferred in ESRD because they have inactive metabolites; their half-lives in ESRD show that they are not short acting.[29] In fact, their half-lives almost quadruple, exceeding that of clonazepam in medically healthy patients:[21]

	Half-life (hours)	
	Normal	ESRD
Lorazepam	9–16	32–70
Oxazepam	6–25	25–90
Clonazepam	5–30	Not known

Remember the rule of two-thirds when prescribing these agents. Neither lorazepam nor oxazepam is removed by dialysis.[21]

Other benzodiazepines with inactive metabolites include clonazepam (Klonopin) and temazepam (Restoril),[29] but changes in half-life during ESRD are not yet known. Keep in mind that dialysis patients were shown to have greater sensitivity to the sedative, memory, and psychomotor effects of alprazolam (Xanax), which does have active metabolites.[197,234–236] The following anxiolytics also have active metabolites, making them less desirable: diazepam (Valium), chlordiazepoxide (Librium), clorazepate (Tranxene), prazepam (Centrax), halazepam (Paxipam), and flurazepam (Dalmane).

Buspirone

Buspirone (BuSpar), like other psychotropics, is hepatically metabolized. It has several advantages as an anxiolytic: it is unassociated with sedation, the development of tolerance, dependency, or withdrawal symptoms. There is little information available about using buspirone in renal failure, nor are details of its protein-binding affinity fully known.[168] According to Bennett et al.,[21] it is not necessary to adjust the dose or interval of buspirone for changes of GFR.

Chloral Hydrate

Chloral hydrate, although not contraindicated, should be avoided once GFR drops below 50 ml/minute, as it may cause excessive sedation and/or encephalopathy in chronic hemodialysis patients.[21]

Barbiturates

Barbiturates, such as sodium amytal, secobarbital, and the like, should be avoided because of excessive sedation and because they may increase osteomalacia in patients with renal failure.[168]

⚜ KIDNEY TRANSPLANTATION

We will briefly review some of the highlights of the transplantation literature. Refer to the excellent collection of papers edited by Craven et al.,[51a,53] the recent review by Levy,[170] and the series on psychopharmacology by Trzepacz et al.[276–278]

Only successful kidney transplantation offers hope for a return to normal life.[167,222] Currently, more than 90% of kidney transplant recipients are alive at 1 year after transplantation.[267] Improved quality of life for successful transplant recipients has been amply demonstrated.[67,86,124,139a,187,203,228,305] Kidney transplantation also improves sexual functioning.[232,244] The majority of patients returned to pre-illness sexual functioning in one study.[232]

Candidates for Organ Transplantation

Soos[249] has commented,

> Although some patients may experience the decision to undergo evaluation for transplantation as an expected progression of their illness, this event may disrupt the psychological equilibrium of many others. *A physician's recommendation of a transplant is a potent validation of illness severity and may interfere with common defenses, such as minimization and denial.* The applicant may become acutely aware of previously unacknowledged fears concerning invalidism or death. Death anxiety may underlie worries about being found unsuitable for a transplant and be manifested clinically as performance anxiety during assessment procedures. (p. 90, italics added)

A patient's refusal of kidney transplantation is usually multifaceted, encompassing such factors as psychological reactions to dialysis, socioeconomic status, age, phase of life, educational level, and cognitive status.[36] Basch[18] has written,

> By the time the patient is ready for transplantation, he may be disheartened by the duration or repetitive nature of hemodialysis, by the restriction of physical activities, weakness, or by complications, such as peripheral neuropathy or renal osteodystrophy. He may have had to relocate his residence, change jobs, adjust to a lower income, and alter his basic routines, diet, and life habits. Malaise may arise from his general condition, uremia, the treatment and its complications, and psychological enervation. He has to adopt a new identity which includes his hemodialysis and transplant experiences and has to accept new dependencies on family, medical staff, and medical technology. (p. 120)

Social[174] and psychological factors influence the success of organ transplantation;[197a] patients must be able to tolerate close collaboration with the transplant team; comply with the medical regimen, follow-up appointments, and rehabilitation; and deal with changes in body image. Compliance is crucial;[98a,273a] for example, Rodriguez and colleagues[224] found that most of a small sample ($N = 12$) of noncompliant patients lost their transplanted kidneys, unlike their compliant counterparts. They suggested that *pre*transplant noncompliance be used as a marker to identify those patients at risk for posttransplant noncompliance. Supportive psychotherapy with behavior modification before surgery may improve postsurgical outcome. (Pike and Dimsdale[204] have recommended that neuropsychological functioning also be assessed, tailoring an approach that allows for the patient's possible cognitive deficits.)

The number of psychiatric exclusion criteria for transplantation has dwindled.[103] The greatest risk factors for late graft loss from psychological causes appear to be the following:[268]

◆ Age under 30 years
◆ History of substance abuse
◆ Untreated major depression

Although predicting long-term graft survival from psychosocial determinants cannot be done with accuracy,[268] Garcia et al.[114] have established the following list of psychological contraindications for transplantation:

◆ **Absolute contraindications:**
  • Inability to recognize the implications of the transplantation procedure
  • Dementia
  • Irreversible psychosis
  • Profound depression
◆ **Relative contraindications:**
  • Reversible psychopathological symptoms

The survival of personality disorder patients undergoing transplant surgery may be jeopardized by their behavioral problems, and such patients make significantly greater demands on staff time.[151] Patients with these risk factors, however, have been successfully transplanted.[253,267,269]

At present, any motivated patient who can medically tolerate kidney transplantation and has a reasonable chance of benefiting is a potential candidate.[268]

Finally, cultural and religious factors play an important role in the psychology of transplantation.[71] Fricchione[103] has written,

> From a cultural standpoint, the transplant team must pay particular attention to the mores and philosophies espoused by the racial and ethnic groups it is caring for in regard to removal and transplantation of bodily organs. A technically successful operation does not ensure a successful transplant in that the recipient may psychologically or spiritually "reject" the organ. This may ultimately result in physical rejection. Also, maladaptive behaviors may reflect cultural unrest in an individual who feels involved in something "unnatural." Specifically trained counselors from the same ethnic and cultural background might be helpful in enabling the patient to address some of these issues. (p. 415)

The role of the psychiatric consultant on the transplantation team has been detailed in several good reviews.[103,130,268,297]

Medical Risks of Transplantation

Unfortunately, Mr. Barry's fears about developing cancer are not unfounded. There is a higher incidence of certain types of tumors in this population, most notably non-Hodgkin's lymphoma, Kaposi's sarcoma, and various skin cancers.[131] Incidence ranges between 1% and 16%, with a 4% average.[201,256] The etiology may be related to disturbed immunoregulation and/or to a direct oncogenic effect on certain cells.[201] Immunosuppressant treatment must be discontinued and chemotherapy begun for this complication.

Organ Donation

For living kidney donors, serious postoperative complications are uncommon,[51] with mortality at less than 0.1% and life expectancy unaffected.[186,212,251] A 5- to 10-year follow-up study showed that the majority of donors expressed positive feelings about kidney donation, irrespective of the transplantation outcome, and kidney donation was shown to cause no long-term adverse psychological sequelae.[240,243] Psychological factors associated with living transplant donors (relatives, distant relatives, and nonrelatives) have been discussed in several papers and reviews.[18,90,95,103,131,191,244,266–268] At this writing, it is not standard practice to accept kidneys from living anonymous donors.[268] Brain death following catastrophic accidents is the usual source of anonymous cadaveric transplant kidneys.[39,175,265,302,303]

Refer to Appendix F for a brief explanation of living wills and durable power of attorney and a concise outline for assessing competency.

Psychotherapeutic Issues

Uncertainty haunts the transplantation candidate. Will he or she receive a kidney in time?[162] Will there be graft rejection? Discharge home may also be stressful, as the patient leaves the protected environment of the transplant team and "goes it alone." Not surprisingly, the emotional well-being of transplant recipients often runs in parallel to the success of allograft function. Most psychiatric disturbances posttransplantation are related to depressive states—especially, but not exclusively, in the context of organ rejection.[107] Morris and Jones[187] have written,

> While the general impression is that renal transplant recipients are much improved physically in the longer term, this neglects the high levels of physical and psychological stress that are endured by some patients for extended periods during episodes of acute and chronic rejection. (p. 431)

Psychiatric consultation is often requested to help patients cope with a failed transplanted kidney.[287]

Patients may theoretically return to work by 4–6 months, and should anticipate increasingly normal function and appearance by 1 year in the absence of major complications.[268] Be cautious, however, about predicting the success of vocational rehabilitation; while nearly 75% of the kidney transplant recipients in the National Kidney Dialysis Kidney Transplantation Study indicated that they were able to work, only 46% were actively working.[87] More recently, 55% of kidney transplant recipients were able to work 3 months after transplant, yet only 29% were actually in the labor force.[88] As previously mentioned, the catch-22 of disability insurance probably affects these statistics.

Psychodynamic Concerns

Most surgical patients must psychologically process the repair or removal of a diseased body part during the postoperative period.[41] The psychological task of the posttransplant patient is different; transplant surgery involves addition of a foreign body part, which must be intrapsychically integrated into a changed body image that incorporates the transplanted kidney as part of oneself.[17,18,41,42,158]

There may be an initial sense of euphoria, a feeling of being granted a chance for a new life.[131] This sense of well-being may be short lived, however, if complications or side effects occur.[130] Disillusionment with the actual emotional and physical burdens imposed by life after transplantation may result in increased feelings of vulnerability and despondency.[108,185] *Some patients feel "Frankenstein-like," and wonder how their personality will change with the addition of an organ from another person.*[131] For example, a male patient who received a liver from a woman expressed the fantasy that he was becoming "part woman."[79] A white man who had belonged to the Ku Klux Klan joined the National Association for the Advancement of Colored People upon learning that his kidney donor had been black.[1] Some patients must make peace with their cadaver donor's anonymity, which is fertile ground for many fantasies. Most people, however, adapt well when they learn demographic information about their organ donor.[131]

The return to health is stressful in ways that are often unanticipated by patient and family. Individuals who had been totally dependent for financial, emotional, or physical support may have difficulty making the transition toward health after successful transplantation. Ancient issues of identity and self-esteem may be rekindled as identity once again must shift, this time away from adaptive acceptance of patienthood and toward health and normalcy—with all its demands, rewards, and expectations. The specter of seeking and holding employment, with the loss of disability payments and coverage, complicates the vocational rehabilitation of many transplantation candidates. This concern secondarily influences many psychodynamic issues, such as feelings of passivity, self-perceptions of not being genuine, and fears of abandonment. As one patient put it, "Becoming healthy is disorienting. I should have known it; in life, there is no free lunch."

◆ An interesting case report described the development of polydipsia and extreme anxiety in an 18-year-old male after a successful kidney transplant.[281] A course of family psychotherapy was directed toward allowing the patient to become more independent; his polydipsia also disappeared. The author of the report concluded that patients and families need psychological assistance to face becoming healthy as well as becoming ill.

There are several papers in the psychoanalytic literature that explore the psychodynamic process of adapting to organ transplantation.[17,41,42,99] These papers provide helpful insights into psychically integrating a foreign organ and reidentifying with health. Several other papers discuss these issues further.[5,20]

Psychological Preparation for Surgery

Several early studies of general surgery patients demonstrated correlations between preoperative teaching and decreased postoperative requests for analgesics, shorter hospital stays,[82,83,136] and decreased postoperative delirium[156,157] and postoperative vomiting.[80] Preoperative preparation for cardiac surgery has been shown to facilitate recovery and reduce psychological distress.[10] Alberts and colleagues[4] extensively reviewed this literature and identified several methodological problems, such as lack of controls and inadequate sample size. They offered the following guidelines:[4]

1. The appropriate intervention should be selected based on the patient's own method of coping and his or her locus of control (internal versus external). Allowing patients to ask questions and to voice their fears with other patients can be reassuring.
2. Information-based interventions that lessen anticipatory fear are helpful, especially in the context of a supportive and trusting relationship between the patient and treatment team member.
3. Behaviorally oriented interventions should be tailored to the anxiety level and coping style of the pa-

tient. For example, highly anxious patients often benefit from relaxation techniques. Internally controlled patients do well when given knowledge that allows them to assume some control of their situation.
4. All patients should have a chance to discuss their feelings about the upcoming surgery with an empathic member of the treatment team. Since presurgical fear often centers on anticipation of anesthesia, the anesthesiologist's participation in such a discussion can be quite effective.

Fear or worry before a surgical procedure may actually *strengthen* the coping skills needed to deal with the surgical experience.[217] The right "dose" of anxiety may allow the patient to visualize the different outcomes of the surgery and postoperative course, with the goal of greater mastery and control of the potential outcome.

◆ Fifty patients about to undergo various surgical procedures were assessed to determine their preoperative fears.[229] The results showed that the possibility of having cancer was the predominant fear, that women expressed their fears more openly than did men, but that *none* had previously mentioned their fears to their surgeon or anesthesiologist *unless specifically asked*.

Preoperative anxiety is not a predictable entity, but depends on the patient's personality and coping style.[72] Patients often do not understand basic anatomy or physiology:

◆ For example, a fascinating study of 81 patients showed that 23% had only a vague understanding of basic anatomy, believing that the stomach and abdominal cavity were the same, and that the duodenum was the term for an ulcer and not part of the gastrointestinal tract.[200] Six percent confused rectum and anus with the vagina and uterus.

One way to explore patients' fantasies about their operations is to ask them to draw a picture of what they imagine the procedure involves.[217] This provides an opportunity to correct misinformation and to offer a clearer understanding of the proposed procedure. However, patients are not always able to incorporate what is being said to them preoperatively.

◆ For example, in a study of cardiac patients undergoing open-heart surgery, all the patients "forgot" significant portions of the preoperative discussion, which had been tape-recorded.[218] Four to 6 months later, some denied hearing certain details regarding the procedure or surgical risk. Such poor recall can be related to anxiety, fear, repression, denial, lack of attention, depression, or cognitive impairment.[131]

Self-administered anxiolytics are useful preoperatively[112] as well as postoperatively.[81] The classic book by Strain and Grossman[261] further discusses the psychology of the surgical patient. Blacher's[27] volume details the psychological experience of anesthesia, various types of surgeries, and brief psychotherapy with the surgical patient.

Cadaver Versus Family Organ Recipients

Pillay and colleagues[205] compared the psychological adjustment between cadaver and family organ recipients. They found few long-term, statistically significant differences postoperatively between the two groups of patients. Several items, however, were significantly related to post-transplant psychological adjustment *for both groups:*

◆ Feelings of inadequacy
◆ The renal graft seeming "alien"
◆ An inability to cope with the transplant
◆ Feeling the transplant to be an external imposition beyond personal control
◆ Accepting the transplant as a responsibility and a "gain"
◆ Feeling culpable for what had happened
◆ Being anxiously preoccupied with long-term prognosis and dependence on others

Basch[18] has speculated on the potential psychodynamic differences between cadaver and family organ recipients:

> The recipient of a family donated kidney enters the transplantation situation with the cumulative complexities of the preceding relationship. Since only consanguineous relatives are donors, elements of the family drama may be compounded by the new factors in the transplantation situation. The recipient of the cadaver kidney, on the other hand, has no previous relationship with the donor. The inert quality of the cadaver, however, *offers ample opportunity for the recipient to fantasize about the donor or to transfer preconceived attitudes and feelings onto the cadaver or its organ.* In addition, the recipient's associations to the life-

less state of the donor can affect his integration of the new organ . . . The cadaver donor is not present to serve as a reminder of dependency, indebtedness, or other conflicts, and the recipient does not have to contend with the donor's reaction to sacrificing his organ. The donor's being dead and unknown, therefore, paves the way for an intense elaboration of fantasies which, in turn, may be colored by the recipient's previous beliefs about death and dying. They [may be] imposed on the feeling of death attached to the organ the recipient now has within him. (p. 127, italics added)

Soos[249] points out that although the psychological benefits of donating a kidney to a family member far outweigh any negative psychosocial outcome, the symbolic implications of saving a family member by sacrificing one's own healthy organ has intrapsychic and interpersonal sequelae for both parties. What happens if a family member feels pressured to donate or refuses to donate?[29a] How is the dilemma of interpersonal closeness and distance negotiated if one feels dependent on the donor's kidney? Might the "gift of life" be used manipulatively by the donor to influence the recipient?

In families with more severe psychopathology, the implications for both the potential donor and the recipient are especially complex. For example, the donation of an organ from an overly controlling parent may further impair a child recipient's attempts at separation-individuation. Remarks made by a young woman during evaluation for a living-related kidney transplant from her mother illustrates this phenomenon. "I don't want my mother to have that control over me. It's like I'll owe her something for the rest of my life. It hurts me when she uses the kidney as leverage." Later in the same interview, the potential recipient voiced the reverse side of her conflicted and ambivalent relationship with her mother. "It feels like I would finally be really bonding with my mother. I can't get closer to her than by having part of her in me" (pp. 92–93).[249]

Family and individual therapy might be necessary to examine such conflicts, and to help each family member communicate his or her respective feelings.[126a]

Suicide

The risk of suicide is higher in transplant patients than in the general population;[119,291] suicide accounts for 15% of deaths among kidney transplant patients.[291] Suicidal behavior is not always direct, but can take the form of noncompliance with the medical regimen. *Noncompliance is most often a reflection of a psychiatric problem, such as depression, anxiety, or a memory disturbance.*[98a,119] Some of the more serious side effects of the immunosuppressant medications, such as cataracts, muscle wasting, impotence, and steroid-induced body image changes, may exacerbate noncompliance and morbidity.[131]

Psychotherapy

The enhanced mobility and freedom from the encumbrance of dialysis may make the transplant recipient more available—at least logistically—for psychotherapy. We were most impressed by the overview of psychotherapy and counseling with transplant patients written by Soos.[249] The specific therapy most commonly used for the psychological complications of dialysis and transplantation is individual psychotherapy, with or without the use of psychotropic medications. Hypnotherapy may be useful for reducing anxiety and developing psychotherapeutic rapport,[268] especially for pain management and for those patients who want to enhance self-care.[270] Being able to visualize him- or herself healthy, enjoying a long-sought-after goal, may help buoy the patient during periods of extended waiting and a difficult postoperative course.[249] Group therapy also has an established place in the psychosocial treatment of transplant patients.[32,249] Behavioral therapy of sexual dysfunction may be indicated.[91]

For the reader interested in additional details on the psychotherapeutic issues arising in working with medical patients, several good papers exist.[3,101,143,149,219–221,239,255,260,261,283,284,301]

Neuropsychiatric Complications

Mental status disorders occur in about 25% of patients postoperatively.[100,293] These include drug-induced neurotoxicity, infection, electrolyte abnormalities, hypertensive encephalopathy, cerebrovascular events, rejection encephalopathy, and central nervous system (CNS) tumors.[61] Note that the immunosuppressant drugs may cause *tremor* that can be easily mistaken for the extrapyramidal side effects of neuroleptics or selective serotonin reuptake inhibitors (SSRIs).

We found that the best recent review of the psychopharmacological issues in organ transplantation was by Trzepacz et al.[276,277] Also consult the volume on drug interactions by Ciraulo et al.[48a] A few highlights follow.

Infection

Immunosuppression predisposes to infection, which has a high rate of morbidity and mortality in this group. Meningitis, brain abscess, septic emboli, hemorrhage, fever, and encephalitis are high in the differential diagnosis of altered mental status.[278] Tip-offs as to the medical etiology of mental status changes include cognitive impairments and, for depressive states, the absence of feelings of worthlessness, hopelessness, or suicidal ideation that are the hallmark of endogenous depression. *Cryptococcus neoformans*, *Listeria monocytogenes*, and *Aspergillus fumigatus* account for more than 80% of the CNS infections in transplantation recipients.[50] Other common systemic infections include *Cytomegalovirus*, *Herpesvirus*, *Candida*, *Staphylococcus*, and *Pneumocystis carinii*.[152] Secondary depressive states have been associated with the *Herpes* group viruses.[268]

Antiinfectious agents also cause neuropsychiatric complications. A brief list follows:

- **Acyclovir (Zovirax) (antiviral):** tremor, confusion, lethargy, major depression with psychotic features, seizures, agitation, confusion, abnormal EEG[11,116,155]
- **DHPG (dihydroxy-prooxymethyl guanine; Ganciclovir) (antiviral):** headache, confusion, seizures, hallucinations[58,75,93,155,272]
- **Alpha interferon** (used in liver transplantation patients with recurrent hepatitis): less than 20% of patients experience dose-related irritability, depression, anxiety, and delirium[179,215,216,225]
- **Ciprofloxacin:** restlessness, dizziness, tremor, headache, insomnia, hallucinations, delirium[7,46,48,233]
- **Cephalosporins:** disorientation, restlessness, anxiety, hallucinations[118,247,286]
- **Sulfonamide antibiotics:** depression, ataxia, occasional visual and auditory hallucinations[247]
- **Penicillins:** hallucinations, seizures[118,247]
- **Gentamicin, ketoconazole, erythromycin:** delirium[34,96,280]
- **Amphotericin B (antifungal):** restlessness, confusion, delirium[121,230,296]
- **Metronidazole (antifungal):** depression, hallucinations, agitation[78,115,288]

Neurological Complications

Other neuropsychiatric complications of renal transplantation include brain tumors of the lymphoproliferative type, central pontine myelinolysis (a progressive brain stem demyelinating illness leading to quadriparesis), and progressive multifocal leukencephalopathy (characterized by behavioral, intellectual, speech, and motor changes).[257]

Corticosteroids

Corticosteroids are used in transplantation for immunosuppression. Some centers treat graft rejection by administering a "prednisone recycle" consisting of high-dose corticosteroids with a rapid taper—that is, starting with prednisone 200 mg/day orally and decreasing the dose by 20 mg/day until the daily dose reaches 20 mg.[277] The occurrence of mood disorders in patients treated with corticosteroids is well documented, especially in the setting of certain illnesses.

♦ The initial response may be a sense of well-being or improved appetite.

♦ Only about 6% of all patients develop corticosteroid-induced mental disturbances,[144] whereas altered mood states occur in approximately 15% of transplant recipients.[268]

♦ The full-blown syndrome of steroid-induced psychosis, which presents characteristically as an affective psychosis with mixed manic and depressive features, is relatively *infrequent* in this population,[268] and may be treated with low doses of haloperidol.[268]

♦ Volatility of mood, restlessness, and irritability occur more often than psychosis.

Cushingoid symptoms may develop, consisting of weakness, centripetal obesity, acniform lesions, and other stigmata. Prednisone undermines established diabetic control, causing progression of diabetic morbidity.[268]

Chapter 5 contains a detailed discussion of the neuropsychiatric effects of steroids.

Cyclosporine

Cyclosporine greatly enhances successful organ transplantation, allowing for rapid reductions in prednisone and thus in steroid-linked morbidity. It is a lipophilic cyclic polypeptide derived from the fungus *Tolypocladium inflatum Goma*.[172] Cyclosporine acts as an immunosuppressant mainly by inhibiting the production of interleukin-2 by T-helper cells.[140] Unfortunately, it is nephrotoxic, hepatotoxic, and neurotoxic,[267] at times inducing seizures, tremor, and encephalopathy.[60,208] It may produce mental status changes, such as disruptions in sleep, agitation, anxiety, confusion, disorientation, and psychosis.[59,294] Psychosis may remit with dosage reduction or the addition of haloperidol.[268] Hypomagnesemia may also result,[139] causing secondary anxiety states and cognitive difficulties.[135] Unfortunately, body-image disturbances, secondary to gingival hyperplasia and hirsutism, as well as lymphoproliferative disease, are well documented.[172] Keep in

mind that antidepressants may potentiate the lowered seizure threshold of patients also receiving cyclosporine or the monoclonal antibody OKT3.[131] In addition, cyclosporine increases lithium resorption by the proximal tubule, so that serum lithium levels may increase.[285]

FK506

FK506, a macrolide produced by *Streptomyces tsukubaensis*, is a novel immunosuppressant currently used after organ transplantation to diminish host rejection. It appears to have a better toxicity and side-effect profile compared with cyclosporine.[147,188,271,282]

The most common neuropsychiatric side effects are headache, anxiety, tremor, restlessness, insomnia, and paresthesias.[111,252] Patients report vivid dreams and nightmares.[277] Delirium may be a complication, especially in patients whose plasma levels exceed 3 ng/ml.[69] Fortunately, neurological side effects occurred in only 5.4% of a series of 290 consecutive transplantation recipients.[84] Two recipients had paranoid psychosis, 6 showed signs of akinetic mutism and/or expressive dysphasia, 4 had seizures, and 4 were encephalopathic.

A secondary anxiety disorder, accompanied by akathisia, was recently described in a 39-year-old man who was started on this agent;[25] however, the coadministration of haloperidol may have been the real culprit. Symptoms remitted with low-dose beta-blocker therapy. (FK506-induced tremor has been empirically observed to also respond to clonidine [Catapres].[277]) The precise interactions with psychotropics are unknown.[277] As with the other immunosuppressants, enhanced susceptibility to infection predisposes these patients to delirium.

OKT3

OKT3 is a monoclonal antibody used as an immunosuppressant and to treat organ rejection. Its major side effects are tremor, dyspnea, fever, chills, aseptic meningitis, hemodynamic instability, pulmonary edema, seizures, sepsis, and delirium.[44,49,85,177]

Azathioprine

Azathioprine (Imuran) is not as frequently used for immunosuppression as is cyclosporine or prednisone. There are no particular neuropsychiatric side effects, but the medication could indirectly increase the risk for developing delirium by predisposing to infection.[277]

Cimetidine

Cimetidine (Tagamet) is often used in conjunction with corticosteroid therapy. It can also cause mental status changes, as well as decreasing oxidative metabolism in the liver, leading to increased serum levels of certain drugs.[273]

Psychopharmacology

Principles of pharmacological intervention in transplant patients are similar to those in patients undergoing dialysis.

Neuroleptics

As usual, haloperidol (Haldol) is the neuroleptic of choice.[276] It has essentially no respiratory, cardiac, hepatic, renal, or bone marrow side effects. *Note that neuroleptic-induced tremor or akathisia can be mistaken for agitation or immunosuppressant-induced tremor.*[276] Benztropine (Cogentin) may be given for other extrapyramidal side effects.[276]

Anxiolytics

Adjustment disorders with anxiety are the most common anxiety disorder in posttransplant patients, with an estimated incidence of 2%–14%,[100,275,279] and only a 1% incidence of generalized anxiety disorder.[100] Benzodiazepines present no special problems for kidney transplant patients other than the usual considerations regarding respiratory depression, cognitive dysfunction, and sedation.[276] As always, the short- to intermediate-acting benzodiazepines (e.g., lorazepam, oxazepam) allow for closer titration and ease of administration. Alprazolam (Xanax) is an extremely effective anxiolytic,[197,234–236] but its potentially serious withdrawal side effects[163,199,290] cause lorazepam (Ativan) to be preferred over it in the medical setting.

Buspirone (BuSpar) has not yet been well studied in transplant candidates.

Antidepressants

There is little literature on using antidepressants in transplant patients. Clinical wisdom, however, dictates starting with lower doses and following serum levels whenever possible.[276] Although they are metabolized hepatically, TCAs have metabolites that are excreted renally and can accumulate in renal insufficiency.[173] Surman[268] reports that doxepin (Sinequan) is well tolerated in this population, especially when pain and insomnia predominate. Trazodone (Desyrel) is an alternative if there are problems with urinary retention or other anticholinergic side effects.[268] For patients experiencing depression and lethargy in the absence of prominent sleep impairment, desipramine (Norpramin) is recommended, starting at 25 mg and increasing by 25-mg increments.[268]

There is scant literature on use of the newer agents, such as fluoxetine (Prozac), bupropion (Wellbutrin), sertraline (Zoloft), and paroxetine (Paxil), in transplant patients. Certainly, the akathisia sometimes associated with fluoxetine and other SSRIs could be mistaken for restlessness or could be interpreted as a side effect of immunosuppression or delirium.[276] Moreover, fluoxetine may induce elevated levels of several medications, including cyclosporine.[276] Although we could locate no studies specifically on sertraline in these patients, Trzepacz et al.[276] report that they have successfully used it in several transplant recipients. They also report favorable but limited clinical experience with bupropion in liver and heart transplant patients;[276] we could find nothing specifically on bupropion in kidney transplantation.

A recent case report of two patients with ESRD revealed successful, safe treatment with the psychostimulant methylphenidate (Ritalin).[258] Although specific studies are lacking, Trzepacz and colleagues[276] report no contraindications to using psychostimulants in kidney transplant recipients.

There is consensus that because transplant patients often have an unpredictable clinical course, MAOIs should be avoided in case of emergency surgery, sedation, pain control, and pressor support.[276]

Electroconvulsive therapy. ECT has been successfully administered to transplant recipients.[131] There is little information about its use in advanced organ failure, but the risk posed by anesthesia is likely to be similar to that associated with minor surgical procedures.[278]

Lithium

The use of lithium in kidney transplantation is somewhat controversial. Some feel that lithium should be avoided because of the possibility of damaging the new kidney, and advocate using carbamazepine (Tegretol)[103] or clonazepam (Klonopin)[9] as a substitute. On the other hand, Trzepacz et al.[276] report that low-dose lithium can be used in the stable renal transplantation setting provided that blood levels are frequently monitored (i.e., three times/week). However, since the immediate posttransplant course is often marked by renal function instability and acute tubular necrosis requiring temporary dialysis, electrolyte imbalance and fluid shifts may complicate lithium management. During acute manic episodes in the perioperative period, neuroleptics are usually preferable to lithium.[278] A long lag time is required to achieve effective drug levels in patients with *changing* renal function;[8] calculating lithium dosages for patients with poor renal function using creatinine clearance and a pharmacokinetic model works only for patients with *stable* renal function. The most specific guidelines for lithium dosing in renal transplant patients were found in Koecheler et al.:[148]

◆ Consanguineous allograft recipients can be expected to show *near-normal* renal functioning *within hours* after surgery, requiring increased doses for renally excreted drugs (compared with their prior state of chronic renal failure).[148] Koecheler et al.[148] recommend that lithium be prospectively increased to 900–1,200 mg/day (doses for normal renal function) by the first transplant day in anticipation of the return of normal renal function. Blood levels and further dosage adjustments should be made at least every month.

◆ Cadaver allograft recipients vary widely in the length of time required before their renal function stabilizes after surgery.[148] Postoperative acute tubular necrosis is common, and often requires 1–2 weeks of dialysis treatments. Serum lithium must be frequently checked in order to maintain adequate levels. Koecheler et al.[148] recommend initiating therapy at 300–600 mg after dialysis (i.e., at doses used in renal failure) and measuring lithium concentrations three times per week, combined with patient assessment. They suggest that as renal function returns, a daily or twice-daily 300-mg dosage will maintain therapeutic levels and compensate for improving lithium clearance. Once creatinine clearance stabilizes, a final assessment of maintenance therapy can be made, depending on the final level of renal function.

◆ Transplant patients with changing renal function require close observation for signs of toxicity as well as frequent measuring of serum lithium concentrations.

The following drug interactions with lithium are of particular relevance:

◆ Cyclosporine may increase reabsorption in the proximal tubules,[285] thereby predisposing to lithium toxicity. Impaired fractional excretion of lithium has been reported to be a sensitive marker of cyclosporine toxicity.[285]

◆ Both lithium and cyclosporine (as well as other immunosuppressants) can cause tremors; teasing apart etiologies may be difficult.

◆ Methylprednisolone can decrease the fractional tubular reabsorption of lithium in rats.[133]

The clinical significance of lithium's immune-stimulant properties for transplant recipients is unclear.[35]

SUMMARY

1. End-stage renal failure is a disease of deprivation that affects every life domain—body image, sexuality, life expectancy, family, work, and finances. Psychosocial factors have an unequivocal impact on dietary and fluid compliance, and therefore affect morbidity. The quality of life in end-stage renal disease (ESRD) depends on many variables, such as treatment time requirements, uremic symptoms, intercurrent nonrenal illnesses, fatigue, and difficulties with daily activities. Increased psychosocial well-being correlates with the occurrence of fewer negative life events, richer social networks, involvement in paid employment, and higher annual family income.

2. Hemodialysis and continuous abdominal peritoneal dialysis (CAPD) are time consuming and cumbersome. Quality-of-life comparisons between the two treatments have varied, with some studies showing advantages of CAPD over hemodialysis and others showing no difference in psychosocial outcomes. Methodological problems have confounded quality-of-life studies; ESRD patients are never randomized to receive a particular form of intervention, and treatment-assignment bias is well known. On the other hand, quality of life after successful renal transplantation is unequivocally better than that with all other treatments.

3. Depression is fairly common in ESRD, and may secondarily affect mortality. In addition, accompanying medical conditions such as anemia, electrolyte disturbances, or underlying systemic disease (e.g., systemic lupus erythematosus [SLE]) may mimic depressive states or cause secondary mood disorders. Medications, such as antihypertensives and steroids, also induce depressive side effects. Patients' perception of illness predicts the occurrence of depression better than does the objective illness severity. The psychiatrist may be asked to assist patients in making decisions about medical management, dialysis, transplantation, or treatment termination. Assumptions that "most" dialysis patients "want to commit suicide" can lead to therapeutic nihilism and are not borne out by the statistical facts. Some patients may be seeking reassurance and support, or may be suffering from a treatable psychiatric illness such as psychosis, an anxiety disorder, or major depression.

4. Several factors make ESRD patients particularly challenging to work with—for example, the effects

of uremia and electrolyte imbalance on energy, mental alertness, and the ability to concentrate and remember. The complex, time-consuming regimens required of dialysis patients are probably unparalleled by other chronic illnesses. Consultation-liaison psychiatrists are often asked to intervene when noncompliance has medical consequences. The Health Belief Model predicts that compliance is the result of the interactions among five variables: 1) perceived susceptibility to negative health consequences caused by poor adherence, 2) perceived seriousness of these consequences, 3) perceived costs versus benefits of performing the prescribed adherence behavior, 4) degree of difficulty in incorporating the adherence behavior into the person's lifestyle, and 5) degree of concern about the disease state itself and its consequences.

5. The tricyclic antidepressants (TCAs) have been widely used to medicate depression in renal failure. From the strictly pharmacological point of view, the half-lives of most antidepressants do not change in ESRD, but the rule of two-thirds cautions about the heightened sensitivity of these patients to side effects. The monoamine oxidase inhibitors (MAOIs) have been useful in patients with renal failure but can potentiate the orthostatic hypotension that commonly accompanies dialysis runs. Electroconvulsive therapy (ECT) can be safely used in this population as one would in standard psychiatric care.

6. Among the selective serotonin reuptake inhibitors (SSRIs), fluoxetine (Prozac) has been most widely studied. It is highly protein bound and can displace other highly bound drugs such as digoxin, warfarin, cyclosporine, beta-blockers, some anticonvulsants, several antiarrhythmics, and other psychotropics.

7. With the exception of barbiturates, almost all psychotropic medications can be used in renal failure, including the benzodiazepines. In fact, there may actually be *increased* clearance of some benzodiazepines, with *lowered* plasma levels of active drug and shortened half-life. Lorazepam (Ativan) and oxazepam (Serax) are preferred in ESRD because they have inactive metabolites, even though ESRD causes their half-lives to almost quadruple, exceeding that of clonazepam in medically healthy patients. Remember the *rule of two-thirds* when prescribing them. Neither lorazepam nor oxazepam is removed by dialysis. Other benzodiazepines with inactive metabolites include clonazepam (Klonopin) and temazepam (Restoril), but changes in half-life during ESRD have not yet been defined for these agents.

The following anxiolytics have active metabolites, making them less desirable: alprazolam (Xanax), diazepam (Valium), chlordiazepoxide (Librium), clorazepate (Tranxene), prazepam (Centrax), halazepam (Paxipam), and flurazepam (Dalmane).

8. Buspirone (BuSpar), like other psychotropics, is hepatically metabolized. It has several advantages as an anxiolytic: it is unassociated with sedation, the development of tolerance, dependency, or withdrawal symptoms. There is little information about using buspirone in renal failure, however, nor are details of its protein-binding affinity fully known.

9. Only successful transplantation offers hope to return to normal functioning, although the psychodynamics of integrating a foreign body part and becoming "well" again are complicated. Social and psychological factors influence the success of organ transplantation: patients must be able to tolerate close collaboration with the transplant team; comply with the medical regimen, follow-up appointments, and rehabilitation; and deal with changes in body image. Age under 30 years, a history of substance abuse, and untreated major depression may pose the greatest risk factors for late graft loss from psychological factors, although predicting long-term graft survival from psychosocial determinants cannot be done with accuracy. Note that the number of psychiatric exclusion criteria for transplantation has dwindled, and patients with these risk factors have been successfully transplanted.

10. The risk of suicide is higher in transplant patients than in the general population; suicide accounts for 15% of deaths among kidney transplant patients. Suicidal behavior is not always direct, but can take the form of noncompliance. Noncompliance most often reflects a psychiatric problem, such as depression, anxiety, or a cognitive disturbance.

11. Delirious disorders occur in about 25% of transplant patients postoperatively. Causes include drug-induced neurotoxicity, infection, electrolyte abnormalities, hypertensive encephalopathy, cerebrovascular events, rejection encephalopathy, and central nervous system tumors.

12. Principles of pharmacological intervention in transplant patients are similar to those for dialysis patients. Haloperidol (Haldol) is the neuroleptic of choice, with essentially no respiratory, cardiac, hepatic, renal, or bone marrow side effects. Note that neuroleptic-induced akathisia can be mistaken for agitation or immunosuppressant-induced tremor. Benzodiazepines or beta-blockers may be adminis-

tered safely. Benztropine (Cogentin) may be given for other extrapyramidal side effects.

13. Benzodiazepines present no special problems for kidney recipients other than the usual considerations regarding respiratory depression, cognitive dysfunction, and sedation. As always, the short- to intermediate-acting benzodiazepines (e.g., lorazepam, oxazepam) allow for closer titration and ease of administration. Buspirone (BuSpar) has not yet been well studied in organ recipients.

14. There is little literature on using antidepressants in transplant patients; however, clinical wisdom dictates starting with lower doses and following serum levels whenever possible. Although they are metabolized hepatically, TCAs have metabolites that are excreted renally and can accumulate in renal insufficiency. The akathisia sometimes associated with fluoxetine and other SSRIs can be mistaken for restlessness or interpreted as a side effect of immunosuppressant therapy. Moreover, fluoxetine may induce elevated levels of hepatically metabolized medications, including cyclosporine. There is consensus that MAOIs should be avoided because transplant patients may unpredictably require emergency surgery, sedation, pain control, and pressor support. ECT has been safely and successfully administered to transplant recipients.

15. The use of lithium in kidney transplant patients is somewhat controversial. Some feel that lithium should be avoided because of the possibility of damaging the new kidney, and advocate using carbamazepine or clonazepam as a substitute. On the other hand, others report that low-dose lithium can be used in the stable renal transplantation setting provided that blood levels are frequently monitored (i.e., three times/week). However, since the immediate posttransplant course is often marked by renal function instability and acute tubular necrosis requiring temporary dialysis, electrolyte imbalance and fluid shifts may complicate lithium management. During acute manic episodes in the perioperative period, neuroleptics are usually preferable to lithium. A long lag time is needed to achieve effective drug levels in patients with changing renal function; calculating lithium dosages for patients with poor renal function using creatinine clearance and a pharmacokinetic model works only when renal function is stable. Note that cyclosporine may increase reabsorption in the proximal tubules, predisposing to lithium toxicity. Both lithium and cyclosporine can cause tremors, so that teasing apart etiologies may be difficult.

REFERENCES

1. Abram H: Renal transplantation, in Massachusetts General Hospital Handbook of General Hospital Psychiatry. Edited by Hackett T, Cassem N. St. Louis, MO, CV Mosby, 1978, pp 365–379
2. Abram H, Moore G, Westervelt FJ: Suicidal behavior in chronic dialysis patients. Am J Psychiatry 127:1199–1204, 1971
3. Adler G: Special problems for the therapist. Int J Psychiatry Med 14:91–98, 1984
4. Alberts M, Lyons J, Moretti R, et al: Psychological interventions in the presurgical period. Int J Psychiatry Med 19:91–106, 1989
5. Allender J, Shisslak C, Kasniak A, et al: Stages of psychological adjustment associated with heart transplantation. Heart Transplantation 2:228–231, 1983
6. Alleyne S, Dillard P, McGregor C, et al: Sexual function and mental distress status of patients with end-stage renal disease on hemodialysis. Transplant Proc 21:3895–3898, 1989
7. Alters J, Gasco J, de Antonio J, et al: Ciprofloxacin and delirium. Ann Intern Med 110:170–171, 1989
8. Amdisen A: Lithium, in Applied Pharmacokinetics. Edited by Evans W, Schentag J, Jusko W. San Francisco, CA, Applied Therapeutics, 1980, pp 586–617
9. Amiel M, Bryan S, Herjanic M: Clonazepam in the treatment of bipolar disorder in patients with non-lithium-induced renal insufficiency (letter). J Clin Psychiatry 48:424, 1987
10. Anderson E: Preoperative preparation for cardiac surgery facilitates recovery, reduces psychological distress, and reduces the incidence of acute postoperative hypertension. J Consult Clin Psychol 55:513–520, 1987
11. Ardent H: Adverse reactions to acyclovir: topical, oral, and intravenous. J Am Acad Dermatol 18:188–190, 1988
12. Aronoff G, Bergstrom R, Pottratz S, et al: Fluoxetine kinetics and protein binding in normal and impaired renal function. Clin Pharmacol Ther 36:138–144, 1984
13. Aronow D: Severity-of-illness measurement: applications in quality assurance and utilization review. Medical Care Review 45:339–366, 1988
14. Baile W: Rational suicide or depression: a new dilemma for the C-L psychiatrist. Psycho-Oncology 2:67–68, 1993
15. Baldree K, Murphy S, Powers M: Stress identification and coping patterns in patients on hemodialysis. Nurs Res 31:107–112, 1981
16. Barrett B, Vavasour H, Major A, et al: Clinical and psychological correlates of somatic symptoms in patients on dialysis. Nephron 55:10–15, 1990
17. Basch S: The intrapsychic integration of a new organ: a clinical study of kidney transplantation. Psychoanal Q 42:364–384, 1973
18. Basch S: Psychological adaptation to renal disease and transplantation, in Psychological Experience of Surgery. Edited by Blacher R. New York, Wiley, 1987, pp 116–129

18a. Beck A: Depression Inventory. Philadelphia, PA, Philadelphia Center for Cognitive Therapy, 1978

19. Becker M, Maiman L: Sociobehavioral determinants of compliance with health and medical care recommendations. Med Care 13:10–24, 1975

20. Beidel D: Psychological factors in organ transplantation. Clin Psychol Rev 7:677–694, 1987

21. Bennett W, Aronoff G, Golper T, et al: Drug Prescribing in Renal Failure: Dosing Guidelines for Adults, 3rd Edition. Philadelphia, PA, American College of Physicians, 1994

22. Bennett W, Muther R, Parker R, et al: Drug therapy in renal failure: dosing guidelines for adults. Ann Intern Med 93:286–325, 1980

23. Bergstrom R, Beasley C, Levy N, et al: Fluoxetine pharmacokinetics after daily doses of 20-mg fluoxetine in patients with severely impaired renal function. Pharm Res 8 (10 suppl):S294, 1991

24. Bergstrom R, Beasley C, Levy N, et al: The effect of renal and hepatic disease on the pharmacokinetics, renal tolerance, and risk-benefit profile of fluoxetine. Int Clin Psychopharmacol 8:261–266, 1993

25. Bernstein L, Daviss S: Organic anxiety disorder with symptoms of akathisia in a patient treated with the immunosuppressant FK506. Gen Hosp Psychiatry 14:210–211, 1992

26. Binik Y, Devins G, Barre P, et al: Live and learn: patient education delays the need to initiate renal replacement therapy in end-stage renal disease. J Nerv Ment Dis 181:371–376, 1993

27. Blacher R: General surgery and anesthesia: the emotional experience, in Psychological Experience of Surgery. Edited by Blacher R. New York, Wiley, 1987, pp 1–25

27a. Block S, Billings J: Patient requests for euthanasia and assisted suicide in terminal illness: the role of the psychiatrist. Psychosomatics 36:445–457, 1995

28. Booth-Kewley S, Friedman H: Psychological predictors of heart disease: a quantitative review. Psychol Bull 101:343–362, 1987

29. Brater D: Drug Use in Renal Disease. Sydney, Australia, Aidis Health Science Press, 1985

29a. Bratton L, Griffin L: A kidney donor's dilemma: the sibling who can donate—but doesn't. Soc Work Health Care 20:75–96, 1994

30. Brown J, Henteleff P, Barakat S, et al: Is it normal for terminally ill patients to desire death. Am J Psychiatry 143:208–211, 1986

31. Brynger H, Brunner F, Chantler C, et al: Combined report on regular dialysis and transplantation in Europe, X: 1979. Proceedings of the European Dialysis and Transplant Association 17:2–86, 1980

32. Buchanan D: Group therapy for kidney transplant patients. Int J Psychiatry Med 6:523–531, 1975

33. Burton H, Kline S, Lindsay R, et al: The relationship of depression to survival in chronic renal failure. Psychosom Med 48:261–269, 1986

34. Byrd G: Acute organic brain syndrome associated with gentamicin therapy. JAMA 238:53–54, 1977

35. Calabrese J, Gulledge A, Hahn K, et al: Autoimmune thyroiditis in manic-depressive patients treated with lithium. Am J Psychiatry 142:1318–1321, 1985

36. Callender C, Jennings P, Bayton J, et al: Psychologic factors related to dialysis in kidney transplant decisions. Transplant Proc 21:1976–1978, 1989

37. Campbell A: Strategies for improving dialysis decision making. Perit Dial Int 11:173–178, 1991

38. Campese V, Liu C: Sexual dysfunction in uremia, in Psychological and Physiological Aspects of Chronic Renal Failure (Contributions in Nephrology series, Vol 77). Edited by D'Amico G, Colasanti G. Basel, Karger, 1990, pp 1–14

39. Caplan A: Ethical and policy issues in the procurement of cadaver organs for transplantation. N Engl J Med 311:981–983, 1985

40. Carney R, Wetzel R, Hagberg J, et al: The relationship between depression and aerobic capacity in hemodialysis patients. Psychosom Med 48:143–147, 1986

41. Castelnuovo-Tedesco P: Organ transplant, body image, psychosis. Psychoanal Q 42:349–363, 1973

42. Castelnuovo-Tedesco P: Ego vicissitudes in response to replacement or loss of body parts. Psychoanal Q 47:381–397, 1978

43. Catanese B, Dionisio A, Barillari G, et al: A comparative study of trazodone serum concentrations in patients with normal or impaired renal function. Boll Chim Farm 117:424–427, 1978

44. Chan G, Weinstein S, Wright C, et al: Encephalopathy associated with OKT3 administration: possible interactions with indomethacin. Transplantation 52:148–150, 1991

45. Charmet G: Sexual function in dialysis patients: psychological aspects, in Psychological and Physiological Aspects of Chronic Renal Failure (Contributions in Nephrology series, Vol 77). Edited by D'Amico G, Colasanti G. Basel, Karger, 1990, pp 15–23

45a. Chochinov H, Wilson K, Enns M, et al: Desire for death in the terminally ill. Am J Psychiatry 152:1185–1191, 1995

46. Christ W, Lehnert T, Ulbrich B: Specific toxicologic aspects of quinolones. Reviews of Infectious Diseases 10 (suppl):S141–S146, 1988

47. Christensen A, Smith T, Turner C, et al: Family support, physical impairment, and adherence in hemodialysis: an investigation of main and buffering effects. J Behav Med 15:313–325, 1992

48. Ciprofloxacin. Med Lett Drugs Ther 30:11–13, 1988

48a. Ciraulo D, Shader R, Greenblatt D, et al. (eds): Drug Interactions in Psychiatry, 2nd Edition. Baltimore, MD, Williams & Wilkins, 1995

49. Coleman A, Norman D: OKT3 encephalopathy. Ann Neurol 28:837–838, 1990

50. Conti D, Rubin R: Infection of the central nervous system in organ transplant recipients. Neurol Clin 6:241–260, 1988

51. Cosimi A: The donor and donor nephrectomy, in Renal Transplantation—Principles and Practice. Edited by Morris PP. New York, Grune & Stratton, 1979, pp 69–87

51a. Craven J, Farrow S: Surviving Transplantation: A Personal Guide for Organ Transplant Patients, Their Families, Friends and Caregivers. Toronto, Canada, University of Toronto, 1993

52. Craven J, Littlefield C, Rodin G, et al: The Endstage Renal Disease Severity Index (ESRD-SI). Psychol Med 21:237–243, 1991

53. Craven J, Rodin G (eds): Psychiatric Aspects of Organ Transplantation. Oxford, UK, Oxford University Press, 1992

54. Craven J, Rodin G, Johnson L, et al: The diagnosis of major depression in renal dialysis patients. Psychosom Med 49:482–492, 1987

55. Cummings K, Becker M, Kirscht J, et al: Intervention strategies to improve compliance with medical regimens by ambulatory hemodialysis patients. J Behav Med 4:111–127, 1981

56. Danis J, Garrett J, Harris R, et al: Stability of choices about life-sustaining treatments. Ann Intern Med 120:567–573, 1994

57. Davis B, Krug D, Dean R: MMPI differences for renal, psychiatric, and general medical patients. J Clin Psychol 46:178–184, 1990

58. Davis C, Springmeyer S, Gmerek B: Central nervous system side effects of ganciclovir. N Engl J Med 322:933–934, 1990

59. de Groen P, Aksamit A, Rakela J, et al: Central nervous system toxicity after liver transplantation. N Engl J Med 317:861–866, 1987

60. de Groen P, Aksarit A, Rakela J, et al: Cyclosporine-associated central nervous system toxicity (letter). N Engl J Med 318:789, 1988

61. de Groen P, Craven J: Organic brain syndromes in transplant patients, in Psychiatric Aspects of Organ Transplantation. Edited by Craven J, Rodin G. Oxford, UK, Oxford University Press, 1992, pp 67–88

62. DeNour A: Some notes on the psychological significance of urination. J Nerv Ment Dis 148:615–623, 1969

63. Devins G: Illness intrusiveness and the psychosocial impact of end-stage renal disease. Loss, Grief and Care 5:83–102, 1991

64. Devins G, Binik Y, Hutchinson T, et al: The emotional impact of end-stage renal disease. Int J Psychiatry Med 13:327–343, 1983

65. Devins G, Edworthy S, Paul L, et al: Restless sleep, illness intrusiveness, and depressive symptoms in three chronic illness conditions: rheumatoid arthritis, end-stage renal disease, and multiple sclerosis. J Psychosom Res 37:163–170, 1993

66. Devins G, Edworthy S, Seland T, et al: Differences in illness intrusiveness across rheumatoid arthritis, end-stage renal disease, and multiple sclerosis. J Nerv Ment Dis 181:377–381, 1993

67. Devins G, Mandin H, Hons R, et al: Illness intrusiveness and quality of life in end-stage renal disease: comparison and stability across treatment modalities. Health Psychol 9:117–142, 1990

68. Devins G, Mann J, Mandin H, et al: Psychosocial predictor of survival in end-stage renal disease. J Nerv Ment Dis 178:127–133, 1990

69. DiMartini A, Pajer K, Trzepacz P, et al: Psychiatric morbidity in liver transplant patients. Transplant Proc 23:3179–3180, 1991

70. DiPaolo N, Capotondo L, Gaggiotti E, et al: Sexual function in uremic patients, in Psychological and Physiological Aspects of Chronic Renal Failure (Contributions in Nephrology series, Vol 77). Edited by D'Amico G, Colasanti G. Basel, Karger, 1990, pp 34–44

71. Dixon D: Religious and spiritual perspectives on organ transplantation, in Psychiatric Aspects of Organ Transplantation. Edited by Craven J, Rodin G. Oxford, UK, Oxford University Press, 1992, pp 131–141

72. Domar A, Everett L, Keller M: Preoperative anxiety: is it a predictable entity? Anesth Analg 69:763–767, 1989

73. Doweiko J, Fogel B, Goldberg R: Trazodone and hemodialysis (letter). J Clin Psychiatry 45:361, 1987

74. Doyle G, Laher M, Kelly J, et al: The pharmacokinetics of paroxetine in renal impairment. Acta Psychiatr Scand 80 (suppl 350):89–90, 1989

75. Drew W, Buhles W, Erlich K: Herpesvirus infections (cytomegalovirus, herpes simplex virus, varicella-zoster virus): how to use ganciclovir (DHPG) and acyclovir. Infect Dis Clin North Am 2:495–509, 1988

76. Drueke T: Endocrine disorders in chronic hemodialysis patients (with the exclusion of hypoparathyroidism). Adv Nephrol 10:351–382, 1981

77. Drueke T, Zins B, Naret C, et al: Utilization of erythropoietin in the treatment of the anemia due to chronic renal failure. Adv Nephrol 18:187–206, 1989

78. Drugs that cause psychiatric symptoms. Med Lett Drugs Ther 31:113–118, 1989

79. Dubovsky S, Metzner J, Warner R: Problems with internalization of a transplanted liver. Am J Psychiatry 136:1090–1091, 1979

80. Dumas R: Psychological preparation for surgery. Am J Nurs 8:52–55, 1963

81. Egan K, Ready L, Nessly M, et al: Self-administration of midazolam for postoperative anxiety: a double-blinded study. Pain 49:3–8, 1992

82. Egbert L, Battit G, Turndorf H, et al: Value of preoperative visit by anesthetist: study of doctor-patient rapport. Am J Psychiatry 185:553–555, 1963

83. Egbert L, Battit G, Welch C, et al: Reduction of postoperative pain by encouragement and instruction of patients: a study of doctor-patient rapport. N Engl J Med 270:825–827, 1964

84. Eidelman B, Abu-Elmagd K, Wilson J, et al: Neurologic complications of FK 506. Transplant Proc 23:3175–3178, 1991

85. Emmons C, Smith J, Flanigan M: Cerebrospinal fluid inflammation during OKT3 therapy. Lancet 2:510–511, 1986

86. Evans R, Manninen D, Garrison L, et al: The quality of life of patients with end-stage renal disease. N Engl J Med 312:553–559, 1985

87. Evans R, Manninen D, Garrison LJ, et al: Special report: findings from the National Kidney Dialysis and Kidney Transplantation Study (Publ No 03230). Baltimore, MD, Health Care Financing Administration, 1987

88. Evans R, Manninen D, Thompson C: A Cost and Outcome Analysis of Kidney Transplantation: The Implications of Initial Immunosuppressive Protocol and Diabetes. Seattle, WA, Battelle Human Affairs Research Centers, 1989

89. Evans R, Rader B, Manninen D, et al: The quality of life of hemodialysis recipients treated with recombinant human erythropoietin. JAMA 263:825–830, 1990

90. Fabro A: Legal aspects of organ transplant: Strunk vs. Strunk. Conn Med 34:583, 1970

91. Fagan P: Sexual dysfunction in the medically ill, in Principles of Medical Psychiatry. Edited by Stoudemire A, Fogel B. Orlando, FL, Grune & Stratton, 1987, pp 307–327

92. Fargnoli D: Symbolic equations and impotence in uremia, in Psychological and Physiological Aspects of Chronic Renal Failure (Contributions in Nephrology series, Vol 77). Edited by D'Amico G, Colasanti G. Basel, Karger, 1990, pp 56–64

93. Faulds D, Heel R: Ganciclovir: a review of its antiviral activity, pharmacokinetic properties and therapeutic efficacy in cytomegalovirus infections. Drugs 39:597–638, 1990

94. Fawcett J: Compliance: definitions and key issues. J Clin Psychiatry 56 (suppl 1):4–8, 1995

95. Fellner C, Marshall J: Twelve kidney donors. JAMA 206:2703–2707, 1968

96. Fisch R, Lahad A: Adverse psychiatric reaction to ketoconazole. Am J Psychiatry 146:939–940, 1989

97. Flaherty M, O'Brien M: Family styles of coping in end stage renal disease. ANNA Journal 19:345–350, 366, 1992

98. Fogel B, Mor V: Depressed mood and care preferences in patients with AIDS. Gen Hosp Psychiatry 15:203–207, 1993

98a. Frazier P, Davis-Ali S, Dahl K: Correlates of noncompliance among renal transplant recipients. Clin Transplant 8:550–557, 1994

99. Freedman A: Psychoanalysis of a patient who received a kidney transplant. J Am Psychoanal Assoc 31:917–956, 1983

100. Freeman AI, Folks D, Sokol R: Cardiac transplantation: clinical correlates of psychiatric outcome. Psychosomatics 29:47–54, 1988

100a. Freeman A, Westphal J, Davis L, et al: The future of organ transplant psychiatry. Psychosomatics 36:429–437, 1995

101. Freyberger H: Psychotherapeutic possibilities in medically extreme situations. Psychother Psychosom 26:337–343, 1975

102. Freyberger H: The renal transplant patients: three-stage model and psychotherapeutic strategies, in Psychonephrology 2: Psychological Problems in Kidney Failure and Their Treatment. Edited by Levy N. New York, Plenum, 1983, pp 259–265

103. Fricchione G: Psychiatric aspects of renal transplantation. Aust N Z J Psychiatry 23:407–417, 1989

104. Fricchione G, Howanitz E, Jandorf L, et al: Psychological adjustment to end-stage renal disease and the implications of denial. Psychosomatics 33:85–91, 1992

105. Friedman E: Competence to refuse medical treatment, in Making Choices: Ethics Issues for Health Care Professionals. Edited by Friedman E. Chicago, IL, American Hospital Association, 1986, pp 141–175

106. Friend R, Singletary Y, Mendell N, et al: Group participation and survival among patients with end-stage renal disease. Am J Public Health 76:670–672, 1986

107. Fukunishi I: Psychosomatic problems surrounding kidney transplantation: incidence of alexithymia and psychiatric disturbances. Psychother Psychosom 57:42–49, 1992

108. Fukunishi I: Anxiety associated with kidney transplantation. Psychopathology 26:24–28, 1993

109. Fukunishi I, Saito S, Ozaki S: The influence of defense mechanisms on secondary alexithymia in hemodialysis patients. Psychother Psychosom 57:50–56, 1992

110. Fuller R, Rothbun R, Parli J: Inhibition of drug metabolism by fluoxetine. Res Commun Chem Pathol Pharmacol 13:353–356, 1976

111. Fung J, Todo S, Jain A, et al: Conversion of liver allograft recipients with cyclosporine related complications from cyclosporine to FK 506. Transplant Proc 22:6–12, 1990

112. Galletly D, Short T, Forrest P: Patient-administered anxiolysis—a pilot study. Anaesth Intensive Care 17:144–150, 1989

113. Ganzini L, Lee M, Heintz R, et al: The effect of depression treatment on elderly patients' preferences for life-sustaining medical therapy. Am J Psychiatry 151:1631–1636, 1994

114. Garcia L, Ageru A, Cavalli N, et al: Kidney transplantation: absolute and relative psychological contraindications. Transplant Proc 23:1344–1345, 1991

115. Giannini A: Side effects of metronidazole. Am J Psychiatry 134:329–330, 1977

116. Gill M, Burgess E: Neurotoxicity of acyclovir in end-stage renal disease. J Antimicrob Chemother 25:300–301, 1990

117. Gonsalves-Ebrahim L, Kotz M: The psychological impact of ambulatory peritoneal dialysis on adults and children. Psychiatr Med 5:177–185, 1987

118. Green R, Lewis J, Kraus S, et al: Elevated procaine concentrations after administration of procaine penicillin G. N Engl J Med 291:223–226, 1974

119. Gulledge A, Buszta K, Montague D: Psychological aspects of renal transplantation. Urol Clin North Am 10:327–335, 1983

120. Gutman R, Stead W, Robinson R: Physical activity and employment status of patients on maintenance dialysis. N Engl J Med 304:309–313, 1981

121. Haber R, Joseph M: Neurological manifestations after amphotericin-B therapy. BMJ 1:230–231, 1962

122. Haenel T, Brunner F, Battegay R: Renal dialysis and suicide: occurrence in Switzerland and Europe. Compr Psychiatry 21:140–145, 1980

123. Hart R, Kreutzer J: Renal system, in Medical Neuropsychology: The Impact of Disease on Behavior. Edited by Tarter R, Van Thiel D, Edwards K. New York, Plenum, 1988, pp 99–120

123a. Hathaway S, McKinley J: Minnesota Multiphasic Personality Inventory. Minneapolis, MN, University of Minnesota, 1943

124. Hauser M, Williams J, Strong M, et al: Predicted and actual quality of life changes following renal transplantation. ANNA Journal 18:295–296, 299–304, 304–305, 1991

125. Hegel M, Ayllon T, Thiel G, et al: Improving adherence to fluid restrictions in male hemodialysis patients: a comparison of cognitive and behavioral approaches. Health Psychol 11:324–330, 1992

125a. Henderson M: Facilitating a "good death" in patients with end stage renal disease. ANNA Journal 22:294, 296, 298–300, 1995

126. Hietanen P, Lönnqvist J, Henriksson M, et al: Do cancer suicides differ from others? Psycho-Oncology 3:189–195, 1994

126a. Hilton B, Starzomski R: Family decision making about living related kidney donation. ANNA Journal 21:346–355, 381, 1994

127. Hinrichsen G, Lieberman J, Pollack S, et al: Depression in hemodialysis patients. Psychosomatics 30:284–289, 1989

128. Hitchcock P, Brantley P, Jones G, et al: Stress and social support as predictors of dietary compliance in hemodialysis patients. Behav Med 18:13–20, 1992

129. House A: Psychosocial problems of patients on the renal unit and their relation to treatment outcome. J Psychosom Res 31:441–452, 1987

130. House R, Thompson TI: Psychiatric aspects of organ transplantation. JAMA 260:535–539, 1988

131. House R, Trzepacz P, Thompson T: Psychiatric consultation to organ transplant services, in American Psychiatric Press Review of Psychiatry, Vol 9. Edited by Tasman A, Goldfinger SM, Kaufmann C. Washington, DC, American Psychiatric Press, 1990, pp 515–536

132. Husebye D, Westlie L, Styrovoky T, et al: Psychological, social, and somatic prognostic indicators in old patients undergoing long-term dialysis. Arch Intern Med 147:1921–1924, 1987

133. Imbs J, Singer L, Danian J: Effects of indomethacin and methylprednisolone on renal elimination of lithium in the rat. Rat International Pharmacopsychiatry 5:143–149, 1980

134. Itschaki N: Psychosocial factors in the care of the geriatric nephrology patient. Loss, Grief and Care 5:211–218, 1991

135. Jefferson J, Marshall J (eds): Neuropsychiatric Features of Medical Disorders. New York, Plenum, 1981

136. Johnson J: The influence of purposeful nurse patient interaction on the patient's post-operative course. American Nurses Association Monographs 2:16–22, 1966

137. Johnston A, Lineberry C, Ascher J, et al: A 102-center prospective study of seizure in association with bupropion. J Clin Psychiatry 52:450–456, 1991

138. Julius M, Hawthorne V, Carpenter-Alting P, et al: Independence in activities of daily living for end-stage renal disease patients: biomedical and demographic correlates. Am J Kidney Dis 13:61–69, 1989

139. June C, Thompson C, Kennedy M, et al: Profound hypomagnesemia and renal magnesium wasting associated with the use of cyclosporine for marrow transplantation. Transplantation 39:620–624, 1985

139a. Juneau B: Psychologic and psychosocial aspects of renal transplantation. Critical Care Nursing Quarterly 17:62–66, 1995

140. Kahn B: Pharmacokinetics and pharmacodynamics of cyclosporine. Transplant Proc 21 (3 suppl 1):9–15, 1989

141. Kaplan De-Nour A, Czaczkes J: Personality factors in chronic hemodialysis patients causing noncompliance with the medical regimen. Psychosom Med 34:333–344, 1972

142. Kaplan De-Nour A, Czaczkes J: The influence of patient's personality in adjustment to chronic dialysis: a predictive study. J Nerv Ment Dis 2:323–333, 1976

143. Karasu T: Psychotherapy with physically ill patients, in Specialized Techniques in Individual Psychotherapy. Edited by Karasu T, Bellak L. New York, Brunner/Mazel, 1980, pp 258–276

144. Kershner P, Wang-Cheng R: Psychiatric side effects of steroid therapy. Psychosomatics 30:135–139, 1989

145. Kimmel P, Miller G, Mendleson W: Sleep apnea syndrome in chronic renal failure. Am J Med 86:308–314, 1989

146. Kimmel P, Weihs K, Peterson R: Survival in hemodialysis patients: the role of depression. J Am Soc Nephrol 4:12–27, 1993

147. Kino T, Hatanaka H, Hashimoto M, et al: FK 506, a novel immunosuppressant isolated from streptomyces, I: fermentation, isolation, and physiochemical and biological characteristics. J Antibiot (Tokyo) 40:1249–1255, 1987

148. Koecheler J, Canafax D, Simmons R, et al: Lithium dosing in renal allograft recipients with changing renal function (letter). Drug Intelligence and Clinical Pharmacy 20:623–624, 1986

149. Krausz S: Illness and loss: helping couples cope. Clinical Social Work Journal 16:52–65, 1988

150. Krawczyk J, Raskin V: Psychological distress related to sexual abuse in a patient undergoing hemodialysis. Am J Psychiatry 147:673–674, 1990

151. Kuhn W, Myers B, Brennan A, et al: Psychopathology in heart transplant candidates. Journal of Heart Transplantation 7:223–226, 1988

152. Kusne S, Dummer J, Singh N, et al: Infections after liver transplantation: an analysis of 101 consecutive cases. Medicine (Baltimore) 67:132–143, 1988

153. Kutner N, Fair P, Kutner M: Assessing depression and anxiety in chronic dialysis patients. J Psychosom Res 29:23–31, 1985

154. Kutner N, Lin L, Fielding B, et al: Continued survival of older hemodialysis patients: investigation of psychosocial predictors. Am J Kidney Dis 24:42–49, 1994

155. Larkin O, Cederberg D, Miss J, et al: Ganciclovir for the treatment and suppression of nervous infections caused by cytomegalovirus. Am J Med 83:201–207, 1987

156. Layne O, Yudofsky S: Postoperative psychosis in cardiotomy patients: the role of organic and psychiatric factors. N Engl J Med 284:518–520, 1971

157. Lazarus H, Hagens J: Prevention of psychosis following open heart surgery. Am J Psychiatry 124:1190–1195, 1968

158. Lefebvre P, Crombez J: The "one day at a time" syndrome in post transplant evolution. Can J Psychiatry 25:319–324, 1980

159. Lemberger L, Rowe H, Bosomworth J, et al: The effect of fluoxetine on the pharmacokinetics and psychomotor responses of diazepam. Clin Pharmacol Ther 43:412–419, 1988

160. Levenson J, Colenda C, Larson D, et al: Methodology in consultation-liaison research: a classification of biases. Psychosomatics 31:367–376, 1990

161. Levenson J, Glochieski S: Psychological factors affecting end-stage renal disease. Psychosomatics 32:382–389, 1991

161a. Levenson J, Glocheski S: End-stage renal disease, in Psychological Factors Affecting Medical Conditions. Edited by Stoudemire A. Washington, DC, American Psychiatric Press, 1995, pp 159–172

162. Levenson J, Olbrisch M: Shortage of donor organs and long waits: new sources of stress for transplant patients. Psychosomatics 28:399–403, 1987

163. Levy A: Delirium and seizures due to abrupt alprazolam withdrawal: a case report. J Clin Psychiatry 45:38–39, 1984

164. Levy N: Sexual adjustment to maintenance hemodialysis and transplantation: national survey by questionnaire—preliminary report. Transactions—American Society for Artificial Internal Organs 19:138–142, 1973

165. Levy N: What's new on cause and treatment of sexual dysfunction in end stage renal disease, in Psychonephrology 1: Psychological Factors in Hemodialysis and Transplantation. Edited by Levy N. New York, Plenum, 1981, pp 43–47

166. Levy N: Sexual dysfunctions of hemodialysis. Clinical and Experimental Dialysis and Apheresis 7:275–288, 1983

167. Levy N: Chronic renal disease, dialysis, and transplantation, in Principles of Medical Psychiatry. Edited by Stoudemire A, Fogel B. Orlando, FL, Grune & Stratton, 1987, pp 583–593

168. Levy N: Psychopharmacology in patients with renal failure. Int J Psychiatry Med 20:325–334, 1990

169. Levy N: Chronic renal failure and its treatment: dialysis and transplantation, in Psychiatric Care of the Medical Patient. Edited by Stoudemire A, Fogel B. New York, Oxford University Press, 1993, pp 627–635

170. Levy N: Psychological aspects of renal transplantation. Psychosomatics 35:427–433, 1994

171. Levy N, Wynbrandt G: The quality of life on maintenance hemodialysis. Lancet 1:1328–1330, 1975

172. Li P, Nicholls M, Lai K: The complications of newer transplant anti-rejection drugs: treatment with cyclosporine A, OKT3, and FK506. Adverse Drug Reactions and Acute Poisoning Reviews 9:122–155, 1990

173. Lieberman J, Cooper T, Suckow R: Tricyclic antidepressant and metabolite levels in chronic renal failure. Clin Pharmacol Ther 37:301–307, 1985

174. Littlefield C: Social support and organ transplantation, in Psychiatric Aspects of Organ Transplantation. Edited by Craven J, Rodin G. Oxford, UK, Oxford University Press, 1992, pp 50–66

175. Lowy F, Martin D: Ethical considerations in transplantation, in Psychiatric Aspects of Organ Transplantation. Edited by Craven J, Rodin G. Oxford, UK, Oxford University Press, 1992, pp 108–120

176. Maida C, Katz A, Wolcott D, et al: Psychological and social adaptation to CAPD and center hemodialysis patients. Loss, Grief and Care 5:47–68, 1991

177. Martin M, Massunari M, Nghiem D, et al: Nosocomial aseptic meningitis associated with administration of OKT3. JAMA 259:2002–2005, 1980

178. Martis C, et al: Que peut esperer la nephrologie de la psychanalyse? ou La rencontre "du discours medical" et "du discours psychanalytique" [What can nephrology hope from psychoanalysis? or The meeting of medical language with psychoanalytic language]. Psychologie-Medicale 20:1835–1838, 1988

179. Mattson K, Niiranen A, Iivanainen M, et al: Neurotoxicity of interferon. Cancer Treat Rev 67:958–961, 1983

180. McConnell E: Personal communication. Burroughs Wellcome, Clinical Medicine Section, Drug Information Department, August 1991

181. Menchini-Fabris G, Turchi P, Giorgi P, et al: Diagnosis and treatment of sexual dysfunction in patients affected by chronic renal failure on hemodialysis, in Psychological and Physiological Aspects of Chronic Renal Failure (Contributions in Nephrology series, Vol 77). Edited by D'Amico G, Colasanti G. Basel, Karger, 1990, pp 24–33

182. Mendelson W, Wadhwa N, Greenberg H, et al: Effects of hemodialysis on sleep apnea syndrome in end-stage renal disease. Clin Nephrol 33:247–251, 1990

183. Meyers B: The patient with renal disease, in Treatments of Psychiatric Disorders: A Task Force Report of the American Psychiatric Association, Vol 2. Washington, DC, American Psychiatric Association, 1989, pp 915–929

184. Meyerson A, Lawn B: Psychiatric aspects of medical disability, in Medical Psychiatric Practice, Vol 1. Edited by Stoudemire A, Fogel B. Washington, DC, American Psychiatric Press, 1991, pp 597–614

185. Milano M, Kornfeld D: Psychiatry and surgery, in Psychiatry Update: The American Psychiatric Association Annual Review, Vol 3. Edited by Grinspoon L. Washington, DC, American Psychiatric Press, 1984, pp 256–277

186. Morris P: Kidney Transplantation. New York, Grune & Stratton, 1983

187. Morris P, Jones B: Life satisfaction across treatment methods for patients with end-stage renal failure. Med J Aust 150:42–432, 1989

188. Morris R, Wu J, Shorthouse R, et al: Comparative immuno-pharmacologic effects of FK506 and CyA in in vivo models of organ transplantation. Transplant Proc 22:35–36, 1990

189. Motes C: Discontinuation of dialysis. ANNA Journal 16:413–415, 1989

190. Murphy J, Monson R, Olivier D, et al: Affective disorders and mortality: a general population study. Arch Gen Psychiatry 44:473–480, 1987

191. Najarian J, Van Hook E, Simmons R: Kidney transplant from distant relatives. Am J Surg 135:362–366, 1978

192. Nelson C, Port F, Wolfe R, et al: The association of diabetic status, age, and race to withdrawal from dialysis. J Am Soc Nephrol 4:1608–1614, 1994

193. Neu S, Kjellstrand C: Stopping long-term dialysis. N Engl J Med 314:14–20, 1986

194. Nissenson A: Measuring, managing, and improving quality in the end-stage renal disease treatment setting: peritoneal dialysis. Am J Kidney Dis 24:368–375, 1994

195. Nissenson A, Nimer S, Wolcott D: Recombinant human erythropoietin and renal anemia: molecular biology, clinical efficacy, and nervous system effects. Ann Intern Med 114:402–416, 1991

196. Numan I, Barklind K, Lubin B: Correlates of depression in chronic dialysis patients: morbidity and mortality. Res Nurs Health 4:295–297, 1981

197. Ochs H, Greenblatt D, Labedzki L, et al: Alprazolam kinetics in patients with renal insufficiency. J Clin Psychopharmacol 6:292–294, 1986

197a. Olbrisch M, Levenson J: Psychosocial assessment of organ transplant candidates: current status of methodological and philosophical issues. Psychosomatics 36:236–243, 1995

198. Pacitti A, Segoloni G, Gallone G, et al: An out-patient approach to sexual problems in uremic patients, in Psychological and Physiological Aspects of Chronic Renal Failure (Contributions in Nephrology series, Vol 77). Edited by D'Amico G, Colasanti G. Basel, Karger, 1990, pp 45–55

199. Patterson J: Withdrawal from alprazolam dependency using clonazepam: clinical observations. J Clin Psychiatry 51:47–48, 1990

200. Pearson J, Dudley H: Bodily perceptions in surgical patients. BMJ 284:1545–1546, 1982

201. Penn I: Development of new tumors after transplantation, in Organ Transplantation and Replacement. Edited by Cerilli G. Philadelphia, PA, JB Lippincott, 1988, pp 439–444

202. Perard D: La grand-mere machine-vampire de Marie-Sophie [Marie-Sophie's machine-vampire grandmother]. Perspectives-Psychiatriques 23:386–397, 1985

203. Petrie K: Psychological well-being and psychiatric disturbance in dialysis and renal transplant patients. Br J Med Psychol 62:91–96, 1989

204. Pike J, Dimsdale J: Neuropsychological functioning in renal transplant candidates (letter). Psychosomatics 35:167–168, 1994

205. Pillay B, Schlebusch L, Louw J: Illness behaviour in live-related and cadaver renal transplant recipients. S Afr Med J 81:411–415, 1992

206. Plough A, Salem S: Social and contextual factors in the analyses of mortality in end-stage renal disease: implications for health policy. Am J Public Health 72:1293–1295, 1982

207. Poll I, Kaplan De-Nour A: Locus of control and adjustment to chronic hemodialysis. Psychol Med 10:153–157, 1990

208. Polson R, Powell-Jackson P, Williams R: Convulsions associated with cyclosporine in transplant recipients (letter). N Engl J Med 290:1003, 1985

209. Popovich R, Moncrief J, Nolph K, et al: Continuous ambulatory peritoneal dialysis. Ann Intern Med 88:449–456, 1978

210. Procci W: Psychological factors associated with severe abuse of the hemodialysis diet. Gen Hosp Psychiatry 3:111–118, 1981

211. Procci W, Goldstein D, Kletzky O, et al: Impotence in uremia: preliminary results of a combined medical and psychiatric investigation, in Psychonephrology 2: Psychological Problems in Kidney Failure and Their Treatment. Edited by Levy N. New York, Plenum, 1983, pp 235–246

212. Rapaport F: Living donor kidney transplantation. Transplant Proc 19:169–173, 1987

213. Reichsman F, Levy N: Problems in adaptation to maintenance hemodialysis: a four-year study of 25 patients. Arch Intern Med 130:850–865, 1972

214. Reisinger C: Personal communication. Mead Johnson Pharmaceuticals, Medical Information Consultant, Pharmaceutical Medical Services, 1991

215. Renault P, Hoofnagle J: Side effects of alpha interferon. Semin Liver Dis 9:273–277, 1989

216. Renault P, Hoofnagle J, Park Y, et al: Psychiatric complications of long-term alpha interferon therapy. Arch Intern Med 147:1577–1580, 1987

217. Riether A, Stoudemire A: Surgery and trauma, in Principles of Medical Psychiatry. Edited by Stoudemire A, Fogel B. Orlando, FL, Grune & Stratton, 1987, pp 423–449

218. Robinson J: Patient consent given but forgotten. Medical World News 17:26–28, 1976

219. Rodin G: Expressive psychotherapy in the medically ill: resistance and possibilities. Int J Psychiatry Med 14:99–108, 1984

220. Rodin G: Psychotherapy of the medically ill: introduction and overview. Int J Psychiatry Med 14:87–88, 1984

221. Rodin G: Psychotherapy of patients with chronic medical disorders, in Review of General Psychiatry. Edited by Goldman H. Norwalk, CT, Appleton & Lange, 1990, pp 567–573

222. Rodin G, Abbey S: Kidney transplantation, in Psychiatric Aspects of Organ Transplantation. Edited by Craven J, Rodin G. Oxford, UK, Oxford University Press, 1992, pp 145–163

223. Rodin G, Chmara J, Ennis J, et al: Stopping life-sustaining medical treatment: psychiatric considerations in the termination of renal dialysis. Can J Psychiatry 26:540–544, 1981

224. Rodriguez A, Diaz M, Colon A, et al: Psychosocial profile of noncompliant transplant patients. Transplant Proc 23:1807–1809, 1991

225. Rohatiner A, Prior P, Burton A, et al: Central nervous system toxicity of interferon. Br J Cancer 47:419–422, 1983

226. Rosenbaum M, Ben-Ari Smira K: Cognitive and personality factors in the delay of gratification of hemodialysis patients. J Pers Soc Psychol 51:357–364, 1986

227. Rothchild E: Family dynamics in end-of-life treatment decisions. Gen Hosp Psychiatry 16:251–258, 1994

228. Russell J, Beecroft M, Ludwin D, et al: The quality of life in renal transplantation—a prospective study. Transplantation 54:656–660, 1992

229. Ryan D: A questionnaire survey of preoperative fears. Br J Clin Pract 29:3–6, 1975

230. Sabra R, Branch R: Amphotericin-B nephrotoxicity. Drug Saf 5:94–108, 1990

231. Sacks C, Peterson R, Kimmel P: Perception of illness and depression in chronic renal disease. Am J Kidney Dis 15:31–39, 1990

232. Salvatierra O, Fortmann J, Belzer F: Sexual function in males before and after transplantation. Urology 5:64–66, 1975

233. Sanders W: Efficacy, safety, and potential economic benefits of oral ciprofloxacin in treatment of infection. Reviews of Infectious Diseases 10:528–543, 1988

234. Schmith V, Piraino B, Smith R, et al: Sensitivity of dialysis patients to alprazolam (abstract 155E). Pharmacotherapy 9:196, 1989

235. Schmith V, Piraino B, Smith R, et al: Alprazolam in end-stage renal disease, I: pharmacokinetics. J Clin Pharmacol 31:571–579, 1991

236. Schmith V, Piraino B, Smith R, et al: Alprazolam in end-stage renal disease, II: pharmacodynamics. Clin Pharmacol Ther 51:533–540, 1992

237. Schneider B: Multidimensional health locus of control as partial predictor of serum phosphorus in chronic hemodialysis. Psychol Rep 70 (3 pt 2):1171–1174, 1992

238. Schneider M, Friend R, Whitaker P, et al: Fluid noncompliance and symptomatology in end-stage renal disease: cognitive and emotional variables. Health Psychol 10:209–215, 1991

238a. Schneiderman L, Teetzel H: Who decides who decides? When disagreement occurs between the physician and the patient's appointed proxy about the patient's decision-making capacity. Arch Intern Med 155:793–796, 1995

239. Schultheiss K, Peterson L, Selby V: Preparation for stressful medical procedures by treatment interactions. Clinical Psychology Review 7:329–352, 1987

240. Sharma V, Enoch M: Psychological sequelae of kidney donation: a 5- to 10-year follow-up study. Acta Psychiatr Scand 75:264–267, 1987

241. Shulman R, Price J, Spinelli J: Biopsychosocial aspects of long-term survival on end-stage renal failure therapy. Psychol Med 19:945–954, 1989

242. Siegel K: Psychosocial aspects of rational suicide. Am J Psychother 40:405–417, 1986

243. Simmons R: Psychological reactions to giving a kidney, in Psychonephrology I: Psychological Factors in Hemodialysis and Transplantation. Edited by Levy N. New York, Plenum, 1981, pp 227–245

244. Simmons R, Klein S, Simmons R: Gift of Life: The Social and Psychological Impact of Organ Transplantation. New York, Wiley, 1977

245. Smith M, Hong B, Michelman J, et al: Treatment bias in the management of end-stage renal disease. Am J Kidney Dis 3:21–26, 1983

246. Smith M, Hong B, Robson A: Diagnosis of depression in patients with end-stage renal disease. Am J Med 79:160–165, 1985

247. Snavely S, Hodges G: The neurotoxicity of antibacterial agents. Ann Intern Med 101:92–104, 1984

248. Somer E, Tucker C: Spouse marital adjustment and patient dietary adherence in chronic hemodialysis: a comparison of Afro-Americans and Caucasians. Psychology and Health 6:69–76, 1992

249. Soos J: Psychotherapy and counselling with transplant patients, in Psychiatric Aspects of Organ Transplantation. Edited by Craven J, Rodin G. Oxford, UK, Oxford University Press, 1992, pp 89–107

250. Soskolne V, Kaplan De-Nour A: Psychosocial adjustment of home hemodialysis, continuous ambulatory peritoneal dialysis and hospital dialysis patients and their spouses. Nephron 47:266–273, 1987

250a. Spitzer R, Endicott J, Robins E: Research Diagnostic Criteria: rationale and reliability. Arch Gen Psychiatry 35:773–782, 1978

251. Starzl T: Living donors: con. Transplant Proc 19:174–176, 1987

252. Starzl T, Fung J, Venkataramanan R, et al: FK 506 for liver, kidney, and pancreas transplantation. Lancet 2:1000–1004, 1989

253. Starzl T, Van Thiel D, Tzakis A, et al: Orthotopic liver transplantation for alcoholic cirrhosis. JAMA 260:2542–2544, 1988

254. Steckler K, Selder F: End-stage renal disease: family responses. Loss, Grief and Care 5:5–14, 1991

255. Stein E, Murdaugh J, MacLeod J: Brief psychotherapy of psychiatric reactions to physical illness. Am J Psychiatry 125:76–83, 1969

256. Sterioff S, Eugen D, Zincke H: Current status of renal transplantation. Mayo Clin Proc 61:573–578, 1986

257. Stewart R, Stewart F: Neuropsychiatric aspects of chronic renal disease. Psychosomatics 20:524–531, 1979

258. Stiebel V: Methylphenidate plasma levels in depressed patients with renal failure. Psychosomatics 35:498–500, 1994

259. Storrow A: Bupropion overdose and seizure. Am J Emerg Med 12:183–184, 1994

260. Strain J: The surgical patient, in Consultation-Liaison Psychiatry and Behavioural Medicine. Edited by Houpt J, Brodie H. New York, Basic Books, 1986, pp 379–389

261. Strain J, Grossman S: Psychological Care of the Medically Ill: A Primer in Liaison Psychiatry. New York, Appleton-Century-Crofts, 1975

262. Streltzer J: Diagnostic and treatment considerations in depressed dialysis patients. Clinical and Experimental Dialysis and Epheresis 7:257–274, 1983

263. Streltzer J, Hassell L: Noncompliant hemodialysis patients: a biopsychosocial approach. Gen Hosp Psychiatry 10:255–259, 1988

264. Sullivan M, Youngner S: Depression, competence, and the right to refuse lifesaving medical treatment. Am J Psychiatry 151:971–978, 1994

265. Surman O: Toward greater donor organ availability for transplantation (letter). N Engl J Med 312:318, 1985

266. Surman O: Participation of living non-related donors in renal transplantation, in Positive Aspects to Living with End Stage Renal Disease: Psychosocial and Thanatological Aspects. Edited by Hardy M, Appel G, Kiernan J, et al. New York, Praeger, 1986, pp 22–31

267. Surman O: Psychiatric aspects of organ transplantation. Am J Psychiatry 146:972–982, 1989

268. Surman O: Hemodialysis and renal transplantation, in Massachusetts General Hospital Handbook of General Hospital Psychiatry, 3rd Edition. Edited by Cassem N. St. Louis, MO, Mosby Year Book, 1991, pp 401–430

269. Surman O, Dienstag J, Cosimi A, et al: Liver transplantation: psychiatric considerations. Psychosomatics 28:615–621, 1987

270. Surman O, Tolkoff-Rubin N: Use of hypnosis in patients receiving hemodialysis for end stage renal disease. Gen Hosp Psychiatry 6:31–35, 1984

271. Thompson A: FK 506: how much potential? Immunol Today 10:6–9, 1989

272. Thompson M, Jeffries D: Ganciclovir therapy in iatrogenically immunosuppressed patients with cytomegalovirus disease. J Antimicrob Chemother 23:61–70, 1989

273. Thompson T, Thompson W: Treating postoperative delirium. Drug Therapy 8:30–40, 1983

273a. Troppmann C, Benedetti E, Gruessner R, et al: Should patients with renal allograft loss due to noncompliance be retransplanted? Transplant Proc 27:1093, 1995

274. Troy S, Schultz R, Parker V, et al: The effect of renal disease on the disposition of venlafaxine. Clin Pharmacol Ther 56:14–21, 1994

275. Trzepacz P, Brenner R, Van Thiel D: A psychiatric study of 247 liver transplantation candidates. Psychosomatics 30:147–153, 1989

276. Trzepacz P, DiMartini A, Tringali R: Psychopharmacologic issues in organ transplantation, II: psychopharmacologic medications. Psychosomatics 34:290–298, 1993

277. Trzepacz P, DiMartini A, Tringali R: Psychopharmacologic issues in organ transplantation, I: pharmacokinetics in organ failure and psychiatric aspects of immunosuppressants and anti-infectious agents. Psychosomatics 34:199–207, 1993

278. Trzepacz P, Levenson J, Tringali R: Psychopharmacology and neuropsychiatric syndromes in organ transplantation. Gen Hosp Psychiatry 13:233–245, 1991

279. Trzepacz P, Maue F, Coffman G, et al: Neuropsychiatric assessment of liver transplantation candidates: delirium and other psychiatric disorders. Int J Psychiatry Med 16:101–111, 1986–1987

280. Umstead G, Neumann K: Erythromycin ototoxicity and acute psychotic reaction in cancer patients with hepatic dysfunction. Arch Intern Med 146:897–899, 1986

281. Velasco M: Symptom formation as resistance to becoming healthy: a case report. Family Systems Medicine 3:45–49, 1985

282. Venkataramanan R, Jain A, Cadoff R, et al: Pharmacokinetics of FK506: preclinical and clinical studies. Transplant Proc 22:52–56, 1990

283. Viederman M: Use of a psychodynamic life narrative in the treatment of depression in the physically ill. Gen Hosp Psychiatry 3:177–181, 1980

284. Viederman M: Psychotherapeutic approaches in the medically ill, in Consultation-Liaison Psychiatry and Behavioural Medicine. Edited by Houpt J, Keith H, Brodie H. New York, Basic Books, 1986, pp 261–272

285. Vincent H, Wenting G, Schalekamp M, et al: Impaired fractional excretion of lithium: a very early marker of cyclosporine toxicity. Transplant Proc 19:4147–4148, 1987

286. Vincken W: Psychiatric reactions to cefuroxine (letter). Lancet 1:965, 1984

287. Viswanathan R: Helping patients cope with the loss of a renal transplant. Loss, Grief and Care 5:103–113, 1991

288. Voth A: Possible association between metronidazole and agitated depression. Can Med Assoc J 100:1012–1013, 1969

289. Wadhwa N, Seliger M, Greenberg H, et al: Sleep related respiratory disorders in end-stage renal disease patients on peritoneal dialysis. Perit Dial Int 12:51–56, 1992

290. Warner M, Peabody C, Boutros N: Alprazolam and withdrawal seizures. J Nerv Ment Dis 178:208–209, 1990

291. Washer G, Schroter G, Starzl T, et al: Causes of death after kidney transplantation. JAMA 250:49–58, 1983

292. Watson A: Adverse effects of therapy for the correction of anemia in hemodialysis patients. Semin Nephrol 9:30–34, 1989

293. Watts D, Freeman A, McGriffin D, et al: Psychiatric aspects of cardiac transplantation. Heart Transplantation 3:243–247, 1984

294. Wilczek H, Ringden O, Tyden G: Cyclosporine-associated central nervous system toxicity after renal transplantation. Transplantation 39:110, 1985

295. Wilson P: Psychological risk factors in kidney transplantation. Paper presented at the First Working Conference on the Psychiatric, Psychosocial and Ethical Aspects of Organ Transplantation, Toronto, Ontario, June 9, 1990

296. Winn R, Bower J, Richards J: Acute toxic delirium: neurotoxicity of intrathecal administration of amphotericin-B. Arch Intern Med 139:706–707, 1979

297. Wolcott D: Organ transplant psychiatry: psychiatry's role in the second gift of life. Psychosomatics 31:91–97, 1990

298. Wolcott D, Maida C, Diamond R, et al: Treatment compliance in end-stage renal disease patients on dialysis. Am J Nephrol 6:329–338, 1986

299. Wolcott D, Marsh J, Asenath L, et al: Recombinant human erythropoietin treatment may improve quality of life and cognitive function in chronic hemodialysis patients. Am J Kidney Dis 14:478–485, 1989

300. Wolcott D, Wellisch D, Marsh J, et al: Relationship of dialysis modality and other factors to cognitive function in chronic dialysis patients. Am J Kidney Dis 12:275–284, 1988

301. Wyszynski A: Managing noncompliance in the "difficult" medical patient: the contributions of insight. Psychother Psychosom 54:181–186, 1990

302. Youngner S: Organ donation and procurement, in Psychiatric Aspects of Organ Transplantation. Edited by Craven J, Rodin G. Oxford, UK, Oxford University Press, 1992, pp 121–130

303. Youngner S, Allen M, Bartlett E, et al: Psychosocial and ethical implications of organ retrieval. N Engl J Med 313:321–323, 1985

304. Ziarnik J, Freeman C, Sherrard D, et al: Psychological correlates of survival on renal dialysis. J Nerv Ment Dis 164:210–213, 1977

305. Zimmermann E: Lebensqualitat wahrend Nierenersatztherapie [Quality of life in artificial kidney therapy]. Wien Klin Wochenschr 101:780–784, 1989

The Patient on Steroids

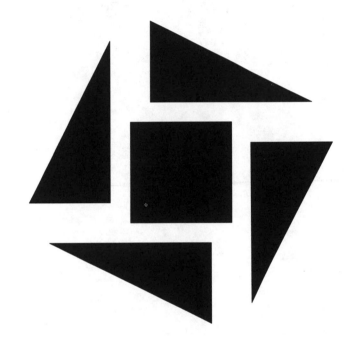

C H A P T E R 5

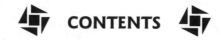 CONTENTS

■ Introduction to Chapter 5 195
■ Case Presentations 196
■ Questions 197
■ Answers 200
■ Discussion 201
   ◆ Corticosteroids and Psychotoxicity 201
     Risk Factors 201
       Prior Psychiatric History 202
     Incidence 202
     Prodrome, Presentation, and Course of
       Steroid Psychosis 203
     Steroid-Related Cognitive Difficulties 203
     Steroid Withdrawal Syndromes 204

Secondary Adrenocortical Insufficiency 205
Alternate-Day Steroids 205
Patient Education 206
Treatment 206
   Antidepressants 206
   Electroconvulsive Therapy 206
   Neuroleptics 206
   Antimanic Agents 206
   Benzodiazepines 207
Anabolic Steroids 207
◆ Summary 208
◆ References 209

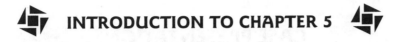

Consultation-liaison psychiatry is often like good detective work, piecing together clues about mental status changes based on timing and "fingerprints." Steroid medication can be a formidable adversary, staging unpredictable, hit-and-run assaults on mood, cognition, and perception. "Throw the punch, but hide the fist" aptly describes steroids and the mental status. Once again, the primarily biological emphasis in this chapter is not intended to minimize the importance of psychosocial issues. The case writeups have been intentionally simplified to simulate the kind of presenting data—usually medical, often telegraphic—typically encountered when a consultation-liaison psychiatrist initially reads a patient's chart. Rather than present cases in depth, we tried to construct a review exercise to help the reader identify misconceptions and gaps in knowledge.

PATIENT A

A 40-year-old woman is admitted to the medical service in acute status asthmaticus and is placed on albuterol inhalation, intravenous fluids, and prednisone 60 mg/day. Psychiatric consultation is requested because the patient is tearful and depressed. She has a history of asthma since age 14 and has been admitted at least 20 times over the years, with worsening respiratory function. She required intubation on one occasion 4 years ago, and has had a several-month course of oral prednisone at least eight times in the past 10 years. This most recent exacerbation occurs 3 months after tapering a 2-month course of prednisone, when her only maintenance medication had been theophylline. The patient has no previous psychiatric or substance abuse history. There is a family history of depression in her mother (which required electroconvulsive therapy [ECT]), and of substance abuse in two brothers.

At the time of mental status testing, her electrolytes are normal, and arterial blood gases have improved (Po_2 70, Pco_2 32, pH 7.39). On examination, she is cooperative although markedly depressed, with labile affect, pressured speech, and mild tangentiality. She claims that she is upset because her parents have recently separated after 41 years of marriage. She believes that her mother's church group has been accusing her father of sexual liaisons. She feels that this group wants to kill her father in order to save her mother's soul. She says that she herself has received the "breath of God" and knows that God is communicating with her by changing her breathing pattern. She denies suicidal ideation. At times she is silly and childish in manner. She is oriented in all three spheres, but her concentration—as tested by reciting the months of the year in reverse—is markedly impaired, with perseverations. She has trouble calculating and can remember only one word after a 5-minute interval, with no improvement on word recognition. Her long-term memory seems unaffected, but it is difficult for her to remain focused during the interview. Naming, repetition, and praxis are normal.

Further history obtained from the family indicate that the patient had been doing well until this admission. They deny vegetative disturbances or changes in affect or personality. They feel that she is having a "nervous breakdown" because of all the difficulties with her asthma in recent years.

PATIENT B

A 27-year-old woman is referred for evaluation of depression. She has a history of sarcoidosis, discovered at the age of 23, when she developed erythema nodosum, fevers, blurred vision, and uveitis and was found to have hilar adenopathy on chest X ray. Bronchoscopy and biopsy revealed noncaseating granulomas typical of sarcoid. She was treated with prednisone (60 mg/day over a period of 4 weeks), which was tapered over 2 months. She has had no other recurrence since that time.

Two months ago, she developed shortness of breath and was found to have diffuse interstitial infiltrates on her chest X ray, increased sedimentation rate, mild elevation of temperature, elevated angiotensin-converting enzyme, and abnormal gallium scan with increased uptake in the lung. Her Po_2 was 80 mm Hg on room air. She was given prednisone 120 mg/day for $3\frac{1}{2}$ weeks, to which she responded well, with less dyspnea, resolution of her fever, and improved pulmonary function and blood gases. The patient reports that within days of starting prednisone on this admission she brightened, experiencing a sense of well-being and hopefulness. She was discharged after 4 weeks on prednisone 80 mg/day, which continued to be tapered.

She has worked as a secretary for the past 3 years in a law office, and enjoys her job. It was not until she was asked by her employer to remain home (on disability) that she finally realized that her illness might be interfering with her work and social life. She recently began noticing increasing sadness, tearfulness, self-deprecatory thoughts, social withdrawal, and even feelings of persecution. She returned to her pulmonologist 1 week ago, who confirmed that she was doing well on her pulmonary function testing, and had a normal sedimentation rate and electrolytes. He recommended decreasing her prednisone from 50 mg/day to 40 mg/day. When he told her she had improved, she became quite tearful, prompting him to suggest a psychiatric consultation.

The patient is taking no other medications. She denies substance abuse. There is no prior history of psychiatric illness. There is no family history of affective disorder. The patient grew up in a family of four and has one older sister in good health. She lived with both parents until the age of 22. She attended college for 2 years, with an interrupted semester when she first became ill. She did not return to school but decided to work and found her own apartment. She has never been married but has been seeing someone steadily for the past year. She is frightened that her boyfriend will reject her on the basis of her illness, and is afraid that he will never marry her.

On mental status testing she is alert, oriented, and has good memory and concentration. She is tearful and constricted in affect, and admits to progressively worsening depression. She has no formal thought disorder. She wonders whether her friends think that she is incompetent, worries that they might talk about her behind her back, but is not entirely convinced that they are doing so. There is no other expressed paranoid or bizarre ideation. She is not suicidal.

🔹 PATIENT C

A 34-year-old woman was admitted to the hospital after a fainting episode. When she arrived in the emergency room, her hemoglobin was 7.1 and hematocrit was 21.8. She was guaiac negative. A workup revealed that her platelet count was 75,000. Her white cell count was normal, as was the differential. On further testing she was found to have a low haptoglobin, elevated indirect and direct bilirubin, and an elevated reticulocyte count. Her antinuclear antibodies test (ANA) was positive at a titer of 1:640, and her sedimentation rate was 120 mm/hour. Recent human immunodeficiency virus (HIV) serology was negative. Arterial blood gases and serum electrolytes were normal. She has no prior medical history. She denied taking any medications or recreational drugs at the time of admission. She does give a history of joint aches and pains, with finger swelling on her right hand about

3 months ago, which resolved spontaneously. On exam she is found to have a butterfly rash, but there are no other signs. Her urinalysis shows hematuria with casts and a negative urine culture. Electrolytes, creatinine, and blood urea nitrogen (BUN) are normal. A Holter monitor and electroencephalogram (EEG) are normal. A computed tomography (CT) scan with contrast is negative. Further workup reveals positive anti–double-stranded DNA. Beta–human chorionic gonadotropin (HCG) is negative. Toxicology screen is negative for alcohol, amphetamines, cocaine, and opiates.

The patient has been seeing a psychotherapist, and 4 years ago was treated for depression with nortriptyline. She has no drug or alcohol history, but her brother and father are alcoholic. Her mother was treated for depression with ECT. The patient is college educated and has been working as a caterer in her own business.

The patient is diagnosed with systemic lupus erythematosus (SLE) and treated with 120 mg daily of prednisone. A psychiatric consultation is requested after the second week of hospitalization when the patient is found decorating her hospital room with torn fragments of bed linens; she has been singing loudly during the night and touching other patients and staff on their genitals. On exam she is loud and belligerent, with flight of ideas and irritability. Her affect is quite labile. She refuses to participate in cognitive mental status testing and is sarcastic and derogatory toward you. She is grandiose and silly, expressing the notion that "All the President's men love Jackie," which is her name. When asked about tearing the hospital sheets, she says that she is the "isthmus ghost of Christmas future with a love more powerful than Zen and Mother Theresa."

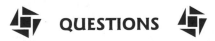

🔹 QUESTIONS 🔹

Choose all that apply.

1. Which of the following are true?
   a. In cases like B and C, in which there may be underlying central nervous system (CNS) complications, prednisone is a more potent inducer of psychiatric side effects and psychosis than are other steroid preparations such as dexamethasone.
   b. In cases B and C, magnetic resonance imaging (MRI) is likely to be diagnostic of the change in mental status.
   c. Persistence or even an increase of psychiatric symptoms during the first few days after initiating or increasing corticosteroids is almost always due to the steroid therapy.

d. The literature shows that psychosis occurs in more than half of all patients treated with steroids.

e. The initial response to corticosteroids in Patient B on the current admission is typical in steroid-treated patients.

2. The two diagnostic groups most at risk for steroid psychosis are patients with . . .
    a. Lymphoma
    b. Multiple sclerosis
    c. SLE
    d. Ulcerative colitis
    e. Pemphigus
    f. Asthma

3. Which of the following is/are *false* regarding steroid-induced mental changes?
    a. The majority of steroid-induced mental changes herald the development of a full-blown psychosis or affective syndrome.
    b. Steroid-induced neuropsychiatric symptoms span the spectrum of psychiatric presentations.
    c. The type of steroid-induced psychiatric disturbance is unpredictable.
    d. The majority of patients with steroid psychosis show affective symptoms at some point.
    e. Steroid-induced psychiatric symptoms tend to shift during the course of the illness.

4. Steroid-associated psychopathology most commonly presents as . . .
    a. Delirium
    b. Depression
    c. Schizophreniform or paranoid psychosis
    d. Mania

5. Which of the following is/are true about the onset of steroid-related psychiatric disturbances?
    a. Onset is usually within the first 2 days.
    b. Onset is usually within the first 2 weeks.
    c. Patient B is atypical in that the majority of steroid-related psychiatric symptoms occur within the first several days of initiating treatment.
    d. Cases A and C are atypical in that steroid-related cognitive changes usually occur in the context of chronic exposure.

6. Which of the following is/are true regarding the role of steroids in systemic lupus erythematosus (SLE)?
    a. Psychological dependence is frequent.
    b. Suicidal actions have not been described.

c. Patient C is atypical in that steroids account for only a small minority of lupus-related psychiatric symptomatology.

d. Severe psychiatric symptoms rarely occurred in SLE before the introduction of steroid therapy.

7. Steroid dosage and treatment duration most consistently forecast . . .
    a. Time of onset of psychiatric side effects.
    b. Duration of psychiatric side effects.
    c. Severity of psychiatric side effects.
    d. Type of mental disturbance.
    e. None of the above.

8. Which of the following statements about the risk of psychotoxicity is correct?
    a. Patients B and C are at greatest risk for psychiatric side effects due to their current prednisone dosage.
    b. Patient B is most at risk for psychiatric side effects because of the chronicity of prednisone treatment.
    c. The type of steroid preparation is probably the best predictor of psychotoxic risk.
    d. Patient C's prior psychiatric history and Patient A's family psychiatric history identify an enhanced risk of psychiatric side effects for them.
    e. Patient A's freedom from steroid-induced psychopathology on at least eight prior occasions should have predicted a lower risk for such side effects now.

9. The 1972 Boston Collaborative Drug Surveillance Program[11] was a landmark study that prospectively examined the development of steroid-related psychiatric side effects. Patients who developed psychosis were receiving approximately how much average daily prednisone (or its equivalent)?
    a. 10 mg
    b. 60 mg
    c. 100 mg
    d. Above 150 mg

10. You are asked to evaluate the psychiatric risks of steroid therapy for a euthymic patient with a bipolar psychiatric history who is about to undergo kidney transplantation. You respond . . .
    a. This patient will be 2–3 times more vulnerable to mental status derangements on steroids than his counterparts with no psychiatric history.

b. A previous history of mania predisposes to steroid-induced psychiatric side effects.

c. Contemporary studies have corroborated that a history of psychotic illness relatively contraindicates steroid treatment.

d. A previous episode of steroid-induced psychotoxicity does not predispose the patient to subsequent episodes.

e. A patient with at least five prior steroid treatments and no psychiatric sequelae is at lowered risk for psychiatric sequelae.

11. The most frequent initial presentation of impending steroid psychosis is . . .

a. Distortions of visual perception

b. Subjective cognitive-motor compromise

c. Hyperexcitability

d. A sense of well-being

12. All of the following are true regarding steroid-related cognitive deficits *except* . . .

a. They occur in patients without obvious CNS involvement.

b. They may occur *independently* of concurrent steroid psychosis or delirium.

c. They have been described with as little as 1 mg of dexamethasone.

d. They are usually noticeable to the patient or family.

13. In Patient B, the depressive symptoms seemed to worsen despite a lowered steroid dosage. Which of the following is a true formulation about this pattern of response?

a. Her symptoms may improve with readministering the steroid.

b. It indicates that she probably has an underlying dementing illness.

c. This pattern is usually indicative of focal right hemispheric or frontal cortical lesions.

d. Worsened depression with *lowered* steroids usually indicates that an underlying primary psychiatric etiology (e.g., endogenous depression) was responsible for what seemed to be caused by steroids.

e. Changing from a more to a less potent steroid preparation should improve psychiatric symptoms, not precipitate them.

14. Which of the following is true?

a. There is nothing characteristic about the presentation of steroid psychosis except its variability.

b. Many patients like Patients A and C evolve a chronic psychiatric syndrome.

c. Alternate-day steroids produce less psychiatric morbidity than daily treatment schedules.

d. A given patient is likely to have consistent steroid-induced psychiatric effects (e.g., the patient with steroid-induced schizophreniform psychosis is likely to present this way again).

15. Neuroleptics that have been found to be *ineffective* in patients like Patient C include . . .

a. Haloperidol (Haldol)

b. Chlorpromazine (Thorazine)

c. Thioridazine (Mellaril)

d. All of the above are ineffective, unless steroids are discontinued before the neuroleptic trial

e. None of the above statements is true

16. Steroid-induced manic states have been *effectively* treated with . . .

a. Lithium carbonate

b. Neuroleptics

c. Clonazepam (Klonopin)

d. Sodium valproate

e. All of the above

17. Which of the following is/are true about neuroleptics for steroid-induced psychosis?

a. Neuroleptics will be ineffective in Patient A unless the steroids are first discontinued.

b. Neuroleptics administered for steroid-induced psychosis improve agitation but do not shorten its duration; the syndrome must run its own course.

c. Haloperidol often precipitates a profound confusional state in patients like Patient C on high doses of steroids.

d. Only a and c above are true.

e. None of the above are true.

18. Psychotropics that have been associated with exacerbating steroid-induced mental status changes include . . .

a. Haloperidol

b. Tricyclic antidepressants

c. Lithium carbonate

d. Lorazepam (Ativan)

19. The most frequently reported adverse side effect(s) reported in athletes who abuse high-dose anabolic steroids include . . .

a. Manic syndromes

b. Schizophreniform episodes

   c. Severe anxiety disorders

   d. Depressive syndromes

   e. Dissociative phenomena

20. The psychiatric side effects of high-dose anabolic steroids . . .

   a. Can for the most part be explained by concurrent abuse of other substances, such as cocaine.

   b. Have been correlated with a higher than expected incidence of personality disorders.

   c. Cannot be predicted by family psychiatric history.

   d. Are relieved by steroid taper.

⚄ Answers

1.	Answer: e (pp. 201–203)	11.	Answer: c (p. 203)
2.	Answer: c, e (p. 202)	12.	Answer: d (pp. 203–204)
3.	Answer: a (pp. 202–203)	13.	Answer: a (pp. 204–205)
4.	Answer: b (p. 203)	14.	Answer: a (pp. 203, 205)
5.	Answer: b (pp. 202–203)	15.	Answer: e (p. 206)
6.	Answer: c (pp. 202–203)	16.	Answer: e (pp. 206–207)
7.	Answer: e (p. 201)	17.	Answer: e (p. 206)
8.	Answer: a (pp. 201–202)	18.	Answer: a (pp. 206–207)
9.	Answer: b (p. 201)	19.	Answer: a, d (pp. 207–208)
10.	Answer: d (pp. 201–203)	20.	Answer: c (pp. 207–208)

✦ CORTICOSTEROIDS AND PSYCHOTOXICITY

Adrenal corticosteroids are classified into two major categories: glucocorticoids and mineralocorticoids. Glucocorticoids affect the function of major organ systems and influence metabolism, immune functions, and inflammatory processes.[63] Mineralocorticoids influence salt and water metabolism. Anabolic steroids are synthetic derivatives of testosterone that were developed to minimize testosterone's masculinizing effects while promoting its effects on protein synthesis and growth.[13] Athletes are increasingly using anabolic steroids to add muscle bulk, and have suffered major psychiatric side effects.[13,18,49,50,54,59,60,74,77,82] Most of the following discussion pertains to the medical uses of corticosteroids, which we will refer to as *steroids*.

Risk Factors

As difficult as the description of the "typical" case of steroid toxicity is the attempt to define risk factors. Pertinent *negatives* tend to prevail; a single dose can surreptitiously disrupt mental status,[58] but *neither **dosage** nor **duration*** (i.e., chronicity) of steroid exposure consistently forecasts[48]

- Time of onset of psychiatric side effects
- Duration of psychiatric side effects
- Severity of psychiatric side effects
- Type of mental disturbance

However, beware of automatically blaming the steroids when psychiatric symptomatology persists or even immediately increases.

- For example, rising fever soon after initiating antibiotics is more likely due to the infection than to the antibiotics. Often the underlying disease (e.g., lupus cerebritis) accounts for the psychiatric symptoms, which slowly dissipate with steroid treatment. This adds, of course, one more diagnostic conundrum.

Nonetheless, steroids have earned continued suspiciousness about their role in mental status disruptions.

The only unambiguous "rule" that can be culled from the research is that higher steroid *dosage* correlates strongly with higher psychotoxic *risk*.[11,15,33,46] The landmark 1972 Boston Collaborative Drug Surveillance Study was based on data derived from 718 consecutively monitored patients in six hospitals in the United States, Canada, and Israel.[11] Prednisone was the most commonly administered glucocorticoid medication, and the analyses were restricted to prednisone recipients who were having their first hospital admission and first reaction attributed to the drug. Patients were monitored for an average of 28 days. The results pertaining to psychiatric reactions were as follows:

- Twenty-one previously stable patients experienced psychiatric reactions: 13 became psychotic, 8 became euphoric. Remission followed reduction in prednisone dosage, supplemented by brief (unspecified) psychopharmacological intervention.
- The mean daily dose for patients with psychiatric reactions was **59.5 mg,** as compared with 31.1 mg/day for patients who did not develop adverse effects.
- The incidence of psychiatric reactions, which varied significantly according to dose, was as follows:

Prednisone dosage (mg/day)	N	Incidence of psychiatric side effects
≤ 40	463	1.3%
41–80	175	4.6%
> 80	38	18.4%

The authors[11] thought that the striking correlation of acute psychiatric reactions with dose suggested a direct relationship between pharmacologically active glucocorticoids and abnormal psychiatric reactions.

Note that once dosage climbed above 80 mg, the incidence of psychotic symptoms increased substantially (18.4%). Moreover, at each dose interval, the frequency of acute reactions was *independent* of the underlying medical diagnosis.

Hall and colleagues'[33] classic 1979 study demonstrated steroid psychosis in 14 patients with variable diagnoses but without CNS lesions. These authors suggested that patients receiving daily doses greater than 40 mg prednisone or its equivalent were at increased risk for developing steroid psychosis.

◆ These reactions are twice as likely to occur during the first 6 days of treatment.

◆ The psychotic state presented as a "spectrum psychosis," ranging from affective through schizophreniform psychoses to delirium.

◆ No characteristic, stable presentation was observed in these 14 patients, leading to the conclusion that nothing typifies the presentation of steroid psychosis except variability.[33]

◆ Upon remission, *none* of the patients showed residual mental status changes of primary affective illness or thought disorder.

No particular synthetic steroid preparation (e.g., cortisone, dexamethasone, adrenocorticotropic hormone [ACTH], prednisone) appears to be more of an offender than the others.[73]

Prior Psychiatric History

Psychiatrists are often asked to screen patients with psychiatric histories before elective procedures that require steroids, such as transplantation. The implicit and quite reasonable assumption is that these patients will be more vulnerable to mental status derangements than their nonpsychiatric counterparts. *Perplexingly contrary to this clinical belief, neither a previous psychiatric history nor current psychiatric disturbance predisposes to steroid-induced psychiatric effects.*[40,70]

This is good news for psychiatric patients, but counterintuitive and downright unbelievable for the medical colleagues who consult us. In their excellent review, Stiefel and colleagues[73] have written,

> Prior psychiatric illness and its relationship to the development of a steroid-induced mental disturbance has been strongly debated. [For example,] some clinicians have excluded patients with prior emotional disturbances from receiving dexamethasone electively as part of antiemetic regimens during chemotherapy.[1,51] Some have viewed psychiatric illness as a contraindication to steroid treatment.[15,68] However, others have found the frequency of psychotic reactions not to be different from that of patients without a previous psychiatric history.[28,30,33,47,72] In our experience, a previous psychiatric history should not deter the clinician from using steroids. (p. 480)

Even more surprising, perhaps, but certainly reassuring to patients and families, is that *a previous episode of steroid-induced psychotoxicity does not predispose a patient to subsequent episodes.*[40] The downside is that patients who have glided through past steroid treatments are not protected from developing psychiatric side effects in the future.[73] The formulation "But Mr. X has had many other steroid treatments before, so his [depression/mania/psychosis] is probably not from the steroids" seems to make good clinical sense, but it is inaccurate. It distracts clinicians from the underlying pharmacotoxic cause of the mental status change (as do prior primary psychiatric episodes). Of course, be sure to rule out other etiologies for mental status changes, as well.

Incidence

The literature is ambiguous about who is the high-risk patient, other than one on high-dose steroids. Remember that the *initial* response to steroids is usually a **sense of well-being** or improved appetite, but these reactions do not predict subsequent events.

Clinical lore suggests that steroid-induced changes are very common, but a look at the research challenges this assumption:

◆ The incidence of a *severe* psychiatric syndrome ranges from 1.6% to 50%, *but with a weighted average of only 5.7%*[31] (of patients on steroids).

◆ The reported incidence of steroid psychosis also varies widely, ranging from 13% to 62%, with a weighted average of 27.6%.[31]

◆ Although no controlled studies exist, the medical illnesses with the highest risk for steroid psychosis are SLE and pemphigus.[31] (However, note that the description of severe psychiatric symptoms in SLE predated the introduction of steroid therapy,[57] and many SLE patients become psychiatrically symptomatic *before* taking steroids.)

◆ The incidence of steroid psychoses in patients with other conditions (e.g., lymphoma, multiple sclerosis, severe intractable asthma, ulcerative colitis, regional enteritis, idiopathic thrombocytopenic purpura, rheumatoid arthritis, severe poison ivy or oak) is estimated at between 3% and 6%.[31]

◆ Psychiatric disturbances *usually occur within the first 2 weeks* of steroid exposure, but can occur as early as the first day to as late as the third month.[73]

◆ Women are at greater risk than men.[31]

◆ Psychological dependence on steroids used for medical indications is rare.[41]

Keep in mind that the vast majority of steroid-induced mental changes are *mild to moderate* and do **not** evolve into full-blown psychotic or affective syndromes.[70] However, suicidal actions based on psychotic and depressive symptomatology do occur.[10,21,45,76] Steroid-associated psychiatric disturbances cover the spectrum, including mild to severe affective disorders (depression and/or mania),[12,20,32,33,40,46] psychotic reactions,[71a] and cognitive disturbances, including delirium.[48]

The type of psychiatric disturbance is **unpredictable,** and symptoms **shift radically** during the course of the illness. *There is no consistent, predictable presentation of steroid-induced psychosis, even for a given patient* (e.g., the patient who presents with schizophreniform psychosis at one point may present with a manic syndrome the next time).

◆ In descending order of frequency, steroid-induced psychiatric symptoms tend to be as follows:
  • depressive > manic > cyclical > agitated schizophreniform or paranoid psychosis > delirium[70]
◆ The majority of patients with steroid psychosis show **affective symptoms** at some point.[70]

Other steroid-associated disturbances include tremor, hyperkinesia, nervousness, sleep disturbances, and subtle alterations in sensation and perception.[73] Obsessive-compulsive behavior[7] and panic attacks[64] have also been associated with steroid administration.

Prodrome, Presentation, and Course of Steroid Psychosis

We quote from Shapiro's[70] concise summary:

The most frequent initial presentation of an impending steroid psychosis is a state of cerebral *hyperexcitability,* clearly perceived and reported by the patient. Patients characterize these states as being marked by increased irritability, lability of mood, profound dysphoria, hyperacusis, and pressured thought processes. These changes often antecede other, more serious disturbances of cognition by 72–96 hours. Once a steroid psychosis has been fully defined, it is likely to present as a spectrum psychosis, with the most prominent symptoms consisting of profound distractibility, pressured speech, anxiety, emotional lability, severe insomnia, sensory flooding, depression, perplexity, auditory and visual hallucinations, agitation, intermittent memory impairment, mutism, delusions, disturbances of body image, apathy, and hypomania. Prior to the advent of treatment with phenothiazines, it was noted that these conditions spontaneously remitted between 2 weeks and 7 months after the discontinuance of steroids, with 80% . . . having remitted untreated by the sixth week. Administration of phenothiazines dramatically reduces this period. The current duration . . . [with neuroleptic treatment] ranges in the literature from 1 to 150 days, with a mean duration until total recovery of 22 days. (p. 390, italics added)

Note that most patients fully recover and do *not* evolve chronic psychiatric syndromes. Persistence of psychiatric symptoms for weeks or months after steroid exposure strongly suggests either another medical etiology (e.g., lupus) or a primary psychiatric syndrome. Steroid-induced syndromes do not imply *focal* CNS lesions, and there is no characteristic MRI pattern.

Steroid-Related Cognitive Difficulties

Both circulating endogenous and exogenous corticosteroids can cause difficulties with attention, concentration, and memory. For example, 6 patients with a variety of medical illnesses (which did not involve the CNS) developed reversible dementia-like syndromes on high-dose steroids.[78] These symptoms included decreased attention, concentration, and retention and slowed mental speed. They were accompanied by psychosis or delirium. Another corroborating study had previously demonstrated a high incidence of intermittent memory impairment in a group of corticosteroid-treated medically ill patients.[33] Chronicity of exposure is not necessary for cognitive difficulties to result.

Researchers have investigated whether there are specific types of steroid-related cognitive effects. In one important study by Wolkowitz et al.,[85] the subjects who became cognitively impaired *were medically healthy.*

◆ This effect *was not limited to the higher dose ranges but also occurred with* **minimal** *steroid exposure* (a single dose of dexamethasone 1 mg; N = 30).
◆ One milligram of dexamethasone increased the rate of intrusions (i.e., self-generated words) into free-recall verbal memory tasks.

◆ Subjects showed a similar inability to discriminate targets from distracters in recognition memory (i.e., incorrectly identifying distracters as target words).

◆ Cognitive deficits were statistically significant *but not grossly discernible*. For example, only 2 of the 11 volunteers receiving high-dose prednisone were aware of their confusion or difficulty concentrating.

The investigators concluded that corticosteroids may impair the ability of subjects to discriminate relevant from irrelevant stimuli, thus altering the signal-to-noise ratio in selective attention and impairing concentration on target information because of irrelevant intrusions into the task.

A number of mechanisms for this effect have been proposed. For example, it is possible that corticosteroids suppress the ability of the hippocampus to filter out irrelevant material (the hippocampus contains the highest concentration of corticosteroid binding sites in the brain); alternatively, corticosteroids may alter the arousal levels that influence cognitive efficiency, especially in selectivity and filtering of internally distracting stimuli.[52,85]

These findings have important clinical implications: even *low*-dose corticosteroids may produce subclinical impairments in processing new information, filtering out distracting information, and responding appropriately to environmental cues. Make it a rule to carefully evaluate cognition, even in patients without subjective cognitive complaints or obvious impairment, including those on minimal short-term steroid therapy.

Steroid Withdrawal Syndromes

The usual treatment for steroid-associated psychiatric disturbances is to reduce or discontinue the medication when possible. However, this treatment strategy may paradoxically *induce* mental disturbances. Steroid withdrawal syndromes can strike unpredictably. Several case examples from the literature follow:

◆ We[86] recently reported on a patient with corticosteroid-dependent Sjögren's disease of the CNS who consistently became depressed in temporal association with the taper of her high-dose corticosteroids, while her CNS disease remained constant. She became profoundly dysphoric, with tearfulness, hopelessness, suicidal ruminations, social withdrawal, anhedonia, autonomy of mood, and diurnal variation of mood (more depressed in the morning). There was no evidence of psychosis, and cognitive functions were intact except for diminished concentration. This patient had no prior psychiatric history. Her depressive syndrome was attributed to exacerbations of Sjögren's disease, complicated by corticosteroid withdrawal. Although steroid-associated affective episodes fare poorly with tricyclic antidepressant medication,[32] our patient responded well to fluoxetine.

◆ Wolkowitz and Rapaport[84] described steroid withdrawal symptoms of dysphoria, depression, anxiety, irritability, emotional lability, fatigue, short-term memory problems, depersonalization, and "spaciness" in two Crohn's disease patients. Both patients were in their early 30s and had no prior psychiatric history. One patient had been treated with a 3-week course of prednisone (30 mg/day), and the other had been administered two courses (8 months and then 3 months) of prednisone (up to 60 mg/day). Taper was as gradual as 2.5 mg every 1–2 weeks. *Of note: these symptoms persisted for up to 6–8 weeks after corticosteroid withdrawal.*

◆ Malone and Dimeff[50] described four patients who suffered major depression upon withdrawal of anabolic steroids. The symptoms were temporally related to anabolic steroid discontinuation, but were long lasting. Like our patient, these patients all improved on fluoxetine.

◆ More dramatically, Campbell and Schubert[14] described a scleroderma patient without previous psychiatric history who developed delirium about 1.5 days *after* discontinuing glucocorticoid therapy. The patient was confused and disoriented, and complained of bugs and germs in the room. He performed bizarre, repetitive behaviors, including spitting into his oxygen mask, picking at his clothing, and attributing special meaning to occurrences. Other causes of delirium were eliminated, and he was restarted on intravenous steroids (hydrocortisone) but no antipsychotics. Within 24 hours, he was calm, attentive, not hallucinating, fully oriented, and cooperative with treatment. It was possible to then taper the steroids without recurrence.

◆ Fricchione et al.[27] similarly reported delirium temporally related to steroid withdrawal, which improved with restoration of steroids, low-dose antipsychotics, and diazepam.

Other well-recognized withdrawal symptoms include anorexia, nausea, lethargy, arthralgia, weakness, and weight loss.[73] Withdrawal is produced not only by dose taper but also by changing to a *less potent* steroid preparation.[44]

There are many of these case reports in the literature.[5,12,26,37,48,66,84,86] Fricchione et al.[27] have comprehensively reviewed steroid withdrawal phenomena:

◆ Steroid-withdrawal syndromes are much less frequent than steroid-induced syndromes.
◆ Depression was the most common symptom, followed by delirium.
◆ Anxiety, psychosis, and catatonia also occurred.
◆ Women were more frequently affected than men, a finding that also holds for steroid-induced psychiatric syndromes.
◆ Asthma and rheumatoid arthritis were among the more frequent diagnoses in this review.
◆ The average peak dose of prednisone or equivalent was 42 mg, but there were patients who were receiving low-dose steroid treatment.
◆ Symptomatic steroid-withdrawal patients appeared to have poorer outcomes, with some patients chronically abusing steroids and developing treatment-resistant depression.
◆ It was unclear whether the poor prognosis in some patients was due to underdiagnosis and undertreatment of depression.
◆ Few data are available on whether steroid-withdrawal depression is more or less likely to respond to tricyclics or other classes of medications, although there are individual reports of success with different agents.
◆ The relationship between steroid-induced syndromes and the predisposition to steroid-withdrawal psychiatric symptoms is unclear from the review.

As mentioned, steroid withdrawal may also exacerbate the underlying medical illness itself (and its associated psychiatric symptoms), resulting in a pathophysiological catch-22. For example, the delirium caused by CNS lupus is often best treated by initiating or increasing steroids; the distinction between steroid-induced versus steroid-deprived symptomatology can become frustratingly obscure.

Moran and Dubester[53] have recommended that when mental status changes precede the steroid increase, the patient should be observed for a few days at the increased dose; for example, most instances of lupus delirium treated with steroids tend to remit. There is no characteristic focal neurological pattern of steroid withdrawal.

Secondary Adrenocortical Insufficiency

There is no question that patients with *primary* adrenal insufficiency (Addison's disease) suffer from fluctuating psychiatric disturbances, often early in the course of the illness; these include apathy, fatigue, irritability, negativism, depression, cognitive impairment, and delirium.[42] Does *secondary* adrenal insufficiency (addisonism) account for steroid-withdrawal psychiatric symptoms?

◆ Exogenous steroids may suppress the pituitary-hypothalamic axis, producing adrenal atrophy secondary to the loss of endogenous ACTH and resulting in *secondary* adrenocortical insufficiency.[81]
◆ Clinical appearances may be deceiving, as the patient may appear cushingoid (e.g., moon facies, acne).

To document secondary adrenocortical insufficiency, it would be necessary to demonstrate abnormal ACTH stimulation in the patients suffering steroid-withdrawal psychiatric symptoms.

◆ Patients who were studied by Amatruda et al.[6] had more general somatic symptoms of steroid withdrawal with normal ACTH challenge; however, psychiatric symptoms were not mentioned.

Be sure to rule out metabolic contributants to changes in mental status in these patients.

Alternate-Day Steroids

Cordess et al.[17] had suggested in 1981 that alternate-day steroids produced less psychiatric morbidity than daily treatment schedules. Joffe and colleagues,[34,36] however, found differently when they assessed mood and cognition on consecutive days in 18 female SLE patients on alternate-day steroid therapy. They demonstrated that substantial alterations in mood, particularly depression and anxiety, occurred between the day-on and the day-off medication in a subgroup of SLE patients. Although the overall mean scores for the mood and cognitive tests were not significantly different between the on-medication and off-medication days, 10 of the 18 patients had substantial changes in their levels of depression or anxiety. The direction of these alterations was not predictable; some improved on drug-free days, whereas others worsened. These data confirmed the clinical findings of Sharfstein et al.,[71] who described three patients who showed mood cycling when treated with 50–60 mg of prednisone on an alternate-day schedule. Joffe et al.'s[34,36] patients, however, took a mean alternating daily dosage of prednisone of only 13.9 mg, suggesting that even low-dose alternate-day corticosteroids may induce psychiatric morbidity.

The underlying mechanism for these changes has remained speculative.[35,83]

Patient Education

Reckart and Eisendrath[65] explored patient preparedness for steroid-induced side effects. They interviewed eight patients who had undergone more than 5 years of intermittent corticosteroid treatments. The patients complained of insomnia, depression, hypomania or euphoria, confusion, and memory problems. Only one patient recalled having been warned by the physician of possible psychiatric side effects. (Because there were no corroborating data from the physicians, it was unclear whether this apparent lack of information was the result of poor preparation by the physician or of poor recall or denial by the patient.) Only three reported the psychiatric side effects to their physician when they occurred. The most common reasons for withholding information were embarrassment or fear of being labeled insane. Upon being informed that corticosteroids could induce such psychiatric side effects, patients felt reassured that they could better manage the emotional disturbances.

Patient resistance to steroid treatment ("steroidphobia")[19,56] often runs high.

Treatment

As with conventional medication side effects, the usual treatment for steroid-induced psychiatric reactions is to discontinue or taper the medication. As mentioned, however, this strategy may have a paradoxical effect if 1) the patient is prone to steroid-withdrawal psychiatric symptoms, or 2) steroid withdrawal exacerbates the underlying medical condition, such as lupus cerebritis (analogous to the rising fever of a septic patient whose antibiotics are prematurely tapered). Fortunately, it is not mandatory to discontinue steroids in order to treat their psychiatric side effects; neuroleptics, antidepressants, ECT, and antimanic agents may be successfully coadministered with steroids. The consultant's approach is often—unavoidably—one of trial and error.

Antidepressants

Treatment recommendations for depression are ambiguous. For example, there are reports suggesting that tricyclic antidepressants are ineffective in corticosteroid-induced depression[40,46] and *may even exacerbate corticosteroid-induced psychosis.*[20,32,33] The mechanism for this effect is unclear; perhaps it is related to the anticholinergic properties of tricyclics. Although Stiefel et al.[73] recommended tricyclic antidepressants in their steroid-treated cancer population, theirs tends to be the mi-

nority view. We agree with Perry and Miller's[57] suggestion that antidepressants without anticholinergic properties, such as the selective serotonin reuptake inhibitors (SSRIs), are worth investigating for this indication.

◆ Steroid-withdrawal depression in our Sjögren's patient repeatedly responded to the SSRI fluoxetine,[86] but this single anecdotal case requires further corroboration.

Certainly, if fluoxetine and other SSRIs proved effective, they would help those patients who require chronic steroid therapy but evolve debilitating depressive syndromes. (Be warned, however, that patients with CNS lupus may be at increased risk of extrapyramidal side effects with fluoxetine.[24] This could be true of other SSRIs as well.)

Electroconvulsive Therapy

ECT has effectively treated severe steroid-associated depression[3,22,67] and catatonia[21] that has been resistant to medications. It has also been useful for treating psychiatric syndromes in the transplantation setting, when steroids cannot be withdrawn without jeopardizing the allograft.[8]

Neuroleptics

There is no well-tried formula for treating secondary psychotic states associated with steroids. Most authors advise rapid taper of steroids whenever possible,[70] although stopping them is *not* a prerequisite for treating steroid psychosis.[29] Neuroleptics both improve steroid-induced psychotic agitation and shorten the duration of the psychotic syndrome. Various neuroleptics have been described in this context, including thioridazine (Mellaril), chlorpromazine (Thorazine), and haloperidol (Haldol).[9,70] In Hall et al.'s[33] classic study, phenothiazines (chlorpromazine or thioridazine) produced an excellent response in all 14 patients.

◆ A good rule of thumb is to apply the principles of managing delirium to these patients, relying on haloperidol because of its efficacy, low anticholinergicity, and minimal cardiovascular side effects. (Additionally, haloperidol has not been implicated in causing a lupus-like syndrome, as have other psychotropic drugs such as the phenothiazines.)

Antimanic Agents

Manic states have also been precipitated by steroid administration.[25,43,80] These can be treated with either lithium carbonate or neuroleptics.[39,70] Prophylactic lithium may also prevent steroid-induced affective (manic and depressive) psychoses.[23,75]

◆ Clonazepam (Klonopin) (1 mg po twice a day) was used in treating steroid-induced mania in a patient after renal transplantation when lithium had to be discontinued.[79]
◆ Sodium valproate has also been useful.[2,38]

Note that carbamazepine (Tegretol), which is another alternative antimanic agent, has been associated with inducing an SLE-like syndrome.[69]

Benzodiazepines

Minor mood disturbances are likely to go unreported but may be quite common. Anxiety, emotional lability, or restlessness simulate adjustment disorders and may be easily missed. Stiefel and colleagues[73] suggest that the sudden onset of such symptoms during steroid treatment is highly suggestive of a steroid-induced etiology. If the symptoms interfere with the patient's quality of life, benzodiazepines with intermediate half-life and no active metabolites, such as lorazepam (Ativan) and oxazepam (Serax), may bring symptomatic relief.

Be sure to rule out other conditions that may mimic minor mood disturbances, such as delirium, respiratory distress, akathisia, and withdrawal syndromes.

Anabolic Steroids

Anabolic steroids are being increasingly used by athletes to add muscle bulk. They produce psychiatric effects (mainly mood disorders) both when administered and when withdrawn. The effects appear subtle when steroids are administered in physiological or mildly supraphysiological doses (as used in most medical and laboratory studies) but become more prominent with markedly supraphysiological doses (as often reported by athletes in naturalistic study designs).[61] Pope and Katz[61] compared 88 steroid-using athletes with 68 nonusers, using the Structured Clinical Interview for DSM-III-R.[71b] In comparison with the nonusers, steroid users were found to have

◆ More frequent gynecomastia, decreased mean testicular length, and higher cholesterol–high-density lipoprotein (HDL) ratios.
◆ Significantly more mood disorders during periods of steroid exposure ($P < .001$).
◆ Significantly more mood disorders ($P < .01$) overall. Strikingly, 23% of steroid users reported major mood

syndromes, often with psychotic features—mania, hypomania, or major depression—associated with steroid use. A highly significant relationship was found between the total weekly dose of steroids and the prevalence of mood disorders.

Additional findings of Pope and Katz[61] included the following:

◆ Users rarely abused other drugs simultaneously with steroids.
◆ Family history of major mood disorders did not predict major mood syndromes among steroid users themselves.
◆ The occurrence of other psychiatric disorders generally did not differ significantly between users and nonusers. Antisocial personality disorder was slightly but not significantly more common among steroid users than nonusers.

Aggressive or violent behavior often accompanies steroid-associated manic or hypomanic episodes:

> For example, one user, using his fists and a metal bar, seriously damaged three cars, all with their drivers cowering inside, because he had become annoyed by a traffic delay. Another was arrested for causing $1,000 of property damage during a fit of anger at a sports event; another was arrested for assaulting a motorist; another rammed his head through a wooden door; another became involved in a nearly successful murder plot; and another beat and almost killed his dog. Several users reported that they were expelled from their homes by parents, wives, or girlfriends because they became intolerably aggressive. Nearly all of these individuals denied comparable behavior before steroid use.[61] (p. 379)

Consistent with prior research,[55] these actions were not explainable by preexisting character traits—such as insecurity or narcissism—that might predispose these individuals to mood disorders. Pope and Katz[61] commented,

> Even if such [personality] traits did exist, they would not explain the relative absence of mood disorders in the nonusers or in the users at times when they were not taking steroids. Antisocial personality disorder . . . was

slightly more common among users than nonusers, but antisocial users did not display any greater prevalence of mood disorders than other users. Similarly, use of other illicit drugs might cause mood syndromes, and many subjects reported substantial use of other drugs, including cannabis, cocaine, amphetamines, opiates, and hallucinogens. But as noted earlier, steroid users largely abstained from other drugs while using steroids, and almost all cases of diagnosable mood disorders occurred in conjunction with steroids and not with other substances. (p. 381)

These findings are in agreement with previous reports.[13,16,18,49,50,55,59,60,74,77,82] Steroid-withdrawal depression further complicates the plight of a subgroup of these individuals, who cannot taper off the drugs without experiencing depression, anhedonia, fatigue, impaired concentration, and even suicidality.[4,16,59,77]

Finally, an unusual body-image disorder, termed *reverse anorexia nervosa*,[61,62] has been described among anabolic steroid users. These individuals were convinced that they looked small and weak, even though they were large and muscular. They refused to be seen in public, turned down invitations to the beach, or wore baggy sweatclothes even in the summer heat to avoid being seen as "small."

✦ SUMMARY

1. Patients are undereducated about the risk of steroid-related psychiatric side effects, and tend to underreport them. Persistence or even an increase of psychiatric symptoms during the first few days after initiating or increasing corticosteroids cannot necessarily be attributed to steroid therapy (e.g., rising fever after initiating antibiotics is not attributable initially to the antibiotics), although it is important to remain suspicious about these agents' potential role.

2. The *initial* response to corticosteroids is often a sense of well-being or improved appetite, which may be misleading in determining etiology retrospectively. Severe steroid-related psychiatric syndromes are relatively rare. The vast majority of mental changes are mild to moderate and do not herald the development of a full-blown psychosis or affective syndrome. Steroid-associated disturbances cover the spectrum of psychiatric symptoms, are unpredictable within a given patient, and shift radically during the course of the illness. Symptoms in descending order of frequency are depressive, manic, cyclical, agitated schizophreniform or paranoid psychosis, and delirium.

3. Psychiatric disturbances *usually occur within the first 2 weeks* of steroid exposure, but this varies. Chronicity of exposure has no predictive value. Psychological dependence is rare. Suicidal actions based on psychotic and depressive symptomatology do occur, so expressed suicidal ideation must be taken very seriously.

4. There is nothing characteristic about the presentation of steroid psychosis except its variability. Neither dosage nor treatment duration consistently forecasts onset, duration, severity, or type of psychiatric side effects. The only unambiguous "rule" is that higher steroid dosage (mean daily dose ≥ 60 mg prednisone) correlates strongly with higher psychotoxic risk. No particular steroid preparation appears to be more of an offender than others. There tends to be no lasting mental status changes once the syndrome remits.

5. Contrary to clinical intuition, neither a primary psychiatric history nor a current psychiatric syndrome predisposes to steroid psychiatric effects. Although still controversial, there is general consensus that psychiatric illness does not contraindicate steroid treatment.

6. Previous steroid-induced psychotoxicity does not predispose to subsequent episodes; conversely, prior freedom from steroid-induced psychiatric side effects does not predict or protect against future side effects.

7. The most frequent initial presentation of an impending steroid psychosis is a state of *hyperexcitability*, clearly perceived and reported by the patient. Increased irritability, labile mood, profound dysphoria, hyperacusis, and pressured thought processes also occur. These changes often antecede other, more serious cognitive disturbances by 72–96 hours. Once a steroid psychosis has been fully defined, it is likely to present with a full spectrum of psychotic symptoms. Alternate-day steroids, even in low doses, do not prevent psychiatric side effects.

8. Cognitive impairment may occur silently, at minuscule doses, and independently of concurrent psychosis or delirium.

9. Steroid withdrawal may paradoxically induce psychiatric disturbances, either immediately or as a delayed reaction. Such reactions include depression, psychosis, anxiety reactions, and delirium.

10. Although high steroid dosage correlates with greater psychotoxic incidence, no relationship has been

found with the severity or type of psychiatric disturbance. Indeed, patients often improve psychiatrically on steroids as the underlying pathophysiological condition is treated.

11. The usual treatment for psychiatric reactions is to discontinue or taper the steroids. General psychopharmacological principles apply, except that tricyclic antidepressants have been associated with worsening steroid psychosis. Fluoxetine (Prozac) appears promising for steroid-withdrawal depression, but selective serotonin reuptake inhibitors (SSRIs) have yet to be adequately explored. Neuroleptics are effective in shortening psychotic episodes once steroids are tapered.

12. High-dose anabolic steroid abuse produces major mood disorders, often with psychotic features, including mania, hypomania, or major depression. These effects cannot be explained by other drug abuse, which rarely occurs simultaneously with steroid exposure. A family history of major mood disorder does not predict major mood syndromes among steroid users themselves. Although presentations of other types of psychiatric disorders generally do not differ significantly between users and nonusers, dangerous aggressive or violent behavior often accompanies steroid-associated manic or hypomanic episodes. These findings are not explainable by preexisting character traits. Steroid-withdrawal depression further complicates management, as there is a subgroup of individuals who cannot taper off of anabolic steroids without experiencing depression, anhedonia, fatigue, impaired concentration, and even suicidality.

🔊 REFERENCES

1. Aapro M, Plezia P, Alberts D, et al: Double-blind crossover study of the antiemetic efficacy of high-dose dexamethasone versus high-dose metoclopramide. J Clin Oncol 2:466–471, 1984

2. Abbas A, Styra R: Valproate prophylaxis against steroid induced psychosis (letter). Can J Psychiatry 39:188–189, 1994

3. Allen R, Pitts FJ: ECT for depressed patients with lupus erythematosus. Am J Psychiatry 135:367–368, 1978

4. Allnutt S, Chaimowitz G: Anabolic steroid withdrawal depression: a case report (letter). Can J Psychiatry 39:317–318, 1994

5. Alpert E, Seigerman C: Steroid withdrawal psychosis in a patient with closed head injury. Arch Phys Med Rehabil 67:766–769, 1986

6. Amatruda T, Hollingsworth D, D'Esopo N: A study of the mechanism of steroid withdrawal syndrome. J Clin Endocrinol Metab 20:339–354, 1960

7. Bick P: Single case study: obsessive-compulsive behavior associated with dexamethasone treatment. J Nerv Ment Dis 171:253–254, 1983

8. Blazer D, Petrie W, Wilson W: Affective psychoses following renal transplant. Diseases of the Nervous System 37:663–667, 1976

9. Bloch M, Gur E, Shalev A: Chlorpromazine prophylaxis of steroid-induced psychosis. Gen Hosp Psychiatry 16:42–44, 1994

10. Borman M, Schmallenberg H: Suicide following cortisone treatment. JAMA 146:337–338, 1951

11. Boston Collaborative Drug Surveillance Program: Acute adverse reactions to prednisone in relation to dosage. Clin Pharmacol Ther 13:694–698, 1972

12. Breitbart W, Stiefel F, Kornblith A, et al: Neuropsychiatric disturbance in cancer patients with epidural spinal cord compression receiving high dose corticosteroids: a prospective comparison study. Psycho-Oncology 2:233–245, 1993

13. Brower K, Blow F, Beresford T, et al: Anabolicandrogenic steroid dependence. J Clin Psychiatry 50:31–33, 1989

14. Campbell K, Schubert D: Delirium after cessation of glucocorticoid therapy. Gen Hosp Psychiatry 13:270–272, 1991

15. Cass L, Alexander L, Enders M: Complications of corticotropin therapy in multiple sclerosis. JAMA 197:105–110, 1966

16. Corcoran J, Longo E: Psychological treatment of anabolic-androgenic steroid-dependent individuals. J Subst Abuse Treat 9:229–235, 1992

17. Cordess C, Folstein M, Drachman D: Psychiatric effects of alternate-day steroid therapy. Br J Psychiatry 138:504–506, 1981

18. Dalby J: Brief anabolic steroid use and sustained behavioral reaction. Am J Psychiatry 149:271–272, 1992

19. Della Bella L: Steroidphobia and the pulmonary patient. Am J Nurs 92:26–29, 1992

20. Dietch J: Steroid psychosis and tricyclic antidepressants (letter). Arch Gen Psychiatry 39:236, 1982

21. Doherty M, Garstin I, McClellan R: A steroid stupor in a surgical ward. Br J Psychiatry 158:125–127, 1991

22. Douglas C, Schwartz H: ECT for depression caused by lupus cerebritis: a case report. Am J Psychiatry 139:1631–1632, 1982

23. Falk W, Mahnke M, Poskanzer D: Lithium prophylaxis of corticotropin-induced psychosis. JAMA 241:1011–1012, 1979

24. Fallon B, Liebowitz M: Fluoxetine and extrapyramidal symptoms in CNS lupus. J Clin Psychopharmacol 11:147–148, 1991

25. Fisher G, Pelonero A, Ferguson C: Mania precipitated by prednisone and bromocriptine (letter). Gen Hosp Psychiatry 13:345–346, 1991

26. Fleishman S, Lesko L: Delirium and dementia, in Handbook of Psychooncology. Edited by Holland J, Rowland J. New York, Oxford University Press, 1990, pp 342–355

27. Fricchione G, Ayyala M, Holmes V: Steroid withdrawal psychiatric syndromes. Annals of Clinical Psychiatry 1:99–108, 1989

28. Glaser G: Psychotic reaction induced by corticotropin (ACTH) and cortisone. Psychosom Med 15:280–291, 1953

29. Glynne-Jones R, Vernon C, et al: Is steroid psychosis preventable by divided doses (letter). Lancet 2:1404, 1986

30. Goolker S, Schein J: Psychic effects of ACTH and cortisone. Psychosom Med 15:589–613, 1953

31. Hall R: Psychiatric adverse drug reactions: steroid psychosis. Clinical Advances in the Treatment of Psychiatric Disorders (A Service of Roerig) (April/May):8–10, 1991

32. Hall R, Popkin M, Kirkpatrick B: Tricyclic exacerbation of steroid psychosis. J Nerv Ment Dis 166:738–742, 1978

33. Hall R, Popkin M, Stickney S, et al: Presentation of the steroid psychoses. J Nerv Ment Dis 167:229–236, 1979

34. Joffe R, Denicoff K, Rubinow D, et al: Mood effects of alternate-day corticosteroid therapy in patients with systemic lupus erythematosus. Gen Hosp Psychiatry 10:56–60, 1988

35. Joffe R, Lippert G, Gray T, et al: Mood disorder and multiple sclerosis. Arch Neurol 44:376–378, 1987

36. Joffe R, Wolkowitz O, Rubinow D, et al: Alternate-day corticosteroid treatment, mood and plasma HVA in patients with systemic lupus erythematosus. Neuropsychobiology 19:17–19, 1988

37. Judd F, Burrows G, Norman T: Psychosis after withdrawal of steroid therapy. Med J Aust 2:350–351, 1983

38. Kahn D, Stevenson E, Douglas C: Effect of sodium valproate in three patients with organic brain syndromes. Am J Psychiatry 145:1010–1011, 1988

39. Kemp K, Lion J, Magram G: Lithium in the treatment of a manic patient with multiple sclerosis: a case report. Diseases of the Nervous System 38:210–211, 1977

40. Kershner P, Wang-Cheng R: Psychiatric side effects of steroid therapy. Psychosomatics 30:135–139, 1989

41. Kimball C: Psychological dependency on steroids? Ann Intern Med 75:111–113, 1971

42. Kornstein S, Gardner D: Endocrine disorders, in Psychiatric Care of the Medical Patient. Edited by Stoudemire A, Fogel B. New York, Oxford University Press, 1993, pp 657–681

43. Krauthammer C, Klerman G: Secondary mania. Arch Gen Psychiatry 35:1333–1339, 1978

44. Kreus K, Viljanen A, Kujala E, et al: Treatment of steroid-dependent asthma patients with beclomethasone dipropionate aerosol. Scandinavian Journal of Respiratory Diseases 56:47–57, 1975

45. Lewis A, Fleminger J: The psychiatric risk from corticotrophin and cortisone. Lancet 1:383–386, 1954

46. Lewis D, Smith R: Steroid-induced psychiatric syndromes. J Affect Disord 5:319–332, 1983

47. Lidz T, Carter J, Lewis B: Effects of ACTH and cortisone on mood and mentation. Psychosom Med 14:363–377, 1952

48. Ling M, Perry P, Tsuang M: Side effects of corticosteroid therapy: psychiatric aspects. Arch Gen Psychiatry 38:471–477, 1981

49. Lombardo J, Sickles R: Medical and performance-enhancing effects of anabolic steroids. Psychiatric Annals 22:19–23, 1992

50. Malone D, Dimeff R: The use of fluoxetine in depression associated with anabolic steroid withdrawal: a case series. J Clin Psychiatry 53:130–132, 1992

51. Markman M, Sheidler V, Ettinger D, et al: Antiemetic efficacy of dexamethasone. N Engl J Med 311:549–552, 1984

52. Martignoni E, Costa A, Sinforiani E, et al: The brain as a target for adrenocortical steroids: cognitive implications (special issue: Psychoneuroendocrinology of Aging: The Brain as a Target Organ of Hormones). Psychoneuroendocrinology 17:343–354, 1992

53. Moran M, Dubester S: Connective tissue diseases, in Psychiatric Care of the Medical Patient. Edited by Stoudemire A, Fogel B. New York, Oxford University Press, 1993, pp 739–756

54. Moss H, Panzak G: Steroid use and aggression (letter). Am J Psychiatry 149:1616, 1992

55. Moss H, Panzak G, Tarter R: Personality, mood, and psychiatric symptoms among anabolic steroid users. American Journal of Addictions 1:315–324, 1992

56. Patterson R, Walker C, Greenberger P, et al: Prednisonephobia. Allergy Proc 10:423–428, 1989

57. Perry S, Miller F: Psychiatric aspects of systemic lupus erythematosus, in Systemic Lupus Erythematosus, 2nd Edition. Edited by Lahita R. New York, Churchill Livingstone, 1992, pp 845–863

58. Pies R: Persistent bipolar illness after steroid administration. Arch Intern Med 141:1087, 1981

59. Pope H, Katz D: Affective and psychotic symptoms associated with anabolic steroid use. Am J Psychiatry 145:487–490, 1988

60. Pope H, Katz D: Psychiatric effects of anabolic steroids. Psychiatric Annals 22:24–29, 1992

61. Pope H, Katz D: Psychiatric and medical effects of anabolic-androgenic steroid use: a controlled study of 160 athletes. Arch Gen Psychiatry 51:375–382, 1994

62. Pope HJ, Katz D, Hudson J: Anorexia nervosa and "reverse anorexia" among 108 male bodybuilders. Compr Psychiatry 34:406–409, 1993

63. Quismorio F: Systemic corticosteroid therapy in systemic lupus erythematosus, in Dubois' Lupus Erythematosus, 4th Edition. Edited by Wallace D, Hahn B. Philadelphia, PA, Lea & Febiger, 1993, pp 574–587

64. Raskin D: Steroid-induced panic disorder (letter). Am J Psychiatry 141:1647, 1984

65. Reckart M, Eisendrath S: Exogenous corticosteroid effects on mood and cognition: case presentations. Int J Psychosom 37:58–61, 1990

66. Ritchie E: Toxic psychosis under cortisone and corticotrophin. Journal of Mental Science 102:830–837, 1956

67. Roberts A: The value of ECT in delirium. Br J Psychiatry 109:653–655, 1963

68. Rome H, Braceland F: Psychological response to cortico-tropin, cortisone, and related steroid substances. JAMA 148:27–30, 1952

69. Schmidt S, Welcker M, Greil W, et al: Carbamazepine-induced systemic lupus erythematosus. Br J Psychiatry 161:560–561, 1992

70. Shapiro H: Psychopathology in the lupus patient, in Dubois' Lupus Erythematosus, 4th Edition. Edited by Wallace D, Hahn B. Philadelphia, PA, Lea & Febiger, 1993, pp 386–402

71. Sharfstein S, Sack D, Fauci A: Relationship between alternate-day corticosteroid therapy and behavioral abnormalities. JAMA 248:2987–2989, 1982

71a. Silva R, Tolstunov L: Steroid-induced psychosis: report of case. J Oral Maxillofac Surg 53:183–186, 1995

71b. Spitzer R, Williams J, Gibbon M, et al: The structured clinical interview for DSM-III-R (SCID): history, rationale and description. Arch Gen Psychiatry 49:624–629, 1992

72. Stern M, Robbins E: Psychoses in systemic lupus erythematosus. Arch Gen Psychiatry 3:205–212, 1960

73. Stiefel F, Breitbart W, Holland J: Corticosteroids in cancer: neuropsychiatric complications. Cancer Invest 7:479–491, 1989

74. Su T-P, Pagliaro M, Schmidt P, et al: Neuropsychiatric effects of anabolic steroids in male normal volunteers. JAMA 269:2760–2764, 1993

75. Terao T, Mizuki T, Ohji T, et al: Antidepressant effect of lithium in patients with systemic lupus erythematosus and cerebral infarction, treated with corticosteroid. Br J Psychiatry 164:109–110, 1994

76. Train G, Winkler E: Homicidal psychosis while under ACTH. Psychosomatics 3:317–322, 1962

77. Uzych L: Anabolic-androgenic steroids and psychiatric-related effects: a review. Can J Psychiatry 37:23–28, 1992

78. Varney N, Alexander B, MacIndoe J: Reversible steroid dementia in patients without steroid psychosis. Am J Psychiatry 141:369–372, 1984

79. Viswanathan R, Glickman L: Clonazepam in the treatment of steroid-induced mania in a patient after renal transplantation (letter). N Engl J Med 320:319–320, 1989

80. Watanabe T, Sylvester C, Manaligod J: Mania or panic associated with dexamethasone chemotherapy in adolescents. J Adolesc Health 15:345–347, 1994

81. Williams G, Dluhy R: Diseases of the adrenal cortex, in Harrison's Principles of Internal Medicine, 12th Edition. Edited by Wilson J, Braunwald E, Isselbacher K, et al. New York, McGraw-Hill, Health Professions Division, 1991, pp 1713–1739

82. Williamson D, Young A: Psychiatric effects of androgenic and anabolic-androgenic steroid abuse in men: a brief review of the literature. Journal of Psychopharmacology 6:20–26, 1992

83. Wolkowitz O: Prospective controlled studies of the behavioral and biological effects of exogenous corticosteroids. Psychoneuroendocrinology 19:233–255, 1994

84. Wolkowitz O, Rapaport M: Long-lasting behavioral changes following prednisone withdrawal (letter). JAMA 261:1731–1732, 1989

85. Wolkowitz O, Reus V, Weingartner H, et al: Cognitive effects of corticosteroids. Am J Psychiatry 147:1297–1303, 1990

86. Wyszynski A, Wyszynski B: Treatment of depression with fluoxetine in corticosteroid-dependent central nervous system Sjögren's syndrome. Psychosomatics 34:173–176, 1993

The HIV-Infected Patient

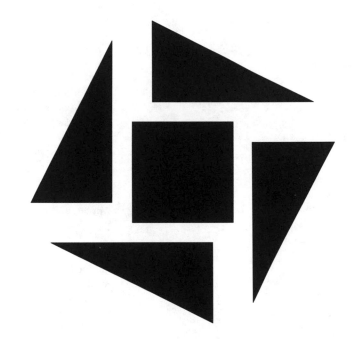

CHAPTER 6

◣◢ CONTENTS ◣◢

■ Introduction to Chapter 6 215
■ Case Presentation: Mr. Lowe: The Depressed
   HIV Patient 216
■ Questions 216
■ Answers 219
■ Discussion 220
  ◆ Classification of HIV Illness 220
  ◆ AIDS Dementia Complex (ADC) 220
    Features 220
    Clinical Course 221
    Differential Diagnosis 221
      ADC Versus Senile Dementia of the
        Alzheimer Type 222
        Controversy: asymptomatic
        seropositive individuals and
        cognitive decline 222
    Assessment 222
    Treatment 223
      Pharmacological 223
      Nonpharmacological Management Strategies 224
    Neurological Correlates of ADC 225
      Neuropathology 225
      Significance of Laboratory Studies 225
      Proposed Pathophysiological Mechanisms . . 225
  ◆ Psychiatric Morbidity, Part I 226
    AIDS Anxiety Versus AIDS Phobia 226
      Prodromal Symptoms and Seroconversion . . 226
    Major Depression in HIV Infection 226
      Prevalence 226
        Risk factors 227
      Suicide, Ethical Issues, and Competency . . . 227
      Differential Diagnosis 228
      Treatment 228
        Tricyclic antidepressants 229
        Psychostimulants 229
        Alprazolam for depression 230
        Monoamine oxidase inhibitors 230
        Newer agents 230
        Zidovudine and antidepressants . . . 231
        Electroconvulsive therapy 231
    HIV and the Psychiatric Patient 231
      The Psychiatric Inpatient Setting 231
      The Chronically Mentally Ill 231
      AIDS Incorporated Into Other
        Psychopathology 232
      The Intravenous Drug User 232

    Caregiver Issues 233
      Family, Friends, and Significant Others . . . 233
      Staff 233
      Burnout 234
  ◆ Summary 235
  ◆ References 236
■ Case Presentation: Ms. Newman: The Female
   HIV Patient 247
■ Questions 247
■ Answers 250
■ Discussion 251
  ◆ Antibody Testing: To Know, or Not to Know? . . 251
    Serotesting and Psychiatric Morbidity 251
    Delayed Reactions to Seropositivity 252
    The Knowledge-Behavior Gap 252
    Countertransference 253
  ◆ Psychotherapy 253
    Psychotherapy and Safer Sex 253
    Health Locus of Control 253
    Survivors of Childhood Sexual Abuse 254
    Psychotherapy and AIDS 255
    Psychoneuroimmunology 256
  ◆ Sex, Culture, and Stereotype 257
    Ethnic Minorities and Risk 258
    Gay Men 259
    Women and Children 259
      Heterosexual HIV Transmission 259
      Maternal HIV Transmission 260
      Conclusion 261
  ◆ Psychiatric Morbidity, Part II 261
    Anxiety and Adjustment Disorders 261
      Treatment 261
        Benzodiazepines 261
        Buspirone 261
        Propranolol 261
        Trazodone 261
        Antihistamines 262
    Mania 262
    Psychosis 262
      Features 262
      Differential Diagnosis 263
      Neuroleptics 263
    Delirium 263
  ◆ Summary 264
  ◆ References 266

As soon as the ink dries on the latest human immunodeficiency virus (HIV) review, it is outdated; the literature on acquired immunodeficiency syndrome (AIDS) is a burgeoning one. We have tried to construct a basic framework that the reader may continue to update according to personal interest and clinical relevance.

AIDS dementia complex (ADC) appears in more detail than perhaps would interest many psychiatric readers. We feel its clinical relevance justifies this emphasis. Although management is often relegated to neurologists, early ADC—the new "great imitator"[257]—may resemble conditions as varied as neurosyphilis,[251] Alzheimer's disease, depression, anxiety disorders, psychotic disorders, and substance abuse. Furthermore, ADC patients often evolve complications, such as depression, mania, anxiety, and psychosis, that prompt psychiatric consultation. It is the only type of dementia to be discussed in this volume; additional topics will appear in the *Casebook of Neuropsychiatry*.

The cases have been taken from our clinical practice. Legal issues are briefly summarized in Appendix F ("A Mini-Outline of Competency and Informed Consent"). Use the questions as you find useful.

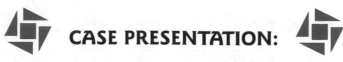

CASE PRESENTATION:

Mr. Lowe: The Depressed HIV Patient

Mr. Lowe is a 32-year-old attorney who has been in psychotherapy for help dealing with the death of his lover, Mark, and several close friends from AIDS. Most distressing has been the intellectual decline of his friends, many quite accomplished in their respective fields. Family history is notable for senile dementia of the Alzheimer type in his mother. She has been institutionalized for the past 5 years. The patient connects his grief about "losing her" to a dementing illness with his experience of losing Mark and his friends to AIDS. He is on no medication. There is no personal or family history of psychiatric illness. He drinks socially. There is no substance abuse. Although he

engaged in "the bathhouse scene" in his early 20s, sometimes having as many as four sexual partners in one evening, he has practiced safe sex for the past 5 years. He does not know his serological status.

Mental status exam reveals a handsome, conservatively dressed man. His speech is goal directed, coherent, and logical. His affect is full. Mood is depressed and appropriate to expressed thought. There are no delusions or hallucinations. There is no suicidal ideation. At the time of cognitive testing 18 months ago, he was alert, fully oriented, and cognitively intact.

 QUESTIONS

Choose all that apply.

1. Mr. Lowe misses several therapy sessions because of fever, sore throat, myalgia, and malaise. He completely recuperates but becomes preoccupied with the fear that he has AIDS. In trying to assess how realistic his concerns are, you consider:
    a. Mr. Lowe's concerns are realistic, since this presentation is characteristic of the syndrome that occurs soon after exposure to the AIDS virus.
    b. The initial presentation of AIDS is usually inexorable and leads to rapid deterioration, unlike these symptoms, which have resolved.
    c. Mr. Lowe is among the "worried well" described in the literature.
    d. Mr. Lowe's concerns about the flulike symptoms are along the lines of obsessional symptoms, and are not rational.

2. Several months later, Mr. Lowe is confirmed to be HIV positive. He states categorically that he is not afraid to die, but admits to difficulty sleeping because it reminds him of death. He is concerned about possible effects on his memory and intellectual functioning, given the nature

of his job and the agony of having watched his mother's deterioration from Alzheimer's disease. What are true statements about AIDS dementia complex (ADC)?
    a. The presence of Mr. Lowe's defensive denial of fearing death argues in favor of intact cognition.
    b. The appearance of ADC would herald a rapidly progressive downhill medical course in a patient like Mr. Lowe.
    c. Were he to develop ADC, initial symptoms would more likely be apathy or social withdrawal than psychotic ideation.
    d. ADC cannot be diagnosed unless there are other *systemic* manifestations AIDS.

3. Mr. Lowe wants to begin zidovudine (formerly azidothymidine [AZT]) immediately, as he feels it to be his "only hope." He becomes exasperated and impatient that his physician wants him "to undergo a lot of tests that waste time" before starting the medication. He scores 30 out of 30 on the Mini-Mental State Exam (MMSE). Which of the following are true?
    a. Once present, the neurological and cognitive abnormalities of HIV infection are resistant to improvement with zidovudine.

b. ADC-related abnormalities on positron-emission tomography (PET) scans in HIV-positive individuals improve with zidovudine.

c. Magnetic resonance imaging (MRI) studies have proven most helpful in diagnosing preclinical ADC.

d. Mr. Lowe's normal MMSE effectively rules out ADC for the time being.

4. Mr. Lowe agrees to a complete neurological and neuropsychological workup before beginning zidovudine. Results are pending. Which of the following is true?

a. Most of the literature shows that an asymptomatic, seropositive person like Mr. Lowe would be likely to demonstrate significant cognitive deficits on neuropsychological testing.

b. Most of the literature shows that an asymptomatic, seropositive person like Mr. Lowe would be *unlikely* to demonstrate significant cognitive deficits on neuropsychological testing.

c. Mr. Lowe's association of ADC with the dementia of Alzheimer's disease is fairly accurate, as the clinical picture in both conditions is similar.

d. Aphasic disorders occur early in ADC.

5. The *initial* cognitive disturbance of HIV infection produces . . .

a. Anterograde amnesia.

b. Disorientation.

c. Slowed mentation.

d. Language disturbance.

6. Which of the following are characteristic neuropathological changes of HIV infection?

a. Cortical changes predominating over subcortical changes

b. Relative neocortical sparing

c. Vacuolar changes of the spinal cord

d. Relative sparing of the spinal cord

e. Relative sparing of cerebral white matter

7. The routine neurological and neuropsychological workups show no abnormalities. Within the next 8 months, Mr. Lowe experiences increasing dysphoria, diminished concentration, and guilty ruminations about whom he may have infected with the virus. He begins to withdraw from social gatherings and feels apathetic about his work, stating that "it doesn't really matter in the overall scheme of things." He acknowledges that he has begun to think about taking his own life. Which of the following

are true regarding the diagnosis of depression in HIV-positive and AIDS patients?

a. Major depression and ADC overlap symptomatically.

b. Persistent suicidal ideation after serological testing is limited to individuals who learn they are seropositive.

c. Most *completed* suicides among terminally ill patients are rational decisions made independently of clinical depression.

d. Patients in the stage of full-blown AIDS have suicide rates that are higher than those of individuals who are HIV positive and asymptomatic.

8. Mr. Lowe's suicidal ruminations increase. He cannot get out of bed in the morning, and feels "paralyzed" by depression. His internist reports that medically he is asymptomatic and doing well. He is not yet on any medication. You decide to admit him to the psychiatry service, but encounter staff resistance to the admission of "yet another" HIV-positive patient. The unit chief confides in you that the staff is exhausted and still grieving the recent deaths of two young, well-known patients from AIDS. Which of the following is/are true regarding the impact of AIDS patients on caregivers?

a. Conclusions about the psychological toll of AIDS on caregivers come mainly from controlled studies appearing in the psychiatric literature.

b. Caregivers were found to frequently express aversion to AIDS as a disease, but not aversion to AIDS patients themselves.

c. AIDS phobia is positively correlated with homophobia in hospital workers.

d. Psychiatrists and family physicians have been found to be the physician groups *least* comfortable with the communicability of AIDS.

e. All of the above.

9. Mr. Lowe is admitted to the psychiatric service. He settles into the ward routine, but is frightened by several psychotic patients who are also on the service. Which of the following are true regarding HIV infection and the chronically mentally ill?

a. Despite assumptions to the contrary, chronic psychiatric patients who do not use intravenous (IV) drugs are at minimally greater risk for HIV infection than the general population.

b. Chronically mentally ill patients have surprisingly good concrete understanding of AIDS and risk-reduction measures, but have difficulty implementing them.

c. A diagnosis of bipolar disorder is significantly correlated with increased risk of HIV infection.

d. Patients with borderline personality disorder are at heightened risk for HIV infection.

10. On psychiatry, Mr. Lowe attends an HIV support group, where several members are IV drug users. He befriends a man who is now abstinent. Which of the following is/are true regarding IV drug use and HIV infection?

a. High-risk drug use behavior is more likely to change than high-risk sexual behavior in IV drug users.

b. High-risk sexual behavior is more likely to change than high-risk drug use in IV drug users.

c. Smoking, sniffing, or orally ingesting drugs are not yet associated with the spread of HIV.

d. Data corroborate the clinical observation that substance abusers are unwilling or unable to change high-risk behaviors, even when confronted with the threat of AIDS.

11. Substance-abusing patients most likely to seek treatment are those who . . .

a. Abuse *non*IV drugs.

b. Abuse IV drugs.

c. Are not distinguishable on the basis of drug-use route.

d. None of the above.

12. Substance-abusing patients who are *most* likely to modify their *sexual* risk behavior . . .

a. Abuse *non*IV drugs.

b. Abuse IV drugs.

c. Are not distinguishable on the basis of drug-use route.

d. None of the above.

13. Syringe sharers differ significantly from nonsharers on the basis of . . .

a. Self-reported HIV antibody status.

b. Number of sexual partners.

c. Attendance at syringe-exchange programs.

d. Recent involvement in crime.

e. Few, if any, characteristics.

14. Which of the following is/are valid to consider in formulating a treatment plan for Mr. Lowe?

a. Agitation predicts those patients likely to improve on tricyclic antidepressant (TCA) treatment.

b. Alprazolam (Xanax) has been shown to exacerbate depression in AIDS patients.

c. Tricyclic medications have greater antidepressant efficacy in patients with more advanced disease compared with their more physically robust counterparts.

d. Cognitive deficits predispose to adverse tricyclic side effects.

15. All of the following are valid considerations *except* . . .

a. Agents such as amitriptyline (Elavil) or doxepin (Sinequan) should be avoided in cognitively impaired HIV patients.

b. The drying of mucous membranes may be a helpful side effect in AIDS patients with opportunistic infections.

c. Zidovudine has been associated with improvement in depressive symptoms.

d. Fluoxetine (Prozac) interacts adversely with zidovudine.

e. Monoamine oxidase inhibitors (MAOIs) interact adversely with zidovudine.

16. Mr. Lowe is unable to tolerate the anticholinergic side effects of the TCAs. He refuses alprazolam (Xanax) and will not consider electroconvulsive therapy (ECT) because of the possible risk of cognitive impairment. What are valid considerations in choosing either bupropion (Wellbutrin) or fluoxetine (Prozac) to treat this patient?

a. Fluoxetine is poorly tolerated.

b. Both fluoxetine and bupropion are effective in cognitively intact HIV patients but not in those with dementia.

c. The most serious side effect of bupropion in HIV-infected individuals is its propensity to produce hypertension.

d. HIV patients who develop seizures on bupropion may be rechallenged later with the same medication.

17. Mr. Lowe's depression markedly improves and he is discharged home on zidovudine 250 mg tid and fluoxetine 20 mg daily. He returns to work and resumes weekly psychotherapy. In the context of making appropriate arrangements about getting his affairs in order, including writing a will, he queries you on what treatment options are available if he develops ADC or his depression no longer responds to fluoxetine. Which are valid?

a. In cognitively impaired AIDS patients, psychostimulants improve mood but not apathy or anorexia.

b. Psychostimulants improve mood, but not the cognitive performance of patients with ADC.

c. TCAs are not as effective as psychostimulants in patients with advanced HIV disease.

d. Psychostimulants are not as effective as TCAs in patients with advanced HIV disease.

e. A major drawback of psychostimulants is that they should not be coadministered with narcotic analgesics.

f. Dextroamphetamine is preferred over methylphenidate.

⟐ Answers

1. Answer: a (p. 226)
2. Answer: c (pp. 220–221)
3. Answer: b (pp. 222–225)
4. Answer: b (pp. 220–222)
5. Answer: c (p. 220)
6. Answer: b, c (p. 225)
7. Answer: a (pp. 221, 227–228)
8. Answer: c, d (pp. 233–235)
9. Answer: c, d (pp. 231–232)
10. Answer: a (pp. 232–233)
11. Answer: b (pp. 232–233)
12. Answer: a (pp. 232–233)
13. Answer: b, d (pp. 232–233)
14. Answer: d (pp. 228–231)
15. Answer: b, d (pp. 228–231)
16. Answer: d (pp. 230–231)
17. Answer: c (pp. 229–230)

🔷 CLASSIFICATION OF HIV ILLNESS

The HIV nosology has mutated quickly over the years and it is a struggle to keep pace. Some notes:

◆ The older terminology formerly distinguished between ARC (AIDS-related complex) and AIDS. Much of the psychosocial literature of the late 1980s investigated ARC patients, who had generalized lymphadenopathy but no other systemic signs of HIV infection. ARC no longer exists in the current terminology.

◆ The term *human immunodeficiency virus* has been supplanted by *human immunodeficiency viruses*; most relevant to our discussion is the HIV-1 strain.

◆ The American Academy of Neurology[6] has suggested categorizing HIV-related central nervous system (CNS) disease into three groups for purposes of research:

   1. **HIV-1–associated dementia complex (HAD)** (AIDS dementia complex [ADC]) (see Appendix I)
   2. **HIV-1–associated minor cognitive-motor disorder** (reserved for individuals who demonstrate cognitive or motor dysfunction not severe enough to interfere with activities of daily living or to qualify for a full-blown dementia syndrome)
   3. **HIV-1–associated myelopathy**

◆ **Synonyms:**
   HIV-1–associated dementia complex (HAD) =
   AIDS dementia complex (ADC) =
   AIDS encephalopathy =
   HIV encephalopathy
   (Brew[42] has suggested that *HIV encephalitis* be reserved as a histopathological term referring to the demonstration of productive HIV-1 infection of the brain. *HIV encephalitis* is sometimes used synonymously with *HIV encephalopathy.*)

◆ The Centers for Disease Control and Prevention (CDC) have revised the classification system for HIV infection to emphasize the clinical importance of the $CD4^+$ T-lymphocyte count in categorizing HIV-related clinical conditions. The current classification system is listed in Appendix J.

See also the excellent 1995 review by Wallack et al.[308a]

🔷 AIDS DEMENTIA COMPLEX (ADC)

Although the diagnostic criteria and nomenclature of ADC is still evolving, ADC's estimated prevalence, unfortunately, continues to mount:

◆ ADC was found in approximately 7.3% of people with AIDS in a recent large-scale epidemiological study, with prevalence highest in patients less than 15 years old or more than 75 years old.[151]

◆ The incidence of *minor* cognitive impairments was higher than 7.3%, at about 20% of systemically *symptomatic* patients.[54] The relationship between these minor deficits and the subsequent development of dementia is not known.

We will summarize ADC in some detail below, and include a brief survey of its neurological features.

Features

ADC is a multifaceted syndrome consisting of cognitive, affective, motor, and behavioral abnormalities. The symptoms are often subtle and insidious in onset, with *slowed decision making* most prominent. This description differs from the amnesia, language disturbance, and agnosia typifying the early stages of *senile dementia of the Alzheimer type* (SDAT), which would be considered a "cortical"-type dementia. DSM-IV[6b] specifically describes *dementia due to HIV disease* (code 294.9).

◆ ADC follows a different pattern than SDAT. It is closer to "subcortical dementia," which has been described in Parkinson's disease, Huntington's disease, Wilson's disease, and others.[69] Although cognitive functioning is eventually globally impaired, *insight is often preserved* until late in the illness.[42] Depression is not uncommon.

◆ The deficits of ADC are concentrated in the following areas:[180,187a,270,271,299,304]
   Cognitive:
   • Mental slowing (less verbal, less spontaneous, not as quick)
   • Poor concentration and attention (e.g., losing track of conversations)
   • Forgetfulness (appointments, names, historical details)

- Confusion (time, place)
- Difficulties in abstraction, problem solving, or manipulating acquired knowledge

Behavior:
- Apathy, social withdrawal
- Personality changes
- Agitated psychosis

Motor:
- Loss of coordination
- Fine motor difficulties (e.g., impaired handwriting)
- Eye movement abnormalities
- Unsteady gait
- Leg weakness
- Tremor

Clinical Course

ADC is a dementia of variable progress and duration. Some ADC patients develop other systemic AIDS manifestations during the course of the dementia. Others have a more indolent, prolonged, and relatively stable course. There are some patients who may compensate for cognitive loss, while others deteriorate rapidly to a severe vegetative dementia over a period of weeks.[25,226] It is not possible to predict the clinical course for a given patient.

Brew[42] has noted that patients with ADC complain of their thinking being slowed and their concentration diminished.

- They report, for example, losing track of the conversation while speaking to people and having to reread a paragraph or page to get it to "sink in."
- Additionally, they complain of forgetfulness, usually for day-to-day events.
- Patients in the early stages may report that they cannot keep up with their personal finances or business activities, describing a constant state of "befuddlement."[77]
- Neurobehavioral abnormalities may soon follow,[23] such as motor complaints of clumsiness, sloppy handwriting, tremor, and poor balance, especially with rapid head turns.

Finally, the apathy and social withdrawal of insidious-onset ADC *may resemble and coincide with psychodynamically motivated phenomena like resistance, denial, and repression.* ADC-related cognitive changes are distinguished by "forgetfulness" that is not limited to psychotherapy or psychodynamically valent material. Such memory and problem-solving deficits will adversely affect the patient's ability to follow through and maintain continuity in psychotherapy.[27] Fortunately, there have been only moderate[170] to weak[281,282] correlations between neuropsychological impairment and frank depressive disorders. *Since insight regarding their intellectual decline is usually preserved until late in the illness, these patients often experience reactions of fear and grief.*

Differential Diagnosis

ADC is in the differential diagnosis of any psychiatric symptom occurring in an HIV-infected individual. Advanced cases are easy to spot, and are characterized by global cognitive deterioration, gross impairment of social functioning, disorientation, agitation, mutism, vacant stare, spasticity and myoclonus, bowel and bladder incontinence, and, rarely, coma.[113] *The symptoms of early ADC, however, may be easily misdiagnosed as depression,[103] particularly in the initial phases when symptoms coincide with affective changes of depression, including dysphoria, anxiety, irritability, apathy, and social withdrawal.*[25] Perry[226] has suggested that dysphoric thought content, such as low self-esteem, irrational guilt, and self-denigration, marks depressive syndromes but not ADC. However, these negative self-perceptions may also reflect patients' awareness of their declining cognitive abilities.

Psychotic ideation and inappropriate behavior are relatively *uncommon* early features of ADC.[113] More typical is the insidious onset of **apathy or social withdrawal** in a previously healthy seropositive individual. Nonetheless, ADC has also been mistaken for primary psychotic disorders,[84,131,133,134,155,226,255,295] mania,[34,72,81,82,108,238,262] Alzheimer's disease,[163] and anxiety and adjustment disorders.[216,298] El-Mallakh[83] has speculated that a window of vulnerability to psychosis or mania may occur relatively early in the dementing process.

- **CAUTION!** *The diagnosis of ADC is one of exclusion. Changes in mental status should prompt* **urgent** *evaluation, as they may herald other conditions, such as new neurological or infectious complications.*[18,180a]

It is critical to distinguish HIV dementia from infections such as cytomegalovirus (CMV) encephalitis, cerebral toxoplasmosis, neurosyphilis, and cryptococcal or tuberculous meningitis. One frequent CNS opportunistic infection that is easily mistaken for HIV dementia is CMV encephalitis. Distinguishing features from HIV dementia include coexisting CMV infection (e.g., retinitis, colitis), electrolyte abnormalities reflecting CMV adrenalitis, and periventricular abnormalities on MRI consistent with periventriculitis.[196]

ADC Versus Senile Dementia of the Alzheimer Type

Kernutt et al.[163] and others[55,208,248] have emphasized that early ADC may be overlooked in the differential diagnosis of dementia in older patients, especially when systemic symptoms or obvious risk factors are absent. Pointing out that AIDS has been called the new "great imitator" of neurological disease,[257] they reviewed five published case reports[13,107,206,256,310] describing patients ranging in age from 57 to 76 years.

- These patients sought medical attention because of significant decline in short-term memory and concentration, personality changes, weight loss, incontinence, or falls. Their rate of deterioration before medical assessment varied from 6 weeks to 5 years.
- Risk factors for HIV infection (blood transfusion[310] and homosexual orientation[107]) were initially obvious in only two of the patients at the time of presentation. In the remaining three, homosexuality was later established in one patient,[256] bisexuality suspected in another,[206] and heterosexual transmission presumed in the last (from a deceased spouse with non-Hodgkin's lymphoma after open-heart surgery).[256]
- All five cases were diagnosed as "dementia," with three specified as senile dementia of the Alzheimer type.[206,256,310]
- The most common computed tomography (CT) findings were cerebral atrophy and ventricular dilatation.
- Concurrent systemic illness was initially absent, although two patients later developed opportunistic infections.

Kernutt et al.[163] have recommended guidelines for diagnosing HIV/AIDS in the older person:

- Patient in a known risk group (i.e., homosexual or bisexual, or having received a *blood transfusion before 1985*)
- Spouse/partner in a known risk group (as above)
- Presentation of dementia with a predominantly "subcortical" pattern of cognitive deficits
- Dementia with atypical features (e.g., rapid progression, focal neurological signs)
- Presence of significant systemic symptoms, especially weight loss, opportunistic infections, pneumonia

Controversy: asymptomatic seropositive individuals and cognitive decline. Like so many other areas in the study of HIV, the neuropsychological impairment of asymptomatic, seropositive individuals has been controversial. Several studies have reported frightening evidence that neuropsychological impairment occurred at all stages of HIV illness, including the asymptomatic stage.[49a,121,180,281,282,315] *Fortunately, most studies have failed to find statistically significant differences between asymptomatic seropositive subjects and comparable seronegative control subjects.*[33,61,80,102,116,152,158,185,192,194,195,203,204,217,235a,238a,267,268,305] When subtle cognitive deficits do occur in the asymptomatic stages of HIV infection, they are not always accompanied by neurological changes and do not seem to affect subjects' social functioning.[184] The prevalence of neurobehavioral abnormalities steadily increases, however, with duration of illness[38] and advancing stages of infection.[37,283a]

- There is some small comfort in the knowledge that the cognitive abnormalities occurring with asymptomatic HIV infection appear to be minimal—a finding recently corroborated by the World Health Organization Neuropsychiatric AIDS Study[183,184] and longitudinal data from the Multicenter AIDS Cohort Study.[267] It is still not known whether these minor abnormalities constitute the same disorder as ADC, why they occur, or whether they will progress to a more severe condition. We advise the clinician to make no assumptions about cognitive status, but to evaluate each patient individually.
- Some of the confounding factors in assessing cognition across subject groups have included differences in neuropsychological instruments, drug and alcohol use, lifestyle, medications, educational level, and previous neurological and/or psychiatric illness.[49]

Assessment

It has been clinically observed that the Mini-Mental State Exam (MMSE),[100] which does *not* assess response time, is not sufficiently sensitive for detecting ADC.[87] Even late in the dementing disease, MMSE scores may underestimate ADC cognitive dysfunction.[249] As mentioned, *cognitive slowing* appears to be the first cognitive disturbance of HIV infection. Most useful are test batteries[204] that assess the following:

- Psychomotor speed
- Information encoding
- Information retrieval
- Concentration
- Attention

Such batteries include the Symbol Digit Modalities Test,[309a] Part B of the Trail Making Test,[246a] and tests of visuoconstructional abilities.

◆ The Trail Making Test is particularly sensitive for identifying and monitoring HIV-related neurocognitive impairment.[113] It assesses changes in psychomotor speed, concentration, and attention.

The literature abounds with neuropsychological batteries and bedside screening instruments of ADC, although rigorous, controlled studies to validate them tend to be lacking. One example notable for its succinctness and ease of administration follows:

◆ Jones et al.[154] developed a new rapid bedside test of cognition targeted for HIV-infected patients with slowed mentation, poor concentration, and impaired psychomotor speed. The test requires timed performance of a sequencing and category-switching task. Patients were asked to count to 20, say the alphabet, and then to alternate between the numbers and letters: 1-A, 2-B, 3-C, and so forth. The number of correct alternation pairs in 30 seconds defines the score, with the maximum score being 52. The test takes less than 1 minute to administer, and correlates with deficits on the MMSE and Trail Making B. A cutoff score of 15 on this test correlated with an abnormal MMSE. **Comment:** As mentioned, the MMSE has questionable sensitivity in detected early ADC. Thus, it is unclear if this bedside screen will prove to be useful after more controlled studies in this population.

Sidtis[270] has described a more detailed 30-minute test battery that requires minimal instrumentation and is highly sensitive to ADC. The vocabulary subtest of the Wechsler Adult Intelligence Scale—Revised (WAIS-R)[309a] is given first, correlated with education level to provide an estimate of premorbid intellectual function. Several brief tests then follow:

◆ **Timed Gait:** This test assesses walking speed. A 10-yard distance is clearly marked, and the subject is instructed to walk as quickly as possible (without running) to the 10-yard marker, step over it with one foot, turn around, and return, still walking as quickly as possible.
◆ **Grooved Pegboard:** Administered for both dominant and nondominant hands, this test is timed and requires fine motor control, rapid eye-hand coordination, as well as the use of somatosensory and visual feedback.

◆ **Trail Making A and B; Digit Symbol (subtest of the WAIS-R):** These instruments require visual search, performance on sequential tasks, and the ability to switch mental set rapidly. They add perceptual and cognitive components to the battery.
◆ **Finger Tapping Test:** Also administered for both dominant and nondominant hands, this test assesses the speed of simple, repetitive movements.
◆ **Auditory Verbal Learning Test:** This instrument measures learning and memory over five repetitions of a 15-item word list. Immediate recall of the word list is challenged using an interference procedure, and recall after a 20-minute delay is also obtained.
◆ **Profile of Mood States:** This self-report questionnaire addresses several psychological states, including depression, anger, fatigue, and "vigor."

The results of this group of tests are then summarized by creating an average normalized score.[270] The test battery serves as a complement to thorough neurological evaluation.

Robertson and Hall[249] advise against routine formal neuropsychological testing when the diagnosis is clinically obvious, because of costliness and the distress caused to the patient. They recommend restricting testing to instances in which the diagnosis is ambiguous.

Additional methods for neuropsychological assessment are reviewed by others.[283]

Treatment

Pharmacological Treatment

Antiviral agents used to treat HIV-1 CNS infection include zidovudine (Retrovir; formerly azidothymidine [AZT]), dideoxycytidine (Hivid; ddC), stavudine (d4T), and dideoxyinosine (Videx; ddI). These agents are nucleoside antagonists of the HIV-1 reverse transcriptase (an enzyme critical in HIV's life cycle) and are able to cross the blood-brain barrier. Many of the side effects are unpleasant, even at therapeutic doses; they include headache, malaise, nausea, and insomnia. The most experience has accrued with zidovudine.

Although not unanimous,[120,167,168] encouraging preliminary evidence shows that zidovudine may reduce the incidence and severity of ADC, as well as improve neurological and neuropsychological performance in AIDS patients.[158a,305a]

◆ Clinical improvement was shown in three out of four and in six out of seven patients with HIV-associated neurological disease in two studies.[319,320] An increased, more homogeneous pattern of cerebral glucose metabolism was found on PET scanning in two patients treated with zidovudine.[320] There were also improvements in nerve conduction studies and neuropsychological tests of attention, fine motor coordination, and memory.[320]

- Zidovudine was found to significantly reduce the occurrence of productive HIV infection of the brain in AIDS.[122]
- A double-blind, placebo-controlled trial reported significant differences between zidovudine and placebo groups on measures of cognition, motor skills, attention, and memory.[263]
- Cognitive scores, gait, and coordination were markedly improved with zidovudine in children with HIV encephalopathy.[235]
- The incidence of ADC has declined with the introduction of zidovudine.[237]
- There was significant neurological improvement in 61.2% of patients treated daily with 600–1,500 mg of zidovudine.[294] The mechanism for this improvement was unclear; there was no correlation between cerebrospinal fluid (CSF) zidovudine concentration and HIV isolated from the CSF.
- An open, prospective study in 30 consecutive ADC patients showed neuropsychological improvement in the majority with zidovudine.[297] Even more encouraging, the severity of ADC at study entry did not correlate with response to treatment; improvements occurred in patients with deficits ranging from mild to end-stage ADC. Brain MRI and single photon emission computed tomography (SPECT) scanning improved in 6 out of 13 and in 9 out of 14 patients, respectively. In several patients, however, the benefit was only transient.
- Less encouragingly, zidovudine-related improvement occurring at 4–6 months had disappeared at 9–12 months in a sample of 11 patients.[246]

Zidovudine is not without neuropsychiatric complications; it has been reported to cause mania,[193,215,260] confusion, anxiety, seizures, a Wernicke's-like encephalopathy,[291] and coma.[247] Zidovudine also causes fatigue and a depressionlike syndrome that may be indistinguishable from either psychological reactions or HIV's systemic effects.[187] (Conversely, zidovudine has also been credited with remitting what appeared to be major depressive symptoms.[224])

There are other limitations. The nucleoside analogues are active only against *replicating* HIV, not latent provirus, and resistance can develop within 6–12 months of use.[196] In addition, many patients who are sick enough to have severe cognitive dysfunction either do not tolerate zidovudine or have already ceased to derive benefit from it. A recent study[173] showed that for asymptomatic patients treated with 500 mg of zidovudine, delayed progression of HIV disease was counterbalanced by an erosion of quality of life secondary to severe side effects of zidovudine therapy.

Note that zidovudine may induce withdrawal in methadone maintenance patients because of induction of hepatic P450 microsomal enzymes.[44]

Unfortunately, ADC still remains essentially incurable.

Nonpharmacological Management Strategies

The demands of a dementing illness require flexibility and stamina on the part of all caregivers, including health care providers.

> For most health providers, [ADC requires] a dramatically different approach to patient care. For example, in the field of psychotherapy, patients enter treatment to make changes in their lives. Psychotherapists expect and encourage this, but the responsibility for change is seen to lie with the patient. In medicine, the idealized patient-doctor model involves a physician who tries to benefit the patient, while respecting the patient's autonomy and competent decision making. A partnership of sorts develops around the offering and receiving of treatment. In the later stages of HIV dementia, however, these approaches are no longer viable. Dementia patients are no longer able to change or monitor their own behavior, nor at times are they able to make reasonable decisions about their own needs. It is, therefore, the health provider who must adapt, taking a more directive role in the patient's life.[35] (p. 189)

Note that the distractibility of mild cognitive impairment may be ascribed to boredom or anxiety, and the apathy misattributed to depression. Mental inflexibility is often characteristic of a dementing illness, but may appear to caregivers to be stubbornness.[35] Caregivers often need to be educated that these behaviors are not deliberate, and that the patient may have little control over them.

Two extremes may occur in relating to cognitively impaired patients:[35]

- One is that of denial, where both caregiver and patient minimize the cognitive deficits: "[S]he's always been like this, it's nothing new." Interventions are difficult in this setting because recommendations usually are seen as unnecessary.
- The other extreme is when the patient is treated as incapable of any independent activity, and the caregiver takes complete charge before it is necessary. This leaves the patient feeling even more powerless and hopeless.

One of the more practical discussions on the non-pharmacological management of ADC is by Boccellari and Zeifert.[35] They have outlined helpful management strategies for the patient with HIV-associated minor cognitive-motor impairment and ADC (see Appendix K).

Neurological Correlates of ADC

A brief survey of the vast neurological literature on ADC follows. Consult also the excellent reviews by Brew,[42] Geleziunias et al.,[112] and McArthur et al.[196]

Neuropathology

Although HIV can attack every level of the neuraxis, it appears to have a proclivity for the deep structures of the brain and the spinal cord.[7,159,232,233] It has been estimated that more than 65% of patients exhibit overt neurological morbidity,[112] with only about 10% showing neurological dysfunction as the *presenting* feature of the disease.[112] Robertson and Hall[249] have summarized the neuropathological changes of HIV infection as follows:

- Most HIV-infected brains show nonspecific changes of patchy pallor and gliosis in the *deep white matter,* whether or not neurological illness is clinically evident.
- Microglial nodules composed of macrophages occur in the deep white and subcortical gray matter (including the basal ganglia).
- In the later stages of the illness, extensive perivascular chronic inflammation in the white matter may appear, and characteristic multinucleated giant cells are found in most ADC brains.
- Although the neocortex is relatively spared, there does appear to be some degree of neuronal loss.[10,164]
- The spinal cord may show marked vacuolar changes that resemble those found in subacute combined degeneration of the cord due to vitamin B_{12} deficiency.[234]

Significance of Laboratory Studies

Laboratory tests have yet to yield definitive diagnostic or prognostic markers of HIV-related cognitive deficits. MRI and CSF examinations are used mainly to provide information for detecting and excluding the secondary effects of HIV infection.

Neither MRI nor CT scanning appears sensitive enough at present for early detection of HIV effects on the CNS, or to follow subtle disease progression. As extensively reviewed by Syndulko et al.,[293] several CSF variables are being explored as preclinical indicators for treatment, including quinolinic acid (an excitotoxic metabolite) levels, p24 antigen (a serum marker of active viral replication) levels, neopterin or β_2-microglobulin (markers of immune response) levels, intrathecal IgG (a marker of humoral immunity) synthesis rate, and quantitated polymerase chain reaction (PCR; permits detection of viral RNA or DNA) levels of HIV-1 viral load. SPECT, PET, computerized electroencephalogram (EEG), evoked potentials, and event-related potentials appear to be promising candidates for early detection of HIV-related brain dysfunction, but remain primarily research tools.

Readers can refer to the 1994 review by Syndulko et al.[293] for a comprehensive list of recent research in this area.

Proposed Pathophysiological Mechanisms

Many questions remain about how the virus invades the CNS. Johnson[153] has written,

> The question that has received the most discussion and laboratory inquiry is, What mediates the disease? Since HIV appears to infect predominantly macrophages and microglial cells of the central nervous system, what causes the clinical signs and symptoms and what causes the proliferation of microglia, the attenuation of neuronal processes and loss of neurons, and the diffuse pallor of myelin? These clinical and pathological changes may represent indirect damage mediated by viral proteins, excitotoxins, or cytokines. Changes could result from a direct effect of proteins or cytokines released by infected macrophages on the target cells, or, quite possibly, via a more indirect mechanism whereby cytokines released from macrophages affect glial cells and endothelial cells while their functional changes adversely affect neuronal function.

Finally, we must not overlook an early hypothesis. Before recognition that HIV infected the nervous system, attempts were made to explain all pathological changes on the basis of opportunistic infections. The role of opportunistic infections as either cofactors or primary factors in some of the HIV-associated neurological syndromes must be kept in consideration. Possibilities range from opportunistic infection with relatively ubiquitous agents such as cytomegalovirus, to the possible pathogenic role of *Mycobacterium avium intracellulare,* to the more exotic possibilities of a new mycoplasma, to the odd agent associated with cat scratch fever, *Rochalimaea henselae.* (p. 319)

🜀 PSYCHIATRIC MORBIDITY, PART I

AIDS Anxiety Versus AIDS Phobia

Realistic fear of AIDS and irrational panic often overlap. Patients with "AIDS anxiety" are reasonably worried about infection but are able to derive reassurance from negative clinical and laboratory findings.[201] The "worried well" are a subgroup who may have HIV risk factors but who remain convinced that they are infected despite negative medical findings, including serological testing.[101,199,201,202] This conviction constitutes a type of "AIDS phobia."

◆ These patients remain chronically ruminative about HIV infection despite counseling, physical examination, and repeated negative antibody screening. They are unshakably convinced that certain somatic complaints are due to HIV, and may complain of nonspecific symptoms (e.g., fatigue, sweating, skin rashes, muscle pains, diarrhea, slight intermittent lymphadenopathy, sore throat, slight weight loss, minor mouth infections, dizziness).[201]

◆ The "worried well" often exhibit obsessive-compulsive behaviors and ruminative states concerning AIDS contagion and death, guilt over high-risk sexual practices, and preoccupation with the dirtiness or infectivity of body fluid.[201] Their distress can be functionally debilitating. Frequent trips to a primary care physician for reassurance and repeated antibody testing are common.

These psychiatric symptoms may indicate underlying obsessive-compulsive disorder,[45,179,201] delusional disorder with somatic symptoms,[182,296] hypochondriasis, Mun-chausen syndrome (factitious disorder),[14,30,67a,205,300,322] or major depression with somatic preoccupations.[60]

Prodromal Symptoms and Seroconversion

Disease course and pathology are variable in early HIV infection. A mononucleosis-like illness may occur within days to weeks of presumed HIV exposure,[63,140] with symptoms such as fatigue, fever, lymphadenopathy, and occasionally a rash. These symptoms usually resolve relatively quickly and may go unnoticed; most patients who present years later with the clinical syndrome of AIDS do not recall such a prodrome.[187]

◆ The time from exposure to HIV and the onset of flulike symptoms ranges from as short as 6 days[63] to as long as 6 weeks.[140] (In one series, seroconversion occurred 8–12 weeks after presumed exposure.[140])

The occurrence of this symptom constellation in an individual with known or high risk of exposure to HIV should raise the question of the primary infection syndrome;[25] Mr. Lowe's fears are realistic and should not be interpreted as irrational or phobic. Frank neurological symptoms usually occur much later.

Major Depression in HIV Infection

Prevalence

Prevalence data on major depressive syndromes in the HIV-spectrum population vary. During the early years of the AIDS epidemic, many reports reflected the impression that depression was an inevitable consequence of living with a stigmatizing and ultimately fatal disease. More recent studies, which have substituted self-report measures and standardized diagnostic interviews for clinical impression or chart reviews, have modified that view.

◆ Self-report studies have yielded prevalence ratings of between 20% and 30%,[135,228] while those using the more cumbersome (but more accurate) standardized diagnostic interviews show results in the 6%–11% range.[11,227,242,317]

Factors such as the underrepresentation of minorities, IV drug users, and women limit the generalizability of these data. Perry[231] has summarized,

Available data indicate that while low-grade depressive symptoms are common among HIV-positive adults, depressive disorders are the exception and not the rule. This tentative conclusion is consistent with studies of other fatal illnesses, such as cancer.[74] Furthermore, this conclusion is supported both by Rabkin et al.,[244] who found that a sample of 124 HIV-positive gay men maintained reasonable hopefulness over time, and by Joseph et al.,[156] who found in a sample of 436 gay and bisexual men that psychiatric symptoms did not increase over 3 years. *The clinical point is that physicians should not assume that severe depressive symptoms in an HIV-infected adult are understandable and justified. Depressive disorder is never "normal." Rather, it is an indication for evaluation and treatment.* (pp. 224–225, italics added)

Risk factors. A pre-HIV history of depression,[225,230,317] the presence of an Axis II personality disorder,[150] and lower perceived social support [95,135] are associated with higher risk of HIV-associated depression. Contrary to early concerns, knowledge of positive antibody status is at best a relatively weak predictor of profound depression.[135,228]

The stage of the illness also does not strongly predict severe depression:

◆ Chuang et al.[57] have suggested that patients in the early or *asymptomatic* stages of HIV infection may experience *higher* levels of psychosocial distress than do those with full-blown AIDS.

◆ Another study confirmed that psychological distress correlated with self-reported *nonspecific* physical symptoms (e.g., fatigue, new skin rash, night sweats, unusual cough) that were *possibly* related to HIV.[219] Seropositive or seronegative subjects were not discernible on the basis of self-reported physical symptoms or measures of psychological distress.

◆ The San Francisco–based Center for AIDS Prevention Study (CAPS)[135] found significant but relatively weak correlations between self-reported depressive symptoms and the number of HIV physical symptoms ($r = .19–.25$).

◆ Perry et al.[227] found somewhat higher correlations between the severity of HIV symptoms and severity of depressive symptoms ($r = .35–.50$), although most subjects with HIV physical symptoms did not have a score associated with clinical depression.

Chuang et al.[57] have advised clinicians that different psychosocial issues and adaptive demands emerge over the course of the illness, and that the critical issues may differ across clinical milestones. For example, end-stage AIDS may force the issues of death, dying, and the resolution of unfinished business, whereas earlier stages may introduce equally—if not more—threatening stressors, such as uncertainties about the progression of the illness, fears of pain and suffering, social isolation and rejection, and more general fears of the unknown.

These data support the clinical maxim that, relative to developing depression, "it may be less important what illness the person has and more important what person has the illness" (p. 229).[231] The etiological role of HIV's direct brain effects in depression remains speculative.[172]

Suicide, Ethical Issues, and Competency

Consulting psychiatrists regularly encounter HIV patients who are refusing medical treatment, bringing into question the patient's capacity to make decisions consistent with informed consent. The potential for ADC sometimes complicates this assessment. Accurate competency and suicidal assessments are crucial. While it is beyond the scope of this chapter to review these issues in detail, several clinically relevant highlights follow. The references and Appendix F ("A Mini-Outline of Competency and Informed Consent") are provided as resources for further study.

◆ Estimates of the suicide rate among individuals who are seropositive and those who have frank AIDS have varied across studies; one of the first studies reported a 36-fold increased relative risk for suicide;[188] a later study revised that figure down to a 7.4-fold increased risk,[64] and several studies yielded estimates in between.[4,46,114,166] Suffice it to say that the risk of suicide must be taken **very** seriously in this population, but the presence of suicidal thoughts should not routinely be considered "normal."

◆ Perry et al.[229] found persistent suicidal ideation in over 15% of *both the seropositive and **seronegative** groups* who underwent HIV testing, suggesting that a sizable subgroup experiences serious emotional distress both before and after HIV testing, regardless of outcome.

◆ Suicidal ideation does not necessarily increase proportionately with clinical stages. McKegney and O'Dowd[197] found that patients with *frank* AIDS ($n = 322$) were significantly *less* suicidal than patients who were "only" HIV positive ($n = 82$). (The AIDS group had suicidality rates comparable with those of patients with negative or unknown HIV status.) The finding of less suicidality in AIDS patients compared with ARC and other HIV-positive patients was corroborated by the same authors in a study of demographically similar medical outpatients.[214] The authors speculated that the psychological changes related to CNS impairment, denial, and/or refocusing of life goals prompted by full-blown AIDS may have mitigated suicidality.

◆ Risk factors for suicide attempts were defined in one study to include social isolation, perceived lack of social support, adjustment disorder, personality disorder, alcohol abuse, HIV-related interpersonal or occupational problems, and a history of depression.[254]

◆ Previous psychiatric treatment and a diagnosis of antisocial personality disorder in HIV-positive individuals have been positively correlated with suicidality.

◆ Delirium and confusion in hospitalized patients may enhance the risk of suicide, especially in those with ADC.[3]

The erosion of cognitive, social, vocational, and family resources overwhelmingly predisposes to depression. Thoughts of rational suicide—an enormously controversial issue[17,22,47,71,111,132,250,253,272,289]—may emerge throughout the illness course, especially when loved ones have suffered and died from HIV. Clinicians have personal reactions to patients wishing to escape a slow and miserable death by committing suicide. *Beware of therapeutic nihilism: most completed suicides among terminally ill patients occur in the setting of clinical depression or impaired judgment.*[47,56a,289] Depression affects decision making;[111,138] for example, the acceptability of life-sustaining interventions was significantly lower in clinically depressed patients, who showed a change of heart when depression was no longer present.[98] A postmortem review of HIV-infected patients who committed suicide confirmed that most suffered from a concomitant psychiatric disorder.[188] These issues overlap with euthanasia (which some consider assisted suicide).[149,165,191,239,278] The therapist must thoughtfully consider the countertransference reactions that arise from working with such patients[52] (see also Chapter 9 and Appendix L).

The treatment of HIV-infected patients also brings a number of other ethical, legal, and clinical dilemmas both in the outpatient[2,123] and the inpatient[32] settings. These issues span the obligation to treat HIV-infected patients, the duty to warn endangered third parties (and thereby break confidentiality), the ethics of mandatory testing, and the questions raised by rational suicide, euthanasia, and "do not resuscitate" orders.[41,70,71,130,162,171,263a,273,275]

◆ An innovative paper by Haas and colleagues[129] explored predictors of failure in patient-physician communication regarding preferences for life-sustaining care. Disturbingly, they found that less than half of AIDS patients had discussed their preferences for resuscitation with their physicians. Moreover, patients were less likely to have discussed resuscitation if they were nonwhite, had never been hospitalized, or were cared for in a health maintenance organization (HMO) facility rather than a private teaching hospital. Among nonwhites, those with a nonwhite physician were more likely to have discussed resuscitation. Of those who had not discussed their preferences, 72% wanted to do so. Patient desire for such discussion did not vary by race, severity of illness, hospitalization status, use of zidovudine, or site of care.

We found particularly helpful the review papers of Rosmarin,[252] Auerbach and Banja,[12] Overman,[220] and Strain et al.[288] on the general legal and ethical aspects of medical illness; of Beckett and Shenson[28] and Starace[280] on suicide in HIV patients; and of Beckett et al.[26] on treating the mentally ill HIV-seropositive patient.

Differential Diagnosis

The psychomotor agitation of depression may be difficult to distinguish from the agitation of ADC.[31] The distinction is important, since antidepressants improve the former but may exacerbate the latter. Acute onset precipitation by a clear medical or neurological event, mood lability, absence of previous affective history, and nocturnal worsening tends to argue in favor of ADC.[277]

Treatment

We will focus on pharmacological interventions in the next section. Issues in psychotherapy of HIV-infected patients will be discussed in the next case, that of Ms. Newman.

We agree that depressive symptoms in HIV patients should be treated whether or not the full diagnostic criteria for major depression are met.[89] Doing so avoids underdiagnosis and potentially improves quality of life. *In the absence of delirium, a trial of antidepressants is appropriate for any depressed HIV patient, regardless of disease stage or symptomatology.*[90] References such as Ciraulo et al.[58a] provide up-to-date information on drug interactions.

Fernandez and Levy[91] recommend maintaining the patient for 3–4 months at the antidepressant dose used for remission. They then lower this dose gradually to a maintenance level (i.e., usually half of the maximum dose used) for an additional 3 months.

Tricyclic antidepressants. There is no antidepressant of choice for HIV-infected patients, but the selective serotonin reuptake inhibitors (SSRIs) have largely replaced TCAs as first-line medications for medically ill patients. Occasionally, however, one meets those patients who either do not respond to or cannot tolerate the SSRIs. For them, the TCAs remain faithful standbys. They should be chosen on the basis of their side-effect profile.

Psychopharmacological management of medically ill patients has been discussed in previous chapters, and in detail by Stoudemire and Fogel.[286] The same principles apply to HIV patients. A few reminders follow:

◆ Tricyclics
- Depressed HIV patients often respond to lower doses than are usually required for physically healthy individuals. Adverse effects may occur more frequently at standard doses.[186,240,285,290]
- Desipramine (Norpramin) and protriptyline (Vivactil) are the most activating of the TCAs, and may be useful for anergic, lethargic patients.
- Avoid highly anticholinergic medications (e.g., amitriptyline [Elavil], doxepin [Sinequan], protriptyline [Vivactil], trimipramine [Surmontil]) in cognitively impaired or demented HIV patients; anticholinergic side effects can aggravate cognitive difficulties or delirium.[89] In addition, the associated drying of mucous membranes may predispose to or worsen the discomfort of oral candidiasis.[90]
- Trazodone (Desyrel) has also been successfully used in HIV patients,[91] and assists in sleep. It is not a tricyclic, so has little anticholinergic or antihistaminic activity. Priapism is a rare but serious complication.

◆ Antituberculars
- As the incidence of tuberculosis continues to rise, especially in immunocompromised patients, note a case report of the interaction between nortriptyline (Pamelor, Aventyl) and the antituberculous drug *rifampin*.[24] Higher than expected doses of nortriptyline were required to obtain therapeutic drug levels while the patient was receiving rifampin; after its discontinuation, serum nortriptyline levels rose to the toxic range. It is not known whether this interaction also occurs between rifampin and other TCAs.
- Note also that rifampin may induce withdrawal in drug abusers at previously well-tolerated

methadone levels because of hepatic P450 microsomal enzyme induction.[44,144]
- Isoniazid (INH), used as a first-line treatment for tuberculosis, has a number of psychiatric complications, including affective disturbance and psychosis.[115,302] Patients from an Afro-Caribbean background may be especially susceptible to toxic psychosis resulting from INH.[19]

◆ Antifungals
- The antifungal drug fluconazole (Diflucan) inhibits the cytochrome P450 enzyme system of the liver, and has been associated with causing toxic serum concentrations of nortriptyline.[110]

TCA efficacy. The less debilitated patients do better on tricyclics than do their sicker counterparts:

◆ The imipramine (Tofranil)-responsive HIV-positive outpatients reported by Rabkin and Harrison[240] were medically asymptomatic (or in the early stages of AIDS), were cognitively intact, and mostly had previous histories of depression.
◆ Similarly, desipramine (Norpramin) and amitriptyline (Elavil) had greater efficacy in the healthier patients (i.e., only those in the very early stages of AIDS experienced a statistically significant improvement in mood).[93]
◆ The sicker patients (i.e., those with AIDS or with AIDS/Kaposi's sarcoma) at best experienced minimal or moderate mood improvement; none of these patients showed marked improvement on either medication.

These data confirm clinical impressions that patients with full-blown AIDS suffer more severe side effects and have fewer therapeutic gains with tricyclics than do healthier HIV-infected individuals.[139]

Fernandez and Levy[90] reserve TCAs for three subgroups: 1) asymptomatic, seropositive individuals; 2) those who have limited symptomatic disease (i.e., those who have progressive generalized lymphadenopathy); and 3) patients who have limited symptomatic disease and no significant cognitive decline.

Although the SSRIs have replaced TCAs as first-line treatment for depressed medical patients, there is good documentation that sicker AIDS patients respond preferentially to the psychostimulants, which we discuss next.

Psychostimulants. Although psychostimulants are extensively reviewed in Chapter 1, a few points deserve emphasis for HIV patients.

Efficacy. The psychostimulants have not yet been compared with SSRIs, but are unambiguously more effective than tricyclics in *advanced* HIV disease.[88,90,92,94] Methylphenidate (Ritalin), dextroamphetamine (Dexedrine), and pemoline (Cylert) have been used in cognitively impaired, medically ill, depressed HIV patients, as well as in terminally ill patients.[50,145,307a,312a,313] They have been shown[8,88,89,92,94,146] to improve

◆ Cognitive performance (with or without accompanying depression)
◆ Apathy
◆ Withdrawal
◆ Anorexia
◆ Suicidal ideation
◆ Self-care

Moreover, these medications can potentiate the effects of narcotic analgesics, reduce narcotic requirements, and oppose the CNS-depressant effect of narcotics.[89]

Fernandez and Levy[91] now recommend that dextroamphetamine be avoided, based on reports on the development of irreversible abnormal involuntary movements in depressed ADC patients.

The efficacy of pemoline is less well documented. Its longer half-life, which may interfere with sleep, may make it less useful than methylphenidate in this population.[113] For patients on npo restrictions, pemoline does have the advantage of a tablet form that can be dissolved in the mouth and absorbed through the buccal mucosa, thereby bypassing the gastrointestinal tract.

Dosing. The initial dose is 5–10 mg of methylphenidate (or its equivalent) by mouth, feeding tube, or suppository.[91,145] Blood pressure and heart rate should be initially monitored, as well as adverse side effects like agitation, restlessness, nausea, or psychosis. The medication should be gradually increased, given in three doses, before 1:00 P.M. (so as not to disturb sleep), until achieving maximum clinical response. Maintenance treatment can continue for several weeks or months with little risk of dependence or abuse,[90,113] although research is needed to explore potential risks in patients with substance abuse histories.

Side effects. Monitor patients for movement disorders, as a significant number of patients have developed involuntary dyskinetic movements, particularly while taking dextroamphetamine[92] or daily doses of methylphenidate above 60 mg.[86] In addition, psychosis is a rare side effect, described with methylphenidate doses exceeding 25 mg or in patients with a history of psychotic symptoms,[113] leading some to recommend against using it in patients with a history of psychosis.

Alprazolam for depression. In recent years, alprazolam (Xanax) has fallen into disfavor because of several disadvantages, including a short duration of action, a propensity to produce rebound anxiety between doses, and difficulties with withdrawal. Nonetheless, it still has a strong following for treating oncological and HIV-infected patients[89,143,245,309] because of its combined anxiolytic and antidepressant properties.

◆ Starting doses should be 0.25 mg po four times daily, gradually increased to an optimally effective antidepressant dose, usually ranging between 4 and 10 mg daily.[190]
◆ Patients must be warned not to skip doses and may require a gradual withdrawal regimen using clonazepam (Klonopin) to end alprazolam treatment.[221]

Monoamine oxidase inhibitors. There is little literature on the use of MAOIs in HIV-infected patients. The dietary restrictions, propensity for hypotension, and potential for adverse drug interactions limit their usefulness compared with other available agents.[91]

Newer agents. There is not enough experience to assess the risks and benefits of many of the newer agents. Early reports on fluoxetine (Prozac)[20,139,175,223,241] and bupropion (Wellbutrin)[20] in HIV patients have been promising. In one study, retrospective analysis of HIV patients receiving either fluoxetine or bupropion revealed that both agents were successful for major depression with or without cognitive impairment.[90] Patients with major depressive episodes and no cognitive impairment fared better on bupropion than on fluoxetine; the reverse was true for patients with CNS dysfunction, but neither trend reached statistical significance.

◆ Although bupropion appeared superior to fluoxetine in activating anhedonic patients, the potential risk for seizures in neurologically compromised HIV patients was of concern.[91]
◆ The 3 (out of 49) patients who developed seizures had DSM-III-R[6a]–defined organic mental disorders and developed seizures when their dosages were increased from 200 to 300 mg/day, or from 300 to 400 mg/day. When the timing of the doses was changed to a fixed schedule (tid at 8 A.M.–2 P.M.–8 P.M., or qid at 6 A.M.–10 A.M.–2 P.M.–6 P.M.) and the patients were rechallenged, seizures did not recur.
◆ To avoid this complication, the authors recommended limiting bupropion to no more than 300 mg/day in fixed divided doses.

Although fluoxetine brings a lower risk of seizures, it is not without side effects. Some patients may be highly sensitive to headache, nausea, diarrhea, and tremor. Fluoxetine's activating effects may potentiate the agitation and confusion that often accompany disease progression.[51] Also, fluoxetine can elevate the serum levels of other hepatically metabolized medications,[58] wreaking potential havoc with HIV's inevitable polypharmacy.

Sertraline (Zoloft) appears to be effective in HIV-infected patients.[243] We await reports on use of the newer agents, such as paroxetine (Paxil) and venlafaxine (Effexor), specifically in HIV patients.

Zidovudine and antidepressants.   Fluoxetine and the TCAs can be coadministered with zidovudine.[90] Be cautious when combining MAOIs with zidovudine, however, because zidovudine's catecholamine-O-methyltransferase–inhibiting effects might potentiate hypertensive responses to tyramine-containing substances.[91]

◆   Interestingly, a recent case report described an HIV-positive patient whose major depressive episode remitted concurrently with zidovudine treatment.[224] The authors speculated that, just as correction of thyroid dysfunction improves hypothyroid-induced depression, so, too, might depressive HIV symptoms remit with zidovudine treatment. They recommend checking for zidovudine-related improvement in depression before initiating antidepressant treatment, although the pathophysiological basis for these recommendations remains speculative.

Electroconvulsive therapy.   ECT has been used safely in HIV-positive depressed inpatients.[163a,259]

HIV and the Psychiatric Patient

The Psychiatric Inpatient Setting

Wiener et al.[314] found that the most common reason for psychiatric admission of HIV-infected patients was suicidal thoughts or attempts; the two most common diagnostic categories were "organic mental syndrome" and substance abuse/dependence. These are themselves difficult-to-treat illnesses and are complicated by additional issues of staff countertransference, confidentiality, isolation of bodily secretions, and management of HIV-related medical illness. Patients who attempt to harm themselves or others by exposure to bodily fluids and who are cognitively impaired due to ADC bring up difficult ethical, legal, and clinical dilemmas foreign to most conventional psychiatric inpatient units. The staff members themselves may feel

personally vulnerable to AIDS, quite apart from their contact with the patient. These issues inevitably interfere with staff's flexibility and emotional availability to the needs of the patient.[5,15,16,32,65,132,141,258]

The Chronically Mentally Ill

There is mounting evidence that psychiatric patients have a high prevalence of HIV infection and risk behaviors,[157,258,292a] yet are not adequately assessed or counseled for HIV during the course of their psychiatric assessment.[137] Many patients with HIV illness have a premorbid diagnosis of schizophrenia, bipolar disorder, or schizoaffective disorder.[66] They may present with anxiety and/or overt delusions about AIDS, making it difficult to determine where psychosis ends and realistic concern begins. The statistics are sobering:

◆   The number of dual-diagnosis (psychiatric disorder and substance abuse) patients entering state hospitals is increasing.[40,65,66,147,292] These patients suffer twin risks of contracting HIV.

◆   In a review of 135 inpatient and 87 outpatient consultations for patients with HIV-related illness, approximately 9% of inpatients and 4% of outpatients received a diagnosis of schizophrenia according to history or presentation.[31]

◆   The findings of two studies that tested unlabeled blood samples of all patients admitted to a psychiatry ward indicated an HIV seroprevalence of approximately 6% in this population.[258,321]

◆   A state hospital survey used a 13-item questionnaire to assess statistical prevalence of seropositivity in hospitalized psychiatric patients.[306] HIV seroprevalence was 0.6% among the low-risk patients *but 14.4% among the high-risk patients.*

◆   A related study reported that 19% of psychiatric inpatients had a history of one or more HIV-related risk behaviors.[258] *A diagnosis of bipolar disorder significantly correlated with the presence of risk-taking behavior.*

◆   IV drug abuse constituted the major risk behavior in 60% of inpatient and outpatient psychiatric consultations.[31]

◆   Personality disorders usually pose special problems in the medical management of nonpsychiatric illness,[97,125,209] and HIV infection is no exception. Enduring patterns such as emotional lability, impulsivity, or predisposition for brief psychotic episodes can complicate evaluation and management.[31] Although relatively little data are available on personality disorders in this population, at least two studies have cited a prevalence of personality disorders in seropositive samples of at least 33%.[222,316] (It is not possible to assess whether this statistic also indicates a higher HIV risk in personality disorder patients.) In a study of the sexual practices of patients with borderline personality disorder, 53% of the men reported engaging in sexual practices that placed them at risk for HIV infection.[323] This has been corroborated by others.[148] Not surprisingly, HIV-positive patients with personality disorders are more likely to cope with AIDS in a dysfunctional way, showing significantly more mood disturbance, greater use of denial and helplessness when coping with the threat of AIDS, and increased social conflict.[222]

◆ A substantial proportion of schizophrenic patients have been found to engage in high-risk behaviors.[67] Sexual activity was associated with younger age, a lower level of functioning, the presence of delusions, and more positive symptoms.

Recently, Kelly et al.[161] surveyed 60 chronically mentally ill outpatients attending an inner-city community health clinic. Although IV drug use was uncommon in this group, *patients showed substantial deficits in their practical understanding of AIDS and risk-reduction measures.* The specifics are chilling:

◆ Many subjects reported engaging in high-risk behaviors, such as trading sex for money, drugs, or a place to stay; submitting to coercion to engage in unwanted sex; and having sexual encounters casually or after using drugs or intoxicants. These findings have been corroborated by subsequent researchers.[157]

◆ Twenty percent of the subjects had met their sexual partners on the streets, in parks, or in other public places.

◆ One-third had been treated for sexually transmitted diseases other than HIV infection.

The chronically mentally ill are at grave risk during the present epidemic, even if they do not abuse drugs. Very often, psychiatrists are the only physicians who treat these patients, underscoring our opportunity to intervene on their behalf regarding HIV risk assessment and counseling.[66,161] Remember that ADC may be **superimposed** on a preexisting psychiatric disorder, and should be considered in the differential diagnosis of psychiatric exacerbations or the onset of continued cognitive and physical deterioration in a psychiatric patient. Beckett et al.[26] and Searight and Pound[266a] have reviewed some of the legal and ethical issues arising in this setting.

AIDS Incorporated Into Other Psychopathology

There is a growing literature on AIDS as it is incorporated into the psychopathology of psychiatric conditions, such as Munchausen syndrome (factitious disorder),[14,30,57a,67a,205,276,278a,300,322] obsessional disorders,[45,179,196a,201] affective disorders,[60] and psychotic illness.[177,182,236,296]

The Intravenous Drug User

It is well known that substance abusers are at high risk in the HIV epidemic.[301] IV drug use accounted for 20% of the cumulative HIV-infected cases in the United States in mid-1989.[56] Although the treatment of substance abuse is beyond the scope of this chapter, several points are worthy of emphasis for the consultation-liaison clinician:

◆ Drug abusers represent a major portal of infection to heterosexuals and children. *Over half of all pediatric HIV-infected cases occur among children of IV drug users, and 60% of heterosexually infected adults are partners of IV drug users.*[76]

◆ The risk is not limited to IV use; smoking, sniffing, or orally ingesting drugs also promote the spread of HIV, since users may trade sex for drugs, employ stimulants to enhance sexual desire, or allow hypnotics to reduce sexual inhibition.[59,169]

◆ Crack cocaine users reported more sexual partners than nonusers, despite adequate knowledge about HIV transmission.[39]

◆ Drug or alcohol use has been found to enhance the likelihood of risky sexual behavior in gay, bisexual, and heterosexual men.[127,279]

◆ Recent serological testing of discarded admission blood samples of 300 patients admitted to an alcohol rehabilitation unit showed that 10.3% had HIV infection.[181] Chart records showed that 4 patients were known to be HIV infected upon admission, and another 3 patients were detected during hospitalization; however, 77% of the HIV-positive sample were discharged with their HIV infection still undetected.

For many psychiatrists, there is often a therapeutic nihilism about the ability or willingness of substance abusers to change, even when confronted with HIV infection. This is a dangerous assumption, and is refuted by a growing body of data. A few samples from this literature follow:

◆ Guydish et al.[128] reported on an outcome and needs-assessment evaluation conducted by the AIDS and Substance Abuse Program (ASAP) of the San Francisco AIDS Health Project. More than half of a sample of 86 drug users were interested in drug treatment and made initial contact with referral sources.

◆ *Most* participants reported at least some modification of high-risk sexual (81%) and drug use (67%) behavior. Participants with an IV drug history were *more* interested in treatment than were non–IV users.

◆ IV drug users *reported more change in drug behavior.*

◆ There was, however, comparatively less *sexual* behavioral change in IV compared with non–IV drug users, consistent with previous reports.[75]

◆ Significant predictors of outcome in this study included source of referral (inpatient referrals were less successful than outpatient), interest level in treatment, and prior sexual-risk behavioral change. The most frequently reported obstacles to treatment were personal unreadiness and waiting lists for treatment programs.

Results like these challenge pessimistic assumptions about the willingness of substance abusers to change. Unfortunately, motivation to change is a start, but not enough. Interventions that are not informed by psychological and cultural understanding will become shipwrecked on the specifics of the subculture, which has its own definition and perception of risk.[62,211]

◆ For example, Donoghoe et al.[78] were curious about what distinguished persistent syringe sharers from nonsharers—information useful for shaping potential interventions. They found that persistent syringe sharers differed on preferred drug (preferring heroin, temazepam, and prescribed methadone); social factors (they had more contact with other injectors); more recent involvement in crime; and greater number of sexual partners, who also injected drugs.

◆ Notably, syringe sharers and nonsharers did *not* differ significantly in attendance at syringe-exchange programs or self-reported HIV antibody status.

Never underestimate the power of denial:

◆ Kelaher and Ross[160] found that high-risk drug users tended to *underestimate* the prevalence of HIV infection compared with their low-risk counterparts, and also underestimated their personal susceptibility.

◆ Friedman et al.[105] culled questionnaire data from almost 12,000 street-recruited drug injectors in 19 U.S. cities. They found differences in self-reported sexual behaviors across cultures. Each racial/gender group averaged 15 or more episodes of unprotected vaginal sex per month, and 10% of most subgroups reported having anal sex within the past 6 months. At least 45% of subjects reported heterosexual sex with non-injectors.

These data highlight the role of lifestyle and culture: Interventions that only provide accessibility to safer behaviors (e.g., syringe exchange programs) or that are solely educative (e.g., assessing serostatus) will not change high-risk behaviors.[18,21,48,53,96,105,207,210,216,269,287]

Ostrow[218] has provided a good recent review of additional issues. See also the section "Sex, Culture, and Stereotype" (p. 257).

Caregiver Issues

Family, Friends, and Significant Others

As reviewed by Folkman et al.,[99] the literature on caregiver stress is derived mainly from studies of patients with Alzheimer's disease, cancer, Parkinson's disease, or stroke. These caregivers are usually female, and the people they care for are usually older adults. As the number of HIV-infected individuals increases, so do the demands on caregivers, but support services *for caregivers* has not kept pace.[78a,104,117,118,136,142,178,198,260,261,265,307,308,311] Folkman et al.[99] suggest three techniques to support and sustain these individuals:

◆ Work with caregivers to define what is personally meaningful by helping to identify values that are activated by caregiving (e.g., the importance of providing good care; of conferring dignity on a sick partner who might otherwise be humiliated by the effects of the illness on his body; of creating a safe, trusting atmosphere so that the person with AIDS can discuss feelings about the illness).

◆ Encourage caregivers and their partners to develop a dialogue about their reactions to the illness. When appropriate, encourage the person with AIDS to acknowledge the efforts of the caregiving partner. These strategies help stem the erosion of intimacy that often attends a progressive, chronic illness.

◆ Help caregivers develop an appreciation for small, intimate moments with their loved one (e.g., a shared sunset; hearing expressions of love and affection) that can be drawn upon for sustenance at later times.

Staff

It becomes quickly obvious that interventions should not be limited to significant others and families, but also must consider an often overtaxed staff.[164a] For example:

♦ A study of the psychological responses of hospital workers showed that misperceptions and fears about HIV patients are common among hospital staff.[213] Workers reported concerns about the potential health risks of job-related exposure, exaggerated the actual time spent in AIDS care, felt a loss of control over their work environment, and were dissatisfied with how they responded to their patients' emotional needs. Interestingly, AIDS phobia was positively correlated with homophobia and *less* contact with AIDS patients; "perceived AIDS stress" (a measure derived from the perceived level of risk of infection and discomfort in working with HIV-infected patients) *was reduced with increased exposure to AIDS care.* These data highlight the importance of in-service education for all hospital workers, especially those with limited contact with HIV-infected patients.

Sometimes insights into complex issues may be derived from studies that are innovative, if not methodologically rigorous:

♦ Stevens and Muskin[284] explored possible psychodynamic explanations for the hatred and fear of AIDS patients that often impedes empathy toward them. They posited that unconscious conflict (i.e., identification with the HIV-infected victim—a symbol of forbidden sexual wishes) interferes with normal compassion and empathy. Using this thesis, they made videotaped vignettes using professional actors, who portrayed nurses caring for HIV-infected patients. The tapes were used to stimulate staff discussion and promote education. This creative intervention proved quite helpful to staff and allowed further liaison work with other hospital personnel (e.g., dietary, housekeeping, transport).

While the inferences from this study must remain speculative, the possibilities are potentially helpful in tailoring interventions. For example, is it possible that minimal patient contact fosters the projection of frightening fantasies onto AIDS patients? Does minimal realistic contact with AIDS patients lead to relating to them as unconscious symbols rather than as real people? Staff's unconscious identification with the AIDS patient[68,284] demonstrates that countertransference is not limited to psychotherapists, but arises for anyone who works with seriously ill people,[68,126] and is complicated by issues such as homosexuality, substance abuse, and close participation in the progressive deterioration of an often young, terminally ill patient.[2,79,109,212,264] (Countertransference

is discussed at greater length in Chapter 9.) Unfortunately, with few exceptions,[1,261a] the psychoanalytic literature on HIV remains meager, with little guidance for the clinician.

Burnout

Many who work with HIV patients experience the "burnout syndrome."[29,36,43,73,189,200,213,266] Symptoms include the following:

♦ Diminished psychological reserve and emotional exhaustion (experienced as a lack of capacity to offer psychological support to others)
♦ Somatic symptoms (fatigue, insomnia, headache, appetite changes)
♦ Emotional numbness, apathy, or boredom
♦ Helplessness/hopelessness
♦ Proneness to anger and frustration
♦ Feeling a lack of personal accomplishment

Some feel that no particular personality pattern or work style predisposes to burnout;[266] rather, health care workers' *attitudes* and *expectations* affect their level of stress.

> Faulty beliefs, such as the need to be constantly available to patients, the need to cure or the denial of one's personal feelings, increases work stress. Such expectations lead health care workers to deny or withhold their personal feelings, not just from patients but from each other. This leads to a work setting where strong emotional issues are not dealt with, increasing the staff's inner tension, and leading to burnout.[318] (p. 53)

The consulting psychiatrist may be asked to help other health professionals cope with their responses to working in the AIDS epidemic.[9,73,77,85,124,176,266,303,312,318]

Comment. Silverman,[274] in his recent comprehensive review, made a surprising observation: few of the current publications concerning HIV caregiver stress come from the psychiatric literature. (Nursing, medical, public health, and health education journals offer the most resources.) Amazingly, "psychiatry appears to lack a strong clinical, educational, research, or policy presence regarding psychosocial stress in HIV care providers" (p. 705).[274] Moreover, he observed that there have been no controlled investigations into the incidence and prevalence of mental, physical, interpersonal, or occupational symptoms in HIV caregivers. *Even more disturbingly, he remarked on the frequency and consistency with which caregivers reveal their aversion not only to the disease but also to the patients themselves, their lifestyles, and the caregiving.* He quoted one study[106] that reported that while psychiatrists conveyed nonjudgmental attitudes about the sexual orientation of AIDS patients, they were (along with family physicians) the *least* comfortable with the communicable aspects of AIDS. Gorman[119] has commented in response to this article:

> Is it possible that health professionals, including psychiatrists, defend themselves against stress and burnout when dealing with HIV-infected patients by adopting . . . irrational fears of becoming infected and self-righteous aversions to the people who actually are infected? Patients with AIDS must live with constant ostracism and societal rejection, but . . . perhaps [their caregivers], by some perverse psychological mechanism of identification, come to fear that family and friends will reject them for treating infected patients . . . [Here] we are no longer talking about the caregivers' level of stress, but about the caregivers' psychological ability to render proper treatment. *Stress and burnout may be dealt with by some individuals through a host of negative attitudes aimed at the patient.* If this is true, then merely condemning the "wrong-thinking" clinician is beside the point; our job as psychiatrists is to recognize the psychological defenses producing the aberrant attitudes and to identify ways to "treat" such attitudes in the clinician as well as the patient. (p. 689, italics added)

Clearly, these findings have important implications for treatment staff interventions and the direction of future research.

🗝 SUMMARY

1. Most cognitive disorders in HIV patients can be classified as either HIV-1–associated minor cognitive-motor disorder or AIDS dementia complex (ADC). The two are not synonymous. Asymptomatic seropositive individuals do not differ from seronegative control subjects in most studies. When subtle cognitive deficits do occur in the otherwise asymptomatic stages of HIV infection, they are often mild and unaccompanied by other neurological changes. It is still not known whether minor abnormalities lie on the same spectrum as ADC, share the same etiology, or eventually progress to more severe conditions.

2. *ADC must be considered as a possible etiology for any psychiatric symptoms occurring in an HIV-infected individual.* Be alert to the insidious onset of apathy or social withdrawal in a previously healthy seropositive individual. It may be easily misdiagnosed as depression, particularly when early symptoms coincide with dysphoria, anxiety, irritability, apathy, or social withdrawal. More obvious disturbances, such as emotional lability, inappropriate behavior, and psychotic features, are relatively uncommon *early* features of ADC.

3. The symptoms of ADC are often subtle and insidious in onset, with *slowed decision making* most prominent. This is different from the disorientation, amnesia, and language disturbance that typify the dementia of the Alzheimer type. ADC has been misdiagnosed as Alzheimer's disease, especially in older patients. It is a dementia of variable progression and unpredictable duration. In the early stages, patients report that they cannot keep up with their personal finances or business activities, describing a constant state of "befuddlement." Since insight is usually preserved until late in the illness, patients often need help working through reactions of grief and fear regarding their intellectual decline. The apathy and social withdrawal of ADC may resemble and coincide with psychodynamically motivated phenomena, such as resistance, denial, and repression.

4. Early ADC may be sometimes misdiagnosed as other dementias in older patients. The features that might bring these patients to medical attention include significant decline in short-term memory and concentration, personality changes, weight loss, incontinence, and falls. HIV risk factors are not always obvious; assess whether the patient *or spouse* is in a known risk group, regardless of age, and be sure to ask about *blood transfusions before 1985.* Concurrent systemic illness (especially if marked by opportunistic infections) should raise suspicion of ADC, as should dementia with atypical features, such as rapid progression or focal neurological signs.

5. The ADC diagnosis is one of exclusion. Changes in mental status require **urgent** evaluation, as they may herald new neurological or infectious complications.

6. No specific tests are pathognomonic of ADC. The Mini-Mental State Exam (MMSE), which does not

assess response time, is not sufficiently sensitive in evaluating patients for ADC. The Trail Making Test (Part B) is particularly sensitive to changes in psychomotor speed, concentration, and attention. It is useful in brief bedside screening of HIV-related neurocognitive impairment.

7. Although not unanimous, encouraging preliminary evidence suggests that zidovudine may reduce the incidence and severity of ADC. It may also improve neurological and neuropsychological performance in patients with AIDS.

8. HIV can attack anywhere in the nervous system, but has a proclivity for the spinal cord and the deep structures of the brain. The spinal cord may show marked vacuolar changes that resemble those found in subacute combined degeneration of the cord due to vitamin B_{12} deficiency. Most HIV-infected brains show nonspecific changes of patchy pallor and gliosis in the deep white matter, whether or not there is clinical evidence of neurological disease. Microglial nodules composed of macrophages occur in the deep white and subcortical gray matter (including the basal ganglia). The neocortex is relatively spared.

9. The risk of suicide must be taken seriously in this population. Persistent suicidal ideation has been found in *both seropositive and seronegative* individuals undergoing HIV testing. Suicidal ideation does not necessarily increase proportionately with clinical stages; research has shown that patients with *frank* AIDS may be *less* suicidal than patients who are "only" HIV positive. Delirium and confusion in hospitalized patients enhance risk. *Beware of therapeutic nihilism: most completed suicides among terminally ill patients occur in the setting of clinical depression or impaired judgment.*

10. Agitated depression may be difficult to distinguish from agitation in ADC. The distinction is an important one; antidepressants improve the former but may exacerbate the latter. Acute onset, precipitation by a clear medical or neurological inciting factor, mood lability, absence of a previous history of mood disorder, and nocturnal worsening tend to argue in favor of ADC. In the absence of delirium, antidepressants may be tried for any depressed HIV patient, regardless of stage of disease or symptomatology.

11. There is no specific antidepressant of choice, but the selective serotonin reuptake inhibitors (SSRIs) have largely replaced tricyclic antidepressants (TCAs) as first-line medications for depressed, medically ill patients. Electroconvulsive therapy (ECT) may also be safely used. Avoid highly anticholinergic medications in cognitively impaired or demented HIV patients; these can aggravate cognitive difficulties or delirium. The efficacy of TCAs is greatest for the less debilitated patients, while medically sicker AIDS patients respond preferentially to the psychostimulants. Psychostimulants improve apathy, withdrawal, anorexia, and cognitive performance, with or without accompanying depression. Most of the psychotropics, with the exception of the monoamine oxidase inhibitors (MAOIs), can be coadministered with zidovudine.

12. Antituberculous drugs may interact with hepatically metabolized medications such as antidepressants, and have been associated with toxic psychoses.

13. Psychiatric patients have a high prevalence of HIV infection and risk behaviors, yet are not adequately assessed or counseled for HIV as part of their psychiatric assessment. The chronically mentally ill and those with personality disorders are at risk during the present epidemic, even if they do not abuse drugs. Very often, the psychiatrist is the only physician who treats these patients, underscoring our opportunity to intervene on their behalf regarding the HIV risk assessment and counseling. Remember that ADC may be superimposed upon a preexisting chronic psychiatric disorder; it should be considered in the differential diagnosis of psychiatric exacerbations, cognitive decline, and/or physical deterioration.

14. Drug abusers are the major portal of infection to heterosexuals and children. The risk is not limited to IV drug use; smoking, sniffing, or orally ingesting drugs spreads HIV indirectly, since users may trade sex for drugs, ingest stimulants to enhance sexual desire, or use hypnotics to reduce sexual inhibition. Crack cocaine users, in particular, report more sexual partners than nonusers, despite adequate knowledge about HIV transmission. Not surprisingly, many drug users underestimate both the prevalence of HIV infection and their personal susceptibility to infection.

15. The attention given in the psychiatric literature to caregiver stress is incongruous with its clinical impact. This has important implications for future research and the psychodynamics of treating HIV disease.

❧ REFERENCES

1. Abramowitz S, Cohen J: The psychodynamics of AIDS: a view from self psychology, in Therapists on the Front Line: Psychotherapy with Gay Men in the Age of AIDS. Edited by Cadwell S, Burnham R Jr, Forstein M. Washington, DC, American Psychiatric Press, 1994, pp 205–221

2. Adler C, Beckett A: Psychotherapy of the patient with an HIV infection: some ethical and therapeutic dilemmas. Psychosomatics 30:203–208, 1989

3. Alfonso C, Cohen M: HIV-dementia and suicide. Gen Hosp Psychiatry 16:45–46, 1994

4. Alfonso C, Cohen M, Aladjem A, et al: HIV seropositivity as a major risk factor for suicide in the general hospital. Psychosomatics 35:368–373, 1994

5. Amchin J, Polan H: A longitudinal account of staff adaptation to AIDS patients on a psychiatric unit. Hosp Community Psychiatry 37:1235–1238, 1986

6. American Academy of Neurology: Nomenclature and research case definitions for neurological manifestations of human immunodeficiency virus type 1 (HIV-1) infection. Report of a Working Group of the American Academy of Neurology AIDS Task Force, 1991

6a. American Psychiatric Association: Diagnostic and Statistical Manual of Mental Disorders, 3rd Edition, Revised. Washington, DC, American Psychiatric Association, 1987

6b. American Psychiatric Association: Diagnostic and Statistical Manual of Mental Disorders, 4th Edition. Washington, DC, American Psychiatric Association, 1994

7. Anders K, Guerra W, Tomiyasu U, et al: The neuropathology of AIDS: UCLA experience and review. Am J Pathol 124:537–558, 1986

8. Angrist B, D'Hollosy M, Sanfilipo M, et al: Central nervous stimulants as symptomatic treatments for AIDS-related neuropsychiatric impairment. J Clin Psychopharmacol 12:268–272, 1992

9. Anoun H: When a house officer gets AIDS. N Engl J Med 321:693–696, 1989

10. Artigas J, Niedobitex F, Gross G, et al: Spongiform encephalopathy in AIDS dementia complex: report of 5 cases. J Acquir Immune Defic Syndr 2:374–381, 1989

11. Atkinson J, Grant I, Kennedy C, et al: Prevalence of psychiatric disorders among men infected with human immunodeficiency virus: a controlled study. Arch Gen Psychiatry 45:859–864, 1988

12. Auerbach V, Banja J: Competency determinations, in Medical Psychiatric Practice, Vol 2. Edited by Stoudemire A, Fogel B. Washington, DC, American Psychiatric Press, 1993, pp 515–535

13. Bach M, Boothby J: Dementia associated with human immunodeficiency virus with a negative ELISA. N Engl J Med 315:891–892, 1986

14. Baer J: Munchausen's AIDS. Gen Hosp Psychiatry 9:75–76, 1987

15. Baer J: Study of 60 patients with AIDS or AIDS related complex requiring psychiatric hospitalization. Am J Psychiatry 146:1285–1288, 1989

16. Baer J, Hall J, Holm K, et al: Challenges in developing an inpatient psychiatric program for patients with AIDS and ARC. Hosp Community Psychiatry 38:1299–1303, 1987

17. Baile W: Rational suicide or depression: a new dilemma for the C-L psychiatrist. Psycho-Oncology 2:67–68, 1993

18. Baker A, Heather N, Wodak A, et al: Evaluation of a cognitive-behavioural intervention for HIV prevention among injecting drug users. AIDS 7:247–256, 1993

18a. Baker J, Ruiz-Rodriguez R, Whitfeld M, et al: Bacillary angiomatosis: a treatable cause of acute psychiatric symptoms in human immunodeficiency virus infection. J Clin Psychiatry 56:161–166, 1995

19. Ball R, Rosser R: Psychosis and antituberculosis therapy (letter). Lancet 2:105, 1989

20. Barlow I: Fluoxetine in HIV-related depression. Workshop 36, presented at the 142nd annual meeting of the American Psychiatric Association, San Francisco, CA, May 1989

21. Batki S, Sorensen J, Faltz B, et al: Psychiatric aspects of treatment of IV drug abusers with AIDS. Hosp Community Psychiatry 39:439–441, 1988

22. Battin M: Physicians, partners, and people with AIDS: deciding about suicide. Crisis 15:15–21, 43, 1994

23. Beason-Hazen S, Nasrallah H, Bornstein R: Self-report of symptoms and neuropsychological performance in asymptomatic HIV-positive individuals. J Neuropsychiatry Clin Neurosci 6:43–49, 1994

24. Bebchuk J, Stewart D: Drug interaction between rifampin and nortriptyline: a case report. Int J Psychiatry Med 21:183–187, 1991

25. Beckett A: The neurobiology of human immunodeficiency virus infection, in American Psychiatric Press Review of Psychiatry, Vol 9. Edited by Tasman A, Goldfinger SM, Kaufman C. Washington, DC, American Psychiatric Press, 1990, pp 593–613

26. Beckett A, Birnbaum R, Gutheil T: Straining the limits of clinical, legal, and ethical standards: the mentally ill HIV-seropositive patient. Harvard Review of Psychiatry 1:345–349, 1994

27. Beckett A, Kassel P: Neuropsychiatric dysfunction: impact on psychotherapy with HIV-infected gay men, in Therapists on the Front Line: Psychotherapy With Gay Men in the Age of AIDS. Edited by Cadwell S, Burnham R Jr, Forstein M. Washington, DC, American Psychiatric Press, 1994, pp 147–162

28. Beckett A, Shenson D: Suicide risk in patients with human immunodeficiency virus infection and acquired immunodeficiency syndrome. Harvard Review of Psychiatry 1:27–35, 1993

29. Bennett C, Miche P, Kippax S: Quantitative analysis of burnout and its associated factors in AIDS nursing. AIDS Care 3:181–192, 1991

30. Bialer P, Wallack J: Mixed factitious disorder presenting as AIDS. Hosp Community Psychiatry 41:552–553, 1990

31. Bialer P, Wallack J, Snyder S: Psychiatric diagnosis in HIV-spectrum disorders. Psychiatr Med 9:361–375, 1991

32. Binder R: AIDS antibody tests on inpatient psychiatric units. Am J Psychiatry 144:176–181, 1987

33. Boccellari A, Dilley J, Chambers D, et al: Immune function and neuropsychological performance in HIV-1–infected homosexual men. J Acquir Immune Defic Syndr 6:592–601, 1993

34. Boccellari A, Dilley J, Shore M: Neuropsychiatric aspects of AIDS dementia complex: a report on a clinical series. Neurotoxicology 9:381–390, 1988

35. Boccellari A, Zeifert P: Management of neurobehavioral impairment in HIV-1 infection. Psychiatr Clin North Am 17:183–203, 1994

36. Bolle J: Supporting the deliverers of care: strategies to support nurses and prevent burnout. Nurs Clin North Am 23:843–850, 1988

37. Bornstein R, Nasrallah H, Para M, et al: Neuropsychological performance in symptomatic and asymptomatic HIV infection. AIDS 7:519–524, 1993

38. Bornstein R, Nasrallah H, Para M, et al: Duration of illness and neuropsychological performance in asymptomatic HIV infection. J Neuropsychiatry Clin Neurosci 6:160–164, 1994

39. Bowser B: Crack cocaine and HIV risk. Paper presented at the Community Forum on Cocaine and AIDS, San Francisco, CA, October 1988 (available from author)

40. Breakey W, Fischer P, Kramer M, et al: Health and mental health problems of homeless men and women in Baltimore. JAMA 262:1352–1357, 1989

41. Brennan T: AIDS and the limits of confidentiality: the physician's duty to warn contacts of seropositive individuals. J Gen Intern Med 4:242–246, 1989

42. Brew B: HIV-1 related neurologic disease. J Acquir Immun Defic Syndr 6 (suppl 1):S10–S15, 1993

43. Brewington J: The AIDS epidemic: caring for caregivers. Nursing Administration Quarterly 18:22–29, 1994

44. Brockmeyer N, Mertins L, Goos M: Pharmacokinetic interaction of antimicrobial agents with levomethadon in drug-addicted AIDS patients. Klin Wochenschr 69:16–18, 1991

45. Brotman A, Forstein M: AIDS obsessions in depressed heterosexuals. Psychosomatics 29:428–431, 1988

46. Brown G, Rundell J: Suicidal tendencies in women with human immunodeficiency virus infection. Am J Psychiatry 146:556–557, 1989

47. Brown J, Henteleff P, Barakat S, et al: Is it normal for terminally ill patients to desire death. Am J Psychiatry 143:208–211, 1986

48. Brown L: Black intravenous drug user: prospects for intervening in the transmission of human immunodeficiency virus infection. NIDA Res Monogr 93:53–67, 1990

49. Burgess A, Riccio M: Cognitive impairment and dementia in HIV-1. Baillieres Clinical Neurology 1:155–174, 1992

49a. Burgess A, Riccio M, Jadresic D, et al: A longitudinal study of the neuropsychiatric consequences of HIV-1 infection in gay men, I: neuropsychological performance and neurological status at baseline and at 12-month follow-up. Psychol Med 24:885–889, 1994

50. Burns M, Eisendrath S: Dextroamphetamine treatment for depression in terminally ill patients. Psychosomatics 35:80–83, 1994

51. Busch K, Maxwell S: Somatic treatment of psychiatric symptoms in HIV disease, in Behavioral Aspects of AIDS. Edited by Ostrow D. New York, Plenum Medical Book, 1990, pp 267–278

52. Cadwell S, Burnham R Jr, Forstein M (eds): Therapists on the Front Line: Psychotherapy With Gay Men in the Age of AIDS. Washington, DC, American Psychiatric Press, 1994

53. Casadonte P, Des Jarlais D, Friedman S, et al: Psychological and behavioral impact among intravenous drug users of learning HIV test results. Int J Addict 25:409–426, 1990

54. Catalan J, Thornton S: Whatever happened to HIV dementia? (editorial). Int J STD AIDS 4:1–4, 1993

55. Catania J, Turner H, Kegeles S, et al: HIV transmission risks of older heterosexuals and gays, in AIDS in an Aging Society—What We Need To Know. Edited by Riley M, Ory M, Zablotsky D. New York, Springer, 1989, pp 77–95

56. Centers for Disease Control: Classification system for human T-lymphotropic virus type III/lymphadenopathy-associated virus infections. MMWR Morb Mortal Wkly Rep 35:334–339, 1986

56a. Chochinov H, Wilson K, Enns M, et al: Desire for death in the terminally ill. Am J Psychiatry 152:1185–1191, 1995

57. Chuang H, Devins G, Hunsley J, et al: Psychosocial distress and well-being among gay and bisexual men with human immunodeficiency virus infection. Am J Psychiatry 146:876–880, 1989

57a. Churchill D, De Cock K, Miller R: Feigned HIV infection/AIDS: malingering and Munchausen's syndrome. Genitourin Med 70:314–316, 1994

58. Ciraulo D, Shader R: Fluoxetine drug-drug interactions, I: antidepressants and antipsychotics. J Clin Psychopharmacol 10:48–50, 1990

58a. Ciraulo D, Shader R, Greenblatt D, et al. (eds): Drug Interactions in Psychiatry, 2nd Edition. Baltimore, MD, Williams & Wilkins, 1995

59. Clark H, Washburn P: Testing for human immunodeficiency virus in substance abuse treatment. Psychoactive Drugs 20:203–211, 1988

60. Colenda C, Kryzanowski L, Klinger R: Major depression in late life with AIDS delusions (letter). Gen Hosp Psychiatry 12:207–209, 1990

61. Connolly S, Manji H, McAllister R, et al: Long-latency event-related potentials in asymptomatic human immunodeficiency virus type 1 infection. Ann Neurol 35:189–196, 1994

62. Connors M: Risk perception, risk taking and risk management among intravenous drug users: implications for AIDS prevention. Soc Sci Med 34:591–601, 1992

63. Cooper D, Gold J, MacLean P, et al: Acute AIDS retrovirus infection: definition of a clinical illness associated with seroconversion. Lancet 1:537–540, 1985

64. Cote T, Biggar R, Dannenberg A: Risk of suicide among persons with AIDS: a national assessment. JAMA 268:2066–2068, 1992

65. Cournos F, Empfield M, Horwath E, et al: Clinical presentations of AIDS and HIV infection in state psychiatric facilities. Hosp Community Psychiatry 40:153–157, 1989

66. Cournos F, Empfield M, Horwath E, et al: HIV infection in state hospitals: case reports and long-term management strategies. Hosp Community Psychiatry 41:163–166, 1990

67. Cournos F, Guido J, Coomaraswamy S, et al: Sexual activity and risk of HIV infection among patients with schizophrenia. Am J Psychiatry 151:228–232, 1994

67a. Craven D, Steger K, LaChapelle R, et al: Factitious HIV infection: the importance of documenting infection. Ann Intern Med 121:763–766, 1994

68. Crawford R: The boundaries of the self and the unhealthy other: reflections on health, culture and AIDS. Soc Sci Med 38:1347–1365, 1994

69. Cummings J, Benson D: Dementia: A Clinical Approach. Boston, MA, Butterworths, 1983

70. Daniolos P, Holmes V: HIV public policy and psychiatry. Psychosomatics 36:12–21, 1995

71. Danis J, Garrett J, Harris R, et al: Stability of choices about life-sustaining treatments. Ann Intern Med 120:567–573, 1994

72. Dauncey K: Mania in early stages of AIDS. Br J Psychiatry 152:716–717, 1988

73. Dworkin S, Pincu L: Counseling in the era of AIDS. Journal of Counseling and Development 73:275–281, 1993

74. Derogatis L, Morrow G, Fetting J, et al: The prevalence of psychiatric disorders among cancer patients. JAMA 249:751–757, 1983

75. Des Jarlais D, Friedman S: The psychology of preventing AIDS among intravenous drug users: a social learning conceptualization. Am Psychol 43:865–870, 1988

76. Des Jarlais D, Friedman S, Casriel C, et al: AIDS and preventing initiation into intravenous (IV) drug use. Psychology and Health 1:179–194, 1987

77. Dilley J, Forstein M: Psychosocial aspects of the human immunodeficiency virus (HIV) epidemic, in American Psychiatric Press Review of Psychiatry, Vol 9. Edited by Tasman A, Goldfinger SM, Kaufmann C. Washington, DC, American Psychiatric Press, 1990, pp 631–655

78. Donoghoe M, Dolan K, Stimson G: Life-style factors and social circumstances of syringe sharing in injecting drug users. Br J Addict 87:993–1003, 1992

78a. Doyle D: Caring for a Dying Relative. Oxford, UK, Oxford University Press, 1994

79. Dunkel J, Hatfield S: Countertransference issues in working with persons with AIDS. Soc Work 31:114–117, 1986

80. Egan V, Crawford J, Brettle R, et al: The Edinburgh cohort of HIV-positive drug users: current intellectual function is impaired, but not due to early AIDS dementia complex. AIDS 4:651–656, 1990

81. El-Mallakh R: Mania and paranoid psychosis in AIDS (letter). Psychosomatics 32:362, 1991

82. El-Mallakh R: Mania in AIDS: Clinical significance and theoretical considerations. Int J Psychiatry Med 21:383–391, 1991

83. El-Mallakh R: AIDS dementia-related psychosis: is there a window of vulnerability? AIDS Care 4:381–387, 1992

84. El-Mallakh R: AIDS-related psychosis. J Clin Psychiatry 53:293–294, 1992

85. Feigenberg L: Terminal Care: Friendship Contracts with Dying Cancer Patients. New York, Brunner/Mazel, 1980

86. Fernandez F: Psychiatric aspects of HIV 2. Paper presented at the 142nd annual meeting of the American Psychiatric Association, San Francisco, CA, May 1989

87. Fernandez F, Adams F, Levy J: Cognitive impairment due to AIDS-related complex and its response to psychostimulants. Psychosomatics 29:38–46, 1988

88. Fernandez F, Holmes V, Adams F, et al: Treatment of severe, refractory agitation with a haloperidol drip. J Clin Psychiatry 49:239–241, 1988

89. Fernandez F, Levy J: Psychiatric diagnosis and pharmacotherapy of patients with HIV infection, in American Psychiatric Press Review of Psychiatry, Vol 9. Edited by Tasman A, Goldfinger SM, Kaufmann C. Washington, DC, American Psychiatric Press, 1990, pp 614–628

90. Fernandez F, Levy J: Psychopharmacotherapy of psychiatric syndromes in asymptomatic and symptomatic HIV infection. Psychiatr Med 9:377–394, 1991

91. Fernandez F, Levy J: Psychopharmacology in HIV spectrum disorders. Psychiatr Clin North Am 17:135–148, 1994

92. Fernandez F, Levy J, Galizzi H: Response of HIV-related depression to psychostimulants: case reports. Hosp Community Psychiatry 39:628–631, 1988

93. Fernandez F, Levy J, Mansell P: Response to antidepressant therapy in depressed persons with advanced HIV infection (W.B.P. 191), in Abstracts of the Fifth International Conference on AIDS. Montreal, Canada, International Development Research Center, 1989, p 383

94. Fernandez F, Levy J: Psychopharmacology in HIV spectrum disorders. Psychiatr Clin North Am 17:135–148, 1994

95. Fishman B, Perry S, Jacobsberg L, et al: Psychological factors predicting distress after HIV testing. Paper presented at the Fifth International Conference on AIDS, Montreal, Canada, June 1989

96. Flavin D, Frances R: Risk-taking behavior, substance abuse disorders, and the acquired immune deficiency syndrome. Advances in Alcohol and Substance Abuse 6:23–32, 1987

97. Fogel B: Personality disorders in the medical setting, in Psychiatric Care of the Medical Patient. Edited by Stoudemire A, Fogel B, Gulley L, et al. New York, Oxford University Press, 1993, pp 289–305

98. Fogel B, Mor V: Depressed mood and care preferences in patients with AIDS. Gen Hosp Psychiatry 15:203–207, 1993

99. Folkman S, Chesney M, Christopher-Richards A: Stress and coping in caregiving partners of men with AIDS. Psychiatr Clin North Am 17:35–53, 1994

100. Folstein M, Folstein S, McHugh P: "Mini-Mental State," a practical method for grading the cognitive state of patients for the clinician. J Psychiatr Res 12:189–198, 1975

101. Forstein M: AIDS anxiety in the "worried well," in Psychiatric Implications of Acquired Immune Deficiency Syndrome. Edited by Nichols S, Ostrow D. Washington, DC, American Psychiatric Press, 1984, pp 50–60

102. Franzblau A, Letz R, Hershman D, et al: Quantitative neurologic and neurobehavioral testing of persons infected with HIV-1. Arch Neurol 48:263–268, 1991

103. Freedman J, O'Dowd M, Wyszynski B, et al: Depression, HIV dementia, delirium, posttraumatic stress disorder (or all of the above). Gen Hosp Psychiatry 16:426–434, 1994

104. Friedland G: Clinical care in the AIDS epidemic, in Living with AIDS. Edited by Graubard S. Cambridge, MA, MIT Press, 1990, pp 125–149

105. Friedman S, Young P, Synder F, et al: Racial differences in sexual behaviors related to AIDS in a 19-city sample of street-recruited drug injectors. NADR Consortium. AIDS Educ Prev 5:196–211, 1993

106. Frierson R, Lippmann S: Stresses on physicians treating AIDS. Am Fam Physician 35:153–159, 1987

107. Fuller G, Guiloff R, Garzzard B, et al: Neurological presentations of AIDS—when to test for HIV. J R Soc Med 82:717–720, 1989

108. Gabel R, Barnar N, Norko M, et al: AIDS presenting as mania. Compr Psychiatry 27:251–254, 1986

109. Gabriel M: Group therapists' countertransference reactions to multiple deaths from AIDS. Clin Soc Work J 19:279–292, 1991

110. Gannon R, Anderson M: Fluconazole-nortriptyline drug interaction. Ann Pharmacother 26:1456–1457, 1992

111. Ganzini L, Lee M, Heintz R, et al: The effect of depression treatment on elderly patients' preferences for life-sustaining medical therapy. Am J Psychiatry 151:1631–1636, 1994

112. Geleziunias R, Schipper H, Wainberg M: Pathogenesis and therapy of HIV-1 infection of the central nervous system. AIDS 6:1411–1426, 1992

113. Gilmer W, Busch K: Neuropsychiatric aspects of AIDS and psychopharmacologic management. Psychiatr Med 9:313–329, 1991

114. Glass R: AIDS and suicide. JAMA 259:1369–1370, 1988

115. Gnam W, Flint A, Goldbloom D: Isoniazid-induced hallucinosis: response to pyridoxine (letter). Psychosomatics 34:537–539, 1993

116. Goethe K, Mitchell J, Marshall D, et al: Neuropsychological and neurological function of human immunodeficiency virus seropositive asymptomatic individuals. Ann Neurol 46:129–133, 1989

117. Goldblum P: Professional facing the AIDS epidemic: who helps the helpers? Paper presented at the annual meeting of the American Psychological Association, Washington, DC, August 1986

118. Gordin F, Willoughby A, Levine L, et al: Knowledge of AIDS among hospital workers: behavioral correlates and consequences. AIDS 1:183–188, 1987

119. Gorman J: Caring for the AIDS victim: What can we learn? (editorial). Am J Psychiatry 150:689–690, 1993

120. Gorman J, Mayeux R, Stern Y, et al: The effect of zidovudine on neuropsychiatric measures in HIV-infected men. Am J Psychiatry 150:505–507, 1993

121. Grant I, Atkinson J, Hesselink J, et al: Evidence for early central nervous system involvement in AIDS and other HIV infections. Ann Intern Med 107:828–836, 1987

122. Gray F, Belec L, Keohane C, et al: Zidovudine therapy and HIV encephalitis: a 10-year neuropathological survey. AIDS 8:489–493, 1994

123. Greif G, Porembski E: Implications for therapy with significant others of persons with AIDS. Journal of Gay and Lesbian Psychotherapy 1:79–86, 1989

124. Grossman A, Silverstein C: Facilitating support groups for professionals working with people with AIDS. Soc Work 38:144–151, 1993

125. Groves J: Taking care of the hateful patient. N Engl J Med 298:883–887, 1978

126. Gunther M: Countertransference issues in staff caregivers who work to rehabilitate catastrophic-injury survivors. Am J Psychother 48:208–220, 1994

127. Guydish J, Coates T, Ekstrand M: Changes in AIDS-related high-risk behavior among heterosexual men. Paper presented at the Fourth International Conference on AIDS, Stockholm, Sweden, July 1988

128. Guydish T, Temoshok L, Dilley J, et al: Evaluation of a hospital based substance abuse intervention and referral service for HIV affected patients. Gen Hosp Psychiatry 12:1–7, 1990

129. Haas J, Weissman J, Cleary P, et al: Discussion of preferences for life-sustaining care by persons with AIDS: predictors of failure in patient-physician communication. Arch Intern Med 153:1241–1248, 1993

130. Haimowitz S: HIV and the mentally ill: an approach to the legal issues. Hosp Community Psychiatry 40:732–736, 1989

131. Halevie-Goldman B, Potkin S, Poyourow P: AIDS-related complex presenting as psychosis (letter). Am J Psychiatry 144:964, 1987

132. Hall J, Stevens P: AIDS: a guide to suicide assessment. Arch Psychiatr Nurs 1:115–120, 1988

133. Halstead S, Riccio M, Harlow P: Psychosis associated with HIV infection. Br J Psychiatry 153:618–623, 1988

134. Harris M, Jeste D, Gleghorn A, et al: New-onset psychosis in HIV-infected patients. J Clin Psychiatry 52:369–376, 1991

135. Hays R, Turner H, Coates T: Social support, AIDS-related symptoms, and depression among gay men. J Consult Clin Psychol 60:463–469, 1992

136. Hayward R, Weissfeld J: Coming to terms with the era of AIDS: attitudes of physicians in U.S. residency programs. J Gen Intern Med 8:10–18, 1993

137. Hellerstein D, Prager M: Assessing HIV risk in the general hospital psychiatric clinic. Gen Hosp Psychiatry 14:3–6, 1992

138. Hietanen P, Lnnqvist J, Henriksson M, et al: Do cancer suicides differ from others? Psycho-Oncology 3:189–195, 1994

139. Hintz S, Kuck J, Peterkin J, et al: Depression in the context of human immunodeficiency virus infection: implications for treatment. J Clin Psychiatry 51:497–501, 1990

140. Ho D, Sarngadharan M, Resnick L, et al: Primary human T-lymphotropic virus type III infection. Ann Intern Med 103 (no 6 pt 1):880–883, 1985

141. Hoffman B, Arthurs K, Lunn S, et al: AIDS: clinical and ethical issues on a psychiatric unit. Can J Psychiatry 34:847–851, 1989

142. Hoffman T, Rhodes L, Reed J: Impact of human immunodeficiency virus on medical and surgical residents. Arch Intern Med 152:1788–1796, 1992

143. Holland J, Morrow G, Schmale A, et al: A randomized clinical trial of alprazolam versus progressive muscle relaxation in cancer patients with anxiety and depressive symptoms. J Clin Oncol 9:1004–1011, 1991

144. Holmes F: Rifampin-induced methadone withdrawal in AIDS (letter). J Clin Psychopharmacol 10:443–444, 1990

145. Holmes T, Sabaawi M, Fragala M: Psychostimulant suppository treatment for depression in the gravely ill (letter). J Clin Psychiatry 55:265–266, 1994

146. Holmes V, Fernandez F, Levy J: Psychostimulant response in AIDS-related complex patients. J Clin Psychiatry 50:5–8, 1989

147. Horwath E, Kramer M, Cournos F, et al: Clinical presentations of AIDS and HIV infection in state psychiatric facilities. Hosp Community Psychiatry 40:502–506, 1989

148. Hull J, Clarkin J, Yeomans F: Borderline personality disorder and impulsive sexual behavior. Hosp Community Psychiatry 44:1000–1002, 1993

149. Huyse F, van Tilburg W: Euthanasia policy in The Netherlands: the role of consultation-liaison psychiatrists. Hosp Community Psychiatry 44:733–738, 1993

150. Jacobsberg L, Perry S, Fishman B, et al: Psychiatric diagnoses among volunteers for HIV testing. Paper presented at the Fifth International Conference on AIDS, Montreal, Canada, June 1989

151. Janssen R, Nwanyanwu O, Selik R, et al: Epidemiology of human immunodeficiency virus encephalopathy in the United States. Neurology 42:1472–1476, 1992

152. Janssen R, Saykin A, Cannon L, et al: Neurological and neuropsychological manifestations of HIV-1 infection: association with AIDS-related complex but not asymptomatic HIV-1 infection. Ann Neurol 26:592–600, 1989

153. Johnson R: Questions and prospects related to HIV-1 and the brain, in HIV, AIDS and the Brain. Edited by Price R, Perry S. New York, Raven, 1994, pp 311–323

154. Jones B, Teng E, Folstein M, et al: A new bedside test of cognition for patients with HIV infection. Ann Intern Med 119:1001–1004, 1993

155. Jones G, Kelly C, Davis J: HIV and onset of schizophrenia (letter). Lancet 1:982, 1987

156. Joseph J, Caumartin S, Tal M, et al: Psychological functioning in a cohort of gay men at risk for AIDS. J Nerv Ment Dis 178:607–614, 1990

157. Kalichman S, Kelly J, Johnson J, et al: Factors associated with risk for HIV infection among chronic mentally ill adults. Am J Psychiatry 151:221–227, 1994

158. Karlsen N, Reinvang I, Froland S: A follow-up study of neuropsychological function in asymptomatic HIV-infected patients. Acta Neurol Scand 87:83–87, 1993

158a. Karlsen N, Reinvang I, Froland S: A follow-up study of neuropsychological functioning in AIDS-patients: prognostic significance and effect of zidovudine therapy. Acta Neurol Scand 91:215–221, 1995

159. Kato T, Hirano A, Llena H, et al: Neuropathology of acquired immune deficiency syndrome (AIDS) in 53 autopsy cases with particular emphasis on microglial nodules and multinucleated giant cells. Acta Neuropathol (Berl) 73:287–294, 1987

160. Kelaher M, Ross M: Sources of bias in perception of HIV risk by injecting drug-users. Psychol Rep 70 (3 pt 1):771–774, 1992

161. Kelly J, Murphy D, Bahr G, et al: AIDS/HIV risk behavior among the chronic mentally ill. Am J Psychiatry 149:886–889, 1992

162. Kermani E, Weiss B: AIDS and confidentiality: legal concept and its application in psychotherapy. Am J Psychother 43:25–31, 1989

163. Kernutt G, Price A, Judd F, et al: Human immunodeficiency virus infection, dementia and the older patient. Aust N Z J Psychiatry 27:9–19, 1993

163a. Kessing L, LaBianca J, Bolwig T: HIV-induced stupor treated with ECT. Convuls Ther 10:232–235, 1994

164. Ketzler S, Weis S, Huag H, et al: Loss of neurons in frontal cortex in AIDS brains. Acta Neuropathol (Berl) 80:92–94, 1990

164a. King M: AIDS, HIV and Mental Health. New York, Cambridge University Press, 1993

165. King S: Assisted suicide: sheer cliff or clinical reality? (letter). JAMA 271:23, 1994

166. Kizer K, Green M, Perkins C, et al: AIDS suicide in California (letter). JAMA 260:1881, 1988

167. Kocsis A, Winwood M, Hopper C, et al: Evaluation of the effects of zidovudine and amoxil on neuropsychological functioning and mood (Th.B. 92), in Abstracts, Seventh International Conference on AIDS. Los Angeles, CA, American Foundation for AIDS Research, 1991, p 79

168. Koralnik I, Burkhard P, Ruiz-Scrignari V, et al: Effect of zidovudine (ZID) on early neurological manifestations of HIV infection (M.B. 2023), in Abstracts, Seventh International Conference on AIDS. Los Angeles, CA, American Foundation for AIDS Research, 1991, p 187

169. Kramer T, Ottomanelli G, Bihari B: IV versus non-IV drug use and selected patient variables related to AIDS risk behaviors. Int J Addict 27:477–485, 1992

170. Krikorian R, Wrobel A: Cognitive impairment in HIV infection. AIDS 5:1501–1507, 1991

171. Lamb D, Clark C, Drumheller P, et al: Applying *Tarasoff* to AIDS-related psychotherapy issues. Professional Psychology: Research and Practice 20:37–43, 1989

172. Law W, Martin A, Salazar A, et al: Symptoms of depression in HIV-infected individuals: etiological considerations. Neuropsychiatry, Neuropsychology, and Behavioral Neurology 6:181–186, 1993

173. Lenderking W, Gelber R, Cotton D, et al: Evaluation of the quality of life associated with zidovudine treatment in asymptomatic human immunodeficiency virus infection: the AIDS Clinical Trials Group. N Engl J Med 330:738–743, 1994

174. Lester D: Sexual versus psychiatric predictors of suicide in men with AIDS-related illnesses. Am J Drug Alcohol Abuse 19:139–140, 1993

175. Levine S, Anderson D, Bystritsky A, et al: A report of eight HIV-seropositive patients with major depression responding to fluoxetine. J Acquir Immune Defic Syndr 3:1074–1077, 1990

176. Lewis J: Dying with friends: implications for the psychotherapist. Am J Psychiatry 139:261–266, 1982

177. Lewis M, Jagger R: Delusion of having AIDS (letter). Br Dent J 175:278–279, 1993

178. Link N, Feingold A, Charap M, et al: Concerns of medical and pediatric house officers about acquiring AIDS from their patients. Am J Public Health 78:455–459, 1988

179. Lippert G: Excessive concern about AIDS in two bisexual men. Can J Psychiatry 31:63–65, 1986

179a. Lipton S, Gendelman H: Seminars in medicine of the Beth Israel Hospital, Boston: dementia associated with the acquired immunodeficiency syndrome. N Engl J Med 332:934–940, 1995

180. Lunn S, Skydsbjerg M, Schulsinger H, et al: A preliminary report on the neuropsychological sequelae of human immunodeficiency virus. Arch Gen Psychiatry 48:139–142, 1991

180a. Lyketsos C, Fishman M, Treisman G: Psychiatric issues and emergencies in HIV infection. Emerg Med Clin North Am 13:163–177, 1995

181. Mahler J, Yi D, Sacks M, et al: Undetected HIV infection among patients admitted to an alcohol rehabilitation unit. Am J Psychiatry 151:439–440, 1994

182. Mahorney S, Cavenar J: A new and timely delusion: the complaint of having AIDS. Am J Psychiatry 145:1130–1132, 1988

183. Maj M, Janssen R, Starace F, et al: WHO Neuropsychiatric AIDS Study, cross-sectional phase I: study design and psychiatric findings. Arch Gen Psychiatry 51:39–49, 1994

184. Maj M, Satz P, Janssen R, et al: WHO Neuropsychiatric AIDS Study, cross-sectional phase II: neuropsychological and neurological findings. Arch Gen Psychiatry 51:51–61, 1994

185. Manji H, Connolly S, McAllister R, et al: Serial MRI of the brain in asymptomatic patients infected with HIV: results from the UCMSM/Medical Research Council neurology cohort. J Neurol Neurosurg Psychiatry 57:144–149, 1994

186. Manning D, Jacobsberg L, Erhart S, et al: Efficacy of imipramine in the treatment of HIV-related depression (Th.B. 32), in Program and Abstracts of the VIth International Conference on AIDS, San Francisco, CA, 1990, p 141

187. Markowitz J, Perry S: AIDS: a medical overview for psychiatrists, in American Psychiatric Press Review of Psychiatry, Vol 9. Edited by Tasman A, Goldfinger SM, Kaufmann C. Washington, DC, American Psychiatric Press, 1990, pp 574–592

187a. Maruff P, Currie J, Malone V, et al: Neuropsychological characterization of the AIDS dementia complex and rationalization of a test battery. Arch Neurol 51:689–695, 1994

188. Marzuk P, Tierney H, Tardiff K, et al: Increased risk of suicide in persons with AIDS. JAMA 259:1333–1337, 1988

189. Maslach C: Burned-out. Canadian Journal of Psychiatric Nursing 20:5–9, 1979

190. Massie M, Holland J: The cancer patient with pain. Med Clin North Am 71:243–258, 1987

191. Mathews M: Suicidal competence and the patient's right to refuse lifesaving treatment. Cal Law Review 75:709–758, 1987

192. Mauri M, Sinforiani E, Muratori S, et al: Three-year neuropsychological follow-up in a selected group of HIV-infected homosexual/bisexual men. AIDS 7:241–245, 1993

193. Maxwell S, Scheftner W, Kessler H, et al: Manic syndrome associated with zidovudine treatment. JAMA 259:3406–3407, 1988

194. McAllister R, Herns M, Harrison M, et al: Neurological and neuropsychological performance in HIV-seropositive men without symptoms. J Neurol Neurosurg Psychiatry 55:143–148, 1992

195. McArthur J, Cohen B, Selnes O, et al: Low prevalence of neurological and neuropsychological abnormalities in otherwise healthy HIV-1-infected individuals: results from the Multicenter AIDS Cohort Study. Ann Neurol 26:601–611, 1989

196. McArthur J, Selnes O, Glass J, et al: HIV dementia: incidence and risk factors (review), in HIV, AIDS and the Brain. Edited by Price R, Perry S. New York, Raven, 1994, pp 251–272

196a. McDaniel J, Johnson K: Obsessive-compulsive disorder in HIV disease: response to fluoxetine. Psychosomatics 36:147–150, 1995

197. McKegney F, O'Dowd M: Suicidality and HIV status. Am J Psychiatry 149:396–398, 1992

198. McShane R, Bumbalo J, Patsdaughter C: Psychological distress in family members living with human immunodeficiency virus/acquired immune deficiency syndrome. Arch Psychiatr Nurs 8:53–61, 1994

199. Miller D: Predictors of chronic psychosocial disturbance arising from the threat of HIV infection: lessons from heterosexual, bisexual and homosexual worried well patients. Poster presented at the Third International Conference on AIDS, Washington, DC, June 1–6, 1987

200. Miller D: Occupational morbidity and burnout: lessons and warnings for HIV/AIDS carers. International Review of Psychiatry 3:439–449, 1991

201. Miller D, Acton T, Hedge B: The worried well: their identification and management. J R Coll Physicians Lond 22:158–165, 1988

202. Miller D, Green J, Farmer R, et al: A "pseudo-AIDS" syndrome following from a fear of AIDS. Br J Psychiatry 146:550–551, 1985

203. Miller E, Satz P, Visscher B: Computerized and conventional neuropsychological assessment of HIV-1-infected homosexual men. Neurology 41:1608–1616, 1991

204. Miller E, Selnes O, McArthur J, et al: Neuropsychological performance in HIV-1 infected homosexual men: the Multicenter AIDS Cohort Study. Neurology 40:197–203, 1990

205. Miller F, Weiden P, Sacks M, et al: Two cases of factitious acquired immune deficiency syndrome (letter). Am J Psychiatry 143:1483, 1986

206. Mirra S, Anand R, Spira T: HTLV-III/LAV infection of the central nervous system in a 57-year-old man with progressive dementia of unknown cause. N Engl J Med 314:1191–1192, 1986

207. Mondanaro J: Community-based AIDS prevention interventions: special issues of women intravenous drug users. NIDA Res Monogr 93:68–82, 1990

208. Moss R, Miles S: AIDS and the geriatrician. J Am Geriatr Soc 35:460–464, 1987

209. Nardo J: The personality in the medical setting: a psychodynamic understanding, in Consultation-Liaison Psychiatry and Behavioral Medicine. Edited by Houpt J, Keith H, Brodie H. New York, Basic Books, 1986, pp 53–63

210. National Research Council: AIDS and IV drug use, in AIDS, Sexual Behavior and Intravenous Drug Use. Edited by Turner C, Miller H, Moses L. Washington, DC, National Academy Press, 1989, pp 186–255

211. Neaigus A, Friedman S, Curtis R, et al: The relevance of drug injectors' social and risk networks for understanding and preventing HIV infection. Soc Sci Med 38:67–78, 1994

212. Norton J: Treatment of a dying patient. Psychoanal Study Child 18:541–560, 1963

213. O'Donnell C, O'Donnell L, Pleck J, et al: Psychosocial responses of hospital workers to acquired immunodeficiency syndrome (AIDS). J Appl Soc Psychol 17:269–285, 1987

214. O'Dowd M, Biderman D, McKegney F: Incidence of suicidality in AIDS and HIV-positive patients attending a psychiatry outpatient program. Psychosomatics 34:33–40, 1993

215. O'Dowd M, McKegney F: Manic syndrome associated with zidovudine. JAMA 260:3587–3588, 1988

216. O'Dowd M, Natali C, Orr D, et al: Characteristics of patients attending an HIV-related psychiatric clinic. Hosp Community Psychiatry 42:615–619, 1991

217. Oechsner M, Moller A, Zaudig M: Cognitive impairment, dementia and psychosocial functioning in human immunodeficiency virus infection: a prospective study based on DSM-III-R and ICD-10. Acta Psychiatr Scand 87:13–17, 1993

218. Ostrow D: Substance abuse and HIV infection. Psychiatr Clin North Am 17:69–89, 1994

219. Ostrow D, Monjan A, Joseph J, et al: HIV-related symptoms and psychological functioning in a cohort of homosexual men. Am J Psychiatry 146:737–742, 1989

220. Overman W: Living wills and advance medical treatment directives, in Medical Psychiatric Practice, Vol 2. Edited by Stoudemire A, Fogel B. Washington, DC, American Psychiatric Press, 1993, pp 537–560

221. Patterson J: Alprazolam dependency: Use of clonazepam for withdrawal. South Med J 81:830–836, 1988

222. Perkins D, Davidson E, Lesserman J, et al: Personality disorder in patients infected with HIV: a controlled study with implications for clinical care. Am J Psychiatry 150:309–315, 1993

223. Perkins D, Evans D: Fluoxetine treatment of depression in patients with HIV infection. Am J Psychiatry 148:807–808, 1991

224. Perkins D, Evans D: HIV-related major depression: response to zidovudine treatment. Psychosomatics 32:451–454, 1991

225. Perkins D, Stern R, Golden R, et al: Mood disorders in HIV infection: prevalence and risk factors in a nonepicenter of the AIDS epidemic. Am J Psychiatry 151:233–236, 1994

226. Perry S: Organic mental disorders caused by HIV: update on early diagnosis and treatment. Am J Psychiatry 147:696–710, 1990

227. Perry S, Fishman B, Jacobsberg L, et al: Relationships over one year between lymphocyte subsets and psychosocial variables among adults infected by HIV. Arch Gen Psychiatry 49:396–401, 1992

228. Perry S, Jacobsberg L, Card C, et al: Severity of psychiatric symptoms after HIV testing. Am J Psychiatry 150:775–779, 1993

229. Perry S, Jacobsberg L, Fishman B: Suicidal ideation and HIV testing. JAMA 263:679–682, 1990

230. Perry S, Jacobsberg L, Fishman B, et al: Psychiatric diagnosis before serological testing for human immunodeficiency virus. Am J Psychiatry 147:89–93, 1990

231. Perry S: HIV-related depression, in HIV, AIDS and the Brain. Edited by Price R, Perry S. New York, Raven, 1994, pp 223–238

232. Petito C: Review of central nervous system pathology in human immunodeficiency virus infection. Ann Neurol 23 (suppl):554–557, 1988

233. Petito C, Cho E, Lemann W, et al: Neuropathology of acquired immunodeficiency syndrome (AIDS): an autopsy review. J Neuropathol Exp Neurol 45:635–646, 1986

234. Petito C, Navia B, Cho E, et al: Vacuolar myelopathy pathologically resembling subacute combined degeneration in patients with acquired immunodeficiency syndrome (AIDS). N Engl J Med 312:874–879, 1985

235. Pizzo P, Eddy J, Falloon J, et al: Effect of continuous infusion of zidovudine (AZT) in children with symptomatic HIV infection. N Engl J Med 319:889–896, 1988

235a. Podraza A, Bornstein R, Whitacre C, et al: Neuropsychological performance and CD4 levels in HIV-1 asymptomatic infection. J Clin Exp Neuropsychol 16:777–783, 1994

236. Pogrel M: Delusion of having AIDS (letter). Br Dent J 176:248, 1994

237. Portegies P, de Gans J, Lang J, et al: Declining incidence of AIDS-dementia complex after introduction of zidovudine treatment. BMJ 299:819–821, 1989

238. Price W, Forejt J: Neuropsychiatric aspects of AIDS: a case report. Gen Hosp Psychiatry 8:7–10, 1986

238a. Pugh K, Riccio M, Jadresic D, et al: A longitudinal study of the neuropsychiatric consequences of HIV-1 infection in gay men, II: psychological and health status at baseline and at 12-month follow-up. Psychol Med 24:897–904, 1994

239. Quill T: Doctor, I want to die. Will you help me? JAMA 270:870–873, 1993

240. Rabkin J, Harrison W: Effect of imipramine on depression and immune status in a sample of men with HIV infection. Am J Psychiatry 147:495–497, 1990

241. Rabkin J, Rabkin R, Wagner G: Effects of fluoxetine on mood and immune status in depressed patients with HIV illness. J Clin Psychiatry 55:92–97, 1994

242. Rabkin J, Remien R, Katoff L, et al: Resilience in adversity among long-term survivors of AIDS. Hosp Community Psychiatry 44:162–167, 1993

243. Rabkin J, Wagner G, Rabkin R: Effects of sertraline on mood and immune status in patients with major depression and HIV illness: an open trial. J Clin Psychiatry 55:433–439, 1994

244. Rabkin J, Williams J, Neugebauer R, et al: Maintenance of hope in HIV-spectrum homosexual men. Am J Psychiatry 147:1322–1326, 1990

245. Razavi D, Delvaux N, Fravacques C, et al: Prevention of adjustment disorders and anticipatory nausea secondary to adjuvant chemotherapy: a double-blind, placebo-controlled study assessing the usefulness of alprazolam. J Clin Oncol 11:1384–1390, 1993

246. Reinvang I, Frland S, Karlsen N, et al: Only temporary improvement in impaired neuropsychological function in AIDS patients with zidovudine (letter). AIDS 5:228–229, 1991

246a. Reitan R: Validity of the Trail Making Test as an indicator of organic brain damage. Percept Mot Skills 8:271–276, 1958

247. Riedel R, Clarenbach P, Reetz K: Coma during azidothymidine therapy for AIDS (letter). J Neurol 236:185, 1989

248. Riley M: AIDS and older people: the overlooked segment of the population, in AIDS in an Aging Society—What We Need To Know. Edited by Riley M, Ory M, Zablotsky D. New York, Springer, 1989, pp 3–26

249. Robertson K, Hall C: Human immunodeficiency virus-related cognitive impairment and the acquired immunodeficiency syndrome dementia complex. Semin Neurol 12:18–27, 1992

250. Rogers J, Britton P: AIDS and rational suicide: a counseling psychology perspective or a slide on the slippery slope. Counseling Psychologist 22:171–178, 1994

251. Rosenbaum M: Similarities of psychiatric disorders of AIDS and syphilis: history repeats itself. Bull Menninger Clin 58:375–382, 1994

252. Rosmarin D: Legal and ethical aspects of HIV disease, in AIDS Primer. Edited by American Psychiatric Association AIDS Education Project. Washington, DC, American Psychiatric Association, 1990, pp 63–76

253. Rothchild E: Family dynamics in end-of-life treatment decisions. Gen Hosp Psychiatry 16:251–258, 1994

254. Rundell J, Kyle K, Brown G: Risk factors for suicide attempts in a human immunodeficiency virus screening program. Psychosomatics 33:24–27, 1992

255. Rundell J, Wise M, Ursano R: Three cases of AIDS related psychiatric disorders. Am J Psychiatry 143:777–778, 1986

256. Ryan F: AIDS as a cause of dementia in the elderly. Md Med J 38:251–254, 1989

257. Sabin T: AIDS: the new "Great Imitator." J Am Geriatr Soc 35:467–471, 1987

258. Sacks M, Silberstein C, Weiler P, et al: HIV-related risk factors in acute psychiatric inpatients. Hosp Community Psychiatry 41:449–451, 1990

259. Schaerf F, Miller R, Lipsey J, et al: ECT for major depression in four patients infected with human immunodeficiency virus. Am J Psychiatry 146:782–784, 1989

260. Schaffner B: Reactions of medical personnel and intimates to persons with AIDS. Psychotherapy Patient 2:67–80, 1986

261. Schaffner B: Psychotherapy with HIV-infected persons, in New Dir Ment Health Serv 48:5–20, 1990

261a. Schaffner B: The crucial and difficult role of the psychotherapist in the treatment of the HIV-positive patient. J Am Acad Psychoanal 22:505–518, 1994

262. Schmidt U, Miller D: Two cases of hypomania in AIDS. Br J Psychiatry 152:839–842, 1988

263. Schmitt F, Bigley J, McKinnis R, et al: Neuropsychological outcome of zidovudine (AZT) treatment of patients with AIDS and AIDS related complex. N Engl J Med 319:1573–1578, 1988

263a. Schneiderman L, Teetzel H: Who decides who decides? when disagreement occurs between the physician and the patient's appointed proxy about the patient's decision-making capacity. Arch Intern Med 155:793–796, 1995

264. Schwartz A, Karasu T: Psychotherapy with the dying patient. Am J Psychother 21:19–35, 1977

265. Schwarz M: Physicians' attitudes toward AIDS, in Public and Professional Attitudes Toward AIDS Patients. Edited by Rogers D, Ginzberg E. Boulder, CO, Westview Press, 1989, pp 31–41

266. Scott C, Jaffe D: Managing occupational stress associated with HIV infection: self-care and management skills. Occup Med 4:85–93, 1989

266a. Searight H, Pound P: The HIV-positive psychiatric patient and the duty to protect: ethical and legal issues. Int J Psychiatry Med 24:259–270, 1994

267. Selnes O, Galai N, Bacellar H, et al: Cognitive performance after progression to AIDS: a longitudinal study from the Multicenter AIDS Cohort Study. Neurology 45:267–275, 1995

268. Selnes O, Miller E, McArthur J, et al: HIV-1 infection: no evidence of cognitive decline during the asymptomatic stages. Neurology 40:204–208, 1990

269. Serrano Y: The Puerto Rican intravenous drug user. NIDA Res Monogr 93:24–34, 1990

270. Sidtis J: Evaluation of the AIDS dementia complex in adults, in HIV, AIDS and the Brain. Edited by Price R, Perry S. New York, Raven, 1994, pp 273–287

271. Sidtis J: Evaluation of the AIDS dementia complex in adults. Research Publications—Association for Research in Nervous and Mental Disease 72:273–287, 1994

272. Siegel K: Psychosocial aspects of rational suicide. Am J Psychother 40:405–417, 1986

273. Silva J, Leong G, Weinstock R: An HIV-infected psychiatric patient: some clinicolegal dilemmas. Bull Am Acad Psychiatry Law 17:33–43, 1989

274. Silverman D: Psychosocial impact of HIV-related caregiving on health providers: a review of recommendations for the role of psychiatry. Am J Psychiatry 150:705–712, 1993

275. Simberkoff M: Ethical aspects in the care of patients with AIDS. Neurol Clin 7:871–882, 1989

276. Sno H, Storosum J, Wortel C: Psychogenic "HIV infection." Int J Psychiatr Med 21:93–98, 1991

277. Snyder S, Strain J, Fulop G: Evaluation and treatment of mental disorders in patients with AIDS. Compr Ther 16:34–41, 1990

278. Solomon M, O'Donnell L, Jennings B, et al: Decisions near the end of life: professional views on life-sustaining treatments. Am J Public Health 83:14–23, 1993

278a. Songer D: Factitious AIDS: A case report and literature review. Psychosomatics 36:406–411, 1995

279. Stall R, McKusick L, Wiley J, et al: Alcohol and drug use during sexual activity and compliance with safe sex guidelines for AIDS: the AIDS Behavioral Research Project. Health Educ Q 13:359–371, 1986

280. Starace F: Suicidal behaviour in people infected with human immunodeficiency virus: a literature review. Int J Soc Psychiatry 39:64–70, 1993

281. Stern R, Marder K, Bell K, et al: Multidisciplinary baseline assessment of homosexual men with and without human immunodeficiency virus infection, III: neurologic and neuropsychological findings. Arch Gen Psychiatry 48:131–138, 1991

282. Stern Y, Singer N, Silver S, et al: Neurobehavioral functioning in a nonconfounded group of asymptomatic HIV-seropositive homosexual men. Am J Psychiatry 149:1099–1102, 1992

283. Stern Y: Neuropsychological evaluation of the HIV patient. Psychiatr Clin North Am 17:125–134, 1994

283a. Stern Y, Liu X, Marder K, et al: Neuropsychological changes in a prospectively followed cohort of homosexual and bisexual men with and without HIV infection. Neurology 45:467–472, 1995

284. Stevens L, Muskin P: Techniques for reversing the failure of empathy towards AIDS patients. J Am Acad Psychoanal 15:539–551, 1987

285. Storch D: Caution with use of tricyclics in patients with AIDS (letter). Am J Psychiatry 148:1750, 1991

286. Stoudemire A, Fogel B: Psychopharmacology in the medical patient, in Psychiatric Care of the Medical Patient. Edited by Stoudemire A, Fogel B, Gulley L, et al. New York, Oxford University Press, 1993, pp 155–206

287. Stowe A, Ross M, Wodak A, et al: Significant relationships and social supports of injecting drug users and their implications for HIV/AIDS services. AIDS Care 5:23–33, 1993

288. Strain J, Rhodes R, Moros D, et al: Ethics in medical-psychiatric practice, in Medical Psychiatric Practice, Vol 2. Edited by Stoudemire A, Fogel B. Washington, DC, American Psychiatric Press, 1993, pp 585–607

289. Sullivan M, Youngner S: Depression, competence, and the right to refuse lifesaving medical treatment. Am J Psychiatry 151:971–978, 1994

290. Sullivan P, Carra J, Musgrave J, et al: Pharmacotherapy and psychotherapy for major depression in a man with AIDS (letter). Am J Psychiatry 149:138, 1992

291. Summergrad P, Glassman R: Human immunodeficiency virus and other infectious disorders affecting the nervous system, in Medical Psychiatric Practice, Vol 1. Edited by Stoudemire A, Fogel B. Washington, DC, American Psychiatric Press, 1991, pp 243–285

292. Susser E, Struening E, Conover S: Psychiatric problems in homeless men: lifetime psychosis, substance use, and current distress in new arrivals at New York City shelters. Arch Gen Psychiatry 46:845–850, 1989

292a. Susser E, Valencia E, Miller M, et al: Sexual behavior of homeless mentally ill men at risk for HIV. Am J Psychiatry 152:583–587, 1995

293. Syndulko K, Singer E, Nogales-Gaete J, et al: Laboratory evaluations in HIV-1-associated cognitive/motor complex. Psychiatr Clin North Am 17:91–123, 1994

294. Tartiglione T, Collier A, Coombs R, et al: Acquired immunodeficiency syndrome: cerebrospinal fluid findings in patients before and during long-term oral zidovudine therapy. Arch Neurol 48:695–699, 1991

295. Thomas C, Szabadi E: Paranoid psychosis as the 1st presentation of a fulminating lethal case of AIDS. Br J Psychiatry 151:693–694, 1987

296. Todd J: AIDS as a current psychopathological theme: a report on five heterosexual patients. Br J Psychiatry 154:253–255, 1989

297. Tozzi V, Narciso P, Galgani S, et al: Effects of zidovudine in 30 patients with mild to end-stage AIDS dementia complex. AIDS 7:683–692, 1993

298. Tross S: Acquired immunodeficiency syndrome, in Handbook of Psychooncology. Edited by Holland J, Rowland J. New York, Oxford University Press, 1990, pp 254–270

299. Tross S, Price R, Navia B, et al: Neuropsychological characterization of the AIDS dementia complex: a preliminary report. AIDS 2:81–88, 1988

300. Tyson E, Fortenberry J: Fraudulent AIDS: a variant on Munchausen's syndrome. JAMA 258:1889–1890, 1987

301. Uldall K, Koutsky L, Bradshaw D, et al: Psychiatric comorbidity and length of stay in hospitalized AIDS patients. Am J Psychiatry 151:1475–1478, 1994

302. Upadhyaya M, Chaturvedi S: Psychosis and antituberculosis therapy. Lancet 2:735–736, 1989

303. Vachon M, Dennis J: HIV, stress, and the health care professional, in Face to Face: A Guide to AIDS Counselling. Edited by Dilley J, Pies C, Helquist M. San Francisco, CA, AIDS Health Project, University of California, 1989, pp 2–14

304. Van Gorp W, Moller E, Satz P, et al: Neuropsychological performance in HIV-1 immunocompromised patients: a preliminary report. J Clin Exp Neuropsychol 11:763–773, 1989

305. Villa G, Monteleone D, Marra C, et al: Neuropsychological abnormalities in AIDS and asymptomatic HIV seropositive patients. J Neurol Neurosurg Psychiatry 56:878–884, 1993

305a. Vion-Dury J, Nicoli F, Salvan A, et al: Reversal of brain metabolic alterations with zidovudine detected by proton localised magnetic resonance spectroscopy (letter). Lancet 345:60–61, 1995

306. Volavka J, Convit A, O'Donnell J, et al: Assessment of risk behaviors for HIV infection among psychiatric inpatients. Hosp Community Psychiatry 43:482–485, 1992

307. Wachter R: The impact of the acquired immunodeficiency syndrome on medical residency training. N Engl J Med 314:177–180, 1986

307a. Wallace A, Kofoed L, West A: Double-blind, placebo-controlled trial of methylphenidate in older, depressed, medically ill patients. Am J Psychiatry 152:929–931, 1995

308. Wallack J: AIDS anxiety among health care professionals. Hosp Community Psychiatry 40:507–510, 1989

308a. Wallack J, Bialer P, Prenzlauer S: Psychiatric aspects of HIV infection and AIDS: an overview and update, in Medical-Psychiatric Practice, Vol 3. Edited by Stoudemire A, Fogel B. Washington, DC, American Psychiatric Press, 1995, pp 257–302

309. Warner M, Peabody C, Whiteford H, et al: Alprazolam as an antidepressant. J Clin Psychiatry 49:148–150, 1988

309a. Wechsler D: WAIS-R Manual. New York, Psychological Corporation, 1981

310. Weiler P, Mungas D, Pomerantz S: AIDS as a cause of dementia in the elderly. J Am Geriatr Soc 36:139–141, 1988

311. Weinberger M, Conover C, Samsa G, et al: Physicians' attitudes and practices regarding treatment of HIV-infected patients. South Med J 85:683–686, 1992

312. Weisman A: On Dying and Denying: A Psychiatric Study of Terminality. New York, Behavioral Press, 1972

312a. Weitzner M, Meyers C, Valentine A: Methylphenidate in the treatment of neurobehavioral slowing associated with cancer and cancer treatment. J Neuropsychiatry Clin Neurosci 7:347–349, 1995

313. White J, Christensen J, Singer C: Methylphenidate as a treatment for depression in acquired immunodeficiency syndrome: an n-of-1 trial. J Clin Psychiatry 53:153–156, 1992

314. Wiener P, Schwartz M, O'Connell R: Characteristics of HIV-infected patients in an inpatient psychiatric setting. Psychosomatics 35:59–65, 1994

315. Wilkie F, Eisdorfer C, Morgan R, et al: Cognition in early human immunodeficiency virus infection. Arch Neurol 47:433–440, 1990

316. William J, Rabkin J, Remien R, et al: The prevalence of personality disorders in HIV+ and HIV- gay men (S.B. 364), in Program and Abstracts of the Sixth International Conference on AIDS, San Francisco, CA, June 1990, p 177

317. Williams B, Rabkin J, Remien R, et al: Multidisciplinary baseline assessment of homosexual men with and without human immunodeficiency virus infection. Arch Gen Psychiatry 48:124–130, 1991

318. Woo S, Levine S, Anderson D: The impact of HIV on the health care provider, in AIDS Primer. Edited by American Psychiatric Association AIDS Education Project. Washington, DC, American Psychiatric Association, 1990, pp 51–55

319. Yarchoan R, Berg G, Brouwers P, et al: Response of human immunodeficiency virus-associated neurological disease to 3'-azido-2',3'-dideoxythymidine. Lancet 1:132–135, 1987

320. Yarchoan R, Thomas R, Grafman J, et al: Long-term administration of 3'-azido-2',3'-dideoxythymidine to patients with AIDS-related neurological disease. Ann Neurol 23 (suppl):S82–S87, 1988

321. Zamperetti M, Goldwurm G, Abbate E, et al: Attempted suicide: epidemiological aspects in a psychiatric ward (S.B. 287), in Program and Abstracts of the Sixth International Conference on AIDS, San Francisco, CA, June 1990, p 182

322. Zuger A, O'Dowd M: The baron has AIDS: a case of factitious human immunodeficiency virus infection and review. Clin Infect Dis 14:211–216, 1992

323. Zybenko G, Anselm G, Soloff P, et al: Sexual practices among patients with borderline personality disorder. Am J Psychiatry 144:748–753, 1987

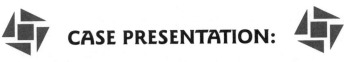

CASE PRESENTATION:

Ms. Newman: The Female HIV Patient

This 25-year-old African-American woman is self-referred and seeks help with her romantic relationships with men. She has always been considered attractive and works as a photographer's model intermittently, but has been trying to complete her B.A. at night. Ms. Newman states that while she enjoys romantic relationships, it is "difficult to take sex seriously" enough to consider ever settling down with one man. She thinks this may have something to do with early sexual abuse between the ages of 6 and 8 by an uncle, which she maintains is painful to talk about, "but I'm over it." On closer questioning, she acknowledges that she cannot bring herself to ask men to wear condoms, even though she knows that they have many other sexual contacts and she is placing herself at risk for

AIDS. Although she denies dysphoria or anxiety, she states that if she were HIV positive, she would kill herself. There is no history of drug or alcohol use. There is no prior personal or family psychiatric history. She has never attempted suicide, nor have any family members. She is on no medications and has no past medical history.

Mental status exam reveals an attractive young woman, neatly and stylishly dressed. Rapport is warmly engaging. Her speech is goal-directed, coherent, and logical. Her affect is full, and mood is euthymic. She sheepishly admits that she does not practice safe sex "in any respect." There are no delusions or hallucinations. She is alert and oriented, and higher cognitive functions are intact.

 QUESTIONS

Choose all that apply.

1. What approach would you take concerning antibody testing for someone like Ms. Newman?
   a. The most effective way to modify her high-risk behavior would be antibody testing.
   b. It has been established that suicidal ideation does *not* uniformly increase in patients discovered to be seropositive.
   c. The use of informed consent as a model for discussing serological testing tends to predispose to adverse psychological reactions.
   d. Patients who react adversely to their uncertain serological status should have antibody testing as a way of lessening their discomfort.

2. Ms. Newman confides that she engages in a full range of sexual activities with her various boyfriends. Which of the following statements are accurate regarding relative risk (i.e., safe, probably safe, unsafe)?
   a. Performing fellatio to climax and swallowing semen is considered "probably safe," because the AIDS virus is inactivated by gastric acid.

   b. Both cunnilingus and fellatio (without swallowing semen) are considered unsafe without a condom or dental dam.
   c. *Insertive* anal intercourse without a condom is considered unsafe to *both* partners.
   d. Mouth-to-mouth kissing is considered safe.
   e. Any genital contact will not be safe if either partner has a genital irritation or rash.

3. Ms. Newman is relieved to be able to discuss with you questions that are "too embarrassing" to ask even her gynecologist. Which of her beliefs below are valid?
   a. Natural-membrane condoms confer better protection than latex against HIV transmission.
   b. If K-Y Jelly is not available, saliva is an acceptable substitute.
   c. Vasectomy protects against HIV infection.
   d. The *only* contraceptive strategy (other than abstinence) that reliably protects against HIV infection is condom use.
   e. Condoms, like diaphragms, should be carefully inspected for defects by unrolling them and gently stretching them.

f. If a sexual activity can result in pregnancy, it can result in HIV infection.

4. As her therapy progresses, Ms. Newman maintains that AIDS is an illness of gay white males. She has little information about the statistics in women or minority communities. Which of the following are accurate?

a. The numbers of African-Americans and Latinos (Hispanics) infected with HIV are roughly proportional to their numbers in the U.S. population.

b. The proportion of infected African-American and Latino men who are IV drug users is about equivalent to the proportion of infected white male IV drug users.

c. The notion that African-American or Latino men are less likely to acknowledge their homosexual behavior is mainly based on stereotype and has little realistic basis.

d. Some gay African-American and Latino men believe that they can safely have unprotected sex, as long as it is only with nonwhite men.

5. The percentage of infected men with bisexual behavior (who are therefore more likely to serve as disease vectors to females) has been reported as . . .

a. Roughly equivalent in African-Americans, Latinos, and whites

b. Lowest in African-Americans

c. Higher in Haitians than in African-American blacks

d. Highest in Latinos born in the United States

e. Higher in African-Americans than in whites

6. The epidemiology of bisexuality in men has shown that . . .

a. Married men who engage in homosexual activity are more likely than unmarried men to inform their regular female partner of their behavior.

b. Bisexual men have higher rates of prostitution than homosexual men.

c. The rates of bisexual activity among Latinos who are born and live *outside* the United States are lower than among those who are born here.

d. The rates of bisexual behavior in black men with AIDS who are Haitian are significantly higher than those in black men with AIDS who are born in the United States.

e. Behaviorally bisexual men who are *self-identified* as heterosexual use condoms at lower rates than do self-identified homosexual or bisexual men.

7. What are valid concerns regarding HIV's impact on women, according to a recent study[25]?

a. Only a minority of *educated*, seropositive women engaged in unprotected heterosexual intercourse.

b. Most educated seropositive women (who knew they were HIV positive) had unprotected intercourse only with seropositive men.

c. Females are at *higher* risk than males for HIV transmission through intercourse with an infected male bisexual partner.

d. No seronegative men had unprotected intercourse with educated, seropositive women without having been informed of their partners' seropositive status.

8. Factors that place economically disadvantaged African-American and Latina women at greater risk for HIV infection compared with their white counterparts include . . .

a. Greater likelihood of having sexual contact with bisexual men.

b. Lack of control over sexual decision making relative to their male partners.

c. Earlier age of onset of sexual activity.

d. Lack of knowledge regarding HIV infection.

9. Over the next several months, Ms. Newman reveals that the uncle who sexually abused her died of AIDS about 2 years ago. The sexual contact with him had been limited to fondling. She states, "I never really thought about it this way before, but I guess I feel like I 'paid my dues,' and that my uncle getting AIDS was his punishment for what he did to me. I was innocent—how could God have something as bad happen to me again?" She also is able to admit that her professional successes have given her a sense of "being invincible, as if nothing can stop me." She begins to see that her reluctance to ask men to use condoms concerns her fears of undermining the sophisticated image she so desperately wishes to promote. Having multiple lovers makes her believe she's desirable—very different from the defective person she feels herself to be. Ms. Newman decides to undergo serological testing, and learns she is HIV positive. She is devastated, with episodes of tearfulness and fear. All of the following are true about the adaptation to HIV infection except . . .

a. A fighting spirit toward the illness often occurs at some point in its course.

b. It is therapeutically unrealistic to expect that Ms. Newman could evolve a new identity with the acceptance of AIDS.

c. Prior personal or family psychiatric history increases the risk for HIV-associated psychopathology.

d. Childhood sexual abuse is a risk factor for adult HIV infection even though there was no exchange of body fluids.

10. Ms. Newman misses one menstrual period about 1 week after learning that she is seropositive. Her pregnancy test comes back positive. She agonizes over whether to have the baby, given her strong religious prohibitions against abortion. She also shares that she has held a secret belief that she could never conceive a child—a reflection of her inner sense of being defective as a woman. Sex with multiple partners that never before resulted in "accidental" pregnancy appeared to confirm her conviction. Which of the following is/are true?

a. Seropositive women are less likely to deliver live babies than are seronegative women.

b. The progression of HIV infection is slower in women than in men.

c. The virus is transmitted in breast milk.

d. There is consensus that pregnancy protects against symptomatic progression in seropositive women.

11. The risk of a seropositive woman having an infected baby . . .

a. Approaches 75%

b. Is largely independent of maternal lymphocyte counts

c. Is significantly affected by placental factors

d. None of the above

12. The *majority* of HIV-infected children have at least one parent with a history of . . .

a. IV drug abuse

b. Male-to-male anal sex

c. Blood transfusion

d. Prostitution

13. Ms. Newman elects to terminate the pregnancy. Several months later, she is hospitalized with her first bout of PCP (*Pneumocystis carinii* pneumonia), which presents with fever, cough, shortness of breath, and weight loss. Although her dyspnea has improved, the nursing staff reports that she is increasingly anxious, often unable to eat or cooperate with the rigors of inpatient treatment. She talks about fears that she will die alone, even though her sister regularly visits and is quite supportive. Which of the following are true?

a. Propranolol (Inderal) is a helpful anxiolytic in PCP patients because it does not depress respiration.

b. Sleeping medications should not be used.

c. Diphenhydramine (Benadryl) is particularly effective when anxiety occurs with PCP, since it does not depress respirations.

d. Buspirone (BuSpar) may increase the risk for dyskinesias.

14. Ms. Newman's friends have introduced her to holistic medicine, adding a nutritional regime and "healing crystals" to her traditional medical treatment. Her physician has told her that she should do what makes her feel better. Ms. Newman knows that psychotherapy brings her relief, and asks about the impact of psychological factors on her illness.

a. Stressful life events are associated with symptom onset in HIV infection.

b. Psychosocial stressors do not correlate with individual measures of HIV illness, but do correlate with a cumulative index of HIV illness stage.

c. Depressive disorders appear to bear no consistent relationship to immune status as measured by CD4 and CD8 cell subsets.

d. All of the above.

15. Ms. Newman is discharged home on zidovudine 1000 mg daily. She is brought to the emergency service about 2 months later with flight of ideas, euphoric affect, psychomotor agitation, and grandiose delusions. Which factors are relevant to this clinical picture?

a. Zidovudine must be discontinued when it precipitates mania, since it cannot be combined with lithium.

b. Ganciclovir (DHPG) has been associated with secondary mania.

c. A cryptosporidial infection is more likely to limit treatment of this psychiatric condition than to be etiological.

d. Secondary mania occurs almost exclusively in the late stages of HIV infection.

e. The cognitive changes that accompany secondary mania in HIV are akin to the "pseudodementia" of depression and remit with clearing of the affective symptoms.

16. Ms. Newman's agitation makes it impossible to complete the necessary workup of her changed mental status. She insists that "I am the World, I am the Children," empowered by Jesus to read the minds of the staff. She "has

seen the face of the Lord" in the radiology suite and at the nurses' station. She is alert, but disoriented for place and time. Concentration is severely impaired, and it is not possible to accurately test other cognitive functions. Which of the following are true regarding the occurrence of psychosis in the setting of HIV infection?

    a. A delusional state without affective changes is the most common psychotic presentation.

    b. Neurological evaluation reveals focal abnormalities in the majority of patients with new-onset HIV psychosis.

    c. Psychosis has been described without coexistent cognitive deterioration in these patients.

    d. A prodromal phase usually precedes the onset of psychosis.

    e. Psychosis is usually accompanied by a seizure disorder.

17. What is true about the occurrence of hallucinations in new-onset HIV psychosis?

    a. Hallucinations are less frequent than delusions.

    b. Hallucinations are usually visual.

    c. Hallucinations usually occur in the absence of an identifiable mood disturbance.

    d. Computed tomography (CT) scan abnormalities are almost always evident when hallucinations are the initial presentation.

18. What are important factors in treating psychotic AIDS patients like Ms. Newman?

    a. Benztropine (Cogentin) is the antiparkinsonian of choice for extrapyramidal side effects.

    b. AIDS patients are more likely to develop extrapyramidal side effects on neuroleptics than are other medically ill patients.

    c. AIDS patients are more likely to develop neuroleptic malignant syndrome than are other medically ill patients.

    d. The psychosis of HIV requires neuroleptic doses at the high end of the therapeutic range.

19. A side effect that would be more likely with amantadine (Symmetrel) than with benztropine (Cogentin) is . . .

    a. Psychosis

    b. Dry mouth

    c. Sedation

    d. Anticholinergic toxicity

20. Ms. Newman has to be restrained and begins haloperidol (Haldol), with fairly good resolution of agitation. It becomes clear, however, that her level of alertness fluctuates throughout the day. Which of the following are likely etiologies for delirium in Ms. Newman?

    a. Herpes encephalitis

    b. Cryptococcal meningitis

    c. CNS lymphoma

    d. Zidovudine

    e. All of the above

✦ Answers

1.	Answer: b (pp. 251–253)	12.	Answer: a (pp. 260–261)
2.	Answer: b, c, e (p. 254)	13.	Answer: d (pp. 261–262)
3.	Answer: d, f (p. 254)	14.	Answer: c (pp. 256–257)
4.	Answer: d (pp. 257–259)	15.	Answer: b, c (p. 262)
5.	Answer: e (p. 258)	16.	Answer: c (pp. 262–263)
6.	Answer: b, e (pp. 257–259)	17.	Answer: a (pp. 262–263)
7.	Answer: c (pp. 259–260)	18.	Answer: b, c (p. 263)
8.	Answer: a, c (pp. 258–259)	19.	Answer: a (p. 263)
9.	Answer: b (pp. 254–256)	20.	Answer: e (p. 264)
10.	Answer: c (pp. 260–261)		
11.	Answer: c (pp. 260–261)		

◆ ANTIBODY TESTING: TO KNOW, OR NOT TO KNOW?

It is a common misconception that serological testing solves the problem of high-risk drug or sexual behavior. Think about other examples of medical noncompliance—smoking cessation, breast self-examination, seat-belt use, low-fat diets, the benefits of exercise—and the knowledge-behavior gap emerges as a familiar landmark. Compliance with medical advice is multidetermined and not simply achieved.

A few years back, Marshall Forstein[74] argued against mandatory HIV testing and counseling for all psychiatric inpatients, which had been proposed[205] to help modify high-risk behavior. Even for patients who *requested* testing, Dr. Forstein warned against shortcuts around the complex psychological issues of serological testing, such as the realistic versus fantasied effects of antiviral medication and the repercussions of knowing that one is HIV positive.

◆ For example, consistent with the psyche's unpredictability, *suicidal ideation has been reported as a result of both **negative** and **positive** tests.*[167,168]

Forstein[74,75] has urged clinicians to *use the model of **informed consent**, framing HIV testing as a medical procedure with benefits but also potential psychological risks.* This approach enhances the likelihood that the patient will receive thorough preparation before potentially devastating news, and provides a framework to which he or she can later return—if necessary—for comfort, support, and further exploration.

Serotesting and Psychiatric Morbidity

The research of Perry et al.[167,168] has shown that suicidal ideation does not invariably increase after HIV testing. Several points are worth noting from their 1990 study:

◆ During the week after result notification, rates of self-reported suicidal ideation decreased significantly among the seronegative subjects ($n = 252$) and did *not* significantly *increase* among the seropositive subjects ($n = 49$).[168] *Two months later, suicidal ideation had also significantly decreased in the seropositive sample.*

◆ These patients were given pretest and posttest counseling[168] that emphasized that seropositivity was not

synonymous with AIDS and should not be viewed as an imminent death sentence (e.g., patients were given information about the prolonged average latency of HIV infection before symptoms develop, the decreasing annual mortality rate of AIDS patients, the efficacy of current maintenance antiviral medications, the promise of future drugs).

◆ Of concern, however, was the finding of *persistent* suicidal ideation in over 15% of *both seropositive and seronegative groups*, suggesting that a subgroup of at-risk subjects is experiencing notable emotional distress regardless of test results.[167,168] This is consonant with the high *lifetime* (i.e., premorbid, pre-HIV) rates of mood disorders in a sample of physically asymptomatic adults seeking HIV serological testing.[169]

Clearly, uncertainty about one's serological status takes an emotional toll; even though most seronegative individuals believed at intake that they would receive good news, they nevertheless experienced significant relief when their correct predictions were confirmed.[170] Also notable is that *suicidal ideation is not an inevitable consequence of the news of seropositivity.*

> Our findings may help reduce the fear of at-risk adults about voluntarily seeking the HIV tests and may also buffer the more general concern that knowledge of HIV infection inevitably will have adverse emotional consequences. The reduced distress over time supports the maxim that "the devil that you see may be less frightening than the devil you don't." Our results are consistent with non-HIV studies that have found that *most adults, when informed of potentially fatal illnesses, do not have psychopathological reactions.*[167] (p. 778, italics added)

Of concern, however, is the group at risk for significant distress *regardless* of serological outcome.[100a] This finding highlights the need for clinicians to be familiar with the general issues surrounding serological testing, and to tailor an approach that recognizes each patient's unique psychodynamics and vulnerabilities. Finally, when considering reports of relatively benign reactions to news of seropositivity, remember that many of these study subjects received excellent pre- and posttest counseling.[167,170] Unfortunately, such preparation may be absent when testing occurs in other contexts.

Factors that do increase risk for HIV-associated psychopathology include the following:[51,186]

◆   Personal or family psychiatric history
◆   Recent bereavement
◆   History of trauma
◆   Few social supports

Delayed Reactions to Seropositivity

There are often *delayed* reactions of disillusionment, despair, or frank depression to a seropositive diagnosis after a period of relatively good psychological and behavioral adjustment.[53] Some studies have reported adverse sexual behavioral change (i.e., from low-risk before disclosure to high-risk afterward).[12] There are often feelings that death is imminent, or that sexuality and intimacy are no longer possible. Understanding the particular character structure, coping mechanisms, and premorbid history helps guide your approach to the patient.

The Knowledge-Behavior Gap

To repeat, there is no shortcut to behavioral change. A growing literature indicates that many individuals continue to be ill informed about HIV,[106,178] or persist in high-risk sexual practices despite adequate information.[25,84,123,140,150,176,198,231] Relevant factors include how personal risk is perceived with specific partners in specific situations, how it is weighed against expectations of potential discomfort or reduced sexual pleasure, and how strong the denial is.[117] For example,

◆   Data from more than 1,000 sexually active young males in the National Survey of Adolescent Males (interviewed in 1988 at ages 15–19 and reinterviewed in 1990–1991 at ages 17–22) showed that as the respondents grew older, their condom use *declined*, as did their degree of worry about AIDS and their perceived likelihood of getting AIDS.[172] Change in condom use was partially affected by perceived reduction in sexual pleasure.

Sometimes negative antibody status makes it *more* difficult to change high-risk sexual behavior.[73,74,209] Higher levels of recreational drug use and the presence of depression correlate with ongoing high-risk sexual practices in seropositive individuals.[107] Forstein[74] reported

that individuals most likely to make appropriate behavioral changes had suspected themselves to be HIV positive and tested positive; those who tested negative failed to make such changes. Dilley and Forstein[53] have written,

> Antibody testing cannot substitute for the exploration of *why it is difficult to engage in safer practices even without knowing antibody status.* Helping a patient to see the self-destructive impulses in the continuation of unsafe sexual practices and/or drug behaviors can be a major part of the work before testing is considered . . . Before testing, the therapist and patient must confront the realistic possibility that the test could be positive, and anticipate whether the information would be more or less difficult to deal with than the uncertainty of knowing the antibody status. (p. 646, italics added)

Forstein's[74] outline of these issues is clinically helpful:

◆   Does the individual perceive that he or she is at risk for HIV infection? If there is no perception of risk, there is no lasting motivation to make behavioral changes.
◆   If the individual believes that he or she is positive, is there the belief that the condition can be worsened by reexposure? Does the person have the capacity to care about infecting others?
◆   Does the individual believe that changing high-risk behavior will have an impact on the outcome of being HIV positive, or will confer some protection from getting infected?
◆   How would either a positive or a negative test affect the way the individual lives his or her life now?
◆   How well does the individual contain ambiguity? Is it acted out behaviorally or managed in an internal, psychological manner?
◆   Has there been any prior experience in the person's life to suggest that knowing his or her antibody status will contribute to the capacity to change behavior?

Psychiatrists are in a unique position to help promote life-saving behavioral change through understanding the psychology of noncompliance for a particular individual. Persistent high-risk sexual behavior should be viewed as a form of noncompliance with medical advice. To repeat, noncompliant behavior is multidetermined; unconscious factors may interfere with modifying actions despite intellectual understanding about a disease and its prevention. Patients like Ms. Newman may deny their infection even while acknowledging that they are having unsafe sex and jeopardizing the health of an unsuspecting partner.[134,197] These attitudes are crucial to explore in psychotherapy.

Countertransference

As mentioned, the caregiver's psychology affects the quality of the caregiving. AIDS is unique; it is a lethal disease spread through sexual contact. Childhood fantasies about sexuality persist in all adults and may influence the adaptation to HIV in both patient and caregiver. The physician must remain alert to his or her personal reactions of anger, condemnation, identification, panic, and denial. Countertransference is discussed in greater detail in Chapter 9 and Appendix L ("The Questions Patients Ask: A Pretest of Countertransference").

✥ PSYCHOTHERAPY

Psychotherapy and Safer Sex

Sexuality and relationships are the subjects of many psychotherapies, providing opportunities to expand HIV education. Very often, the psychotherapist is the only medical professional to hear about specific sexual practices that seem too intimate and embarrassing to tell anyone else.

The concept of *relative risk* becomes particularly meaningful.[31] The goal of education is to help individuals clarify their willingness to tolerate the relative risk of particular sexual behaviors. For heterosexual couples, if an activity can result in pregnancy, it can produce HIV infection. (Frost[76] reviews how to take a sexual history specifically with gay patients in psychotherapy.) Psychiatrists must know some details in order to be of help (see Table 6–1).

Health Locus of Control

The Health Locus of Control (HLOC) scale[221,222] was designed to measure whether people believe that they themselves, powerful others, or chance controls their health. People with a greater "internal HLOC" are more autonomous relative to their health—that is, they believe that they can influence life events affecting their health. Individuals with a high "chance HLOC" perceive that events are influenced by fate alone. Those with a power "external" or "other-oriented HLOC" believe that health events are influenced by an external source beyond their control.

An intriguing paper by Arrufo et al.[5] explored cultural differences relative to this concept. Subjects were asked to endorse items on a scale from "strongly agree" to "strongly disagree." We have listed their study questions because they are easily adapted to clinical interviews and provide a simple way to elicit certain health beliefs for further discussion.

- "If I take care of myself, I can avoid illness" (internally worded)
- "Whenever I get sick, it is because of something I've done or not done" (internally worded)
- "Good health is largely a matter of good fortune" (externally worded)
- "No matter what I do, if I am going to get sick I will get sick" (externally worded)
- "Most people do not realize the extent to which their illnesses are controlled by accidental happenings" (externally worded)
- "I can only do what my doctor tells me to do" (externally worded)
- "There are so many strange diseases around that you can never know how or when you might pick one up" (externally worded)
- "When I feel ill, I know it is because I have not been getting the proper exercise or eating right" (internally worded)
- "People who never get sick are just plain lucky" (externally worded)
- "People's ill health results from their own carelessness" (internally worded)
- "I am directly responsible for my health" (internally worded)

They found that HLOC score was a strong independent predictor of AIDS knowledge, with high "externality" associated with less knowledge. Hispanic and black individuals had a higher external orientation than whites. Another study reported a small, but statistically significant, positive relationship between higher "chance HLOC" and unprotected anal intercourse in a sample of predominantly white, well-educated men attending gay bars.[109]

Comment. Individuals from outside the majority culture are often already burdened by problems of limited financial resources, racism, prejudice, language barriers, illiteracy, and limited access to health-related information. It is plausible that their sense of limited personal autonomy creates a passive stance relative to disease prevention, including AIDS. Other studies have corroborated that a denial-fatalism coping style may exacerbate high-risk behavior, even with adequate educational information.[12] We discuss these issues further in the section "Sex, Culture, and Stereotype" (p. 257).

Survivors of Childhood Sexual Abuse

The association between childhood traumatization (either physical or sexual abuse) and high-risk behaviors is becoming increasingly apparent.[2,3,30,105,230] The profile of sexual compulsivity, revictimization, substance abuse, and chronic depression characterizes many adult survivors of sexual abuse and predisposes them to become infected with HIV. Ms. Newman showed several of these symptoms. In addition, covert symptoms of childhood sexual or physical trauma may confound subsequent HIV health care management:

> Physicians, nurses, and social workers [may be] largely unaware that the abuse survivor issues of chronic depression, anxiety or dissociation may lead to (a) increased hostility and/or passivity in the patient's interaction with medical personnel; (b) medical noncompliance; and (c) misdiagnosis of HIV-related dementia [as an explanation for noncompliant behavior] . . . Additionally, survivors are more likely to [feel] revictimized or retraumatized as a result of physically intrusive diagnostic/treatment procedures.[2] . . . The majority of persons working in AIDS service organizations are not trained to recognize the common characteristics of abuse survivors. Frequently unrecognized survivor characteristics include trauma intrusion phenomena, dissociative phenomena, somatization, and sexual dysfunction. Lack of adequate training leads to medical/psychological misdiagnosis, insufficient treatment strategies, and the HIV-infected adult survivor's continuation of self-destructive, high-risk behaviors.[3] (pp. 295–296)

Table 6–1. Safer sex guidelines

Safe: abstinence, fantasizing, erotic conversation, self-masturbation, separate sex toys, phone sex, voyeurism, social kissing (dry), body massage, hugging

Safe if skin is intact: Mutual masturbation (male or female,) body-to-body rubbing (frottage), light S&M activities (without bruising or bleeding), body licking (excluding genital and anus)

Probably safe: mouth-to-mouth ("wet") kissing, urine contact ("water sports")

Probably safe **only with latex** *condom or latex barrier (e.g., condom split open to lie flat):* vaginal intercourse, anal intercourse (with a doubled or extra-strong latex condom), fellatio, oral-vaginal contact (cunnilingus), heavy petting (if an activity can result in pregnancy, it can result in HIV infection), sharing sex toys

Unsafe: receptive or insertive anal intercourse without a condom, manual-anal intercourse ("fisting"), fellatio without a condom (especially swallowing semen; stopping before climax is not safe either, because an erect penis can ooze fluid containing HIV),[14] oral-anal contact ("rimming") or cunnilingus without latex barrier, any activities involving bruising or bleeding ("heavy" S&M), sharing sex toys without a latex condom

The following do not reliably protect against HIV infection:[14]

- Having sex with only one person, regardless of his or her risk history or healthy appearance
- Douching or urinating after sex
- Coitus interruptus
- Contraceptives other than *latex* condoms (including diaphragms, birth-control pills, intrauterine devices, contraceptive sponges, implantable contraceptives such as Norplant, pre-/postcoital application of spermicidal jelly such as nonoxynol-9 alone)
- Sterilization (including vasectomy, tubal ligation, hysterectomy)

Notes:[14]

- Only *latex* condoms are adequate, not lambskin or other natural membranes.
- Condoms should not be unrolled to inspect for defects; unrolling, stretching, or blowing up condoms before using them correlates with high rates of condom breakage.
- Use only water-based lubricants like K-Y or spermicidal jelly (e.g., nonoxynol-9 may also have virucidal activity against HIV and may be used to lubricate the outside of condoms); oil-based lubricants such as Vaseline, vegetable oil, cold cream, mineral oil, or oil-based vaginal medications are associated with disintegration of condom integrity within 60 seconds of exposure.
- Saliva should not be used as lubricant because it may contain infectious material.
- If the condom or barrier fails (breaks, leaks, or falls off), "probably safe" activities become *unsafe.*
- Condom failure is more likely with vaginal and particularly anal intercourse than with oral sex.
- If either partner currently has genital irritation or rash, any genital contact, including frottage, will not be safe.

Source. Adapted from Cabaj et al. 1990,[31] Berger and Vizgirda 1993,[14] Anastos et al. 1991,[4] and Raisler 1990.[177]

Once again, psychiatrists and psychotherapists of all theoretical perspectives are in a unique position to foster lifesaving behavioral change.

Psychotherapy and AIDS

Many papers have appeared on the psychotherapy of individuals with HIV disease. Rather than survey them here, we will present the important principles and refer the reader to several recent comprehensive reviews.[33,79,108,179,213,225,229]

Psychotherapy with HIV patients is complex and requires flexibility, adaptability, and knowledge of the illness's medical, psychiatric, and psychodynamic impact.[189a] Issues seemingly resolved at one phase of treatment may emerge again with a vengeance as changes in physical and cognitive status occur. Several treatment goals should be considered for AIDS and HIV-infected individuals:[229]

- Help patients maintain control of their lives.
- Assist in finding healthy coping skills, especially when confronting the many stresses of their illness.
- Vigorously work to mitigate feelings of anger, denial, panic, and despair.
- Enable patients to establish and maintain feelings of self-respect by working through issues connected with guilt, shame, and self-blame, particularly regarding homophobia and sexuality.
- Facilitate communication with family, partners, and friends about the disease.[70a,90a] Also address fears of rejection and abandonment in the context of terminal illness.
- Assist the patient in maintaining good interpersonal and sexual relationships, whenever possible.
- Collaborate in developing strategies to deal with real and anticipated crises in the health and socioeconomic spheres.
- Help identify and address the "unfinished business" in patients' lives.
- Work together with the patient to explore the meaning of death.

Four stages have been defined in the psychosocial adaptation to AIDS.[72,151] Although they may occur simultaneously or in any order, they are helpful in orienting the therapist who works with these patients. They are briefly summarized as follows:

- **Initial crisis.** The catastrophic effects the HIV-positive diagnosis registers on the patient and supportive relationships. Denial predominates, sometimes alter-

nating with intense emotions (shock, anxiety, guilt, fear, anger, sadness). Denial may be so intense that the patient may adopt an attitude of indifference. As long as medical advice is being followed, the denial should be considered an equilibrium-preserving response to the crisis and no attempt made to dislodge it.[69] Patients typically have difficulty retaining information and may distort what they are told regarding their illness. The reactions are similar to patients' reactions to other serious diseases like cancer, but may be more intense due to the fear of contagion and the need to maintain risk behaviors associated with seropositivity.

- **Transitional state.** Begins when denial is superseded by alternating waves of guilt, anger, self-pity, and anxiety, often with ruminations about past behavior. This is a period of distress, confusion, and disruption. Depression, suicidal ideation, and lashing out at family and caregivers might ensue, sometimes leading to drug use and/or sexual acting-out. Because of frequently impaired comprehension, accompanied medical visits are advised to be sure that patients understand and adhere to instructions.

- **Acceptance.** This has been described as forming a new identity with the acceptance of AIDS and its implications.[151] Patients may describe appreciating the quality of life rather than quantity, develop a fighting spirit toward the illness, reassess former values, and sometimes feel a new sense of spirituality and concern for others. They feel less victimized by life, become less egocentric, and find satisfaction in altruistic and community activities.[69] "Acceptance is a deficiency state, however, as is evidenced by losses of health, energy, income, and independence. Under these circumstances, the human spirit's ability to marshal such inner resources is remarkable" (p. 31).[69]

- **Preparatory stage.** Characterized by the fear of becoming totally dependent on others. Patients take care of unfinished practical business (e.g., making wills, taking care of finances) as well as unfinished emotional business with loved ones. It is crucial for patients to have opportunities to discuss their feelings about dying and death. Although suicidal ideation occurs fleetingly throughout all stages, and many consider suicide as an alternative to intolerable dependency, most patients continue to fight for life.[69] Rabkin et al.[173] found extraordinary psychological resiliency in a cohort of patients who had suffered at least one life-threatening complication; they "shared the conviction that good times lay ahead and that life continued to be worthwhile" (p. 162).

The specter of an early death, the unpredictability of the illness, and the stigma attached to the illness and the lifestyles of many patients are unique to AIDS. J. Easton (personal communication, October 1993) has written,

> A unique problem faced by HIV positive persons is the "pseudo-reality" that HIV-positivity lends to any preexisting negative fantasies about the self. The patient easily believes that he is absolutely right to hate himself for being awful in all the ways he has always felt he was awful—here, it seems, is the *proof*. The HIV-positive diagnosis gives these fantasies the stamp of reality. This presents many technical difficulties in psychotherapy, since the patient has difficulty recognizing his fantasies as fantasies, making self-reflection seem irrelevant. Therapists and other helpers tend to emphasize the problems faced by HIV-positive persons as a result of *external* factors, especially the painful ostracism and shocking rejections by family and friends. These surely are burdens that no one should have to bear, losses that no one should have to grieve; but what makes these traumas far worse (and what tends to be overlooked) is the *internal* factor—the person's reactivated hatred of himself. The HIV-positive person tends to see AIDS as a proper punishment for fantasied sins, or if not aware of his guilt, will unconsciously view himself as a punishable person. This unconscious conflict results in all kinds of self-injurious behavior and, commonly, failure to get the help and other decent things in life that are actually available.

Good practical papers include those by Landau-Stanton et al.[122] (who illustrate psychotherapeutic interventions using case presentations), Chesney and Folkman[42] (who have summarized a group-based intervention based on cognitive theory), and the volume on the specific issues of gay men by Cadwell et al.[33]

The struggle to maintain hope is a central dilemma faced by both clinicians and patients.[125,174] Countertransference issues can be difficult to manage, particularly if the therapist feels personally vulnerable to the virus.[70] The shifting needs of the patient creates stress for the therapist[189a] as well as other caretakers. Zegans et al.[229] have outlined the following areas that may hinder clinical effectiveness:

1. There is a tendency for the therapist to create distance from the patient because of the discomfort of facing the potential loss of that person through death or serious illness.
2. The therapist may have difficulty addressing issues of death and dying directly with the patient.
3. The therapist may find him- or herself unable to face the patient's physical deterioration.
4. The therapist may disapprove of the patient's lifestyle choices, and this attitude may negatively affect the therapeutic alliance. Feelings of disapproval may include anger toward the patient if he or she continues to have unsafe sex, thereby jeopardizing another person.
5. The clinician may harbor unexamined fears of him- or herself being exposed to and contracting AIDS.
6. The clinician may be worried about the patient's use of "unauthorized" and potentially dangerous drugs.
7. The clinician may be disturbed by the patient's sense of hopelessness and possible wish to commit suicide. The clinician should think through his or her own position on "rational suicide" before facing it clinically.
8. It may be difficult for the therapist to know whether or not to confront the patient's use of denial as a coping mechanism.
9. Working with HIV patients challenges the therapist's need for effective restoration of function of the patient.
10. Working with HIV patients may force the therapist to confront his or her own fears of loss of cognitive and emotional control.

Winiarski[225] has constructed a 12-question exercise to help therapists anticipate questions that are often asked by HIV-positive patients. Since we have also found these questions useful in working with other seriously ill people, we have included them in Appendix L. We discuss countertransference in greater detail in Chapter 9.

Psychoneuroimmunology

The role of psychosocial factors in HIV immune function has been of great interest. These factors could influence the natural history of the HIV illness at several points, including behaviors predisposing to the initial infection with HIV, effects on subsequent immunopathology and symptomatic illness, and survival after diagnosis.[110,111,165,188] Unfortunately, the heterogeneity of HIV's clinical course makes it difficult to construct a natural history of the psychological response to this illness.

- Kessler and colleagues[113,114] found no relationship between certain stressful life events and either decrease in percentage of CD4 cells or symptom onset in HIV infection.
- Rabkin and colleagues[175] similarly found no relationships between depressive disorders, psychiatric distress, and psychosocial stressors on measures of HIV illness (immune status measured by CD4 and CD8 cell subsets, number of signs and symptoms associated with HIV infection, and cumulative index of HIV illness stage).
- Kertzner and Gorman[112] attempted to link psychosocial factors to immune measures and health in HIV-associated disease, with contradictory results.

Emerging reports continue to show contradictory findings of the relationship between depression, lymphocyte counts, and prognosis,[28,130,164] and there is debate over the meaning of these findings.[83]

Kertzner[111] has summarized:

Two uncertainties limit the present application of psychoneuroimmunology to HIV infection. First, the temporal and quantitative relationship between stress, effects on the immune system, and changes in actual health is poorly understood. Further research is needed to determine if stress-related changes in mitogen stimulation response or lymphocyte subsets are of sufficient duration or magnitude to influence actual health. Second, given the complexity of basic HIV immunopathology, it may be difficult to pinpoint the significance of changes in immune function attributable specifically to stress or psychosocial factors. In the absence of more definitive findings, there are still several clear messages for clinicians and patients. *Psychiatric interventions can and do have a highly beneficial effect on the quality of life experienced by HIV-infected persons, regardless of immunological effects. In contrast, premature or misguided interpretations of psychoneuroimmunologic research may lead patients to blame themselves for becoming ill due to "the wrong state of mind."* (p. 38, italics added)

Perry and colleagues[164,165] cite evidence for a relationship between emotional distress and behaviors that transmit HIV.[109] Moreover, they have shown that reducing emotional distress in HIV-positive individuals might increase hope and therefore compliance with medical care, promoting early medical intervention for treatable opportunistic infections and tumors.[166] These are indirect but tangible benefits that could affect the course of HIV in a given individual. Surely these patients deserve every therapeutic intervention that may be of benefit, however indirect.

The interested reader should consult other, more detailed surveys of this important literature.[99,110,202]

SEX, CULTURE, AND STEREOTYPE

Culture influences behavior, attitudes, and therefore potential vulnerability to HIV infection. Denial and disavowal of personal risk often attaches itself to homophobia; some individuals still cling to the belief (which often is culturally syntonic) that AIDS is a disease of gay white males. This is a bit like bird-watching on the good ship Titanic: there is frightening evidence that HIV infection is spreading in ever-growing numbers of nonwhite, nonmale, and nongay populations. For example, recent worldwide estimates[81] by the World Health Organization cited that *85% of adults infected with HIV-1 live outside Western industrialized countries, with over 75% of adult HIV infection transmitted through heterosexual intercourse, and with women representing more than 45% of HIV-infected people.* A sampling of the data in the United States alone is chilling:

- According to the Centers for Disease Control,[38] in the United States in 1986, the proportion of infected blacks and Hispanics was approximately **double** their proportion in the general population: blacks represented 27% of infected individuals, but only 12% of the general population; Hispanics represented 15% of infected individuals but only 6% of the general population.[214]
- There are higher rates of IV drug use—and therefore greater risk of spreading the virus to uninfected members of these groups—in infected African-American and Latino men as compared with infected white men (39% versus 7%, respectively).[39] The patterns of IV drug use in these groups, such as injecting in "shooting galleries" and sharing needles, place these individuals at even greater peril than their white counterparts.[17]
- Socioeconomically disadvantaged women from ethnic minorities are more likely to engage in sexual intercourse early and are less likely to use contraceptives, such as condoms, that would confer protection against HIV.[227]

◆ A study of young African-American men and women showed that although this group is knowledgeable about HIV infection, knowledge does not always lead to behavioral change.[103]

In fact, the model for successful HIV prevention strategies may be found in the gay community, which was the first group to be stricken.

Ethnic Minorities and Risk

Ethnocultural factors interact with sexual orientation[54a,57,162] and may heighten risk. For example, sexual behaviors of bisexual men differ from those of heterosexual and homosexual men,[44,55,56,91,127] and also vary across ethnicities.

◆ Bisexual men have higher rates of prostitution than heterosexual or homosexual men, and approximately one-half of them do *not* use condoms with their clients.[52]

◆ There are higher rates of prostitution among bisexual men who inject drugs.[52]

◆ In a study of male prostitutes in Georgia, most male prostitutes who had sex with both men and women had recreational sex with women only and favored sex with women.[60a]

◆ Another study in New Orleans found that male prostitutes reported having sex with men, but 39% self-identified as heterosexual.[146]

◆ Studies have found higher rates of bisexual activity among U.S.-born infected black[52,119,127] and Hispanic[9] men compared with infected white men. Bing[17] has postulated that since homosexuality is particularly taboo in African-American and Latino cultures, these men may be less likely to acknowledge their high-risk homosexual activity to female partners. Others have speculated that black men may adopt a bisexual lifestyle because being homosexual in the black community is difficult, and an alliance with the gay, predominantly white community may be seen as a betrayal of blacks.[55]

◆ Aruffo et al.[5] found that the Health Locus of Control score was a strong independent predictor of AIDS knowledge, with high externality in Hispanic and black individuals associated with less knowledge. (This study was discussed in more detail above.)

Beware of generalities and stereotypes; there are important differences within the larger racial or ethnic groups:

◆ Diaz et al.[52] found that infected black Haitian men reported less bisexual behavior as compared with U.S.-born infected black men. It is not clear whether this reflected underreporting of bisexual behavior or the predominance of heterosexual transmission of HIV among Haitians.[36,161,210] Similarly, infected Hispanic men of Latin American and Puerto Rican ancestry born in the United States (excluding Puerto Rico) had lower rates of bisexual activity than Hispanic men born outside the United States and living here less than 10 years (most of whom were Mexican). Studies conducted in Mexico have estimated that as many of 30% of Mexican men aged 15–25 years engage in bisexual activity.[35]

◆ Kline and colleagues[117] tested the hypothesis that cultural factors caused economically disadvantaged minority women to lack the necessary power in their relationships with men to influence the course of sexual decision making (i.e., to insist on safer sexual practices). They used a qualitative, focus-group methodology to assess sexual decision making among groups of high-risk African-American and Hispanic women. Contrary to assumptions about the impact of gender inequality on condom use, they found that passivity relative to sexual decision making was not the key factor; more important was how the women *assessed their risk with specific partners in specific situations,* and how they weighed it against their own expectations of potential physical discomfort or reduced sexual pleasure.

Sexual *self-identification* also influences risk behaviors:

◆ Behaviorally bisexual men who self-identified as *heterosexual* were found to use condoms at *lower* rates than self-identified homosexual or bisexual men.[40]

◆ Diaz et al.[52] found that bisexual Hispanic men, regardless of birthplace, were more likely to be currently married (i.e., engaging in heterosexual intercourse) than were other bisexual men. Some African-American and Hispanic men may believe that their behavior is not risky as long as they themselves are not anally penetrated[171] and/or their male partner is nonwhite.[171] If they also have sex with women, they may view themselves as heterosexual[35] rather than bisexual, fostering the fantasy of greater safety than their behavior realistically warrants.

◆ Finally, it has been shown that married men who engage in homosexual activity are less likely than unmarried men to inform their regular female partner of their behavior.[59]

These epidemiological findings have tragic portent. Female partners who do not suspect the high-risk sexual activity of their partners are less likely to insist on safer sex practices, especially if these men are regular sexual partners. This potentially expands the radius of infection to their unborn children and to other sexual partners. These data are concordant with reports than many women are not aware of their partner's bisexual behavior,[59] particularly among blacks and Hispanics.[141,160] Of additional concern are data indicating that female rates of HIV infection secondary to sexual contact with bisexual men are *highest* among black and Hispanic women.[44]

Know thy patient! Intervention programs must be tailored to specific ethnic communities if they are to be effective.[17,25,26,88,132,133,137,138,155,171,192,203,204,228]

- ◆ Kalichman et al.[104] recruited African-American women from low-income housing projects in Chicago (N = 106) and randomly assigned them to view one of three 20-minute videotapes: a standard public health service tape on AIDS prevention; the same public health service tape, but matching presenter and participant ethnicity and gender; or a tape that included the same content but was framed in a context specifically intended to increase cultural relevance. Participants who viewed tapes with same-gender, same-ethnicity presenters (i.e., other African-American women) were found at follow-up to be significantly more sensitized to AIDS and more likely to have discussed AIDS with friends, to seek testing for HIV, and to request condoms.
- ◆ Significant gender, ethnic, and cultural differences affect the frequency of condom use.[37,152,153]

If you and your patient are from discordant ethnocultural backgrounds, ask for help from other knowledgeable professionals. Generic programs based on the majority culture or ethnic stereotypes are primed to fail.

Gay Men

One focus of this chapter has been to dispel the myth of AIDS as a gay disease, but no single group has suffered as much specific stigmatization as the gay male community.[32,195] Rather than repeat material that is more extensively discussed elsewhere in the current literature,[12,19,22,33,71,121,135,147,154,163,190a,197a,219] we will outline the highlights by Folkman et al.[71] on the specific issues confronted by *caregiving partners* of gay men with AIDS:

- ◆ The literature on caregiver stress is derived mainly from studies of patients with Alzheimer's disease,

cancer, Parkinson's disease, or stroke. These caregivers are usually female, and the people they care for are usually older adults.
- ◆ There are four key dimensions that distinguish caregiving partners of men with AIDS from traditional family caregivers:
  - Individuals with AIDS and their partners are likely to be young or middle-aged rather than elderly. These caregiving partners are "premature" in their caregiving role compared with traditional caregivers, who tend to be in their late 50s or older. At a time when their peers are building relationships as well as careers, these caregivers are forced to prepare for the loss of their partner and must often curtail their own career development.
  - Traditional caregiving adult children, spouses, and parents frequently depend on other family members for support. Gay men and their partners are often physically—and psychologically—distant from their families. Stigma, homophobia, and fear of contagion exacerbate barriers to family support.
  - There are few role models for male caregivers; caregiving is typically viewed as a female's role. The absence of public support or acknowledgment of male caregiving is one more way the gay couple is isolated from the majority culture and support.
  - Many caregiving partners are themselves seropositive for the virus. For these men, the progression of disease in their partner is a nightmarish harbinger of things to come. Who will care for them? Seronegative caregivers face the threat of becoming infected with the virus in the future, as well as the burden of survivor guilt.[157,158]

Folkman et al.[71] suggest three techniques to support and sustain caregivers. These are reviewed in the section on caregivers in the case of Mr. Lowe in the first part of this chapter (p. 233).

Women and Children

Heterosexual HIV Transmission

Infected IV drug users account for much of the increase in heterosexual HIV infection; before 1983, heterosexual transmission accounted for only 1% of all HIV-infected cases, but by 1989 this figure had risen to 5%.[39] In women, heterosexual transmission has grown from 14% of female

HIV cases in 1982 to 31% in 1989.[39] In New York City, AIDS has been the leading cause of death in women between the ages of 15 and 44 years since 1986; female AIDS cases have now been reported in all 50 states and the District of Columbia.[45] Several additional epidemiological trends are worth emphasizing:

- High-risk sexual behaviors among IV drug users are *highest in heterosexual males, representing a significant vector of disease to women*.[184]
- Bisexual men practice riskier sex with *female* than with male partners: one study showed that only a minority of bisexual men engaged in unprotected anal sex with their male partners, *whereas a full two-thirds had unprotected vaginal sex with their female partners*.[20] These asymmetrical findings reflect a perception of differential risk based on the partner's gender.

To date, prospective studies of psychiatric morbidity in HIV-seropositive women without active AIDS have been scant. In one, Brown and Rundell[25] conducted a 5-year longitudinal investigation of 20 employed, educated seropositive women who were not IV drug abusers. (Fifty percent of the patients were Caucasian and 50% were black. Sixty-five percent were married, 30% single, and 5% divorced.)

- Heterosexual transmission was the rule, with 20% having HIV-seropositive spouses.
- Fifty percent had an Axis I diagnosis; none developed major depression or became dependent on drugs; 5% abused alcohol.
- Fifteen percent exhibited subtle signs of cognitive decline.
- Suicidal behavior and psychiatric hospitalization were absent.
- Sexual functioning was disrupted in the majority of subjects, with 20% meeting criteria for new-onset *hypoactive sexual desire disorder*.
- Despite intensive and repeated HIV education, 60% *engaged in unprotected intercourse while aware that they were seropositive*. A full two-thirds of this group had *seronegative* sexual partners, some of whom were *unaware* of their partner's seropositivity.
- The rate of HIV progression was three times faster than in a comparable male sample, consistent with other data[185] indicating that men survive 14% longer at the same stage of illness.

Maternal HIV Transmission

While only 2% of HIV-infection cases in 1989 represented female-to-male transmission, the vast majority of pediatric HIV cases are due to mother-to-fetus transmission.[39] Of all children with HIV infection, 75% are born to women who are IV drug users themselves or who are the sexual partners of IV drug users.[39]

- HIV seropositivity in the setting of pregnancy presents many issues,[95,96,101] including controversy over whether pregnancy accelerates disease progression in the mother.[62,118,191] Pregnancy may aggravate the course of HIV infection in women who are in advanced stages of the disease.[62] On the other hand, HIV infection does not appear to increase the risk of obstetrical complications, even though lymphocyte counts might drop.[54] Moreover, zidovudine appears to reduce the transmission of HIV from mother to infant.[41,48]
- As recently reviewed by St. Louis et al.,[201] *most HIV-infected women do not transmit HIV to their children* (rates across studies are 13% to 40%), but factors such as low maternal lymphocyte counts ($< 0.60 \times 10^9$/L) and placental membrane inflammation significantly increase that risk. Burchett[29] and Dinsmoor[54] have recently reviewed these issues in detail.
- The virus can also be transmitted to an infant through breast milk.[191]

Clearly, the scope of the pediatric HIV epidemic will be determined by the reproductive decisions of infected women.[120,127a]

- One study explored the impact of HIV serostatus on reproductive decisions of women. Sunderland and colleagues[207] studied 108 seronegative women and 98 seropositive women through an index pregnancy and for an average of 1.5 years postpartum. Approximately one-third of each group learned their serostatus early enough in pregnancy to have the option of an abortion. About 19% of the seropositive women chose abortion, compared with 3% of the seronegative women.
- During follow-up there were *no significant differences in the numbers of pregnancies or live births between seropositive and seronegative women*, or between drug-using and non–drug-using women. Although positive HIV status did correlate with the decision to terminate pregnancies, *it did not correlate with subsequent fertility*. These findings indicate that seropositive

women continue to be important vectors of pediatric HIV infection, since fertility and fetal viability do not appear to be significantly affected. In addition, for infants whose HIV infection is maternally acquired, the rate of disease progression varies directly with the severity of the mother's disease at the time of delivery.[18]

Conclusion

There is clearly the need for gender-specific research into the sexual beliefs and practices of women so as to better intervene with this group.[34,43,77,93,145,196] Additional issues specific to women, children and HIV/AIDS are detailed in the recent volume by Cohen and Durham,[46] although little is known about female-to-female transmission of HIV.[135a]

⚕ PSYCHIATRIC MORBIDITY, PART II

Anxiety and Adjustment Disorders

"AIDS anxiety" has been described in noninfected individuals,[23,144] but the prevalence of panic disorder and obsessive-compulsive disorder[139a] in the HIV-spectrum population has not yet been calculated. Anxiety usually accompanies other psychiatric disorders such as adjustment disorders or major depression.[16] Secondary anxiety reactions may be precipitated by zidovudine and steroids, as well as withdrawal from narcotics, alcohol, benzodiazepines, and barbiturates. *Drug withdrawal reactions are likely to occur early in a hospitalization and may mimic anxiety reactions.*

Adjustment disorders occur quite frequently, given the succession of stressors and losses. Patients with HIV-related neurocognitive impairment, which further compromises good coping, still retain insight about their deterioration. Social isolation, abandonment by family and friends, shame, and depression may become overwhelming. Patients who have already witnessed HIV's destruction of loved ones must themselves endure a nightmarish encore. The early stages of delirium may resemble adjustment disorders, since both can present with irritability, anxiety, tearfulness, and agitation.[16]

Treatment

Anxiolytic treatment in the setting of lung disease and delirium has been reviewed in Chapter 2. The same general guidelines apply to managing patients with *P. carinii* pneumonia. A brief summary of notes specific to HIV follows.

Benzodiazepines. The same parameters apply to managing anxiety in HIV infection as in other medical illnesses, combining support and appropriate anxiolytics. The intermediate-acting benzodiazepines (lorazepam, alprazolam, oxazepam) in low starting doses are preferred.[67] For insomnia, use oxazepam (Serax; 10–15 mg hs), temazepam (Restoril; 15 mg hs), lorazepam (Ativan; 0.5 mg hs), or trazodone (Desyrel; 25–50 mg hs).[80] Agents with very short half-lives, such as midazolam (Versed) and triazolam (Halcion), or with long-acting metabolites are less well-tolerated in AIDS patients who have significant neurocognitive impairment.[80] Be alert to potential benzodiazepine abuse in cognitively impaired, chronically stressed patients who may also have substance abuse histories.

◆ When agitation approaches panic or accompanies delusions, neuroleptic medication is the treatment of choice.[67] Neuroleptics are also favored over benzodiazepines (which may have a disinhibiting effect) for patients in the early stages of encephalopathy, delirium, or ADC who present with anxiety or restlessness.[65]

◆ Note that midazolam[158a] and triazolam[83a,217] adversely interact with the systemic antimycotics ketoconazole (Nizoral) and itraconazole (Sporanox).

Buspirone. The experience with buspirone (BuSpar) in AIDS patients is limited. Reports of treatment-related dyskinesias in this already vulnerable population are of concern.[181,206] There has also been one report of buspirone-induced psychosis in an HIV-infected patient.[211] However, preliminary experience with buspirone has shown diminution of drug-seeking behavior occurring in a subgroup of HIV-infected patients.[10]

◆ Fernandez and Levy[67] have found that buspirone is best tolerated by patients who either are asymptomatic or have limited disease. When buspirone was coadministered with zidovudine, patients on lower doses of zidovudine (i.e., < 300 mg/day) did better. These patients typically required buspirone in the higher therapeutic range (45–60 mg/day).

Propranolol. The beta-blocker propranolol (Inderal) should be avoided because of the increased incidence of dysautonomia,[49,128] making patients more vulnerable to hypotensive episodes. Propranolol may also induce bronchospasm.

Trazodone. Fernandez and Levy[67] have found that anxious HIV patients with neuropsychiatric and/or neuromuscular complications often respond well to trazo-done (Desyrel) in low doses (i.e., 25–200 mg/day in divided doses) without adverse side effects. They have reported trazodone's usefulness in the long-term treatment of chronic anxiety in HIV disease, irrespective of systemic symptoms or stage of disease. Unlike buspirone, which has no immediate sedative effect, trazodone has a quick-sedating and relaxing effect, mimicking that of the benzodiazepines, but without the complications.

Antihistamines.   Antihistamines like diphenhydramine (Benadryl) or hydroxyzine (Vistaril, Atarax) should be avoided in the setting of delirium because they are anticholinergic.

Mania

Secondary manic syndromes occur *infrequently* in HIV infection. The few case reports have implicated the following presumptive etiologies:

- Ganciclovir (DHPG)[65]
- Zidovudine (AZT)[136,156]
- Didanosine (Videx; ddI)[24]
- Cryptococcal meningitis[102,209]

Mania may also be the *presenting feature* of HIV infection.[27,50,61,78,116,190] These cases have been successfully treated with lithium, which may be coadministered with AZT.

Significant cognitive dysfunction often accompanies secondary mania and may *persist* even after manic symptoms remit, suggesting that it is not merely an epiphenomenon of the mood disorder in this context.[116] Patients without a family or personal history of mood disorder have presented with mania late in the course of HIV infection, and have shown a higher prevalence of comorbid dementia.[129] Unfortunately, Treisman et al.[212] found that demented patients tended to develop delirium on lithium, requiring a switch to low-dose neuroleptics and often remaining chronically manic.

Maintenance lithium may be continued for bipolar patients after the patient tests seropositive.[65] However, dehydration due to severe diarrhea (e.g., such as occurs in cryptosporidial infection, CMV enteritis or colitis) can cause lithium toxicity. Frequent monitoring is appropriate, especially in light of recent suggestions of an HIV-associated nephropathy in some patients.[124]

- Fernandez and Levy[67] have also used lithium to treat several patients with significant agitation secondary to dideoxyinosine.

- Poor lithium and neuroleptic tolerance correlates with abnormal brain MRIs; in these patients, anticonvulsant agents (carbamazepine [Tegretol], clonazepam [Klonopin]) are effective alternatives.[86] Monitor carbamazepine's potential for neutropenia, anemia, and thrombocytopenia, however, as well as the risk of hepatotoxicity in patients also taking zidovudine.

Vamos[216] has urged that the psychodynamics of the manic AIDS patient not be neglected. Rosenbaum[182] has made the interpretation that the manic content may serve to protect the patient "in the face of absolute hopelessness and certain death . . . [as] a denial of impending disintegration" (p. 416).

Psychosis

Features

As the new "great imitator,"[187] early HIV infection may be mistaken for primary psychiatric illness. The relationship between psychosis and HIV, however, is still poorly understood. Several authors have described psychosis as an early presentation of HIV infection,[11,85,87,212] *occurring even in the absence of affective changes or detectable cognitive deterioration.*[27] Psychosis may also be a manifestation of HIV-associated encephalopathy.[193] In a 1989 review of the published literature on psychotic HIV-infected patients, Harris et al.[89] found that 31% of all reported patients with HIV-related psychosis had psychotic symptoms as the initial presentation of their HIV infection. A more recent chart and literature review was conducted by the same authors:[90]

- Surprisingly, the **majority** of patients with new HIV-associated psychosis showed a **normal** initial neurological evaluation (exam, CT scan, CSF).
- The onset of psychotic symptoms was usually *without an apparent prodromal phase*, and the symptoms tended to be severe.
- The most common psychotic symptoms were persecutory, grandiose, or somatic delusions. Hallucinations also occurred, and were usually auditory in nature.
- Mood and/or affective disturbance occurred frequently (81%), as did bizarre behavior (52%).
- Psychotic patients with an abnormal CT and EEG tended to deteriorate rapidly in cognitive and medical status.
- Psychotic symptoms did improve with neuroleptic treatment, although side effects were frequent.

Note that the diagnoses upon hospital admission in this study included undifferentiated schizophrenia, schizophreniform disorder, "reactive psychosis," atypical psychosis, depression with psychotic features, and mania. These diagnoses were later revised to AIDS encephalitis, cryptococcal meningitis, or "organic psychosis." It was not possible to determine the incidence of psychosis in this study because of methodological limitations.

Monosymptomatic hypochondriacal psychosis with the delusion of parasitic infestation,[97] and catatonia have also been described in AIDS delirium and AIDS dementia.[189,200,218]

Differential Diagnosis

The age at onset of idiopathic psychosis and HIV infection overlap, so that the differential diagnosis often includes primary psychiatric disorders, such as schizophrenia and bipolar affective disorder. Other causes of psychosis include substance abuse, antiviral agents such as zidovudine, or agents like steroids. Isoniazid (INH), used as a first-line treatment for tuberculosis, has a number of psychiatric complications, including affective disturbance and psychosis.[82,215] CNS disease, such as cryptococcosis[102] and herpes encephalitis, and space-occupying lesions like lymphoma may also precipitate psychotic states. There have been cases presenting predominantly with psychotic symptoms, which then progressed to AIDS dementia complex (ADC), raising the possibility that CNS viral infection may be etiological in HIV-related psychosis.[149]

Several authors have speculated that HIV affects dopaminergic and catecholaminergic systems preferentially,[92,115,131,148] although it attacks cell lines throughout the central and peripheral nervous systems. Fernandez and Levy[67] have summarized evidence for this hypothesis.

HIV infection should be ruled out in all patients who present with new-onset psychosis, especially if the patient has any risk factors for HIV exposure.[128a] Acute or subacute onset of confusion, memory complaints, affective or mood disturbances, bizarre behavior, abnormal posturing, or symptoms of a medical illness (e.g., fever, weight loss) should raise the possibility of HIV infection.

Neuroleptics

AIDS patients seem consistently *more vulnerable to neuroleptic side effects* such as neuroleptic malignant syndrome (NMS), extrapyramidal side effects (EPS), or other side effects of dopamine-blocking agents.[8,15,21,60,64,94,100,193a,224] There is at least one report of heightened vulnerability to tardive dyskinesia.[194] A retrospective chart review confirmed that the likelihood of developing EPS in AIDS patients was at least 2.4 times higher than that in psychotic patients without AIDS.[98]

♦ For patients who develop EPS, a neuroleptic of intermediate potency, such as molindone (Moban; starting dosage 5 mg two or three times daily), may be preferable, especially in patients also at risk for seizures.[66,80]

♦ Risperidone (Risperdal) was effective in four male AIDS patients with manic psychosis,[199] although it was previously reported to exacerbate manic symptoms in patients with schizoaffective disorder.[58]

Fernandez and Levy[67] have cautioned that while most patients respond rapidly to neuroleptics, there is a subgroup of patients whose psychosis never completely remits and who show residual cognitive impairment consistent with ADC. As with any medically fragile group, start with low-dose neuroleptics, cautiously titrating to minimize the risk of side effects.

The routes of medication administration may be limited by[80]

♦ Poor intestinal absorption
♦ Thrombocytopenia and inadequate muscle mass secondary to wasting
♦ Lack of venous access

In addition, anticholinergic agents such as low-potency antipsychotics (e.g., chlorpromazine [Thorazine]) and antiparkinsonian drugs (e.g., benztropine [Cogentin] and trihexyphenidyl [Artane]) may contribute to delirium.

♦ When antiparkinsonian drugs are required for EPS, amantadine (Symmetrel) is recommended because it is less anticholinergic than either benztropine or trihexyphenidyl.[80] Starting doses are at 50 mg orally bid (up to 100 mg bid).

♦ Since no medication regimen is ever problem free, note that amantadine is a dopamine agonist and has been implicated in causing delusional states in patients with Parkinson's disease[142] and chronic psychosis.[223] If adding amantadine to a neuroleptic regimen increases psychosis, it should be discontinued and the patient reevaluated.

Delirium

The diagnosis and treatment of delirium is discussed in detail in Chapter 2. The following points are specifically relevant to AIDS patients.

◆ Delirium is probably the most commonly occurring mental disorder in hospitalized AIDS patients.[64,226] The true incidence is unknown, but estimates range from 22%[16] to 56%.[64] (The overall incidence of delirium in general medical-surgical patients is in the range of only 10%–15%.[13]) HIV patients are at particularly high risk for delirium both because of the direct impact of the virus on the CNS and as a result of their vulnerability to opportunistic infections and malignancies.

Certain etiologies for delirium are particularly likely in AIDS patients:

◆ Sepsis of any cause (especially CNS opportunistic infections, such as CMV encephalitis, cerebral toxoplasmosis, neurosyphilis, and cryptococcal or tuberculous meningitis[139])

◆ Malignancies

◆ Hypoxia, especially in the setting of *P. carinii* pneumonia[16]

◆ Anemia

◆ Metabolic abnormalities

◆ Almost every medication[44a] used to treat AIDS, including pentamidine,[16] isoniazid, amphotericin B, ganciclovir (DHPG), trimethoprim/sulfamethoxazole, and zidovudine[47,143,159,180]

◆ Repeated doses of analgesics, particularly meperidine (Demerol)

◆ Alcohol or benzodiazepine withdrawal

The treatment of delirium in the setting of HIV infection is based on the same principles used in treating delirium in other medically ill patients (see Chapter 2, Mr. Davis). High-potency neuroleptics, specifically haloperidol (Haldol), have become the treatment of choice. Haloperidol can be administered orally, intramuscularly, or intravenously, either alone or in combination with lorazepam (Ativan), for agitated, delirious patients.[1,6,7,68,208] (Continuous infusion of haloperidol has also been used.[63]) *Beware of misdiagnosing the mood changes of delirium as depression; antidepressants are contraindicated in this setting.*[126,183]

🍳 SUMMARY

1. It is a fallacy that serological testing will solve the problem of high-risk behavior. Shortcuts that bypass the complex psychological issues of serological testing will fail. The paradigm of informed consent is a useful model, and frames HIV testing as a medical procedure with potential benefits but also psychological risks. This prepares the patient for potentially devastating news and provides a framework for comfort, support, and further exploration. Persistent high-risk sexual behavior should be viewed as a form of noncompliance with medical advice. Antibody testing cannot substitute for the exploration of why it is difficult to engage in safer practices even without knowing antibody status. Sometimes negative antibody status may make it *more* difficult to change high-risk sexual behavior.

2. Suicidal ideation and psychiatric distress do not invariably increase after HIV testing, nor are they inevitable for seropositivity. Suicidal ideation has been found in both seropositive and seronegative individuals, suggesting that there is a subgroup at risk for emotional distress regardless of test results. Be alert to delayed reactions to the diagnosis of seropositivity. A period of relatively good psychological and behavioral adjustment to serological status may be followed by disillusionment, despair, or frank depression.

3. Factors that increase risk for adverse psychological reactions are personal or family psychiatric history, recent bereavement, history of trauma, and few social supports.

4. A growing literature indicates that many individuals continue to be ill informed about HIV or to persist in high-risk sexual practices despite adequate information. In order to change, an individual must perceive that he or she is at risk for HIV infection. If there is no perception of risk, there is no lasting motivation to make behavioral changes. The individual must have the belief that a seropositive condition can be worsened by reexposure and/or the capacity to care about infecting others. There must also be the conviction that modifying high-risk behavior will affect the outcome of being HIV positive or will confer some protection from getting infected.

5. Recreational drug use, depression, and a history of childhood sexual or physical abuse have been associated with high-risk sexual practices.

6. Sexuality and relationships are the subjects of many psychotherapies, which offer opportunities to expand HIV education. Individuals must be educated in the concept of *relative risk* regarding sexual activities so that they can clarify their personal willingness to tolerate the relative risk of given behaviors.

7. Psychotherapy with HIV-related disorders is complex and requires flexibility, adaptability, and knowledge. The treatment goals are to reduce anxiety, alleviate depression, mobilize healthy defenses and coping skills, and promote reconciliation and acceptance. The model of psychotherapy with other catastrophi-

cally ill individuals, such as cancer patients, emphasizes the additional goals of decreasing the sense of alienation by communicating with other patients, clarifying misperceptions and misinformation, and lessening isolation, feelings of helplessness, and neglect. The struggle to maintain hope is a central dilemma for doctor and patient alike. Seropositivity may lend the stamp of "apparent reality" to preexisting negative fantasies about the self and predispose to adverse psychological consequences.

8. Attempts to link psychosocial factors to measures of immunity have yielded contradictory results. Premature or misguided interpretations of this research may lead patients to blame themselves for becoming ill due to being in "the wrong state of mind." Psychiatric interventions do benefit the quality of life and improve compliance, regardless of their direct immunological effects.

9. The impact of culture influences behavior, attitudes, and therefore potential vulnerability to HIV infection. Denial and disavowal of personal risk often attaches itself to homophobia; some individuals still cling to the belief that AIDS is a disease of gay white males. This flies in the face of epidemiological evidence, which shows that HIV is spreading most rapidly among nonwhite, nonmale, nongay individuals. In the United States, IV drug users, women, Hispanics, and Afro-Americans are at particular risk.

10. Less reliable than self-identified sexual orientation (i.e., hetero-, homo-, bisexual; married, single; and so forth) are assessments of actual behavior. Behavioral patterns vary according to cultural and social factors. Intervention programs must be tailored to specific communities if they are to be effective. Generic programs based exclusively on the majority culture or on ethnic stereotypes will likely fail.

11. Managing anxiety in HIV-infected patients involves the same techniques used in other medically ill patients, with a combined approach of support and appropriate anxiolytics. The intermediate-acting benzodiazepines (lorazepam [Ativan], alprazolam [Xanax], oxazepam [Serax]) in low starting doses are preferred. When anxiety becomes immobilizing as panic, neuroleptic medication is the treatment of choice. Neuroleptics are also favored over benzodiazepines (which may have a disinhibiting effect) for patients in the early stages of encephalopathy, delirium, or AIDS dementia complex (ADC) who present with anxiety or restlessness.

12. Secondary manic syndromes do occur in HIV infection, but infrequently. They have been successfully treated with lithium, although poor lithium and neuroleptic tolerance appears to be correlated with abnormal brain MRIs. In these patients, anticonvulsants (carbamazepine [Tegretol], clonazepam [Klonopin]) have been effective alternatives. Carbamazepine's potential for neutropenia, anemia, and thrombocytopenia must be monitored, as well as the risk of hepatotoxicity in patients also on zidovudine. Patients without a family or personal history of mood disorder who present with mania later in the course of HIV infection have a higher prevalence of comorbid dementia. Be cautious when prescribing lithium when there is fluid loss or severe diarrhea, such as in cryptosporidial infection. Frequent monitoring for lithium toxicity is necessary, especially in light of recent suggestions of an HIV-associated nephropathy in some patients.

13. *HIV infection should be ruled out in all patients with new-onset psychosis, especially if the patient has any risk factors for HIV exposure.* The new "great imitator," early HIV infection often resembles primary psychiatric illness, especially when psychosis occurs without systemic signs of illness or detectable cognitive deterioration. Acute or subacute onset of confusion, memory complaints, affective or mood disturbances, bizarre behavior, abnormal posturing, or symptoms of a medical illness (e.g., fever, weight loss) should raise the possibility of HIV-associated psychosis. The initial neurological evaluation may be normal, although patients with abnormal computed tomography (CT) scans or electroencephalograms (EEGs) at the time of presentation tend to rapidly deteriorate. Psychotic symptoms are usually without prodrome, and improve with neuroleptic treatment, although there is a heightened risk for side effects.

14. AIDS patients are more likely to experience medication side effects, such as neuroleptic malignant syndrome (NMS) and extrapyramidal side effects (EPS). Although most patients respond rapidly to neuroleptics, there is a subgroup of patients whose psychosis never completely remits and who show residual cognitive impairment consistent with ADC. As with any medically fragile group, low neuroleptic doses are usually effective and minimize the risk of side effects. The route of medication administration may be limited by poor intestinal absorption of oral medications; by thrombocytopenia and inadequate muscle mass secondary to wasting for intramuscular medications; and by lack of venous access for intravenous administration. In addition, anticholinergic agents such as low-potency antipsychotics (e.g., chlorprom-

azine [Thorazine]) and antiparkinsonian drugs (e.g., benztropine [Cogentin] and trihexyphenidyl [Artane]) may contribute to delirium. Amantadine (Symmetrel) has been recommended for EPS because it is less anticholinergic than either benztropine or trihexyphenidyl (however, it has been associated with worsening psychosis).

15. HIV patients are thought to be at particularly high risk for delirium, both because of the direct central nervous system (CNS) impact of the virus itself and because of their vulnerability to opportunistic infections and malignancies. Certain etiologies for delirium are particularly likely in AIDS patients. Sepsis of any cause, malignancies, anemia, hypoxia, and other metabolic abnormalities can cause altered mental status. Repeated doses of analgesics, particularly meperidine (Demerol), can induce delirium, as can alcohol or benzodiazepine withdrawal. As with other medically ill patients, haloperidol (Haldol) is the mainstay of treatment, either alone or in combination with lorazepam (Ativan).

⚜ REFERENCES

1. Adams F, Fernandez F, Andersson B: Emergency pharmacotherapy of delirium in the critically ill cancer patient: intravenous combination drug approach. Psychosomatics 27 (suppl 1):33–37, 1986

2. Allers C, Benjack K: Connections between childhood abuse and HIV infection. Journal of Counseling and Development 70:309–313, 1991

3. Allers C, Benjack K, White J, et al: HIV vulnerability and the adult survivor of childhood sexual abuse. Child Abuse Negl 17:291–298, 1993

4. Anastos K, Palleja S: Caring for women at risk of HIV infection. J Gen Intern Med 6 (suppl):S40–S46, 1991

5. Aruffo J, Coverdale J, Pavlik V, et al: AIDS knowledge in minorities: significance of locus of control. Am J Prev Med 9:15–20, 1993

6. Ayd F: Intravenous haloperidol therapy. International Drug Therapy Newsletter 13:20–23, 1978

7. Ayd JF: Haloperidol: twenty years' clinical experience. J Clin Psychiatry 39:807–814, 1978

8. Baer J: Study of 60 patients with AIDS or AIDS related complex requiring psychiatric hospitalization. Am J Psychiatry 146:1285–1288, 1989

9. Bakeman R, McCray E, Lumb J, et al: The incidence of AIDS among blacks and hispanics. J Natl Med Assoc 79:921–928, 1987

10. Batki S: Buspirone in drug users with AIDS or AIDS-related complex. J Clin Psychopharmacol 10:111S–115S, 1990

11. Beckett A, Summergrad P, Manschreck T, et al: Symptomatic HIV infection of the CNS in a patient without clinical evidence of immune deficiency. Am J Psychiatry 144:1342–1343, 1987

12. Beltran E, Ostrow D, Joseph J: Predictors of sexual behavior change among men requesting their HIV-1 antibody status: the Chicago MACS/CCS cohort of homosexual/bisexual men, 1985–1986. AIDS Educ Prev 5:185–195, 1993

13. Beresin E: Delirium, in Inpatient Psychiatry: Diagnosis and Treatment. Edited by Sederer L. Baltimore, MD, Williams & Wilkins, 1983

14. Berger B, Vizgirda V: Prevention of HIV infection in women and children, in Women, Children, and HIV/AIDS. Edited by Cohen F, Durham J. New York, Springer, 1993, pp 60–82

14a. Bernstein G, Klein R: Countertransference issues in group psychotherapy with HIV-positive and AIDS patients. Int J Group Psychother 45:91–100, 1995

15. Bernstein W, Scherokman B: Neuroleptic malignant syndrome in a patient with acquired immunodeficiency syndrome. Acta Neurol Scand 73:636–637, 1986

16. Bialer P, Wallack J, Snyder S: Psychiatric diagnosis in HIV-spectrum disorders. Psychiatr Med 9:361–375, 1991

17. Bing E: The many faces of AIDS: opportunities for intervention, in AIDS Primer. Edited by American Psychiatric Association AIDS Education Project. Washington, DC, American Psychiatric Association, 1990, pp 45–50

18. Blanche S, Mayaux M, Rouzioux C, et al: Relation of the course of HIV infection in children to the severity of the disease in their mothers at delivery. N Engl J Med 330:308–312, 1994

19. Bochow M, Chiarotti F, Davies P, et al: Sexual behaviour of gay and bisexual men in eight European countries. AIDS Care 6:533–549, 1994

20. Boulton M, Hart G, Fitzpatrick R: The sexual behaviour of bisexual men in relation to HIV transmission. AIDS Care 4:165–175, 1992

21. Breitbart W, Marotta R, Call P: AIDS and neuroleptic malignant syndrome. Lancet 2:1488–1489, 1988

22. Britton P, Zarski J, Hobfoll S: Psychological distress and the role of significant others in a population of gay/bisexual men in the era of HIV. AIDS Care 5:43–54, 1993

23. Brotman A, Forstein M: AIDS obsessions in depressed heterosexuals. Psychosomatics 29:428–431, 1988

24. Brouillette M-J, Chouinard G, Lalonde R: Didanosine-induced mania in HIV infection (letter). Am J Psychiatry 151:1939–1940, 1994

25. Brown G, Rundell J: Prospective study of psychiatric morbidity in HIV-seropositive women without AIDS. Gen Hosp Psychiatry 12:30–35, 1990

26. Brown L: Black intravenous drug user: prospects for intervening in the transmission of human immunodeficiency virus infection. NIDA Res Monogr 93:53–67, 1990

27. Buhrich N, Cooper D, Freed E: HIV infection associated with symptoms indistinguishable from functional psychosis. Br J Psychiatry 152:649–653, 1988

28. Burack J, Barrett D, Stall R, et al: Depressive symptoms and CD4 lymphocyte decline among HIV-infected men. JAMA 270:2568–2573, 1993

29. Burchett S: The placental barrier to HIV-1 transmission. The AIDS Reader (September/October):1663–1665, 1993

30. Burnham R: Trauma revisited: HIV and AIDS in gay male survivors of early sexual abuse, in Therapists on the Front Line: Psychotherapy With Gay Men in the Age of AIDS. Edited by Cadwell S, Burnham R Jr, Forstein M. Washington, DC, American Psychiatric Press, 1994, pp 379–404

31. Cabaj R, Nichols S, Ostrow D: Prevention of HIV infection and disease: a mental health perspective, in AIDS Primer. Edited by American Psychiatric Association AIDS Education Project. Washington, DC, American Psychiatric Association, 1990, pp 41–44

32. Cadwell S: Twice removed: the stigma suffered by gay men with AIDS, in Therapists on the Front Line: Psychotherapy With Gay Men in the Age of AIDS. Edited by Cadwell S, Burnham R Jr, Forstein M. Washington, DC, American Psychiatric Press, 1994, pp 3–24

33. Cadwell S, Burnham R Jr, Forstein M (eds): Therapists on the Front Line: Psychotherapy With Gay Men in the Age of AIDS. Washington, DC, American Psychiatric Press, 1994

34. Campbell C: Women and AIDS. Soc Sci Med 30:407–415, 1990

35. Carrier J: Mexican male bisexuality, in Bisexualities: Theory and Research. Edited by Klein F, Wolf T. New York, Haworth, 1985, pp 75–85

36. Castro K, Lieb S, Jaffe H, et al: Transmission of HIV in Belle Glade, Florida: lessons for other communities in the United States. Science 239:193–197, 1989

37. Catania J, Coates T, Golden E, et al: Correlates of condom use among black, Hispanic, and white heterosexuals in San Francisco: the AMEN longitudinal study. AIDS Educ Prev 6:12–26, 1994

38. Centers for Disease Control: Classification system for human T-lymphotropic virus type III/lymphadenopathy-associated virus infections. MMWR Morb Mortal Wkly Rep 35:334–339, 1986

39. Centers for Disease Control: AIDS associated with IVDU—United States 1988. MMWR Morb Mortal Wkly Rep 38:229–236, 1989

40. Centers for Disease Control and Prevention: Condom use and sexual identity among men who have sex with men. MMWR Morb Mortal Wkly Rep 42:7–14, 1991

41. Centers for Disease Control and Prevention: Zidovudine for the prevention of HIV transmission from mother to infant. MMWR Morb Mortal Wkly Rep 43:285–287, 1994

42. Chesney M, Folkman S: Psychological impact of HIV disease and implications for intervention. Psychiatr Clin North Am 17:163–182, 1994

43. Chiasson M, Marte C, Thomas P, et al: Women and AIDS, in Psychological Aspects of Women's Health Care: The Interface Between Psychiatry and Obstetrics and Gynecology. Edited by Stewart D, Stotland N. Washington, DC, American Psychiatric Press, 1993, pp 313–327

44. Chu S, Peterman T, Dou L, et al: AIDS in bisexual men in the United States: epidemiology and transmission to women. Am J Public Health 82:220–224, 1992

44a. Ciraulo D, Shader R, Greenblatt D, et al. (eds): Drug Interactions in Psychiatry, 2nd Edition. Baltimore, MD, Williams & Wilkins, 1995

45. Cohen F: Epidemiology of HIV infection and AIDS in women, in Women, Children, and HIV/AIDS. Edited by Cohen F, Durham J. New York, Springer, 1993, pp 43–59

46. Cohen F, Durham J (eds): Women, Children, and HIV/AIDS. New York, Springer, 1993

47. Collaborative DHPG Treatment Study Group: Treatment of serious cytomegalovirus infections with 9-(1,3 dihydroxy-2-propoxymethyl)guanine in patients with AIDS and other immunodeficiencies. N Engl J Med 314:801–805, 1986

47a. Collaborative Study Group of AIDS in Haitian-Americans: Risk factors for AIDS among Haitians residing in the United States: evidence of heterosexual transmission. JAMA 257:635–639, 1987

48. Connor E, Sperling R, Gelber R, et al: Reduction of maternal-infant transmission of human immunodeficiency virus 1 with zidovudine treatment: results of AIDS Clinical Trials Group Protocol 076. N Engl J Med 331:1173–1180, 1994

49. Craddock C, Bull R, Pasvol G, et al: Cardiopulmonary arrest and autonomic neuropathy in AIDS. Lancet 2:16–18, 1987

50. Dauncey K: Mania in early stages of AIDS. Br J Psychiatry 152:716–717, 1988

51. Dew M, Ragni V, Nimorwicz P: Infection with human immunodeficiency virus and vulnerability to psychiatric distress. Arch Gen Psychiatry 47:737–744, 1990

52. Diaz T, Chu S, Frederick M, et al: Sociodemographics and HIV risk behaviors of bisexual men with AIDS: results from a multistate interview project. AIDS 7:1227–1232, 1993

53. Dilley J, Forstein M: Psychosocial aspects of the human immunodeficiency virus (HIV) epidemic, in American Psychiatric Press Review of Psychiatry, Vol 9. Edited by Tasman A, Goldfinger SM, Kaufmann C. Washington, DC, American Psychiatric Press, 1990, pp 631–655

54. Dinsmoor M: HIV infection and pregnancy. Clin Perinatol 21:85–94, 1994

54a. Dolcini M, Coates T, Catania J, et al: Multiple sexual partners and their psychosocial correlates: the population-based AIDS in multiethnic neighborhoods (AMEN) study. Health Psychol 14:22–31, 1995

55. Doll L, Peterson J, Magna J, et al: Male bisexuality and AIDS in the United States, in Bisexuality and HIV/AIDS. Edited by Tielman R, Carballo M, Hendriks A. Buffalo, NY, Prometheus Books, 1991, pp 27–39

56. Doll L, Peterson J, White C, et al: Homosexually and non-homosexually identified men who have sex with men: a behavioral comparison. Journal of Sex Research 29:1–14, 1992

57. Dowd S: African American gay men and HIV and AIDS: therapeutic challenges, in Therapists on the Front Line: Psychotherapy With Gay Men in the Age of AIDS. Edited by Cadwell S, Burnham R Jr, Forstein M. Washington, DC, American Psychiatric Press, 1994, pp 319–338

58. Dwight M, et al: Antidepressant activity and mania associated with risperidone treatment of schizoaffective disorder (letter). Lancet 344:554–555, 1994

59. Earl W: Married men and same sex activity: a field study of HIV risk among men who do not identify as gay or bisexual. J Sex Marital Ther 16:251–257, 1990

60. Edelstein H, Knight R: Severe parkinsonism in two AIDS patients taking prochlorperazine (letter). Lancet 2:341–342, 1987

60a. Elifson K, Boles J, Sweat M, et al: Risk factors for HIV infection among male prostitutes in Atlanta (abstract WAP 38). International Conference on AIDS 5:126, 1989

61. El-Mallakh R: Mania and paranoid psychosis in AIDS (letter). Psychosomatics 32:362, 1991

62. Ellerbrock T, Rogers M: Epidemiology of human immunodeficiency virus infection in women in the United States. Obstet Gynecol Clin North Am 17:523–544, 1990

63. Fernandez F, Holmes V, Adams F, et al: Treatment of severe, refractory agitation with a haloperidol drip. J Clin Psychiatry 49:239–241, 1988

64. Fernandez F, Holmes V, Levy J, et al: Consultation-liaison psychiatry and HIV-related disorders. Hosp Community Psychiatry 40:146–153, 1989

65. Fernandez F, Levy J: Psychiatric diagnosis and pharmacotherapy of patients with HIV infection, in American Psychiatric Press Review of Psychiatry, Vol 9. Edited by Tasman A, Goldfinger SM, Kaufmann C. Washington, DC, American Psychiatric Press, 1990, pp 614–628

66. Fernandez F, Levy J: The use of molindone in the treatment of psychotic patients infected with human immunodeficiency virus. Gen Hosp Psychiatry 15:31–35, 1993

67. Fernandez F, Levy J: Psychopharmacology in HIV spectrum disorders. Psychiatr Clin North Am 17:135–148, 1994

68. Fernandez F, Levy J, Mansell P: Management of delirium in terminally ill AIDS patients. Int J Psychiatry Med 19:165–172, 1989

69. Fernandez F, Nichols S: Psychiatric complications of HIV disease, in AIDS Primer. Edited by American Psychiatric Association AIDS Education Project. Washington, DC, American Psychiatric Association, 1990, pp 29–33

70. Fishman J: Countertransference, the therapeutic frame, and AIDS: one psychotherapist's response, in Therapists on the Front Line: Psychotherapy With Gay Men in the Age of AIDS. Edited by Cadwell S, Burnham R Jr, Forstein M. Washington, DC, American Psychiatric Press, 1994, pp 497–516

70a. Foley M, Skurnick J, Kennedy C, et al: Family support for heterosexual partners in HIV-serodiscordant couples. AIDS 8:1483–1487, 1994

71. Folkman S, Chesney M, Christopher-Richards A: Stress and coping in caregiving partners of men with AIDS. Psychiatr Clin North Am 17:35–53, 1994

72. Forstein M: The psychosocial impact of the acquired immunodeficiency syndrome. Semin Oncol 11:77–82, 1984

73. Forstein M: Psychotherapy with gay male couples: loving in the time of AIDS, in Therapists on the Front Line: Psychotherapy With Gay Men in the Age of AIDS. Edited by Cadwell S, Burnham R Jr, Forstein M. Washington, DC, American Psychiatric Press, 1994, pp 293–315

74. Forstein M: HIV testing, in AIDS Primer. Edited by American Psychiatric Association AIDS Education Project. Washington, DC, American Psychiatric Association, 1990, pp 57–61

75. Forstein M: Testing for HIV: psychological and psychotherapeutic considerations, in Therapists on the Front Line: Psychotherapy With Gay Men in the Age of AIDS. Edited by Cadwell S, Burnham R Jr, Forstein M. Washington, DC, American Psychiatric Press, 1994, pp 185–202

76. Frost J: Taking a sexual history with gay patients in psychotherapy, in Therapists on the Front Line: Psychotherapy With Gay Men in the Age of AIDS. Edited by Cadwell S, Burnham R Jr, Forstein M. Washington, DC, American Psychiatric Press, 1994, pp 163–184

77. Fullilove M: Minority women: ecological setting and intercultural dialogue, in Psychological Aspects of Women's Health Care: The Interface between Psychiatry and Obstetrics and Gynecology. Edited by Stewart D, Stotland N. Washington, DC, American Psychiatric Press, 1993, pp 519–539

78. Gabel R, Barnar N, Norko M, et al: AIDS presenting as mania. Compr Psychiatry 27:251–254, 1986

79. Gabriel M: Group therapists' countertransference reactions to multiple deaths from AIDS. Clin Soc Work J 19:279–292, 1991

80. Gilmer W, Busch K: Neuropsychiatric aspects of AIDS and psychopharmacologic management. Psychiatr Med 9:313–329, 1991

81. Global Programme on AIDS: Current and Future Dimensions of the HIV/AIDS Pandemic: A Capsule Summary (January 1992). Geneva, Switzerland, World Health Organization, 1992

82. Gnam W, Flint A, Goldbloom D: Isoniazid-induced hallucinosis: response to pyridoxine (letter). Psychosomatics 34:537–539, 1993

83. Goodkin K, Mulder C, Blaney N, et al: Psychoneuroimmunology and human immunodeficiency virus type 1 infection revisited (letter). Arch Gen Psychiatry 51:246–247, 1994

83a. Greenblatt D, von Moltke L, Harmatz J, et al: Interaction of triazolam and ketoconazole (letter). Lancet 345:191, 1995

84. Greenlee S, Ridley D: AIDS and college students: a survey of knowledge, attitudes and beliefs. Psychol Rep 73:490, 1993

85. Halevie-Goldman B, Potkin S, Poyourow P: AIDS-related complex presenting as psychosis (letter). Am J Psychiatry 144:964, 1987

86. Halman M, Worth J, Sanders K, et al: Anticonvulsant use in the treatment of manic syndromes in patients with HIV-1 infection. J Neuropsychiatry Clin Neurosci 5:430–434, 1993

87. Halstead S, Riccio M, Harlow P: Psychosis associated with HIV infection. Br J Psychiatry 153:618–623, 1988

88. Handler A, Lampman C, Levy S, et al: Attitudes toward people with AIDS and implications for school-based youth AIDS education. AIDS Educ Prev 6:175–183, 1994

89. Harris M, Gleghorn A, Jeste D: HIV-related psychosis. Paper presented at the 142nd annual meeting of the American Psychiatric Association, San Francisco, CA, May 1989

90. Harris M, Jeste D, Gleghorn A, et al: New-onset psychosis in HIV-infected patients. J Clin Psychiatry 52:369–376, 1991

90a. Hays R, Magee R, Chauncey S: Identifying helpful and unhelpful behaviours of loved ones: the PWA's perspective. AIDS Care 6:379–392, 1994

91. Hernandez M, Uribe P, Gortmaker S, et al: Sexual behavior and status for immunodeficiency virus type 1 among homosexual and bisexual males in Mexico City. Am J Epidemiol 135:883–894, 1992

92. Hill J, Farrar W, Pert C: Autoradiographic localization of T4 antigen, the HIV receptor in human brain. Int J Neurosci 32:687–693, 1987

93. Holland J, Ramazanoglu C, Scott S, et al: Risk, power and the possibility of pleasure: young women and safer sex. AIDS Care 4:273–283, 1992

94. Hollander H, Golden J, Mendelson T, et al: Extrapyramidal symptoms in AIDS patients given low-dose metoclopramide or chlorpromazine (letter). Lancet 2:1186, 1985

95. Holman S, Berthaud M, Sunderland A, et al: Women infected with human immunodeficiency virus: counseling and testing during pregnancy. Semin Perinatol 13:7–15, 1989

96. Holman S, Sunderland A, Berthaud M, et al: Prenatal HIV counseling and testing. Clin Obstet Gynecol 32:445–455, 1989

97. Holmes V: Treatment of monosymptomatic hypochondriacal psychosis with pimozide in an AIDS patient (letter). Am J Psychiatry 146:554–555, 1989

98. Hriso E, Kuhn T, Masdeu J, et al: Extrapyramidal symptoms due to dopamine-blocking agents in patients with AIDS encephalopathy. Am J Psychiatry 148:1558–1561, 1991

99. Husband A (ed): Psychoimmunology: CNS-Immune Interactions. Boca Raton, FL, CRC Press, 1993

100. Ioannou C, Viswanathan R: Neuroleptic-induced akathisia in an HIV-infected individual (letter). Gen Hosp Psychiatry 16:57–58, 1994

100a. Jacobsberg L, Frances A, Perry S: Axis II diagnoses among volunteers for HIV testing and counseling. Am J Psychiatry 152:1222–1224, 1995

101. James M: HIV seropositivity diagnosed during pregnancy: psychosocial characterization of patients and their adaptation. Gen Hosp Psychiatry 10:309–316, 1988

102. Johannessen D, Wilson L: Mania with cryptococcal meningitis in two AIDS patients. J Clin Psychiatry 49:200–201, 1988

103. Johnson E, Gant L, Hinkle Y, et al: Do African-American men and women differ in their knowledge about AIDS, attitudes about condoms, and sexual behaviors? J Natl Med Assoc 84:49–64, 1992

104. Kalichman S, Kelly J, Hunter T, et al: Culturally tailored HIV-AIDS risk-reduction messages targeted to African-American urban women: impact on risk sensitization and risk reduction. J Consult Clin Psychol 61:291–295, 1993

105. Kaliski E, Rubinson L, Lawrence L, et al: AIDS, runaways, and self-efficacy. Family and Community Health 13:65–72, 1990

106. Keller M: Why don't young adults protect themselves against sexual transmission of HIV? possible answers to a complex question. AIDS Educ Prev 5:220–233, 1993

107. Kelly J, Murphy D, Bahr G, et al: Factors associated with severity of depression and high-risk sexual behavior among persons diagnosed with human immunodeficiency virus (HIV) infection. Health Psychol 12:215–219, 1993

108. Kelly J, Murphy D, Bahr R, et al: Outcome of cognitive-behavioral and support group brief therapies for depressed, HIV-infected persons. Am J Psychiatry 150:1679–1686, 1993

109. Kelly J, St. Lawrence J, Brasfield T, et al: Psychological factors which predict AIDS high-risk and AIDS precautionary behavior. J Consult Clin Psychol 58:117–120, 1990

110. Kemeny M: Psychoneuroimmunology of HIV infection. Psychiatr Clin North Am 17:55–68, 1994

111. Kertzner R: Psychoneuroimmunology and AIDS, in AIDS Primer. Edited by American Psychiatric Association AIDS Education Project. Washington, DC, American Psychiatric Association, 1990, pp 35–39

112. Kertzner R, Gorman J: Psychoneuroimmunology and HIV infection, in American Psychiatric Press Review of Psychiatry, Vol 11. Edited by Tasman A, Riba M. Washington, DC, American Psychiatric Press, 1992, pp 219–235

113. Kessler R, Foster C, Joseph J, et al: Stressful life events and symptom onset in HIV infection. Am J Psychiatry 148:733–738, 1991

114. Kessler R, Foster C, Joseph J, et al: Stress and HIV infection (letter). Am J Psychiatry 149:417, 1992

115. Kieburtz K, Epstein L, Gelbard H, et al: Excitotoxicity and dopaminergic dysfunction in the acquired immunodeficiency syndrome dementia complex. Arch Neurol 48:1281–1284, 1991

116. Kieburtz K, Zettelmaier A, Ketonen L, et al: Manic syndrome in AIDS. Am J Psychiatry 148:1068–1070, 1991

117. Kline A, Kline E, Oken E: Minority women and sexual choice in the age of AIDS. Soc Sci Med 34:447–457, 1992

118. Koonin L, Ellerbrock T, Atrash H, et al: Pregnancy-associated deaths due to AIDS in the United States. JAMA 261:1306–1309, 1989

119. Kramer M, Aral S, Curran J: Self-reported behavior patterns of patients attending a sexually transmitted disease clinic. Am J Public Health 70:997–1000, 1980

120. Kurth A: Reproductive issues, pregnancy, and childbearing in HIV-infected women, in Women, Children, and HIV/AIDS. Edited by Cohen F, Durham J. New York, Springer, 1993, pp 104–133

121. Lackner J, Joseph J, Ostrow D, et al: A longitudinal study of psychological distress in a cohort of gay men: effects of social support and coping strategies. J Nerv Ment Dis 181:4–12, 1993

122. Landau-Stanton J, Clements C, Stanton M: Psychotherapeutic intervention: from individual through group to extended network, in AIDS Health and Mental Health: A Primary Sourcebook. Edited by Landau-Stanton J, Clements C. New York, Brunner/Mazel, 1993, pp 214–266

123. Landis S, Earp J, Koch G: Impact of HIV testing and counseling on subsequent sexual behavior. AIDS Educ Prev 4:61–70, 1992

124. Langs C, Gallo G, Schacht R, et al: Rapid renal failure in AIDS-associated focal glomerulosclerosis. Arch Intern Med 150:287–292, 1990

125. Lesserman J, Perkins D, Evans D: Coping with the threat of AIDS: the role of social support. Am J Psychiatry 149:1514–1520, 1992

126. Levenson J: Should psychostimulants be used to treat delirious patients with depressed mood? (letter). J Clin Psychiatry 53:69, 1992

127. Lever K, Kanouse D, Rogers W, et al: Behavior patterns and sexual identity of bisexual men. Journal of Sex Research 29:141–167, 1992

127a. Lindsay M, Grant J, Peterson H, et al: The impact of knowledge of human immunodeficiency virus serostatus on contraceptive choice and repeat pregnancy. Obstet Gynecol 85:675–679, 1995

128. Lin-Greenberger A, Taneja-Uppal N: Dysautonomia and infection with the human immunodeficiency virus (letter). Ann Intern Med 106:167, 1987

128a. Lyketsos C, Fishman M, Treisman G: Psychiatric issues and emergencies in HIV infection. Emerg Med Clin North Am 13:163–177, 1995

129. Lyketsos C, Hanson A, Fishman M, et al: Manic syndrome early and late in the course of HIV. Am J Psychiatry 150:326–327, 1993

130. Lyketsos C, Hoover D, Guccione M, et al: Depressive symptoms as predictors of medical outcomes in HIV infection. JAMA 270:2563–2567, 1993

131. Maccario M, Scharre D: HIV and acute onset of psychosis (letter). Lancet 2:342, 1987

132. Marin B: AIDS prevention for non-Puerto Rican Hispanics. NIDA Res Monogr 93:35–52, 1990

133. Marin G: AIDS prevention among Hispanics: needs, risk behaviors and cultural values. Public Health Rep 104:411–415, 1989

134. Marks G, Richardson J, Ruiz M, et al: HIV-infected men's practices in notifying past sexual partners of infection risk. Public Health Rep 107:100–105, 1992

135. Martin J, Dean L: Effects of AIDS-related bereavement and HIV-related illness on psychological distress among gay men: a 7-year longitudinal study, 1985–1991. J Consult Clin Psychol 61:94–103, 1993

135a. Maxwell S: Female homosexuality overlooked (letter). Am J Psychiatry 152:961–962, 1995

136. Maxwell S, Scheftner W, Kessler H, et al: Manic syndrome associated with zidovudine treatment. JAMA 259:3406–3407, 1988

137. Mays V, Cochran S: Acquired immunodeficiency syndrome and black Americans: special psychosocial issues. Public Health Rep 102:224–231, 1987

138. Mays V, Cochran S: Issues in the perception of AIDS risk and risk reduction activities by black and hispanic/latina women. Am Psychol 43:949–957, 1988

139. McArthur J, Selnes O, Glass J, et al: HIV dementia: incidence and risk factors (review), in HIV, AIDS and the Brain. Edited by Price R, Perry S. New York, Raven, 1994, pp 251–272

139a. McDaniel J, Johnson K: Obsessive-compulsive disorder in HIV disease: response to fluoxetine. Psychosomatics 36:147–150, 1995

140. McGuire Ed, Shega J, Nicholls G, et al: Sexual behavior, knowledge, and attitudes about AIDS among college freshmen. Am J Prev Med 8:226–234, 1992

141. McKirnan D, Burzette R, Stokes J: Differences in AIDS risk behavior among black and white bisexual men (abstract MD4042), in Proceedings of the Seventh International Conference on AIDS, Florence, Italy, June 1991, p 400

142. McNamara P, Durso R: Reversible pathologic jealousy (Othello syndrome) associated with amantadine. J Geriatr Psychiatry Neurol 4:157–159, 1991

143. Mermel L, Doro J, Kabadi U: Acute psychosis in a patient receiving trimethoprimsulfamethoxazole intravenously. J Clin Psychiatry 47:269–270, 1986

144. Miller D, Acton T, Hedge B: The worried well: their identification and management. J R Coll Physicians Lond 22:158–165, 1988

145. Mondanaro J: Community-based AIDS prevention interventions: special issues of women intravenous drug users. NIDA Res Monogr 93:68–82, 1990

146. Morse E, Simon P, Osofsky H, et al: The male street prostitute: a vector for transmission of HIV infection into the heterosexual world. Soc Sci Med 32:535–539, 1991

147. Myers T, Orr K, Locker D, et al: Factors affecting gay and bisexual men's decisions and intentions to seek HIV testing. Am J Public Health 83:701–704, 1993

148. Navia B, Cho E, Petito C, et al: The AIDS dementia complex, II: neuropathology. Ann Neurol 19:525–535, 1986

149. Navia B, Jordan B, Price R: The AIDS dementia complex, I: clinical features. Ann Neurol 19:517–524, 1986

150. Nemeroff CJ, Brinkman A, Woodward CK: Magical contagion and AIDS risk perception in a college population. AIDS Educ Prev 6:249–265, 1994

151. Nichols S: Psychosocial reactions of persons with the acquired immunodeficiency syndrome. Ann Intern Med 103:765–767, 1985

152. Norris A, Ford K: Associations between condom experiences and beliefs, intentions, and use in a sample of urban, low-income, African-American and Hispanic youth. AIDS Educ Prev 6:27–39, 1994

153. Norris A, Ford K: Condom beliefs in urban, low income, African American and Hispanic youth. Health Educ Q 21:39–53, 1994

154. O'Brien K, Wortman C, Kessler R, et al: Social relationships of men at risk for AIDS. Soc Sci Med 36:1161–1167, 1993

155. O'Donnell L, San Doval A, Vornfett R, et al: Reducing AIDS and other STDs among inner-city Hispanics: the use of qualitative research in the development of video-based patient education. AIDS Educ Prev 6:140–153, 1994

156. O'Dowd M: Psychosocial issues in HIV infection. AIDS 2 (suppl 1):S201–S205, 1988

157. Odets W: Seronegative gay men and considerations of safe and unsafe sex, in Therapists on the Front Line: Psychotherapy With Gay Men in the Age of AIDS. Edited by Cadwell S, Burnham R Jr, Forstein M. Washington, DC, American Psychiatric Press, 1994, pp 427–452

158. Odets W: Survivor guilt in seronegative gay men, in Therapists on the Front Line: Psychotherapy With Gay Men in the Age of AIDS. Edited by Cadwell S, Burnham R Jr, Forstein M. Washington, DC, American Psychiatric Press, 1994, pp 453–471

158a. Olkkola K, Backman J, Neuvonen P: Midazolam should be avoided in patients receiving the systemic antimycotics ketoconazole or itraconazole. Clin Pharmacol Ther 55:481–485, 1994

159. Ostrow D, Grant I, Atkinson H: Assessment and management of the AIDS patient with neuropsychiatric disturbances. J Clin Psychiatry 49 (suppl):S14–S22, 1988

160. Padian N: Female partners of bisexual men, in CDC Workshop on Bisexuality and AIDS. Atlanta, GA, Centers for Disease Control and Prevention, 1989

161. Pape J, Liautaud B, Thomas F: The acquired immunodeficiency syndrome in Haiti. Ann Intern Med 103:674–678, 1985

162. Parés-Avila J, Montano-López R: Issues in the psychosocial care of Latino gay men with HIV infection, in Therapists on the Front Line: Psychotherapy With Gay Men in the Age of AIDS. Edited by Cadwell S, Burnham R Jr, Forstein M. Washington, DC, American Psychiatric Press, 1994, pp 339–362

163. Perkins D, Leserman J, Murphy C, et al: Psychosocial predictors of high-risk sexual behavior among HIV-negative homosexual men. AIDS Educ Prev 5:141–152, 1993

164. Perry S, Fishman B: Depression and HIV: how does one affect the other? JAMA 270:3609–3610, 1993

165. Perry S, Fishman B, Jacobsberg L: Stress and HIV infection (letter). Am J Psychiatry 149:416–417, 1992

166. Perry S, Fishman B, Jacobsberg L, et al: Effectiveness of psychoeducational interventions in reducing emotional distress after human immunodeficiency virus antibody testing. Arch Gen Psychiatry 48:143–147, 1991

167. Perry S, Jacobsberg L, Card C, et al: Severity of psychiatric symptoms after HIV testing. Am J Psychiatry 150:775–779, 1993

168. Perry S, Jacobsberg L, Fishman B: Suicidal ideation and HIV testing. JAMA 263:679–682, 1990

169. Perry S, Jacobsberg L, Fishman B, et al: Psychiatric diagnosis before serological testing for human immunodeficiency virus. Am J Psychiatry 147:89–93, 1990

170. Perry S, Jacobsberg L, Fishman B, et al: Psychological responses to serological testing for HIV. AIDS 4:145–152, 1990

170a. Peterson J, Coates T, Catania J, et al: Help-seeking for AIDS high-risk sexual behavior among gay and bisexual African-American men. AIDS Educ Prev 7:1–9, 1995

171. Peterson J, Marin G: Issues in the prevention of AIDS among black and Hispanic men. Am Psychol 43:871–877, 1988

172. Pleck J, Sonenstein F, Ku L: Changes in adolescent males' use of and attitudes toward condoms, 1988–1991. Fam Plann Perspect 25:106–110, 117, 1993

173. Rabkin J, Remien R, Katoff L, et al: Resilience in adversity among long-term survivors of AIDS. Hosp Community Psychiatry 44:162–167, 1993

174. Rabkin J, Williams J, Neugebauer R, et al: Maintenance of hope in HIV-spectrum homosexual men. Am J Psychiatry 147:1322–1326, 1990

175. Rabkin J, Williams J, Remien R, et al: Depression, distress, lymphocyte subsets, and human immunodeficiency virus symptoms on two occasions in HIV-positive homosexual men. Arch Gen Psychiatry 48:111–119, 1991

176. Ragni M, Gupta P, Rinaldo C, et al: HIV transmission to female sexual partners of HIV antibody-positive hemophiliacs. Public Health Rep 103:54–57, 1988

177. Raisler J: Safer sex for women. Clinical Issues in Perinatal and Women's Health Nursing 1:28–32, 1990

178. Ralston G, Dow M, Rothwell B: Knowledge of AIDS and HIV among various groups. Br J Addict 87:1663–1668, 1992

179. Ratigan B: On not traumatising the traumatised: the contribution of psychodynamic psychotherapy to work with people with HIV and AIDS. Br J Psychother 8:39–47, 1991

180. Richman D, Fischl M, Grieco M, et al: The toxicity of azidothymidine (AZT) in the treatment of patients with AIDS and AIDS-related complex. N Engl J Med 317:192–197, 1987

181. Ritchie E, Bridenbaugh R, Jabbari B: Acute generalized myoclonus following buspirone administration. J Clin Psychiatry 49:242–243, 1988

182. Rosenbaum M: Mania in AIDS and syphilis (paresis) (letter). Am J Psychiatry 149:416, 1992

183. Rosenberg P, Ahmed I, Hurwitz S: Methylphenidate in depressed medically ill patients. J Clin Psychiatry 52:263–267, 1991

184. Ross M, Wodak A, Gold J, et al: Differences across sexual orientation on HIV risk behaviours in injecting drug users. AIDS Care 4:139–148, 1992

185. Rothenberg R, Woelfel M, Stoneburner R, et al: Survival with the acquired immunodeficiency syndrome. N Engl J Med 317:1297–1302, 1987

186. Rundell J, Brown C, McManis S, et al: Psychiatric predisposition and current psychiatric findings in HIV infected persons (abstract SB362). Abstracts of the Sixth International Conference on AIDS, San Francisco, CA, 1990, p 176

187. Sabin T: AIDS: the new "Great Imitator." J Am Geriatr Soc 35:467–471, 1987

188. Sahs J, Goetz R, Reddy M, et al: Psychological distress and natural killer cells in gay men with and without HIV infection. Am J Psychiatry 151:1479–1484, 1994

189. Scamvougeras A, Rosebush P: AIDS-related psychosis with catatonia responding to low-dose lorazepam (letter). J Clin Psychiatry 53:414–415, 1992

189a. Schaffner B: The crucial and difficult role of the psychotherapist in the treatment of the HIV-positive patient. J Am Acad Psychoanal 22:505–518, 1994

190. Schmidt U, Miller D: Two cases of hypomania in AIDS. Br J Psychiatry 152:839–842, 1988

190a. Schwarzer R, Dunkel-Schetter C, Kemeny M: The multidimensional nature of received social support in gay men at risk of HIV infection and AIDS. Am J Community Psychol 22:319–339, 1994

191. Selwyn P, Carter R, Schoenbaum E, et al: Knowledge of HIV antibody status and decisions to continue or terminate pregnancy among intravenous drug users. JAMA 261:3567–3571, 1989

192. Serrano Y: The Puerto Rican intravenous drug user. NIDA Res Monogr 93:24–34, 1990

193. Sewell D, Jeste D, Atkinson J, et al: HIV-associated psychosis: a study of 20 cases. Am J Psychiatry 151:237–242, 1994

193a. Sewell D, Jeste D, McAdams L, et al: Neuroleptic treatment of HIV-associated psychosis: HNRC group. Neuropsychopharmacology 10:223–229, 1994

194. Shedlack K, Soldato-Couture C, Swanson CJ: Rapidly progressive tardive dyskinesia in AIDS (letter). Biol Psychiatry 35:147–148, 1994

195. Shelby R: Mourning within a culture of mourning, in Therapists on the Front Line: Psychotherapy With Gay Men in the Age of AIDS. Edited by Cadwell S, Burnham R Jr, Forstein M. Washington, DC, American Psychiatric Press, 1994, pp 53–80

196. Sherr L, Strong C: Safe sex and women. Genitourin Med 68:32–35, 1992

197. Shtarkshall R, Awerbuch T: It takes two to tango but one to infect (on the underestimation of the calculated risk for infection with HIV in sexual encounters, arising from nondisclosure of previous risk behavior or seropositivity). J Sex Marital Ther 18:121–127, 1992

197a. Siegel K, Raveis V, Karus D: Psychological well-being of gay men with AIDS: contribution of positive and negative illness-related network interactions to depressive mood. Soc Sci Med 39:1555–1563, 1994

198. Simkins L: Update on AIDS and sexual behavior of college students: seven years later. Psychol Rep 74:208–210, 1994

199. Singh A, Catalan J: Risperidone in HIV-related manic psychosis (letter). Lancet 344:1029–1030, 1994

200. Snyder S, Prenzlauer S, Maruyama N, et al: Catatonia in a patient with AIDS-related dementia (letter). J Clin Psychiatry 53:414, 1992

201. St. Louis M, Kamenga M, Brown C, et al: Risk for perinatal HIV-1 transmission according to maternal immunologic, virologic and placental factors. JAMA 269:2853–2859, 1993

202. Stein M, Miller H, Trestman R: Depression, the immune system, and health and illness: findings in search of meaning. Arch Gen Psychiatry 48:171–177, 1991

203. Stevenson H, Davis G: Impact of culturally sensitive AIDS video education on the AIDS risk knowledge of African-American adolescents. AIDS Educ Prev 6:40–52, 1994

204. Stevenson H, White J: AIDS prevention struggles in ethnocultural neighborhoods: why research partnerships with community based organizations can't wait. AIDS Educ Prev 6:126–139, 1994

205. Strain J, Forstein M: "Yes" and "no." Viewpoints—Crossfire: is it time to require mandatory HIV testing of all hospitalized inpatients? Psychiatric News 26:9, 30, March 15, 1991

206. Strauss A: Oral dyskinesia associated with buspirone use in an elderly woman. J Clin Psychiatry 49:322–323, 1988

207. Sunderland A, Minkoff H, Handte J, et al: The impact of human immunodeficiency virus serostatus on reproductive decisions of women. Obstet Gynecol 79:1027–1031, 1992

208. Tesar G, Murray G, Cassem N: Use of high-dose intravenous haloperidol in the treatment of agitated cardiac patients. J Clin Psychopharmacol 5:344–347, 1985

209. Thienhaus O, Khosla N: Meningeal cryptococcosis misdiagnosed as a manic episode. Am J Psychiatry 141:1459–1460, 1984

210. Thomas C, Szabadi E: Paranoid psychosis as the 1st presentation of a fulminating lethal case of AIDS. Br J Psychiatry 151:693–694, 1987

211. Trachman S: Buspirone-induced psychosis in a human immunodeficiency virus–infected man. Psychosomatics 33:332–335, 1992

212. Treisman G, Fishman M, Lyketsos C, et al: Evaluation and treatment of psychiatric disorders associated with HIV infection, in HIV, AIDS and the Brain. Edited by Price R, Perry S. New York, Raven, 1994, pp 239–250

213. Tunnell G: Complications in group psychotherapy with AIDS patients. Int J Group Psychother 41:481–498, 1991

214. United States Census, 1980

215. Upadhyaya M, Chaturvedi S: Psychosis and antituberculosis therapy. Lancet 2:735–736, 1989

216. Vamos M: Mania and AIDS: a psychodynamic emphasis. Aust N Z J Psychiatry 26:111–118, 1992

217. Varhe A, Olkkola K, Neuvonen P: Oral triazolam is potentially hazardous to patients receiving systemic antimycotics ketoconazole or itraconazole. Clin Pharmacol Ther 56:601–607, 1994

218. Volkow N, Harper A, Munnisteri D, et al: AIDS and catatonia (letter). J Neurol Neurosurg Psychiatry 50:104–118, 1987

219. Wagner G, Rabkin J, Rabkin R: Sexual activity among HIV-seropositive gay men seeking treatment for depression. J Clin Psychiatry 54:470–475, 1993

220. Wallack J, Bialer P, Prenzlauer S: Psychiatric aspects of HIV infection and AIDS: an overview and update, in Medical-Psychiatric Practice, Vol 3. Edited by Stoudemire A, Fogel B. Washington, DC, American Psychiatric Press, 1995, pp 257–302

221. Wallston B, Wallston K, Kaplan G, et al: Development and validation of the health locus of control (HLC) scale. J Consult Clin Psychol 44:580–585, 1976

222. Wallston K, Wallston B, Devellis R: Development of the multi-dimensional health locus of control (MHLC) scales. Health Education Monographs 6:161–170, 1978

223. Wilcox J, Tsuang J: Psychological effects of amantadine on psychotic subjects. Neuropsychobiology 23:144–146, 1990

224. Wilson J, Smith R: Relation between elderly and AIDS patients with drug-induced Parkinson's disease (letter). Lancet 2:686, 1987

225. Winiarski M: AIDS-Related Psychotherapy. Elmsford, NY, Pergamon, 1991

226. Wolcott D, Fawzy F, Pasnau R: Acquired immune deficiency syndrome and consultation-liaison psychiatry. Gen Hosp Psychiatry 7:280–292, 1985

227. Wyatt G: Reexamining factors predictive of African-American and white women's age at first coitus. Arch Sex Behav 18:271–298, 1989

228. Yep GA: HIV/AIDS education and prevention for Asian and Pacific Islander communities: toward the development of general guidelines. AIDS Educ Prev 6:184–186, 1994

229. Zegans L, Gerhard A, Coates T: Psychotherapies for the person with HIV disease. Psychiatr Clin North Am 17:149–162, 1994

230. Zierler S, Feingold L, Laufer D, et al: Adult survivors of childhood sexual abuse and subsequent risk of HIV infection. Am J Public Health 81:572–575, 1991

231. Zimmerman RS, Olson K: AIDS-related risk behavior and behavior change in a sexually active, heterosexual sample: a test of three models of prevention. AIDS Educ Prev 6:189–204, 1994

The Patient With Gastrointestinal Distress and Psychiatric Symptoms

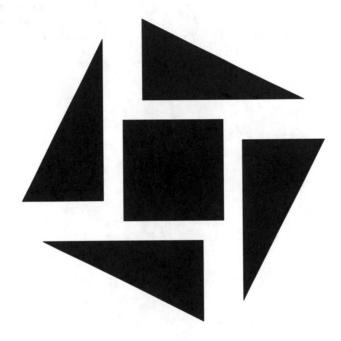

C H A P T E R   7

CONTENTS

■ Introduction to Chapter 7 277
■ Case Presentation: Ms. Mack: The Patient
   With Gastrointestinal Distress and
   Psychiatric Symptoms 278
■ Questions 278
■ Answers 282
■ Discussion 283
   ◆ Medical Conditions With Psychiatric and
      Gastrointestinal Symptoms 283
      Pancreatic Cancer 283
      Acute Intermittent Porphyria 283
      B$_{12}$ (Cobalamin) Deficiency 284
   ◆ Irritable Bowel Syndrome 285
      Definition 285

   Other Symptoms 286
   Epidemiology 286
   Pain 286
◆ The Gut, Stress, and Emotions 287
   Psychiatric Comorbidity: Chicken or Egg? . . . 287
      Psychopathology and the Gut 288
      "Irritable Bowel Personality"? 289
      Method or "Madness"? 289
   Conclusions 289
◆ Treatment 290
   Medications 290
   Psychological Treatments 290
◆ Summary and Recommendations 291
◆ References 291

One of the most common dilemmas in outpatient consultation-liaison psychiatry is the patient with gastrointestinal (GI) symptoms and psychiatric distress. Often the patient has had a normal medical workup, and comes to the initial psychiatric appointment defensive, stating "they're telling me it's all in my head, but these symptoms are *real.*" Knowledge of the differential diagnosis of the co-occurrence of psychological and GI complaints helps triage those patients who require additional workup from those who would benefit from a primarily psychiatric intervention. We use the following case to explore these issues. As with the other cases, some organizational decisions may seem arbitrary, but we hope the questions and discussion provide a practical review for the clinician.

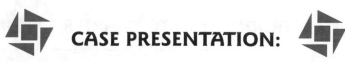

Ms. Mack is a 39-year-old businesswoman with a long history of GI symptoms, which have recently worsened as her job has become more stressful. Her work is a source of almost constant irritation, and a change in company owners has led to unpredictable challenges to her authority. She feels that her boss undermines her well-organized, smoothly running department and that things have become "chaotic." Ms. Mack is able to function well at her job, but experiences bouts of abdominal pain accompanied by frequent, mucousy loose stools. The pain is relieved by defecation. It does not awaken her from sleep, but she often notices transient pins and needles in her fingers and toes when it happens. Ms. Mack also complains of urinary frequency, although she has never had a urinary tract infection. The patient has not lost weight nor had a change in appetite. She is afraid that she might have pancreatic cancer like her mother, who died about 20 years ago at the age of 40. Her internist refers the patient to you for evaluation.

Past medical history is otherwise unremarkable. She is on no medications. The patient denies recent changes in weight or appetite, hopelessness, anhedonia, or persistent depressed mood. She has never been suicidal.

Past psychiatric history is notable for chronic anxiety, tension, intermittent abdominal uneasiness with stress, jumpiness, and irritability for as long as the patient can remember. As a small child, she was afraid of leaving home to go to school, but has never had any formal psychiatric treatment. Her former internist prescribed diazepam (Valium) intermittently in the past for anxiety. There is no drug or alcohol history. Family psychiatric history is reportedly negative.

Mental status exam reveals an attractive, meticulously groomed woman, obviously distraught. Speech is goal-directed, coherent, and logical. Affect is full. Mood is anxious, but appropriate to expressed thought. Thought content shows no delusions or hallucinations. She denies suicidal ideation. The patient is preoccupied with concerns about her health and job, but there are no obsessions or compulsions. She is alert and fully oriented. Cognitive functions are entirely intact.

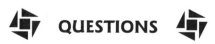

QUESTIONS

Choose all that apply.

1. Ms. Mack reiterates that she is terrified that her symptoms are those of pancreatic cancer and that she will die like her mother. She remembers that her mother had been quite depressed and anxious before the cancer was finally diagnosed, "and then it was too late." Which of the following are true of pancreatic cancer?
   a. It has a bleak 5-year survival rate of < 1%.
   b. It is decreasing in incidence.
   c. Psychiatric problems occur *without* systemic symptoms.
   d. Psychiatric symptoms are almost always in the context of delirium.

2. When psychiatric syndromes occur with pancreatic cancer . . .
   a. Delusions are the most frequent.
   b. The symptoms are usually affective.
   c. They are no more common than those occurring with other GI neoplasms.
   d. None of the above.

3. Although not relevant to Ms. Mack, acute intermittent porphyria is in the differential diagnosis of abdominal pain and psychiatric symptoms. The most common presentation of acute intermittent porphyria is . . .
   a. Depression in the setting of severe diarrhea.
   b. Delirium in the setting of intense abdominal pain.
   c. Psychosis in the setting of bowel obstruction.
   d. Anxiety in the setting of jaundice.

4. Attacks of acute intermittent porphyria may be precipitated by all of the following except . . .
   a. The menstrual cycle.
   b. Alcohol.
   c. Medications oxidized by the cytochrome P450 system.
   d. Medications undergoing hepatic glucuronidation.
   e. Oral contraceptives.
   f. Attacks are precipitated by all of the above.

5. When delusions or hallucinations accompany acute intermittent porphyria . . .
   a. Psychotic symptoms are less typical than depression.
   b. It is late in the course of the illness.
   c. They are almost exclusively in the setting of delirium.
   d. All of the above.

6. What is true of the course of acute intermittent porphyria?
   a. It progresses unremittingly after the initial episode.
   b. It improves with pregnancy.
   c. It is characterized by remissions and exacerbations.
   d. None of the above.

7. Ms. Mack is tearful in the sessions with you as she speaks about her mother's terrible GI symptoms and rapid death. She is otherwise without evidence of endogenous depression. Ms. Mack reveals that she has always been concerned about health and nutrition. She follows a vegetarian diet, supplemented by a vitamin regimen prescribed by a "holistic nutritionist." Her internist feels that the vitamins are unnecessary but benign. You receive a copy of Ms. Mack's laboratory work. Electrocardiogram (ECG) and all lab values are normal, including thyroid function tests and human immunodeficiency virus (HIV) serological testing. Routine urinalysis is negative. Colonoscopy is pending. The internist consults with you and asks if you want any other tests. GI symptoms are not typical, but when psychiatric symptoms accompany B_{12} (cobalamin) deficiency . . .
   a. They are a late complication.
   b. They are accompanied by pathognomonic macrocytic anemia.
   c. They are predated by neurological symptoms.
   d. Serum B_{12} levels are diagnostic.
   e. None of the above.

8. The *prototypical* psychiatric symptom of B_{12} deficiency is . . .
   a. Depression.
   b. Mania.
   c. Schizophreniform psychosis.
   d. Paranoid psychosis.
   e. Not predictable.

9. Which of the following is/are true regarding *clinically significant* B_{12} deficiency?
   a. An abnormal serum B_{12} level is the most reliable test.
   b. Anemia is necessary, by definition.
   c. Macrocytosis may be absent.
   d. A normal Schilling test rules out cobalamin deficiency.

10. The neurological symptoms of B_{12} deficiency classically consist of . . .
    a. Delirium.
    b. Paresthesias in feet and fingers.
    c. Disturbed vibratory sense.
    d. Extrapyramidal features resembling neuroleptic side effects.

11. Ms. Mack's workup is completed and she is diagnosed with irritable bowel syndrome (IBS). She knows little about the condition, except that it is considered "psychosomatic." Which of the following are true regarding IBS?
    a. It is a type of inflammatory bowel disease.
    b. It is a type of structural bowel disease.
    c. It is a type of malabsorption syndrome.
    d. It is associated with urological symptoms.
    e. It is associated with mucus in the stools.

12. All of the following are characteristic of IBS (in the absence of a mood disorder) *except* . . .
    a. Pain relieved by defecation.
    b. Pain interfering with sleep.
    c. Weight loss.
    d. Constipation.
    e. Diarrhea.
    f. Variable pain location.

13. The diagnosis of IBS is made by characteristic changes seen on . . .
    a. Barium enema.
    b. Histopathology.
    c. Colonoscopy.
    d. Autoimmune studies.
    e. None of the above.

14. Ms. Mack believes that *psychosomatic* means "imaginary," a common misconception. What are *physiological* characteristics of IBS?
    a. Abnormal small intestinal motility
    b. Abnormal colonic motility
    c. Normal esophageal motility
    d. There are no physiological changes.

15. Ms. Mack notes that her GI symptoms worsen with anxiety and seem to peak every morning right before she leaves for work. Ms. Mack's husband has observed that her symptoms improve on weekends and vacations. He has urged her to "calm down" at work because she is "giving herself" the symptoms. Your formulation of how bowel physiology interacts with psychological factors will influence how you educate Ms. Mack about IBS and work with her psychiatrically. Which physiological sequelae of strong affective states are found in both IBS patients and "normals"?
    a. Increased colonic pressure
    b. Decreased colonic motility
    c. Increased colonic motor and spike potential activity
    d. Only a and c are true
    e. Only a and b are true

16. Ms. Mack says that she has always been a "nervous person," even as a college student. "I'd worry about my grades. I'd worry about my finances. I liked things to be routine, no changes. I don't do well with change. It makes me very nervous." She also mentions that her father was phobic of bridges and tunnels and was quite hypochondriacal. There is no present or past personal history of depression. What is known about the epidemiology of IBS?
    a. Increased prevalence in first-degree relatives
    b. Increased concordance in monozygotic twins
    c. Male predominance
    d. Highest incidence after age 60
    e. A history of parental reinforcement of childhood somatic complaints

17. What is true about the role of stress for IBS patients?
    a. There is evidence of central alpha-adrenergic receptor dysfunction in response to stressful events.
    b. IBS patients' increased colonic sensitivity to stress can be explained by psychological factors rather than physiological events.
    c. Objectively stressful events are no more common in IBS patients than in control subjects.
    d. The association between IBS exacerbations and stress almost disappears in *controlled* studies.

18. Historical factors found to be more prevalent among IBS patients include . . .
    a. Parental loss.
    b. Sexual or physical abuse.
    c. Impaired reality testing.
    d. All of the above.

19. Which of the following are true?
    a. The most commonly reported pattern is for psychiatric symptoms, when present, to predate the appearance of bowel symptoms.
    b. The most commonly reported pattern is for bowel symptoms to predate psychiatric symptoms.
    c. Crohn's disease, which requires multiple surgeries and often steroid treatment, has a higher prevalence of psychiatric disorders than IBS.
    d. Psychological testing has shown a personality profile that is unique to patients with IBS.

20. In the psychosomatic literature, "illness behavior" refers to . . .
    a. Alterations in lifestyle secondary to a medical condition.
    b. A pattern of multiple somatic complaints and overutilization of health care services.
    c. The perceived intrusiveness of a disease and its treatment.
    d. The combined psychological and behavioral consequences of a disease and its treatment.

21. Which of the following are true?
    a. There is consensus that psychological factors cause IBS.
    b. There is consensus that psychiatric comorbidity occurs with IBS.
    c. Community surveys indicate that individuals with IBS who do *not* consult a physician have rates of psychiatric symptomatology equivalent to those who *do* seek treatment.
    d. The high association between IBS and psychological factors is only minimally explained by patients' multiple somatic complaints and overutilization of health care services.

22. Sexual functioning in IBS . . .
    a. Is unaffected in the majority of patients.
    b. Is disrupted at a rate equivalent to that in patients with inflammatory bowel disease.
    c. Is disrupted at a rate lower than that in patients with peptic ulcer disease.
    d. Is disrupted in the majority of patients.

23. There are many methodological problems in past research on IBS that current studies are attempting to address. The *previous* perspective on the percentage of IBS patients with psychiatric symptomatology has been in the range of . . .
    a. < 10%.
    b. 25%–33%.
    c. 50%–66%.
    d. 70%–90%.

24. How do the lifetime prevalence rates of psychiatric illness in IBS compare with those of other bowel disorders, such as Crohn's disease or ulcerative colitis?
    a. Psychiatric illness in IBS patients is higher.
    b. Psychiatric illness in Crohn's and ulcerative colitis exceeds that in IBS.
    c. They are approximately equal.
    d. All groups are equivalent to patients with other medical illnesses.

25. The current thinking about the association between IBS and psychopathology is that it . . .
    a. Is unlikely to be methodological artifact.
    b. May result from ambiguous diagnostic inclusion criteria.
    c. Indicates an etiological connection.
    d. Has been underestimated.

26. Ms. Mack is lost to follow-up for several months. She returns after having failed several trials of antispasmodic and bulking agents. Her anxiety about her health has skyrocketed. What is true about using medication for IBS?
    a. There is a high placebo response.
    b. The failure of antispasmodic and bulking agents strongly suggests that she was probably noncompliant with treatment.

    c. Except for the relief of diarrhea, tricyclic antidepressants do not benefit other irritable bowel symptoms.
    d. Anxiolytics should be avoided.

27. Ms. Mack feels less anxious on clonazepam (Klonopin) 0.5 mg tid and imipramine (Tofranil) 25 mg. However, her GI symptoms persist, as does her preoccupation with stressful work events. She feels she needs help coping and concedes that she is now "willing to try anything, including psychotherapy." How would you advise Ms. Mack regarding the efficacy of psychological treatments for IBS?
    a. *Controlled* studies have proven psychotherapy's effectiveness in improving IBS symptoms.
    b. The effects of hypnotherapy are no greater than for placebo alone.
    c. A major drawback of psychotherapy is that it requires *at least* 6 months to be effective for IBS symptoms.
    d. If reassurance and symptomatic medical treatment have not been effective, psychological treatments have a low likelihood of helping.

28. What can Ms. Mack expect regarding the course, treatment, and prognosis of her condition?
    a. The prognosis for IBS is poor, with most patients following a progressive, downhill course.
    b. Psychological treatment *alone* may be as effective as drug therapy.
    c. The effectiveness of psychotherapy has been limited to those treatments using psychodynamic techniques.
    d. The effectiveness of psychotherapy has been limited to those treatments using behavioral techniques.

⬧ Answers

1. Answer: a, c (p. 283)
2. Answer: b (p. 283)
3. Answer: b (pp. 283–284)
4. Answer: d (pp. 283–284)
5. Answer: c (pp. 283–284)
6. Answer: c (pp. 283–284)
7. Answer: e (pp. 284–285)
8. Answer: e (p. 284)
9. Answer: c (pp. 284–285)
10. Answer: b, c (p. 285)
11. Answer: d, e (pp. 285–286)
12. Answer: b, c (pp. 285–286)
13. Answer: e (p. 285)
14. Answer: a, b (pp. 286–287)
15. Answer: d (pp. 286–287)
16. Answer: a, e (p. 286)
17. Answer: a (p. 287)
18. Answer: a, b (p. 288)
19. Answer: a (pp. 288–289)
20. Answer: b (p. 288)
21. Answer: b (p. 289)
22. Answer: d (p. 286)
23. Answer: d (p. 288)
24. Answer: a (pp. 287–288)
25. Answer: b (p. 289)
26. Answer: a (p. 290)
27. Answer: a (pp. 290–291)
28. Answer: b (pp. 290–291)

Even psychiatrists who do not concentrate their practice in consultation-liaison psychiatry will eventually encounter a patient with prominent GI symptoms who is psychiatrically symptomatic. We decided to select among the so-called functional GI disorders—irritable bowel syndrome (IBS), globus hystericus, pseudodysphagia, nonulcer dyspepsia—and concentrate on the most common, IBS.[72] IBS has a lifetime prevalence of at least *one-fifth* of the general population.[170] Terms that have been used synonymously with IBS have included spastic colon/colitis, colonic neurosis, dyskinesia of the colon, functional diarrhea/enterocolonopathy, nervous diarrhea, and "unhappy colon."[171]

◆ IBS represented approximately 11% of all GI diagnoses in 1984, with an estimated annual cost approaching 1 billion dollars.[137]

Not everyone with IBS symptoms becomes a patient (i.e., seeks medical care;)[40] the majority "learn to live" with their symptoms; only 5% become patients.[59]

The reader is referred to the excellent text by Kellner[89] for a survey of the other functional GI disorders, as well as other useful review articles.[24,53,113,146,165,179,197]

A tour of medical conditions with GI complaints and psychiatric symptoms follows.

⚜ MEDICAL CONDITIONS WITH PSYCHIATRIC AND GASTRO-INTESTINAL SYMPTOMS

Pancreatic Cancer

Pancreatic cancer has long been known to present with unexplained depression and psychological distress,[65] which may predate more obvious systemic signs, such as anorexia, weight loss, jaundice, and abdominal pain.[86,101,134,143,144,147,201] Adenocarcinoma of the pancreas has an extremely poor prognosis: less than 1% 5-year survival even with treatment. By the time of biopsy or surgical exploration, the disease usually has spread beyond the pancreas in 85%–90% of patients.[83] Its frequency is increasing in the United States, especially in women, with the sex ratio approaching 1:1.[77,114]

The "classical" triad of *depression, anxiety, and premonition of impending doom* was described in many early clinical case reports. Subsequent attention has focused on *depression*. (Schizophreniform psychosis has not been typically associated with pancreatic cancer.) It has been debated whether the pancreatic cancer and depression link is true correlation or medical folklore.[11,17,82,85,142,143]

◆ Two prospective studies[58,91] reported a robust association between a diagnosis of depression and subsequent discovery of pancreatic cancer.

◆ Holland and colleagues[84] studied a large cohort of patients with advanced pancreatic cancer (n = 107) matched to those with advanced gastric cancer (n = 111). Patient self-ratings of depression, tension-anxiety, fatigue, confusion-bewilderment, and total mood disturbance were significantly greater for the pancreatic cancer group, confirming that psychological disturbance occurs more frequently in pancreatic cancer than in other advanced abdominal neoplasms.

The mechanism for this association remains hypothetical.[84]

Acute Intermittent Porphyria

Acute intermittent porphyria is an inborn error of metabolism that leads to a defect in the biosynthesis of porphyrins. (There is a deficiency of the enzyme hydroxymethylbilane synthase.[33]) It is inherited as a dominant autosomal gene with incomplete penetrance, so that the disease often exists in latent form without a contributory family history. Most heterozygotes remain clinically asymptomatic unless exposed to factors that increase the production of porphyrins.[33]

Typical symptoms consist of acute abdominal pain, or pain in the limbs or back, often associated with nausea, vomiting, headache, and severe constipation.[33] Abdominal crises may resemble an acute abdomen and result in laparotomy. Seizures occur in approximately 20% of cases, and status epilepticus may develop.[104] A rapidly developing motor peripheral neuropathy may ensue, with weakness, numbness, paresthesias, or pain in the limbs. This may progress to paralysis with respiratory compromise, resembling acute inflammatory polyradiculopathy (Guillain-Barré syndrome).

Mental disorder accompanies the attacks in 25%–75% of cases,[104] and may dominate the picture.[131]

◆ *Delirium* is the most common neuropsychiatric presentation, with central nervous system (CNS) involvement and diffuse electroencephalogram (EEG) slowing occurring in the great majority of cases.[103]

◆ The patient may initially become acutely depressed, agitated, or violent. Marked emotional lability with histrionic behavior is common. Psychotic and paranoid symptoms may resemble schizophrenia, and the patient may be misdiagnosed as having a primary psychiatric condition. (There was also a recent report of obsessive-compulsive disorder in association with acute intermittent porphyria.[71])

◆ What starts as a nonspecific clouding of consciousness and confusion may progress rapidly to delirium, with hallucinations, delusions, and behavioral abnormalities, at times culminating abruptly in coma.

◆ Exacerbations may *correlate with the menstrual cycle* in some women, and latent porphyria may first express itself during or shortly after pregnancy[119]—factors that could easily be diagnostically misleading.

◆ The syndrome of inappropriate antidiuretic hormone (SIADH) may also be a consequence of acute intermittent porphyria and in itself may cause neuropsychiatric symptoms.[33]

Acute attacks may last from days to months, varying in frequency and severity. Symptoms may be *completely absent* in periods of remission. Episodes are precipitated by drugs oxidized by hemoproteins of the cytochrome P450 system, such as usual therapeutic doses of barbiturates, anticonvulsants, estrogens, contraceptives, or alcohol.[33,141] The diagnosis is made by detecting excess porphobilinogen in the urine[119] *during* the acute episode, because interepisode tests may be inconclusive.

The pattern of Ms. Mack's GI complaints is not consistent with porphyria. However, be sure to screen for this disorder in patients presenting with unexplained intermittent abdominal pain and psychiatric symptomatology, particularly in the emergency room setting. Haloperidol has been used safely.[84a]

B₁₂ (Cobalamin) Deficiency

There are many causes of B_{12} (cobalamin) deficiency, such as subtotal gastrectomy and atrophic gastritis. The most well-known etiology is pernicious anemia, which produces psychiatric symptoms and, occasionally, GI complaints, possibly including diarrhea and paroxysmal abdominal pain.[49] It is an acquired deficiency state, usually characterized by macrocytic anemia, megaloblastic hyperplasia of the bone marrow, gastric achlorhydria

and, frequently, subacute combined degeneration of the spinal cord.[49]

◆ In pernicious anemia, there is inadequate *intrinsic factor* secondary to gastric mucosal atrophy, leading to an inability to absorb vitamin B_{12} from the intestinal tract.[5] Pernicious anemia is currently thought to be caused by an autoimmune reaction against gastric parietal cells.[5]

The onset is usually insidious and is described as gradually increasing weakness, anorexia, soreness of the tongue, and a characteristic yellow pallor.[49] Men and women are equally affected, with the average patient presenting near age 60.[5]

The psychiatric symptoms accompanying cobalamin deficiency span the range of psychiatric pathology. *There is no prototypical psychiatric presentation;* rather, presentations range from mood disorders (depressive or manic) to schizophreniform and paranoid psychoses and dementia.[36,104] Psychiatric symptoms may **predate** and occur **independently** of neurological and hematological abnormalities.[8,104] The literature is filled with case reports of B_{12} deficiency presenting surreptitiously as primary psychiatric syndromes.[3,36,48,63,93,120,151–153,160,175] For example:

◆ We (A. A. Wyszynski and B. Wyszynski, unpublished report) successfully treated a 61-year-old man who had a subtotal gastrectomy 15 years before for bleeding ulcers. The patient had a history of IBS since his early 40s, and had always been "an anxious guy." A second psychiatric opinion was sought for "resistant depression and anxiety." The patient's anxiety and depression had been unresponsive to a series of treatments, including clonazepam (Klonopin) 4 mg/day, lorazepam (Ativan) 4 mg/day, imipramine (Tofranil; discontinued because of constipation), paroxetine (Paxil; trial stopped because of worsened GI distress), fluoxetine (Prozac; trial stopped because of worsened GI distress), and trazodone (Desyrel 350 mg/day; ineffective). Workup (endoscopy, barium swallow) for a persistent "queasy, anxious feeling" was negative for structural GI disease or cardiological illness. Blood work, including complete blood count (CBC) and thyroid function tests, was normal. Results of neurological examination by his family practitioner were reportedly normal. At the psychiatrist's request for a complete workup, thyroid function tests were repeated and a B_{12} level was drawn. A B_{12} level of 202 pg/ml was initially dismissed as "normal" (lower limit of normal 200 pg/ml), especially in light of the normal CBC. Repeat B_{12} was 200. The hematology consultant advised a Schilling test, which came back positive for pernicious anemia. The patient was started on intramuscular B_{12}, doxepin (Sinequan; 100 mg), and diazepam (Valium; 5 mg twice daily), with gradual resolution of the queasy feeling and the psychiatric symptoms. Serum B_{12} returned to within normal limits.

The neurological syndrome of cobalamin deficiency classically consists of symmetric paresthesias in the feet and fingers, with a positive Romberg's sign and associated disturbances of vibratory sense and proprioception,[8] due to vacuolation in the posterior columns.[1] Later there is corticospinal tract involvement, with spastic paresis and ataxia. This combined syndrome is called *subacute combined degeneration* of the spinal cord (i.e., degenerative changes of the dorsal and lateral columns).[1] Neurological symptoms will develop in 80%–95% of patients with untreated pernicious anemia.[49] Like the psychiatric symptoms, they may predate hematological abnormalities.[8]

Neuropsychiatric symptoms were formerly considered to be *late* manifestations of cobalamin deficiency. It was also thought that they always occurred in the setting of *anemia*. This notion was definitively challenged in 1988, however, when a large cohort of patients with neuropsychiatric abnormalities due to cobalamin deficiency was shown to have *no anemia or macrocytosis* (28%; n = 141).[102]

- In this study, serum cobalamin levels were only moderately lower than normal in 16 patients, and 2 were in the low-normal range.
- Serum methylmalonic acid and total homocysteine were markedly abnormal and aided in making the diagnosis.
- *Hallucinations or changes in personality and mood were the chief or only symptom in several cases.*
- Except for one patient who died during the first week of treatment, every patient in this group benefited clinically from cobalamin therapy.
- The authors concluded that neuropsychiatric disorders due to cobalamin deficiency commonly occur *in the* **absence** *of anemia or an elevated mean cell volume* (MCV).

Others have corroborated these findings in clinical case reports.[151] Note that there are etiologies for cobalamin deficiency other than pernicious anemia—for example, ileal or gastric resection. The Schilling test assesses the ability to absorb cobalamin. As recently reviewed,[8] a normal Schilling test does not definitively rule out co-

balamin deficiency,[7,18] but a positive Schilling clinches the diagnosis.

✦ IRRITABLE BOWEL SYNDROME

Definition

Alteration in bowel habits is the most consistent feature of IBS and is required to make the diagnosis according to most definitions.[75] Like Ms. Mack, patients may present with a confusing array of bowel symptoms, such as constipation, diarrhea, or constipation alternating with diarrhea. Those with diarrhea may experience fecal urgency during periods of stress; stools are characteristically loose and frequent but of normal total daily volume.[75] Patients with constipation may have a sense of incomplete fecal evacuation leading to repeated, uncomfortable attempts at stool passage. There are a number of pertinent negatives:

- Many patients report mucus in their stools, but this does not indicate structural or "inflammatory" bowel disease; that is, IBS patients have *histologically normal* colons, unlike patients with ulcerative colitis or Crohn's disease. Rather, IBS is a disorder of intestinal *motility*. (Inflammatory bowel disease, however, is also influenced by psychological factors.[43,46,60–62,126,136,149])

Symptoms that are *not* associated with IBS include the following:[75]

- Nocturnal diarrhea
- Rectal bleeding
- Malabsorption
- Weight loss
- Pain that is progressive in nature, prevents sleep, leads to anorexia or inability to eat, or is associated with systemic findings such as weight loss

Studies of pathogenesis and treatment have yielded ambiguous results because *no clear diagnostic markers for IBS exist.* In addition, symptoms may show wide variation among individuals and even within a given patient on different days.[75] Definitions of IBS have varied, but all include alterations in bowel habits with or without abdominal pain. The International Congress of Gastroenterology attempted to develop a standardized definition of IBS as follows:[37]

1. Abdominal pain relieved by defecation or associated with change in frequency or consistency of stool; and/or
2. Disturbed defecation involving two or more of the following:
   i. Altered stool frequency
   ii. Altered stool form (hard or loose and watery)
   iii. Altered stool passage (straining or urgency, feeling of incomplete evacuation)
   iv. Passage of mucus

Even this schema is controversial, however, given that others have proposed different definitions that are more or less restrictive in their criteria.[115,185]

Other Symptoms

IBS patients also have upper GI symptoms, such as heartburn and dysphagia, that are related to abnormal motility in other parts of the GI tract. Nonspecific symptoms that are also prevalent include fatigue, loss of concentration, insomnia, palpitations, back pain, pruritis, and an unpleasant taste in the mouth.[31,194]

Finally, IBS patients have a significantly greater incidence of sexual dysfunction compared with patients with inflammatory bowel disease or peptic ulcer (83% versus 30% and 16%, respectively).[70] The reasons for this association are unclear, but may be related to correlations that are emerging between the functional GI disorders, somatization, and childhood sexual or physical abuse.[38,39,145,177]

Epidemiology

Although there have been no genetic studies, IBS is more prevalent in first-degree relatives. Two studies found that two-thirds of the parents and half of the siblings of children with recurrent abdominal pain also described abdominal pain themselves.[129,159] However, this association may be the result of learning rather than genetics, since parental attention to bowel problems reinforces this somatic pattern.[107,191] Twin studies on the genetic influences in IBS are not available.

Onset is common during late adolescence to young adulthood, with a prevalence twice as high in females as in males.[51] Most patients are between 20 and 40 years old, and onset is rare after age 60.[54]

◆ Kay et al.[88] found that psychological vulnerability and the presence of stressful problems were strongly associated with the prevalence and incidence of IBS, whereas lifestyle factors showed only a weak or no relationship.

Pain

Irritable bowel pain can be quite variable in intensity and location, occurring in atypical abdominal areas as well as in extraabdominal sites,[121,164] even within the same patient on different days. It can be so severe that it interferes with daily activities, and patients often avoid situations where there is no bathroom readily available. Hasler and Owyang[75] have noted, however, that the pain of IBS rarely interferes with the patient's nutritional status or normal sleep pattern. The character of the pain is either crampy, or a generalized ache with superimposed periods of abdominal cramps. Sharp, dull, gaslike, or nondescript pains are also consistent with IBS.

The normal medical workup can be more of a frustration than a relief to IBS patients, who often infer that they are thought to be "imagining" or "giving themselves" symptoms. Frustrated family members, who often feel ruled by the patient's GI complaints, frequently support this formulation. Interpersonal and self-esteem issues arise, engendering more anxiety, which feeds back to the sensitized gut to produced more GI distress. Even though anxiety affects colonic function in everyone, the increased IBS colonic sensitivity cannot be explained solely by psychological factors or emotional states like anxiety.[95] It is helpful to educate patients that there are *objective* findings producing a *different*—albeit not diseased— physiology:

◆ A significantly lower pain threshold to bowel distention[22,188]

◆ Abnormal motility of both the colon[127] and the small intestine[26,97] (suggesting a sensitive gastrointestinal tract that overresponds to normal stimuli regulating bowel motor activity)[179]

◆ More frequent preprandial and postprandial high-amplitude, prolonged colonic contractions compared with symptom-free control subjects[174]

◆ A higher proportion of "slow" (3 cycles/minute) contractions in the distal colon compared with symptom-free control subjects[155,156,161,168] (These findings appear unrelated to bowel habits or diet, and persist *despite* symptom remission.[167] They are also present in healthy individuals without IBS, but to a much lesser extent.)

◆ More frequent slow contractions under certain conditions, such as following infusions of cholecystokinin and pentagastrin,[156] food ingestion,[161] or balloon distention of the colon[188]

◆ A close parallel between the GI pain and slow-frequency contractions in patients with primarily meal-associated bowel symptoms[74]

◆ Decreased esophageal sphincter pressure as well as other abnormalities of esophageal motility[192]

◆ Abnormal fasting and residual gallbladder volumes[16]

◆ Abnormal bladder function on urodynamic studies[193] (with symptoms of genitourinary dysfunction, including a high incidence of dysmenorrhea, dyspareunia, impotence, urinary frequency, urgency nocturia, and a sensation of incomplete bladder emptying)[23]

◆ In both IBS patients and healthy individuals, a significant increase in baseline colonic motor and spike potential activity with experimentally induced anger[182]

◆ Emotionally charged topics increase colonic pressure and motility in everyone, but *baseline* colonic pressure is higher in people with IBS[89]

Walker et al.[179] believe that these physiological traits confer vulnerability to irritable bowel symptoms when appropriate input occurs from the CNS. Whorwell et al.[192] have speculated that the syndrome may be a widespread disorder of smooth muscle or its innervation.

✦ THE GUT, STRESS, AND EMOTIONS

Psychological stress clearly worsens irritable bowel symptoms.[19,23,44,45,79]

◆ Fifty-one percent of IBS patients have cited a stressful event preceding the onset of their GI condition.[79]

◆ Stress occurring within a 3-month period has been significantly correlated with bowel symptoms in the subsequent 3-month period.[187]

◆ Psychological stress significantly correlates with the number of disability days and medical clinic visits for bowel symptoms.[187]

◆ IBS patients are hypervigilant and more reactive to stress paradigms than are control subjects,[55] but these findings are not unanimous.[133]

◆ Results about IBS and the *number* of stressful life events is conflicting, with some studies finding more,[50,118] others showing less,[42] and still others reporting no relationship between stressful life events and an IBS diagnosis.[55]

In trying to integrate these findings, Crowell and colleagues[32] acknowledged that stress influences the course and possibly the onset of IBS. They cautioned, however, about retrospective attribution (i.e., subjects may explain their physical symptoms by attributing them to psycho-

logical stress). This would artifactually inflate estimates of the IBS-stress link.

Walker and colleagues[179] pointed out that a large percentage of IBS patients have previous diagnoses of anxiety disorder, similar to patients with atypical chest pain. These authors (and others[2]) hypothesize that autonomic dysregulation might produce parallel disorders of anxiety and abnormal motility, resulting in a self-reinforcing cycle of reciprocally worsening anxiety and gut dysfunction. Direct neural and indirect chemical modulation probably mediate GI function in the setting of emotional distress.[64] There is evidence of central alpha-adrenergic receptor dysfunction in IBS,[35] and there are investigations into the role of the locus coeruleus.[163] Lydiard et al.[110] have summarized,

Emerging evidence suggests significant interplay between the brain and the gastrointestinal system. The enteric nervous system, which has been called the "third division" of the autonomic nervous system, resembles the central nervous system in many ways . . . One important link between [them] may be at the level of a pontine noradrenergic nucleus, the locus ceruleus, which has been postulated to mediate some aspects of fear and arousal states, including panic disorder. This nucleus receives afferent input from the gut such that perturbation of the bladder, bowel, or stomach may cause increased neuronal firing of this noradrenergic nucleus. Patients with IBS or certain psychiatric conditions such as anxiety or depression also often complain of numerous autonomic symptoms, suggesting that there may be some common pathophysiology, perhaps in part at the level of this noradrenergic nucleus. (p. 233)

Many neurotransmitters and CNS peptides share behavioral and bowel activity,[94,99,157,199] although the mediator of the brain-bowel link still remains speculative.[179]

Psychiatric Comorbidity: Chicken or Egg?

Unlike IBS, inflammatory bowel conditions like Crohn's disease and ulcerative colitis often require stressful treatments, such as multiple surgeries, colostomy, chronic steroids, and hyperalimentation.[41,179] Although these conditions also respond adversely to psychological stress, *the reported prevalence of psychiatric comorbidity for IBS is far greater than for either of them,*[150] *with estimates ranging from 70% to 90%,*[40,55,100,105,173,180,183,202] including recent estimates.[110]

◆ Structured psychiatric interviews and psychological self-report measures were administered to 28 patients with IBS and to 19 patients with inflammatory bowel disease.[180] Significantly more of the patients with IBS had lifetime diagnoses of major depression, somatization disorder, generalized anxiety disorder, panic disorder, and phobic disorder. In addition, the IBS patients had significantly more medically unexplained somatic symptoms, and most had suffered from psychiatric disorders, particularly anxiety disorder, before the onset of their irritable bowel symptoms.

◆ A comparison study showed that 83% of IBS patients experienced impaired sexual function, compared with only 30% of inflammatory bowel disease patients and 16% of peptic ulcer patients.[70]

◆ Robust correlations have been found between IBS and severity of anxiety and/or depression.[14,115a,171]

◆ Numerous studies have found high self-ratings of anxiety.[12,47,130,138]

◆ These patients are more depressed on numerous rating scales, including the Minnesota Multiphasic Personality Inventory (MMPI),[188] the States of Anxiety and Depression scales,[4] and the Zung Depression Scale.[76]

◆ IBS patients experience symptoms of autonomic arousal resembling those occurring in mood and anxiety disorders.[179] Weakness, fatigue, palpitations, nervousness, dizziness, headache, tremor, back pain, sleep disturbance, and sexual dysfunction show a high concordance with IBS symptoms.

◆ Several authors have noted a substantial overlap with panic disorder.[108,109,111,112,128,200] Resolution of coexisting panic symptoms often results in dramatic relief of irritable bowel symptoms.

Psychopathology and the Gut

Although psychiatric comorbidity has been well established over many years of research,[23,28,42,47,100,105,130,169,185,202] the mechanism for this association remains controversial. There are few data to support IBS as a *precursor* to psychiatric illness.[171,179] On the other hand, psychiatric symptomatology often *predates* IBS.[55,105,202] These patients report a higher prevalence of

◆ Childhood parental loss[78,80,107]

◆ Childhood sexual or physical abuse[38,39,145,177]

◆ Childhood history of frequent doctor's visits, pain syndromes, losses or separations, school absenteeism, and poorer general health[14]

(Defective reality testing and psychosis are *not* components of IBS.)

One hypothesis is that *illness behavior* (a pattern of multiple somatic complaints and overutilization of health care services[191]) is learned during childhood as a result of parental attitudes toward bodily symptoms. Whitehead and colleagues[191] conducted a telephone survey in which they interviewed randomly selected subjects about their gastrointestinal and other symptoms. A subgroup with a probable diagnosis of "functional bowel disorder" was identified:

◆ Compared with control subjects, these subjects endorsed significantly more items about parental rewards (toys, gifts, special foods) during childhood colds or flu. (These findings were replicated in structured interviews of other IBS patients concerning their childhood illness experiences.[107])

◆ They were significantly more likely to report two or more acute physical illnesses and/or colds during the past year, felt that their colds were "more serious" than those of most other people, and were more likely to consult a doctor rather than to treat the cold or flu themselves.[191]

◆ These subjects were also twice as likely as control subjects to have been hospitalized medically.[191]

Psychiatric symptomatology is quite prevalent in this group of patients:

◆ Kumar and colleagues[96] found a predominance of anxiety (but not depression) in these patients compared with healthy control subjects.

◆ Fowlie et al.[56,57] concluded that whereas anxiety may be more important than depression in maintaining the IBS symptom complex, depression may be more important in influencing perceived distress and illness behavior in response to adverse life events. A depressive emotional state also influences the response to medical treatment.[57]

◆ Walker and colleagues[179] have pointed out that their finding of a 61% lifetime prevalence of depression for IBS patients is similar to the 60%–70% lifetime depression rates found in previous studies of chronic pelvic pain,[106] atypical chest pain, chronic fatigue syndrome, tinnitus, and low back pain—all conditions associated with chronic distress.

◆ Tollefson et al.[172] found that IBS was significantly more common in a sample of ambulatory psychiatric clinic patients with generalized anxiety and major depression than in matched control subjects.

"Irritable Bowel Personality"?

Although Ms. Mack shows certain traits of obsessive-compulsive personality disorder, there is no personality profile *unique* to IBS.[29,47,78,100,132,185,188,198] The MMPI "psychosomatic triad" of hysteria, hypochondriasis, and depression described in IBS also occurs in other medical disorders, such as chronic pain syndromes, and is not unique to IBS.[29,100,105,140,186,189,202]

When reading the psychosomatic literature, think critically about the appropriateness of the test instruments. Tests like the MMPI can yield spurious results; chronically ill individuals are more likely to endorse disease-related items because these items *realistically* concern their physical health, but their endorsements of such items are scored as indicating depression and hypochondriasis.[29] Instruments such as the Diagnostic Interview Schedule[139a] and the Present State Examination[196a] seem to be more useful in patients with "functional" bowel symptoms, such as those of IBS[55,173] or "functional" abdominal pain.[25,27,90,116]

Method or "Madness"?

Many investigators are skeptical about the extremely high association of IBS with psychopathology; they are suspicious that poor methodology might account for the results:

◆ **Sample bias:** Psychosocial factors determine *treatment-seeking behavior*,[42,154,185] creating a self-selected population who comes to medical attention and enters the researched world of "patienthood." The high concurrence of IBS symptoms and psychopathology may be the result of sample bias,[166] reflecting characteristics of those who seek out medical care rather than representing the natural history of IBS. Fifteen percent to 20% of the general population have symptoms consistent with IBS, but only 5% go to physicians.[59] Notably, this "nonpatient" subgroup has *no greater prevalence of psychological distress than do symptom-free control subjects.*[185]

◆ **Sample heterogeneity; inclusion criteria:** Subjects reporting "abdominal pain" and "altered bowel habits" *in the absence of any other evidence for IBS* have been included in many study samples.[186] This procedure easily includes patients with somatization disor-

der, thereby confounding an already heterogeneous and vaguely defined population. A potentially inflated psychopathology-IBS association results. For example, Whitehead and co-workers[185] demonstrated that the vague complaint of abdominal pain was significantly correlated with neuroticism on the Hopkins Symptom Checklist.[32a] However, when the pain complaint was made more specific (i.e., pain relieved by defecation and associated with changes in stool frequency or consistency), the correlation with neuroticism disappeared. Future research should use more restrictive diagnostic criteria.

◆ **Clinic contaminants:** Prevalence data based on clinic populations are notoriously spurious when extrapolated to the general community. Attendance at clinics is determined by a complex interaction of personal, social, economic, and cultural factors that can skew the data derived from them. For example, the view that menopause was deleterious to mental health was based on studies using clinic subjects. These data were not substantiated when general population surveys superseded them (see Chapter 9). IBS clinic attendees may be a distinct subgroup of the population suffering irritable bowel symptoms. They may have *premorbid* psychological characteristics that influence their choice of medical venue as well as their processing of physiological cues.[180]

Conclusions

The causal relationship between IBS and psychiatric morbidity remains poorly understood. It appears that the two conditions are reciprocal, not that one clearly precipitates the other.[178] Despite the controversies, one unambiguous conclusion is that individuals with IBS who seek medical attention are in significant distress and may benefit from psychiatric intervention.

> The irritable bowel syndrome remains a clinical conundrum. It is a syndrome that lacks a clear definition or established pathophysiology. There are no known clinical tests that will confirm or refute the diagnosis with certainty, and there is no specific therapy for the condition . . . Given the lack of evidence of organic dysfunction, the idea that it is primarily a psychopathological condition has continued to be attractive . . . [but] there is also a further possibility . . . that the "psychopathological" aspects of IBS have been overemphasized in the past. This might arise from

flaws in the design of psychometric studies in IBS. Comparison of IBS sufferers with healthy control subjects might be expected to reveal differences but these differences may relate more closely to the differences between the well and the unwell rather than to intrinsic psychopathology.[96] (p. 80)

⚛ TREATMENT

Medications

No one drug is consistently effective in treating IBS. Treatment approaches have included bulking agents, diets, antispasmodics, psychotropics, and various psychotherapies. Klein's[92] 1988 critique of 43 placebo-controlled, double-blind studies emphasized that specific entrance criteria (used to define the psychiatric and/or GI syndromes) were missing in approximately 60% of the trials, as were objective markers of clinical IBS improvement. Inadequate sample size (< 30 subjects were used in at least one-third of the trials) and duration of treatment (several days or weeks) were additional limitations.

Given these caveats, a few observations are worth noting:

◆ Placebo response estimates in the IBS literature are variable but high, ranging from 20% to 70%.[81,171,190]

◆ A diagnosable Axis I psychiatric disorder predicted significantly less likelihood of medical improvement in response to cognitive and behavioral treatments.[13]

◆ Controlled studies of tricyclics[66,76,98,122,123,158] suggest that they relieve selected irritable bowel symptoms, such as diarrhea and pain, but not (expectably) constipation. Investigators have shown the effectiveness of medications such as amitriptyline (Elavil),[79] trimipramine (Surmontil),[124] and desipramine (Norpramin),[67,76] but there is no evidence that one tricyclic antidepressant is better than another. The doses required seem to be substantially lower than those for depression.[89] It is unclear whether the tricyclics' benefits are due to their antidepressant or anticholinergic activity.

◆ Anxiolytic medications have been associated with improvement of gastrointestinal symptoms in most studies.[6,21,30,34,52,87,117,135,139,148,181] The bulk of the research has examined alprazolam (Xanax),[112,128,171] lorazepam (Ativan),[112,128] and diazepam (Valium).[128] (Note that remission of panic disorder with anxiolytic treatment also significantly relieved irritable bowel symptoms.[112,128])

The clinical course of IBS is characteristically intermittent, so it may be possible to use anxiolytics temporarily to improve situational anxiety, and thus avoid the risks of habituation or addiction.[59]

Psychological Treatments

Most psychotherapy techniques have been shown to relieve the symptoms of IBS. Several controlled studies have demonstrated psychotherapy's efficacy, even when administered over relatively *brief* periods of time.[73,162,196] There may be a particular profile of psychotherapy-responsive IBS patients, but data are still quite limited.

◆ One sample received standard antispasmodic therapy either with or without dynamic psychotherapy.[69] Those who demonstrated a superior outcome to the combined approach had overt psychiatric symptoms, intermittent pain exacerbated by stress, and GI histories characterized by diarrhea.

It is not possible to recommend one therapy over another, since controlled studies have shown clinical improvement with just about all of them, including short-term, dynamically oriented individual psychotherapy,[69,162] supportive psychotherapy,[196] cognitive therapy,[68,125] relaxation techniques,[10,125,176,184] and hypnotherapy.[20,73,195,196] As with medications, there also appears to be a significant placebo effect for some patients. For example,

◆ Blanchard and co-workers[15] compared a multicomponent treatment for IBS (relaxation, thermal biofeedback, and cognitive therapy) with a placebo intervention (pseudo-meditation and EEG alpha-suppression biofeedback). They found no significant difference between the two interventions, but notable relief of GI symptoms, anxiety, and depression for both groups.

Impressively, psychological treatments *alone* (combining stress management training, education, cognitive therapy, and relaxation) can be comparable in efficacy to medical treatment with drug therapy:[9]

◆ A group of 33 patients with IBS who had not previously responded to reassurance and simple symptomatic medical treatment were randomly assigned to either medical or psychological intervention for 8 weeks.[9] Both groups experienced comparable symptomatic improvement, with those who received the psychological treatments having the added advantage of lessened anxiety.

Comment. Although it is tempting to conclude that psychological treatments have their impact on the psycho-gastrointestinal interface, the same methodological caveats also apply to this segment of the IBS literature.[186] In addition to falling prey to selection bias, none of these studies used restrictive diagnostic inclusion criteria to select patients. Vague diagnostic criteria skewed toward the tendency to somatize may select patients responsive to psychological intervention. The literature is promising, but requires methodological tightening before specific conclusions can be drawn.

SUMMARY AND RECOMMENDATIONS

What practical advice is the clinician to abstract from this ambiguous literature? Walker et al.[179] have written,

Although not all patients with irritable bowel syndrome have psychiatric comorbidity, psychiatric referral may be beneficial in the clinical management of many patients. The psychiatrist may be of assistance by *reframing irritable bowel syndrome as a biological vulnerability that worsens with psychological distress, providing proper diagnosis and treatment of coexisting psychiatric disease and maladaptive illness behaviors, and developing a multimodal treatment plan including psychotherapeutic and pharmacological management* . . . Therapeutic goals should be restricted to symptom reduction rather than cure, since many gastrointestinal symptoms may persist after resolution of the concurrent psychiatric disorder. (pp. 569–570, italics added)

We could not improve on the summary of Whitehead and Crowell,[186] who have recommended the following:

1. An internist may be the most acceptable care provider for patients with IBS who believe that they are physically ill and insist on medical care. They may accept advice more readily from an internist than from a mental health professional.
2. Somatization may be most effectively dealt with by an internist who provides sympathetic attention, educates the patient about the normal range of bowel physiology, and sets firm limits on the frequency of contact and use of invasive treatments.

3. Referral to a psychiatrist or mental health professional is most readily accepted if the internist has already established good rapport with the patient.
4. The patient must be educated to understand that IBS is a disorder of intestinal motility that is chronic, recurrent, and influenced by factors such as stress, food, and drugs. Framing IBS in this way helps the patient to accept recurrences as part of the condition itself, rather than indicating inappropriate diagnosis or inadequate treatment.
5. Fears of alternative diagnoses (e.g., cancer) should be reviewed with the patient as they come up, with explanations about why such options were rejected.
6. Scheduling return appointments offers the reassurance of the physician's continued interest, avoids a sense of abandonment, provides support, and promotes the treatment program.
7. Psychologically oriented treatments have a role in managing IBS. A variety of psychological interventions may produce significant reductions in bowel symptoms and also relieve psychological symptoms. Treatments studied to date emphasize developing coping skills in response to here-and-now stress.
8. Tricyclic antidepressants may be tried as a first-line treatment. They are superior to placebo for managing abdominal pain and diarrhea, but not constipation. It is unclear whether their benefits are due to antidepressant or anticholinergic activity. We await data on the selective serotonin reuptake inhibitors.

Other helpful reviews can be found in the papers by Drossman and co-workers.[19,45]

REFERENCES

1. Adams R, Victor M: Principles of Neurology, 4th Edition. New York, McGraw-Hill Information Services Company, 1989
2. Aggarwal A, Cutts T, Abell T, et al: Predominant symptoms in irritable bowel syndrome correlate with specific autonomic nervous system abnormalities. Gastroenterology 106:945–950, 1994
3. Ambrosino S: Neuropsychiatric aspects of pernicious anemia: report of a case. Psychosomatics 6:24–28, 1966
4. Arapakis G, Lyketsos C, Gerolymatos K, et al: Low dominance and high intropunitiveness in ulcerative colitis and irritable bowel syndrome. Psychother Psychosom 46:171–176, 1986
5. Babior B, Bunn H: Megaloblastic anemias, in Harrison's Principles of Internal Medicine, 12th Edition. Edited by Wilson J, Braunwald E, Isselbacher K, et al. New York, McGraw-Hill, Health Professions Division, 1991, pp 1523–1529

6. Baume P, Cuthbert J: The effect of medazepam in relieving symptoms of functional gastrointestinal distress. Aust N Z J Med 3:457–460, 1973

7. Beck W: The assay of serum cobalamin by Lactobacillus leichmannii and the interpretation of serum cobalamin levels. Methods in Hematology 10:31–50, 1983

8. Beck W: Neuropsychiatric consequences of cobalamin deficiency. Adv Intern Med 36:33–56, 1991

9. Bennett P, Wilkinson S: A comparison of psychological and medical treatment of the irritable bowel syndrome. Br J Clin Psychol 24:215–216, 1985

10. Berndt H, Maercker W: Psychotherapy of irritable colon. Z Gesamte Inn Med 40:107–110, 1985

11. Birnbaum D, Kleesberg J: Carcinoma of the pancreas: a clinical study based on 84 cases. Ann Intern Med 48:1171–1184, 1958

12. Blanchard E, Radnitz C, Evans D, et al: Psychological comparisons of irritable bowel syndrome to chronic tension and migraine headache and nonpatient controls. Biofeedback Self Regul 11:221–230, 1986

13. Blanchard E, Scharff L, Payne A, et al: Prediction of outcome from cognitive-behavioral treatment of irritable bowel syndrome. Behav Res Ther 30:647–650, 1992

14. Blanchard E, Scharff L, Schwarz S, et al: The role of anxiety and depression in the irritable bowel syndrome. Behav Res Ther 28:401–405, 1990

15. Blanchard E, Schwarz S, Suls J, et al: Two controlled evaluations of multicomponent psychological treatment of irritable bowel syndrome. Behav Res Ther 30:175–189, 1992

16. Braverman D: Gallbladder contraction in patients with irritable bowel syndrome. Isr J Med Sci 23:181–184, 1987

17. Brown J, Paraskevas F: Cancer and depression: cancer presenting with depressive illness: an autoimmune disease? Br J Psychiatry 141:227–232, 1982

18. Carmel R, Sinow R, Siegel M, et al: Food cobalamin malabsorption occurs frequently in patients with unexplained low serum cobalamin levels. Arch Intern Med 148:1715–1719, 1988

19. Cassileth B, Drossman D: Psychosocial factors in gastrointestinal illness. Psychother Psychosom 59:131–143, 1993

20. Chantler L, Edwards C: The treatment of irritable bowel syndrome using hypnosis. Australian Journal of Clinical and Experimental Hypnosis 20:39–47, 1992

21. Chaplan A, Vanov S: GI illness: treatment of the anxiety component. Psychosomatics 18:49–54, 1977

22. Chasen R, Tucker H, Palmer D, et al: Colonic motility in irritable bowel syndrome and diverticular disease (abstract). Gastroenterology 82:1031, 1982

23. Chaudhary N, Truelove S: The irritable colon syndrome: a study of the clinical features, predisposing causes, and prognosis in 130 cases. Q J Med 31:307–322, 1962

24. Clouse R: Psychiatric interactions with the esophagus. Psychiatric Annals 22:598–605, 1992

24a. Clouse R, Lustman P, Geisman R, et al: Antidepressant therapy in 138 patients with irritable bowel syndrome: a five-year clinical experience. Aliment Pharmacol Ther 8:409–416, 1994

25. Colgan S, Creed F, Klass S: Psychiatric disorder and abnormal illness behaviour in patients with upper abdominal pain. Psychol Med 18:887–892, 1988

26. Corbett C, Read T, Read N, et al: Electrochemical detector for breath hydrogen determination: measurement of small bowel transit time in normal subjects and patients with the irritable bowel syndrome. Gut 22:836–840, 1981

27. Craig T, Brown G: Goal frustrating aspects of life event stress in the aetiology of gastrointestinal disorder. J Psychosom Res 28:411–421, 1984

27a. Creed F: Irritable bowel or irritable mind? psychological treatment is essential for some. BMJ 309:1647–1648, 1994

28. Creed F, Guthrie E: Psychological factors in the irritable bowel syndrome. Gut 28:1307–1318, 1987

29. Creed F, Guthrie E: Relation among personality and symptoms in nonulcer dyspepsia and the irritable bowel syndrome (letter). Gastroenterology 100:1154–1155, 1991

30. Cromwell H: Double-blind study of a psychotropic-anticholinergic drug in gastric disorders. Medical Times 96:933–938, 1968

31. Crouch M: Irritable bowel syndrome: toward a biopsychosocial systems understanding. Prim Care 15:99–110, 1988

32. Crowell M, Whitehead W, Heller B, et al: Prospective evaluation of stressful life events on bowel symptoms in a large community sample (abstract). Gastroenterology 98:A341, 1990

32a. Derogatis L, Lipman R, Rickels K, et al: The Hopkins Symptom Checklist (HSCL): a self-report symptom inventory. Behav Sci 19:1–15, 1974

33. Desnick R: The porphyrias, in Harrison's Principles of Internal Medicine, 13th Edition. Edited by Isselbacher K, Braunwald E, Wilson J, et al. New York, McGraw-Hill, Health Professions Division, 1994, pp 2073–2079

34. Deutsch E: Relief of anxiety and related emotions in patients with gastrointestinal disorder. Dig Dis 16:1091–1095, 1971

35. Dinan T, Barry S, Ahkion S, et al: Assessment of central noradrenergic functioning in irritable bowel syndrome using a neuroendocrine challenge test. J Psychosom Res 34:575–580, 1990

36. Dommisse J: Subtle vitamin B12 deficiency and psychiatry: a largely unnoticed but devastating relationship? (review). Med Hypotheses 34:131–140, 1991

37. Drossman D: Irritable bowel syndrome. Am Fam Physician 39:159–164, 1989

38. Drossman D: Sexual and physical abuse and GI disorders in women: what is the link? Emerg Med Clin North Am 24:171–175, 1992

38a. Drossman D: The Functional Gastrointestinal Disorders: Diagnosis, Pathophysiology, and Treatment. Boston, MA, Little, Brown, 1994

39. Drossman D, Leserman J, Nachman G, et al: Sexual and physical abuse in women with functional or organic gastrointestinal disorders. Ann Intern Med 113:828–833, 1990

40. Drossman D, Li Z, Andruzzi E, et al: U.S. householder survey of functional gastrointestinal disorders: prevalence, sociodemography, and health impact. Dig Dis Sci 38:1569–1580, 1993

41. Drossman D, Li Z, Leserman J, et al: Ulcerative colitis and Crohn's disease health status scales for research and clinical practice. J Clin Gastroenterol 15:104–112, 1992

42. Drossman D, McKee D, Sandler R, et al: Psychosocial factors in the irritable bowel syndrome: a multivariate analysis of patients and nonpatients with irritable bowel syndrome. Gastroenterology 95:701–708, 1988

43. Drossman D, Patrick D, Mitchell C, et al: Health-related quality of life in inflammatory bowel disease. Dig Dis Sci 34:1379–1386, 1989

44. Drossman D, Sandler R, McKee D, et al: Bowel patterns among subjects not seeking health care. Gastroenterology 83:529–534, 1982

45. Drossman D, Thompson W: The irritable bowel syndrome: review and a graduated multicomponent treatment approach. Ann Intern Med 116:1009–1016, 1992

46. Duffy L, Zielezny M, Marshall J, et al: Relevance of major stress events as an indicator of disease activity prevalence in inflammatory bowel disease. Behav Med 17:101–110, 1991

47. Esler M, Goulston K: Levels of anxiety in colonic disorders. N Engl J Med 288:16–20, 1973

48. Evans D, Edelsohn G, Golden R: Organic psychosis without anemia or spinal cord symptoms in patients with vitamin B_{12} deficiency. Am J Psychiatry 140:218–221, 1983

49. Farmer T: Neurologic complications of vitamin and mineral disorders, in Clinical Neurology, Vol 4. Edited by Joynt R. Philadelphia, PA, JB Lippincott, 1991, pp 1–34

50. Fava G, Pavan L: Large bowel disorders, I: illness configuration and life events. Psychother Psychosom 27:93–99, 1976/1977

51. Fielding J: A year in outpatients with the irritable bowel syndrome. Ir J Med Sci 146:162–166, 1977

52. Fisher J: The treatment of functional and emotional symptoms in patients with gastrointestinal disorder. Current Therapeutic Research 11:247–251, 1969

53. Folks D, Kinney F: The role of psychological factors in gastrointestinal conditions: a review pertinent to DSM-IV. Psychosomatics 33:257–270, 1992

53a. Folks D, Kinney F: Gastrointestinal conditions, in Psychological Factors Affecting Medical Conditions. Edited by Stoudemire A. Washington, DC, American Psychiatric Press, 1995, pp 99–122

54. Ford M: Invited review: the irritable bowel syndrome. J Psychosom Res 30:399–410, 1986

55. Ford M, Miller P, Eastwood J, et al: Life events, psychiatric illness and irritable bowel syndrome. Gut 28:160–165, 1987

56. Fowlie S, Eastwood M, Ford M: Irritable bowel syndrome: the influence of psychological factors on the symptom complex. J Psychosom Res 36:169–173, 1992

57. Fowlie S, Eastwood M, Prescott R: Irritable bowel syndrome: assessment of psychological disturbances and its influence on the response to fibre supplementation. J Psychosom Res 36:175–180, 1992

58. Fras I, Litin E, Pearson J: Comparison of psychiatric symptoms in carcinoma of the pancreas with those in some other intraabdominal neoplasms. Am J Psychiatry 123:1553–1562, 1967

59. Friedman G: Treatment of the irritable bowel syndrome. Gastroenterol Clin North Am 20:325–333, 1991

60. Fuller R, Gordis E: Refining the treatment of alcohol withdrawal. JAMA 272:557–558, 1994

61. Garrett J, Drossman D: Health status in inflammatory bowel disease. Gastroenterology 99:90–104, 1990

62. Gilligan I, Fung L, Piper D, et al: Life event stress and chronic difficulties in duodenal ulcer: a case-control study. J Psychosom Res 31:117–123, 1987

63. Goggans F: A case of mania secondary to vitamin B_{12} deficiency. Am J Psychiatry 141:300–301, 1984

63a. Gorard D, Libby G, Farthing M: Effect of a tricyclic antidepressant on small intestinal motility in health and diarrhea-predominant irritable bowel syndrome. Dig Dis Sci 40:86–95, 1995

64. Gorman J, Liebowitz M, Fyer A, et al: A neuroanatomical hypothesis for panic disorder. Am J Psychiatry 146:148–161, 1989

65. Green A, Austin C: Psychopathology of pancreatic cancer: a psychobiologic probe. Psychosomatics 34:208–221, 1993

66. Greenbaum D: Preliminary report on antidepressant treatment of irritable bowel syndrome: comments on comparison with anxiolytic therapy. Psychopharmacol Bull 20:622–628, 1984

67. Greenbaum D, Mayle J, Vanegeren L, et al: Effects of desipramine on irritable bowel syndrome compared with atropine and placebo. Dig Dis Sci 32:257–266, 1987

68. Greene B, Blanchard E: Cognitive therapy for irritable bowel syndrome. J Consult Clin Psychol 62:576–582, 1994

69. Guthrie E, Creed F, Dawson D, et al: A controlled trial of psychological treatment for the irritable bowel syndrome. Gastroenterology 100:450–457, 1991

70. Guthrie E, Creed F, Whorwell P: Severe sexual dysfunction in women with the irritable bowel syndrome: comparison with inflammatory bowel disease and duodenal ulceration. BMJ 295:577–578, 1987

71. Hamner M: Obsessive-compulsive symptoms associated with acute intermittent porphyria. Psychosomatics 33:329–331, 1992

72. Harper R, Kane F, Stroehlein J: Age, affective distress, and illness detection in patients evaluated for gastrointestinal complaints. Psychosomatics 35:125–131, 1994

73. Harvey R, Hinton R, Gunary R, et al: Individual and group hypnotherapy in treatment of refractory irritable bowel syndrome. Lancet 1:424–425, 1989

74. Harvey R, Read A: Effect of cholecystokinin on colonic motility and symptoms in patients with the irritable bowel syndrome. Lancet 1:1–3, 1973

75. Hasler W, Owyang C: Irritable bowel syndrome, in Textbook of Gastroenterology. Edited by Yamada T, Alpers D, Owyang C, et al. Philadelphia, PA, JB Lippincott, 1991, pp 1696–1714

76. Heefner J, Wilder R, Wilson I: Irritable colon and depression. Psychosomatics 19:540–547, 1978

77. Herman R, Cooperman A: Current concepts in cancer of the pancreas. N Engl J Med 301:482–485, 1979

78. Hill O, Blendis L: Physical and psychological evaluation of "nonorganic" abdominal pain. Gut 8:221–229, 1967

79. Hislop I: Psychological significance of the irritable colon syndrome. Gut 12:452–457, 1971

80. Hislop I: Childhood deprivation: an antecedent of the irritable bowel syndrome. Med J Aust 1:372–374, 1979

81. Holdsworth C: Drug treatment of irritable bowel syndrome, in Irritable Bowel Syndrome. Edited by Read N. New York, Grune & Stratton, 1985, pp 223–232

82. Holland J: Psychological aspects of cancer, in Cancer Medicine, 2nd Edition. Edited by Holland J, Frei E III. Philadelphia, PA, Lea & Febiger, 1982, pp 1175–1203

83. Holland J: Gastrointestinal cancer, in Handbook of Psychooncology. Edited by Holland J, Rowland J. New York, Oxford University Press, 1990, pp 208–217

84. Holland J, Hughes A, Tross S, et al: Comparative psychological disturbance in patients with pancreatic and gastric cancer. Am J Psychiatry 143:982–986, 1986

84a. Ibrahim Z, Carney M: Safe use of haloperidol in acute intermittent porphyria (letter). Ann Pharmacother 29:200, 1995

85. Jacobsen L, Ottoson J: Initial mental disorder in carcinoma of the pancreas and stomach. Acta Psychiatr Scand 220:120–127, 1971

86. Karlinger W: Psychiatric manifestations of cancer of the pancreas. N Engl J Med 56:2251–2252, 1967

87. Kasich A, Fein H, Miller J: Comparative effect of phenaglycodol, meprobamate, and a placebo on the irritable colon. American Journal of Digestive Diseases 4:229–234, 1959

88. Kay L, Jorgensen T, Jensen KH: The epidemiology of irritable bowel syndrome in a random population: prevalence, incidence, natural history and risk factors. J Intern Med 236:23–30, 1994

89. Kellner R: Psychosomatic Syndromes and Somatic Symptoms. Washington, DC, American Psychiatric Press, 1991

90. Kingham J, Dawson A: Origin of chronic right upper quadrant pain. Gut 26:783–788, 1985

91. Klatchko B, Gorzynski J: A prospective controlled study of depression in patients with pancreatic and other intra-abdominal malignancies. Paper presented at the annual meeting of the American Psychosomatic Society, Denver, CO, March 1982

92. Klein K: Controlled treatment trials in the irritable bowel syndrome: a critique. Gastroenterology 95:232–241, 1988

93. Ko S, Liu T: Psychiatric syndromes in pernicious anemia—a case report. Singapore Med J 33:92–94, 1992

94. Krantis A, Harding R: GABA-related action in isolated in vitro preparations of the rat small intestine. Eur J Pharmacol 141:291–298, 1987

95. Kullman G, Fielding J: Rectal distensibility in the irritable bowel syndrome. Ir Med J 74:140–142, 1981

96. Kumar D, Pfeffer J, Wingate D: Role of psychological factors in the irritable bowel syndrome. Digestion 45:80–87, 1990

97. Kumar D, Wingate D: The irritable bowel syndrome: a paroxysmal motor disorder. Lancet 2:973–977, 1985

98. Lancaster-Smith M, Prout B, Pinto T, et al: Influence of drug treatment on the irritable bowel syndrome and its interaction with psychoneurotic morbidity. Acta Psychiatr Scand 66:33–41, 1982

99. Lanfranchi G, Bazzochi G, Fois F, et al: Effect of domperidone and dopamine on colonic motor activity in patients with the irritable bowel syndrome. Eur J Clin Pharmacol 29:307–310, 1985

100. Latimer P, Sarna S, Campbell D, et al: Colonic motor and myoelectrical activity: a comparative study of normal subjects, psychoneurotic patients and patients with irritable bowel syndrome. Gastroenterology 80:893–901, 1981

101. Latter K, Wilbur D: Psychic and neurological manifestations of carcinoma of the pancreas. Proceedings of the Mayo Clinic 12:457–462, 1937

102. Lindenbaum J, Healton E, Savage D, et al: Neuropsychiatric disorders caused by cobalamin deficiency in the absence of anemia or macrocytosis. N Engl J Med 318:1720–1728, 1988

103. Lipowski Z: Delirium: Acute Confusional States. New York, Oxford University Press, 1990

104. Lishman W: Organic Psychiatry, 2nd Edition. London, Blackwell Scientific, 1987

105. Liss J, Alpers D, Woodruff R: The irritable colon syndrome and psychiatric illness. Diseases of the Nervous System 34:151–157, 1973

106. Longstreth G: Irritable bowel syndrome and chronic pelvic pain. Obstet Gynecol Surv 49:505–507, 1994

107. Lowman B, Drossman D, Cramer E, et al: Recollection of childhood events in adults with irritable bowel syndrome. J Clin Gastroenterol 9:324–330, 1987

108. Lydiard R: Anxiety and the irritable bowel syndrome. Psychiatric Annals 22:612–618, 1992

109. Lydiard R, Fossey M, Ballenger J: Irritable bowel syndrome in patients with panic disorder (letter). Am J Psychiatry 148:1614, 1991

110. Lydiard R, Fossey M, Marsh W, et al: Prevalence of psychiatric disorders in patients with irritable bowel syndrome. Psychosomatics 34:229–234, 1993

111. Lydiard R, Greenwald S, Weissman M, et al: Panic disorder and gastrointestinal symptoms: findings from the NIMH epidemiological catchment area project. Am J Psychiatry 151:64–70, 1994

112. Lydiard R, Laraia M, Howell E, et al: Can panic disorder present as irritable bowel syndrome? J Clin Psychiatry 47:470–473, 1986

112a. Lynn R, Friedman L: Irritable bowel syndrome. Managing the patient with abdominal pain and altered bowel habits. Med Clin North Am 79:373–390, 1995

113. Magni G, Bernasconi G, Mauro P, et al: Psychiatric diagnoses in ulcerative colitis. Br J Psychiatry 158:413–415, 1991

114. Malagelada J: Pancreatic cancer: an overview of epidemiology: clinical presentation and diagnosis. Mayo Clin Proc 54:459–467, 1979

115. Manning A, Thompson W, Heaton K, et al: Towards positive diagnosis of the irritable bowel. BMJ 2:653–654, 1978

115a. Masand P, Kaplan D, Gupta S, et al: Major depression and irritable bowel syndrome: is there a relationship? J Clin Psychiatry 56:363–367, 1995

116. McDonald A, Bouchier P: Non-organic gastrointestinal illness: a medical and psychiatric study. Br J Psychiatry 136:276–283, 1980

117. McHardy G, Sekinger D, Balart L, et al: Chlordiazepoxide-clidinium bromide in gastrointestinal disorders: controlled clinical studies. Gastroenterology 54:508–513, 1968

118. Mendeloff A, Monk M, Siegel C, et al: Illness experience and life stresses in patients with irritable colon and with ulcerative colitis: an epidemiologic study of ulcerative colitis and regional enteritis in Baltimore, 1960–1964. N Engl J Med 282:14–17, 1970

119. Meyer U: Porphyrias, in Harrison's Principles of Internal Medicine, 12th Edition. Edited by Wilson J, Braunwald E, Isselbacher K, et al. New York, McGraw-Hill, Health Professions Division, 1991, pp 1829–1834

120. Miller H, Golden R, Evans D: Mental dysfunction and cobalamin deficiency (letter). Arch Intern Med 150:910–911, 1990

121. Moriarty K, Dawson A: Functional abdominal pain: further evidence that whole gut is affected. BMJ 284:1670–1672, 1982

122. Myren J, Groth M, Larssen S, et al: The effects of trimipramine in patients with the irritable bowel syndrome. Scand J Gastroenterol 17:871–875, 1982

123. Myren J, Lövland B, Larssen S, et al: A double-blind study of the effect of trimipramine in patients with the irritable bowel syndrome. Scand J Gastroenterol 19:835–843, 1984

124. Myren J, Lövland B, Larssen S, et al: Psychopharmacologic drugs in the treatment of the irritable bowel syndrome. Ann Gastroenterol Hepatol (Paris) 20:117–123, 1984

125. Neff D, Blanchard E: A multi-component treatment for irritable bowel syndrome. Behavior Therapy 18:70–83, 1987

126. North C, Alpers D, Helzer J, et al: Do life events or depression exacerbate inflammatory bowel disease? Ann Intern Med 114:381–386, 1991

127. Nostrand T, Barnett J: Management of irritable bowel syndrome. Modern Medicine 57:100–102, 111–113, 1989

128. Noyes R, Cook B, Garvey M, et al: Reduction of gastrointestinal symptoms following treatment for panic disorder. Psychosomatics 31:75–79, 1990

129. Oster J: Recurrent abdominal pain, headache and limb pains in children and adolescents. Pediatrics 50:429–436, 1972

129a. Owens D, Nelson D, Talley N: The irritable bowel syndrome: long-term prognosis and the physician-patient interaction. Ann Intern Med 122:107–112, 1995

130. Palmer R, Stonehill E, Crisp A, et al: Psychological characteristics of patients with the irritable bowel syndrome. Postgrad Med J 50:416–419, 1974

131. Patience D, Blackwood D, McColl K, et al: Acute intermittent porphyria and mental illness—a family study. Acta Psychiatr Scand 89:262–267, 1994

132. Paykel E, Prusoff B, Uhlenhuth E: Scaling of life events. Arch Gen Psychiatry 25:340–347, 1971

133. Payne A, Blanchard E, Holt C, et al: Physiological reactivity to stressors in irritable bowel syndrome patients, inflammatory bowel disease patients and non-patient controls. Behav Res Ther 30:293–300, 1992

134. Perlas A, Faillace L: Case reports: psychiatric manifestations of carcinoma of the pancreas. Am J Psychiatry 121:182, 1964

135. Rhodes J, Abrams J, Manning R: Controlled clinical trial of sedative-anticholinergic drugs in patients with the irritable bowel syndrome. J Clin Pharmacol 18:340–345, 1978

136. Richards H, Prendergast M, Booth I: Psychiatric presentation of Crohn's disease: diagnostic delay and increased morbidity. Br J Psychiatry 164:256–260, 1994

137. Richter J: Issues in the treatment of irritable bowel syndrome. Family Practice Recertification 11:58–59, 1989

138. Richter J, Barish C, Castell D: Abnormal sensory perception in patients with esophageal chest pain. Gastroenterology 91:845–852, 1986

139. Ritchie J, Truelove S: Comparison of various treatments for irritable bowel syndrome. BMJ 281:1317–1319, 1980

139a. Robins L, Helzer J, Croughan J, et al: National Institute of Mental Health Diagnostic Interview Schedule: its history, characteristics, and validity. Arch Gen Psychiatry 38:381–389, 1981

140. Robins L, Helzer J, Weissman M, et al: Lifetime prevalence of specific psychiatric disorders in three sites. Arch Gen Psychiatry 41:949–958, 1984

141. Rosenbaum J, Gelenberg A: Anxiety, in The Practitioner's Guide to Psychoactive Drugs, 3rd Edition. Edited by Gelenberg A, Bassuk E, Schoonover S. New York, Plenum Medical Book, 1991, pp 203

142. Sachar E: Evaluating depression in the medical patient, in Psychological Care of the Medically Ill: A Primer in Liaison Psychiatry. Edited by Strain J, Grossman S. New York, Appleton-Century-Crofts, 1975, pp 64–75

143. Savage C, Butcher W, Noble D: Psychiatric manifestations in pancreatic disease. J Clin Psychopathol 13:9–16, 1952

144. Savage C, Noble D: Cancer of the pancreas: two cases simulating psychogenic illness. J Nerv Ment Dis 120:62–65, 1954

145. Scarinci I, McDonald-Haile J, Bradley L, et al: Altered pain perception and psychosocial features among women with gastrointestinal disorders and history of abuse: a preliminary model. Am J Med 97:108–118, 1994

146. Schindler B, Ramchandani D: Psychologic factors associated with peptic ulcer disease. Med Clin North Am 75:865–876, 1991

147. Scholz T, Pfeiffer F: Roentgenologic diagnosis of carcinoma of the tail of the pancreas. JAMA 81:275–277, 1923

148. Schonecke O, Schuffel W: Evaluation of combined pharmacological and psychotherapeutic treatment in patients with functional abdominal disorders. Psychother Psychosom 26:86–92, 1975

149. Schwarz S, Blanchard E: Evaluation of a psychological treatment for inflammatory bowel disease. Behav Res Ther 29:167–177, 1991

150. Schwarz S, Blanchard E, Berreman C, et al: Psychological aspects of irritable bowel syndrome: comparisons with inflammatory bowel disease and nonpatient controls. Behav Res Ther 31:297–304, 1993

151. Shanoudy H, Salem A: Neuropsychiatric manifestations of vitamin B_{12} deficiency in the absence of anemia or macrocytosis: a case report. S D J Med 45:129–131, 1992

152. Shulman R: Psychiatric aspects of pernicious anemia: a prospective controlled investigation. BMJ 3:266–270, 1967

153. Shulman R: Vitamin B_{12} deficiency and psychiatric illness. Br J Psychiatry 113:252–256, 1967

154. Smith R, Greenbaum D, Vancouver J, et al: Psychosocial factors are associated with health care seeking rather than diagnosis in irritable bowel syndrome. Gastroenterology 98:293–301, 1990

155. Snape W, Carlson G, Cohen S: Colonic myoelectric activity in the irritable bowel syndrome. Gastroenterology 70:326–330, 1976

156. Snape W, Carlson G, Matarrazzo S, et al: Evidence that abnormal myoelectric activity produces colonic motor dysfunction in the irritable bowel syndrome. Gastroenterology 72:383–387, 1977

156a. Spiller R: Irritable bowel or irritable mind? medical treatment works for those with clear diagnosis. BMJ 309:1646–1647, 1994

157. Stacher G, Steinringer H, Schmeier G: Stimulatory effects of the synthetic enkephalin analogue FK 33-824 on colonic motor activity antagonized by naloxone. Hepatogastroenterology 28:110–115, 1981

158. Steinhart M, Wong P, Zarr M: Therapeutic usefulness of amitriptyline in spastic colon syndrome. Int J Psychiatry Med 11:45–57, 1982

159. Stone R, Barbero G: Recurrent abdominal pain in children. Pediatrics 45:732–738, 1970

160. Strachan R, Henderson J: Psychiatric syndromes due to avitaminosis B_{12} with normal blood and marrow. Q J Med 34:303–317, 1965

161. Sullivan M, Cohen S, Snape W: Colonic myoelectrical activity in irritable bowel syndrome. N Engl J Med 298:878–883, 1978

162. Svedlund J, Ottosson J, Sjdin I, et al: Controlled study of psychotherapy in irritable bowel syndrome. Lancet 2:589–592, 1983

163. Svensson T: Peripheral, autonomic regulation of locus coeruleus noradrenergic neuron in brain: putative implications for psychiatry and psychopharmacology. Psychopharmacology 92:1–7, 1987

164. Swabrick E, Hegarty J, Bat L, et al: Site of pain from the irritable bowel. Lancet 2:443–446, 1980

164a. Talley N, Fett S, Zinsmeister A: Self-reported abuse and gastrointestinal disease in outpatients: association with irritable bowel-type symptoms. Am J Gastroenterol 90:366–371, 1995

165. Talley N, Phillips S, Bruce B, et al: Relation among personality and symptoms in nonulcer dyspepsia and the irritable bowel syndrome. Gastroenterology 99:327–333, 1990

166. Talley N, Phillips S, Zinmeister A, et al: Relation among personality and symptoms in nonulcer dyspepsia and the irritable bowel syndrome (letter, reply). Gastroenterology 100:1155, 1991

167. Taylor I, Darby C, Hammond P: Comparison of rectosigmoid myoelectrical activity in the irritable colon syndrome during relapses and remissions. Gut 19:923–929, 1978

168. Taylor I, Hammond P, Basu P: Is there a myoelectrical abnormality in the irritable colon syndrome? Gut 19:391–395, 1978

169. Thompson W: The irritable bowel. Gut 25:305–320, 1984

170. Thompson W, Heaton K: Functional bowel disorders in apparently healthy people. Gastroenterology 79:283–288, 1980

170a. Thompson W, The Working Team for Functional Bowel Disorders: Functional bowel disorders and functional abdominal pain, in The Functional Gastrointestinal Disorders: Diagnosis, Pathophysiology, and Treatment. Edited by Drossman D. Boston, MA, Little, Brown, 1994, pp 115–173

171. Tollefson G, Luxenberg M, Valentine R, et al: An open label trial of alprazolam in comorbid irritable bowel syndrome and generalized anxiety disorder. J Clin Psychiatry 52:502–508, 1991

172. Tollefson G, Tollefson S, Pederson M, et al: Comorbid irritable bowel syndrome in patients with generalized anxiety and major depression. Annals of Clinical Psychiatry 3:215–222, 1991

173. Toner B, Garfinkel P, Jeejeebhoy K: Psychological factors in irritable bowel syndrome. Can J Psychiatry 35:158–161, 1990

174. Vassallo M, Camilleri M, Phillips S, et al: Colonic tone and motility in patients with irritable bowel syndrome. Mayo Clin Proc 67:725–731, 1992

175. Verbanck P, LeBon O: Changing psychiatric symptoms in a patient with vitamin B_{12} deficiency (letter). J Clin Psychiatry 52:182–183, 1991

176. Voirol M, Hipolito J: Anthropo-analytical relaxation in irritable bowel syndrome: results 40 months later. Schweiz Med Wochenschr 117:1117–1119, 1987

176a. Walker E, Gelfand A, Gelfand M, et al: Medical and psychiatric syMptoms in female gastroenterology clinic patients with histories of sexual victmization. Gen Hosp Psychiatry 17:85–92, 1995

177. Walker E, Katon W, Roy-Byrne P, et al: Histories of sexual victimization in patients with irritable bowel syndrome or inflammatory bowel disease. Am J Psychiatry 150:1502–1506, 1993

178. Walker E, Roy-Byrne P: Irritable bowel syndrome and anxiety, in Anxiety: New Findings for the Clinician. Edited by Roy-Byrne P. Washington, DC, American Psychiatric Press, 1989, pp 43–70

179. Walker E, Roy-Byrne P, Katon W: Irritable bowel syndrome and psychiatric illness. Am J Psychiatry 147:565–572, 1990

180. Walker E, Roy-Byrne P, Katon W, et al: Psychiatric illness and irritable bowel syndrome: a comparison with inflammatory bowel disease. Am J Psychiatry 147:1656–1661, 1990

180a. Wassif W, Deacon A, Floderus Y, et al: Acute intermittent porphyria: diagnostic conundrums. Eur J Clin Chem Clin Biochem 32:915–921, 1994

181. Wayne H: A tranquilizer-anticholinergic preparation in functional gastrointestinal disorders: a double-blind evaluation. California Medicine 111:79–83, 1969

182. Welgan P, Meshkinpour H, Beeler M: Effect of anger on colon motor and myoelectric activity in irritable bowel syndrome. Gastroenterology 94:1150–1156, 1988

183. Wender P, Kalm M: Prevalence of attention deficit disorder, residual type, and other psychiatric disorders in patients with irritable colon syndrome. Am J Psychiatry 140:1579–1582, 1983

184. Whitehead W: Psychotherapy and biofeedback in the treatment of irritable bowel syndrome, in Irritable Bowel Syndrome. Edited by Read N. New York, Grune & Stratton, 1985, pp 245–266

185. Whitehead W, Bosmajian L, Zorderman A, et al: Symptoms of psychologic distress associated with irritable bowel syndrome: comparison of community and medical clinic samples. Gastroenterology 95:709–714, 1988

186. Whitehead W, Crowell M: Psychologic considerations in the irritable bowel syndrome. Gastroenterol Clin North Am 20:249–267, 1991

187. Whitehead W, Crowell M, Robinson J, et al: Effects of stressful life events on bowel symptoms: subjects with irritable bowel syndrome compared with subjects without bowel dysfunction. Gut 33:825–830, 1992

188. Whitehead W, Engel B, Schuster M: Irritable bowel syndrome: physiological and psychological differences between diarrhea-predominant and constipation-predominant patients. Dig Dis Sci 25:404–412, 1980

189. Whitehead W, Holtkotter B, Enck P, et al: Tolerance for rectosigmoid distention in irritable bowel syndrome. Gastroenterology 98:1187–1192, 1990

190. Whitehead W, Schuster M: Gastrointestinal Disorders: Behavioral and Physiological Basis for Treatment. New York, Academic Press, 1985

191. Whitehead W, Winget C, Fedoravicius A, et al: Learned illness behavior in patients with irritable bowel syndrome and peptic ulcer. Dig Dis Sci 27:202–208, 1982

192. Whorwell P, Clouter C, Smith C: Oesophageal motility in the irritable bowel syndrome. BMJ 282:1101–1102, 1981

193. Whorwell P, Lupton E, Erduran D, et al: Bladder smooth muscle dysfunction in patients with irritable bowel syndrome. Gut 27:1014–1017, 1986

194. Whorwell P, McCallum M, Creed F, et al: Non-colonic features of irritable bowel syndrome. Gut 27:37–40, 1986

195. Whorwell P, Prior A, Colgan S: Hypnotherapy in severe irritable bowel syndrome: further experience. Gut 4:423–425, 1987

196. Whorwell P, Prior A, Faragher E: Controlled trial of hypnotherapy in the treatment of severe refractory irritable bowel syndrome. Lancet 2:1232–1233, 1984

196a. Wing J, Cooper J, Sartorius N: The Description and Classification of Psychiatric Symptoms: An Instruction Manual for the PSE and CATEGO System. Cambridge, UK, Cambridge Univeristy Press, 1974

197. Wise T: Psychiatric management of functional gastrointestinal disorders. Psychiatric Annals 22:606–611, 1992

198. Wise T, Cooper J, Ahmed S: The efficacy of group therapy for patients with irritable bowel syndrome. Psychosomatics 23:465–469, 1982

199. Wood J: Enteric neurophysiology. Am J Physiol 247:G585–G597, 1984

200. Woodman C, Noyes R: The relationship between panic disorder and irritable bowel syndrome: a review. Annals of Clinical Psychiatry 4:175–180, 1992

201. Yaskin J: Nervous symptoms as earliest manifestations of carcinoma of the pancreas. JAMA 96:1664–1668, 1931

202. Young S, Alpers D, Norland C, et al: Psychiatric illness and the irritable bowel syndrome. Gastroenterology 70:162–166, 1976

203. Zighelboim J, Talley N, Phillips S, et al: Visceral perception in irritable bowel syndrome: rectal and gastric responses to distension and serotonin type 3 antagonism. Dig Dis Sci 40:819–827, 1995

The Obstetrics Patient

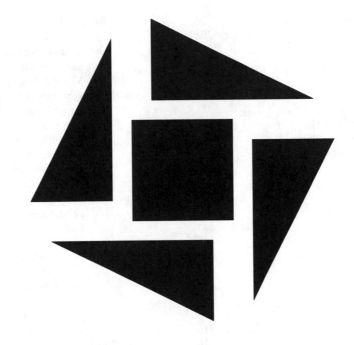

CHAPTER 8

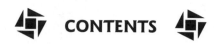

CONTENTS

■ Introduction to Chapter 8 301
■ Case Presentation: Ms. Wright: The Anxious,
   Depressed Pregnant Patient 302
■ Questions 302
■ Answers 306
■ Discussion 307
   ◆ Contraception 307
   ◆ Postpartum Blues and Depression 307
      Postpartum Blues 307
         Features 307
         Psychological Hypotheses 308
         Treatment 308
      Postpartum Depression 308
         Incidence 308
         Suicide 309
         Adverse Effects on Infants 309
      Risk Factors 309
      Physiological Correlates 310
   ◆ Panic Disorder 311
   ◆ Obsessive-Compulsive Disorder 311
   ◆ Psychopharmacology in Pregnancy, Part I . . . 311
      Anxiolytics and Sedatives 312
         Benzodiazepines 312
         Barbiturates 314
      Antidepressants 314
         Tricyclic Antidepressants 314
         Newer Antidepressants 315
            Fluoxetine 315
            Newer SSRIs 315
            Bupropion 315
         Monoamine Oxidase Inhibitors 315
         Electroconvulsive Therapy 315
         Miscellaneous Treatments 316
            Sleep deprivation 316
            Light therapy 316
         Conclusions 316

      Neonatal Toxicity 316
      Breast Feeding 316
   ◆ Summary 318
   ◆ References 318
■ Case Presentation: Ms. Sawyer: The Psychotic,
   Bipolar Pregnant Patient 324
■ Questions 324
■ Answers 327
■ Discussion 328
   ◆ Postpartum Psychosis 328
      Methodological Problems 328
      Features 328
      Risk Factors 329
      Prognosis 329
      Differential Diagnosis 330
      Pregnancy and the Chronically Mentally Ill . . 330
      The Violent Pregnant Patient 330
   ◆ Psychopharmacology in Pregnancy, Part II . . . 331
      Electroconvulsive Therapy 331
      Neuroleptics 331
         Indications in Pregnancy 331
         Teratogenicity 331
         Medications for Neuroleptic Side Effects . . . 332
         Adjuvant Clonazepam 332
      Lithium: When? Why? How? 332
         Before Conception 332
         During Pregnancy 333
            Pregnancy pharmacokinetics and
            lithium 334
            Lithium alternatives 334
         After Childbirth 335
            Neonatal lithium toxicity 336
            Breast feeding 336
            Lithium children 336
   ◆ Summary 336
   ◆ References 337

It was difficult to choose among the many topics on women's health for this volume. So much is relevant, and the literature is always expanding. We decided to select the more medically problematical issues rather than duplicate the comprehensive approach that has already been done so well by others.[155] In this spirit, Chapters 8 and 9 focus selectively on pregnancy, menopause, hysterectomy, chronic pelvic pain, and breast cancer.

Managing a psychiatrically symptomatic pregnant patient sometimes feels like a 9-month "Perils of Pauline." Everyone agrees that medication is best avoided, but its use is sometimes inevitable. That said, then, what can you use? There is a maddening lack of consensus on pharmacological treatments; controlled studies in humans do not exist. How do you present this kind of information to a pregnant, distressed patient, and expect her to agree to your medication recommendations? We struggle with some of these dilemmas in this chapter. Needless to say, the eventual delivery—by an intact mother—of a healthy baby is a time of rejoicing and great relief for all concerned.

The questions following each vignette were designed as an exercise, not a test. There may be more than one correct option.

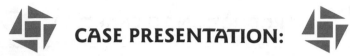

CASE PRESENTATION:

Ms. Wright: The Anxious, Depressed Pregnant Patient

Ms. Wright is a 31-year-old woman who has worked as a successful music teacher for many years. She was referred by her internist 2 years ago with symptoms of insomnia and extreme anxiety, marked by panic attacks, palpitations, dry mouth, fear of going crazy, sweating, and a choking sensation. Panic attacks occurred 2–3 times per week. Ms. Wright was extremely depressed at the time, felt she could "no longer cope," but was at no point suicidal. She acknowledged feelings of guilt, inability to concentrate, and felt worse in the early morning. Cognitive functions were intact except for diminished concentration. Past psychiatric history was negative except for occasional diazepam (Valium) 5 mg before recitals. Family history was negative for psychiatric illness. There was no drug or alcohol history.

Complete medical and neurological workups (including electroencephalogram [EEG] and magnetic resonance imaging [MRI] of the brain) were normal. The dual diagnosis of panic disorder without agoraphobia and major depression was made, and the patient was begun on low-dose alprazolam (Xanax) and nortriptyline (Pamelor, Aventyl) in slowly incremental doses. Panic and depressive symptoms disappeared entirely on 60 mg/day of nortriptyline, with blood levels averaging approximately 90 µg/L. She was tapered off the alprazolam uneventfully. Over the next 2 years, however, efforts to discontinue the nortriptyline, even by slow taper, resulted in a return of panic attacks, insomnia, dysphoria, and diminished concentration.

 QUESTIONS

Choose all that apply.

1. The Wrights have used a diaphragm and condom as their main form of birth control. Ms. Wright would like to try oral contraceptives, which would have the added benefit of lessening her severe menstrual cramping. What statements are true regarding the psychiatric side effects associated with oral contraceptives?
   a. When oral contraceptives produce adverse psychiatric effects, high levels of estrogen are usually the culprit.
   b. Newer preparations containing higher estrogen-to-progestin ratios have fewer of these side effects.
   c. The psychiatric symptoms most commonly associated with oral contraceptives are anxiety states.
   d. The psychiatric side effects of oral contraceptives occur mainly when the woman takes them irregularly, rather than as directed.

2. One year later, Ms. Wright and her husband decide that they want a second child. She wishes to slowly dis-
continue the medication, but is quite concerned about the risk of recurrence of panic disorder. She fears becoming pregnant and "trapped" by the horrible symptoms again, without help available to her. What factors do you consider as you begin to counsel Ms. Wright and her husband?
   a. She is at risk for reemergence of panic symptoms during pregnancy, despite gradual taper of the medication.
   b. They should be aware that if Ms. Wright becomes pregnant and her panic attacks recur, medication would be used only if they became disabling.
   c. If Ms. Wright's panic attacks recur during pregnancy, she should be reassured you will pursue prepregnancy symptom control.
   d. Pregnancy has been shown to confer a protective effect for the majority of women with panic disorder.

3. Mr. Wright wants to know the likelihood of his wife's becoming depressed again during pregnancy. Which of the following is/are true?

a. The risk is greatest *after* delivery.

b. The risk is greatest during pregnancy.

c. The pattern of dysphoric symptoms after childbirth is almost identical to that after gynecological surgery, suggesting a common substrate.

d. She is at no greater risk than someone without an affective history.

4. "Postpartum blues" is a term found throughout the literature on mood disorders in pregnancy. How does DSM-IV[3b] classify this condition?

a. It has created a new category, *brief postpartum dysphoric disorder.*

b. It advises classifying it under *adjustment disorder with depressed mood.*

c. It groups it under *mental disorder due to a general medical condition.*

d. It does not specify.

5. Which of the following correlate(s) with the risk of postpartum blues?

a. Premenstrual dysphoria

b. Depression during pregnancy

c. A prior major depressive episode unassociated with pregnancy

d. Low socioeconomic status

e. All of the above

6. All of the following have been associated with the diagnosis of postpartum blues except . . .

a. Anxiety.

b. Insomnia.

c. Poor appetite.

d. Psychosis.

7. Ms. Wright wants to know if you will be able to see her while she is in the hospital after the delivery. In formulating your potential treatment plan, you consider that she would be most at risk for the blues . . .

a. Within 24 hours of delivery.

b. Between postpartum days 3 and 7.

c. Between postpartum weeks 2 and 3.

d. Between postpartum months 1 and 2.

8. Ms. Wright wants to know if her obstetrical history and course will have anything to do with the likelihood of developing the blues. Which are true?

a. The blues are not related to parity.

b. Easy pregnancies and deliveries, with few obstetric stressors, are less likely to be followed by the blues.

c. Marital discord closely correlates with risk.

d. Stressful life events do not correlate with developing the blues.

e. Women who bottle-feed rather than breast-feed show increased likelihood of developing the blues.

9. Many etiological factors have been studied regarding postpartum blues. What has been found regarding the role of hormonal factors?

a. The peak symptoms of the blues occur during a rapid flux of gonadotropins and hormones.

b. Mood ratings correlate with levels of estrogen and progesterone.

c. Altered thyroid function indices within 3 weeks postpartum identify patients at risk for the blues.

d. Estrogen withdrawal is the major hormonal change implicated in triggering the postpartum blues.

10. What are valid statements concerning psychodynamic findings and the blues?

a. Disappointment in the newborn baby has been found to be the primary affect in "blue" mothers.

b. Older studies conducted when new mothers had longer postpartum stays showed that themes of disappointment with the neonate or delivery were secondary to the more prominent content related to separation from family.

c. The postpartum blues are a hormonally assisted grief reaction.

d. Ambivalence about the pregnancy was found as a risk factor for developing the blues.

11. When assessing any depressed patient, thyroid function tests are useful to check. What would be normal results during and after pregnancy?

a. Thyroid function tests should normally remain at prepregnancy levels throughout.

b. They vary during pregnancy, but should return to baseline by postpartum week 1.

c. They vary during pregnancy, but should return to baseline by postpartum weeks 3–4.

d. None of the above.

12. If Ms. Wright were to develop the postpartum blues, what would be treatment considerations?

a. The condition requires antidepressant treatment (preferably selective serotonin reuptake inhibitors [SSRIs]).

b. Administration of low-dose methylphenidate (Ritalin) is the current standard treatment.

c. It remits spontaneously.

d. It requires no specific pharmacological treatment.

13. Under the supervision of her obstetrician, Ms. Wright decides to continue the nortriptyline until conception is confirmed. She becomes pregnant almost immediately, and the medication is discontinued. By the seventh week of gestation, she notes the return of panic attacks, now daily. She is extremely anxious about what will happen to her and her unborn child. Dysphoric symptoms also return, with insomnia, feelings of guilt, diminished self-esteem, and impaired concentration. There is no psychosis, but she experiences transient suicidal ideation. All of the following statements are true except . . .

a. Women *during* pregnancy have a low risk of suicide in comparison with the general female population.

b. Despite their high rate of psychiatric morbidity, women in the first year *after* childbirth have a low risk of suicide.

c. Pregnant teenagers are at substantially increased risk for suicide compared with other pregnant women.

d. Stillbirth increases the risk of suicide.

e. Women who committed suicide most often did so in the *first* postpartum month, usually using nonviolent methods.

14. Which are *false* statements?

a. The majority of "blue" new mothers do not progress to postpartum depression.

b. The majority of new mothers with major depression start out with the blues within the first week after delivery.

c. The prevalence of major depression *during* pregnancy is < 1% of all pregnant women.

d. Depressive symptoms *during* pregnancy indicate vulnerability to depression *after* delivery.

e. The risk of affective disorders in families is equivalent for pregnancy-related and pregnancy-independent affectively ill patients.

15. Which of the following is true regarding the diagnosis of postpartum depression according to DSM-IV?

a. DSM-IV adds a "postpartum onset" specifier to the *major depressive disorder* diagnosis.

b. DSM-IV terms it *major depressive disorder due to a general medical condition* (i.e., pregnancy).

c. DSM-IV has created a separate category of *postpartum depressive disorder.*

d. DSM-IV segregates it under *mood disorder not otherwise specified.*

16. DSM-IV considers "postpartum" to be within what time interval following delivery?

a. Within 2 weeks

b. Within 1 month

c. Within months

d. Within 1 year

17. Mr. Wright takes some time off from work to stay with his wife and help care for the couple's 3-year-old daughter. Family members take turns helping and monitoring the patient. Ms. Wright's suicidal ideation diminishes but she continues to feels depressed, although reassured by the family support. She does not want to be hospitalized because she would have to leave her child. However, Mr. Wright runs out of sick time and vacation time, and family members eventually have to return home. It is now week 11, with panic attacks occurring about every other day and depressive symptomatology quite profound. Mr. and Ms. Wright are willing to give informed consent to pharmacological treatment and agree to hire help. They want above all else for Ms. Wright to be able to remain at home. Which of the following should you consider in your treatment plan?

a. The teratogenic potential of tricyclic antidepressants (TCAs) has been less controversial than that of the benzodiazepines.

b. Tricyclic ingestion during pregnancy has been associated with significant fetal morbidity.

c. The preferred antidepressants for pregnant patients are the secondary tricyclic amines (i.e., nortriptyline [Pamelor, Aventyl], desipramine [Norpramin]).

d. Electroconvulsive therapy (ECT) significantly increases the incidence of premature labor.

18. Ms. Wright is able to wait until week 14 before starting medication. She begins to feel less depressed on nortriptyline 75 mg/day (blood level 65 μg/L) but still has breakthrough panic symptoms, generalized anxiety, and insomnia. She is unable to tolerate increases in nortriptyline without worsening dysphoria. You reluctantly decide to add an anxiolytic. What factors influence your choice of medication?

a. The teratogenic potential of diazepam (Valium), the oldest, most widely used anxiolytic, makes it the least controversial of the benzodiazepines.

b. Most evidence does not support the teratogenicity of the benzodiazepines.

c. Pregnancy is one of the rare instances in which a low-dose barbiturate (like secobarbital) under close medical supervision is safer for anxiolysis than benzodiazepines.

d. Low-dose diphenhydramine (Benadryl) and temazepam (Restoril) are particularly helpful in restoring sleep in pregnant patients, and may actually reduce daytime medication requirements.

19. Which of the following medications has been rated "absolutely contraindicated" during pregnancy?

a. Lorazepam (Ativan)
b. Alprazolam (Xanax)
c. Temazepam (Restoril)
d. Clonazepam (Klonopin)
e. None of the above

20. Which are true regarding the physiological changes of pregnancy?

a. The tricyclic dose required to achieve symptom remission and adequate serum blood levels *increases* in the second and third trimester.
b. The tricyclic dose required to achieve symptom remission and adequate serum blood levels *decreases* in the second and third trimester.
c. There is reduced hepatic metabolism.
d. There is increased protein-binding capacity of medication.

21. Ms. Wright finally arrives at the ninth month. She is due to deliver in about 10 days. Which of the following are true?

a. Ideally, the medication should be gradually discontinued at this point.
b. Ideally, the medication should be continued up until delivery in order to protect her from recurrent depression.
c. She is at heightened risk for recurrent depression as she approaches her delivery date.
d. The main adverse side effect of continuing medication up until delivery is maternal cardiotoxicity.

22. Infants born to mothers on tricyclics at the time of delivery have been reported to have . . .

a. No greater incidence of side effects than those born to mothers whose tricyclics have been discontinued or decreased.
b. Hypotonia and poor sucking

c. Tachypnea and transient cyanosis
d. Learning disabilities

23. Three-year follow-up of "tricyclic babies" who were exposed to TCAs in utero has shown . . .

a. Normal motor skills.
b. Delayed motor development.
c. Normal behavioral development.
d. No morphological problems, but language lags.
e. Delayed developmental milestones.

24. Ms. Wright delivers a healthy baby girl. She agrees to remain on nortriptyline but wants to breast-feed. How do you advise her?

a. There is consensus that tricyclics are secreted into breast milk, but in very small concentrations.
b. There is consensus that the small concentrations of tricyclics ingested through breast milk are innocuous to the infant.
c. Mothers with a history of unipolar depression who refuse antidepressant therapy while breast feeding are at high risk for relapse.
d. The American Academy of Pediatrics classifies TCAs as compatible with breast feeding.

25. What percentage of maternal TCA concentration crosses to the breast milk?

a. < 1%
b. 10%
c. 25%
d. 50%

26. One must weigh the psychological risks to the neonate of recurrent maternal depression against the pharmacological risks of antidepressants. Which of the following is a *false* statement about the impact of depression on the baby?

a. Depressed mothers consider harming not only themselves, but also their infants.
b. Depressed mothers are more likely to express negative feelings about their babies.
c. The negative affect is usually limited to self-denigration, and does not extend to the baby.
d. Infants of depressed mothers perform worse on object concept tasks.
e. Infants of depressed mothers show more behavioral difficulties.

Answers

1. Answer: b (p. 307)
2. Answer: a, b (p. 311)
3. Answer: a (pp. 309–310)
4. Answer: d (p. 308)
5. Answer: a, b, c (p. 308)
6. Answer: d (pp. 307–308)
7. Answer: b (p. 308)
8. Answer: a, d (pp. 307–308)
9. Answer: a (pp. 310–311)
10. Answer: b, d (p. 308)
11. Answer: c (p. 310)
12. Answer: c, d (p. 308)
13. Answer: e (p. 309)
14. Answer: c (pp. 308–309)
15. Answer: a (p. 308)
16. Answer: b (p. 308)
17. Answer: a, c (pp. 314–316)
18. Answer: b (pp. 312–314)
19. Answer: c (p. 314)
20. Answer: a (pp. 314–315)
21. Answer: a (pp. 314–315)
22. Answer: b, c (p. 316)
23. Answer: a, c (p. 316)
24. Answer: a, c (pp. 316–318)
25. Answer: b (p. 317)
26. Answer: c (p. 309)

The reader looking for easy formulas will find none in this literature; there is no substitute for individual risk-benefit analysis and informed consent. The emphasis away from optimizing pharmacological treatment and toward "making do," often with significant symptomatic residua, is unsatisfying for the consulting psychiatrist, troublesome for the obstetrician, and downright nightmarish for the expectant patient and her family. L. Miller (personal communication, April 1994) has pointed out, however, that

> [although] we have little data about the effects of in utero drug exposure, we have even *fewer* data about effects of in utero exposure to untreated psychiatric disorder. In our Women's Clinic, we see all too often the adverse consequences of hastily discontinuing needed psychotropic medication during pregnancy.

It *is* possible to abstract some guidelines from this ambiguous, uncontrolled literature, which follow.

◢ CONTRACEPTION

First, a word about oral contraceptives. They have been associated with causing symptoms resembling endogenous depression,[94] albeit in a minority of women.[47,91,140,164,167] It appears to be the **progestin** that is the culprit,[30,53] although Petersen[111] points out that some women with premenstrual irritability do better on the more progestational agents. Newer preparations containing lower progestin-to-estrogen ratios have fewer depressive effects.

◆ Note that the relatively new contraceptive Norplant (introduced in 1991) is a progestin-only preparation. So far, there are at least two case reports of women with no psychiatric history who developed major depression and panic disorder within 1–2 months after insertion of Norplant system capsules.[161] The symptoms of anxiety and depression resolved within 1 month of discontinuing the medication. Otherwise, there have been relatively few adverse psychological effects.[138]

We have also seen recurrent depression in menopausal women with depressive histories who were given estrogen replacement therapy, which is combined with progestin to minimize the risk of endometrial cancer.

◆ *Routinely* inquire about contraceptive regimens or estrogen replacement therapy, especially in those women who present with depression. *A trial of discontinuing or switching to a different oral contraceptive preparation may spare antidepressant treatment.*

Pyridoxine, a cofactor in catecholamine synthesis, may be deficient in oral contraceptive users.[108,122] Pyridoxine supplementation (20 mg twice daily) alleviated contraceptive-associated depression in one double-blind study.[2]

◢ POSTPARTUM BLUES AND DEPRESSION

Postpartum Blues

You will undoubtedly hear many etiological speculations about the postpartum blues from obstetricians, staff, families, and the patients themselves. These theories cover the gamut—attributing the blues to difficult deliveries, grief hypotheses, breast feeding, bottle feeding, difficult marriages, low socioeconomic status, "it usually happens with the first child," "it usually happens with the third child," and so on. In fact, the etiology of the postpartum blues has remained elusive and something of a mystery. We present the results of several studies to assist the consultant in sorting out fact from fantasy. Keep in mind, however, that while these confusing data are correlational, they do not explain cause.

Most of the research literature concerns postpartum psychological disturbance, which is classified into three categories: "the blues," postpartum depression, and postpartum psychosis (affective and schizophreniform). Although we discuss these as distinct syndromes, there is overlap and ambiguity about whether they lie along the same biological spectrum.[56]

Features

The "postpartum blues" refers to a common, mild syndrome of tearfulness or sadness typically experienced by women within the first 7 to 10 days after delivery,[101,114,175] with peak symptoms occurring between the third and seventh day.[72] Characteristic symptoms include dysphoria, mood lability, anxiety, crying, insomnia, poor appetite, and irritability.[54,73] Prevalence estimates of the postpartum blues have ranged from 26%[107] to 85%.[149] Several points to note:

♦ There are no well-established criteria for the diagnosis; psychosis is not part of the syndrome, but would signal a more serious condition.

♦ Apart from a brief mention that the "baby blues" occur 3–7 days postpartum, DSM-IV[3b] offers no specific designation for this condition.

♦ Although the blues do not in themselves cause serious impairment, women who experience them may be at increased risk for postpartum depression.[72,110]

♦ It is unclear whether they represent a specific affective syndrome associated with childbirth or a nonspecific response to a major psychosocial stressor.[83,105,175] For example, dysphoric symptoms after childbirth differ from those after gynecological surgery,[64] suggesting that the blues are distinct from nonspecific reactions to physical and emotional stress. However, another study found similarities between the blues and postoperative dysphoria,[83] with the major difference relating to symptom timing: the postoperative dysphoric ratings peaked right after surgery, but postpartum blues were highest days later. Reconciling these disparate findings will require additional research.

Psychological Hypotheses

Several psychological hypotheses have been tested regarding the blues. In a prospective study of 89 women, it was hypothesized that the postpartum blues are a hormonally assisted grief reaction occurring predominantly in women whose antenatal expectation of the baby or delivery fails to be fulfilled by the reality events.[25] Disappointment was posited to be the main affect. The authors found that there was no relationship between the occurrence of the blues and postnatal disappointment. More prominent was content related to separation from family. In addition, over half of those who experienced the blues did not equate the feeling with "sadness," as would have been predicted by the grief hypothesis, corroborating the report of other studies that the women do not define the experience as equivalent to "depression."[33,98,150,175] Four risk factors for the blues were identified by this study:

♦ Severe premenstrual tension

♦ Ambivalence about the pregnancy, as suggested by its having been unplanned or its elective termination considered

♦ Subjective ratings of the pregnancy as moderately to very emotionally stressful

♦ Pessimistic expectations during late pregnancy about the delivery and immediate postpartum period that have a high probability of being fulfilled

We will discuss risk factors further in the section on postpartum depression.

Treatment

The blues are usually transitory[56] and rarely require pharmacological treatment.[46] The key therapeutic interventions are support and reassurance.

Postpartum Depression

Postpartum depression is a major affective disorder, unlike the blues. DSM-IV[3c] adds a "Postpartum Onset" specifier to Major Depressive Disorder for onset within 4 *weeks* (1 month) after delivery. Note that other etiologies for mood disorders in pregnancy should be ruled out first, such as *major depressive disorder due to a general medical condition* (e.g., hypothyroidism) or *substance-induced major depressive disorder.*

Incidence

The factors determining which "blue" women evolve a full-blown major depression remain uncertain.[3,29] A major methodological problem has been the lack of control groups.

♦ Hannah and colleagues[56] showed that 42% of "blue" new mothers had recovered by the sixth week—that is, they did not progress to major depression. However, the majority of women diagnosed with postpartum major depression at the sixth week started out "blue" in the first week after delivery. Bottle feeding, delivery by caesarean section, recollection of low mood after a previous birth, and a high depression score at 5 days postpartum increased the risk of postpartum depression at 6 weeks by 85-fold.

The claim that pregnancy confers protection against the emergence of psychiatric symptoms is not accurate: a prospective study of the development of depression in pregnancy reported that although a greater percentage become depressed *after* delivery, as many as **10%** of women meet criteria for major or "minor" depression (using Research Diagnostic Criteria [RDC][143a] or DSM-III[3c] criteria) *during* pregnancy.[31,78,100,102,113,166,175]

◆ Depressive symptoms during pregnancy predict vulnerability to depression after childbirth.[52,104]

The incidence of postpartum major depression has been estimated at between 4% and 16%.[27,78,100,165,166] Sadly, new mothers often do not seek help from any source, attributing their affective condition to difficulties with motherhood itself.[85]

Suicide

Fortunately, women during pregnancy and in the first year after childbirth have a *low* risk of suicide despite their high rate of psychiatric morbidity—about one-twentieth of the expected rate in the general female population.[5,70,171] Appleby[5] found that while pregnant teens were at less risk than nonpregnant teens, they carried a suicide risk 5 times greater than that for pregnant women as a group. Women after stillbirth were found to have the highest rate among pregnant women, approaching that of the general female population. Women who committed suicide most often did so in the first postpartum month, and there was a tendency to use violent methods (self-incineration, jumping from a height, jumping in front of a train), suggesting that these individuals may have been psychotic. With few exceptions,[39a] the sociocultural factors which contribute to maternal suicide have been relatively neglected in current research.

Adverse Effects on Infants

Major depression before, during, or after pregnancy is never benign. It may adversely affect the newborn by predisposing to poor prenatal compliance, cigarette use, and self-medication with substances like alcohol or drugs.[176] Furthermore, pregnant women who become depressed for the first time in their lives may have persistent psychological problems for up to *4 years after childbirth*.[78] Even if a physically healthy baby is delivered, the effects of maternal depression on infant development are potentially noxious:

◆ Depressed mothers are more likely to express negative or mixed feelings about their 3-month-old babies.[78]

◆ A study of mothers who had suffered depressive disorders in the first postnatal year showed reduced quality of mother-child interaction, such as less facilitation of the children by the mothers, less affective sharing by the children, and less sociability with a stranger.[146]

◆ Postpartum depression may increase the risk for later maternal depression, and in turn exacerbate the risk for childhood behavioral problems.[112]

◆ Infants of postnatally depressed mothers performed worse on object concept tasks, were more insecurely attached to their mothers, and showed more behavioral difficulties.[18,61a,95]

◆ More research is needed into how to provide good aftercare when there has been pregnancy-associated mental illness.[77b]

In a phenomenological study of postpartum depression, Beck[10] has stated,

> Postpartum depression [is] a living nightmare filled with uncontrollable anxiety attacks, consuming guilt, and obsessive thinking. *Mothers contemplated not only harming themselves, but also their infants.* The mothers were enveloped in loneliness and the quality of their lives was further compromised by a lack of emotional and all previous interests. Fear that their lives would never return to normal was all-encompassing. (p. 170, italics added)

We will discuss treatment later.

Risk Factors

The search continues for risk factors and to clarify whether postpartum blues and depression represent distinct affective variants or lie on a continuum with other affective disorders. Results are inconsistent, and methodological problems prevail. Most studies have been retrospective, using heterogeneous assessment instruments and varying definitions of what constitutes the blues or depression. There have been several attempts to develop specific scales for the postpartum blues using systematic psychometric methods.[28,73] Such specificity has been absent in most studies, however, which have relied instead on instruments designed for assessing general depression, rather than postpartum states specifically.

◆ **Affective history:** A recent large prospective study of biological and psychosocial causative factors for the postpartum blues was conducted in 182 women. Women were followed from the second trimester until postpartum week 9.[105] Those at greater risk were women who had
  • Higher levels of depressive symptoms during the pregnancy itself.

- At least one previous episode of depression.
- Self-reported premenstrual depression.

There is corroboratory data that the most consistent predictors of postpartum blues are a history of premenstrual dysphoria[74,98,175] and the woman's mood during the pregnancy.[25,54,57,74,101] Interestingly, there are preliminary findings that hypomania in the first 5 days following childbirth may mark a subset of women who later become clinically depressed.[49]

◆ **Family history:** Studies suggest a high genetic loading for psychiatric disorders, but not specifically for postpartum psychiatric disorders.[34,117,153] The risk of affective disorders in families is *equivalent* for pregnancy-related and pregnancy-independent affectively ill patients.[168] Moreover, there may be a subgroup that is at risk for severe affective episodes only in the postpartum period, even without a predisposition to affective disorders at other times.[132]

◆ **Demographics:** Demographic variables, such as socioeconomic class, are not predictive of the blues.[67,69,74,101,105,148] Some studies found a correlation with marital discord,[7,31,106,133] but not consistently.[105] Thus, do not assume that the blues will be more common, for example, in economically disadvantaged women or in women with difficult marriages. The influence of cultural factors on onset appears weak.[77a]

◆ **Obstetric factors:** There is no clear relationship to parity: the blues have been variously reported as more common in primiparous women,[98,175] more common in multiparous women,[33] and not related to parity at all.[25,54,74,104,105,148] Obstetric stressors (i.e., difficult deliveries) sometimes[14,56] but not always[103–105,110] predict the blues. Similarly, caesarean section,[36,56,71] bottle versus breast feeding,[7,56,57,69,72,159] low birth weight,[56] maternal sleep disruption,[169] and infant feeding difficulties[27,57,72,114] have been found to correlate inconsistently with the blues.

◆ **Stressful life events:** Stressful life events during pregnancy were positively correlated with the onset of blues in several studies,[94a,105,110,118,126,141] but the findings—predictably—have been variable.

Physiological Correlates

The peak symptoms of the blues occur during a rapid flux of gonadotropins and hormones, which has led many investigators to study biochemical variables. Note that there is overlap with investigations into *post-*

partum depression. There are many studies but few positive findings:

◆ **Estrogen and metabolites, follicle-stimulating hormone (FSH), luteinizing hormone (LH), progesterone, prolactin:** No consistent correlation has been found between these hormones and mood ratings.[15,40,42,98,150] In a large prospective study,[105] there was only weak support for the hypothesis that estrogen withdrawal precipitates postpartum blues. *Free estriol* was significantly higher at gestational week 38 in "blue" women than in nondepressed control subjects, and showed a significantly greater decrease from mean prepartum to postpartum levels. *Estradiol* levels, however, showed no significant association with the blues at any time. Furthermore, there were no significant correlations with progesterone or prolactin levels, or with the ratio of prolactin to either progesterone or any of the estrogens. Few significant associations were found between the blues and measurements of urinary free and total plasma cortisol. (Harris et al.,[60] however, recently found that development of maternity blues was associated with higher antenatal levels of progesterone and lower postnatal progesterone levels.)

◆ **Thyroid function:** Altered thyroid function indices ($\uparrow$T4, $\downarrow$T3 resin uptake) persist for about 3–4 weeks after delivery.[151] The role of thyroid dysfunction in the genesis of postpartum depression is unclear.[58]
  - Recently, a positive correlation was found between thyroid dysfunction and postpartum depression, with the incidence of thyroid dysfunction more than twice as high in depressed versus nondepressed women.[115]
  - Autoimmune thyroiditis was associated with postpartum depression, as measured by the Raskin[118a]—but not the Edinburgh[28] and the Montgomery-Äsberg[92a]—depression rating scales.[59]
  - No greater prevalence of thyroid dysfunction was found in women with postpartum affective psychoses compared with matched postpartum control subjects.[152]

◆ **Sleep:** There is preliminary evidence that the sleep systems of women with affective histories may be more sensitive to the psychobiological changes associated with childbearing. Coble et al.[16,17] found that these women showed earlier onset of sleep disruption over the childbearing course and a reduction in rapid eye movement (REM) latency in the final trimester that persisted throughout the eighth postpartum month. Women with prior affective disorder were more likely to be distressed after delivery.

♦ **Miscellaneous markers:**

- Low postpartum plasma *tryptophan* has correlated with the blues,[40,54] but tryptophan supplementation does not effectively treat the condition.[57]
- More *platelet gamma$_2$-adrenoreceptor sites* were found in women with than in those without the blues.[87]
- Abnormal *platelet 5-hydroxytryptamine uptake and imipramine binding* have been correlated with the blues.[55]
- *Platelet monoamine oxidase* levels have correlated with depression ratings during the first postpartum week.[43]
- Changes in *cyclic plasma adenosine monophosphate* (cAMP) were found during the first postpartum week for women who demonstrated postpartum elation, compared with those who were not elated.[8]

♦ The *tyramine test* performed postpartum does not predict vulnerability to postpartum depression.[48]

At present, these are biochemical findings awaiting a clinical application; there is no definitive pattern for either the blues or postpartum depression. Moreover, the positive biochemical findings are as likely to be the *result* of mood changes as they are to be etiological. Gitlin and Pasnau[46] have suggested that women who develop postpartum blues are not biologically different from those who do not, but may respond to the normal physiological postpartum changes with more affective symptoms, reflecting individual vulnerabilities to common changes. Condon and Watson[25] have summarized:

> The implications for future research would seem to be that both psychological and biological variables *already operating* during pregnancy powerfully predispose to the maternity blues. Thus, a shift of emphasis away from the more acute changes occurring in the immediate postnatal period, and a closer scrutiny of pregnancy variables, may prove more rewarding in unraveling the mystery of the blues etiology. (p. 170)

☙ PANIC DISORDER

The effects of pregnancy on preexisting panic disorder are controversial. Some authors have suggested that pregnancy provides a protective effect,[26,44,75,160] while others have documented persistent panic attacks during pregnancy[19,23,97,163] and in the postpartum period.[11,24,97,136,137] Panic attacks themselves are not always benign; there is at least one case report of panic attack–associated placental abruption in a unmedicated pregnant woman.[21] Panic attacks may also occur for the first time postpartum.[86]

Medication should be reserved for those women who are at risk of becoming seriously disabled during pregnancy without treatment.[163] Supportive psychotherapy[121,163] and/or behavioral therapy[20] are helpful adjuvants or substitutes for pharmacotherapy, and can actually mitigate the need for medication.

☙ OBSESSIVE-COMPULSIVE DISORDER

Although not relevant to our discussion, the interested reader may refer to the small but growing literature on the association between pregnancy and obsessive-compulsive disorder.[96,139,147]

☙ PSYCHOPHARMACOLOGY IN PREGNANCY, PART I

Rule: Minimizing risk to the fetus and mother takes precedence over symptom control. Nonpharmacological interventions such as psychotherapy (of varying types[158]), hypnosis,[51] environmental management, and/or hospitalization (on either psychiatry or obstetrics) are preferable to medication, especially for first-trimester patients.

♦ Whenever feasible, we outline a management strategy with a woman who has a previous affective or anxiety disorder history *before* she attempts conception. Such an approach allows the woman (and her partner, if available) to plan for practical matters in advance—for example, by informing the obstetrician, considering the impact on job or income, enlisting helpful family members or friends, and so forth.

♦ Although this approach has the disadvantage of burdening an already anxious patient with potentially too much information, we have found that most couples respond gratefully to having a "safety net"—"a game plan just in case" of a psychiatric recurrence. Reassurance that she won't get depressed again, or statements like "we'll cross that bridge when we come to it" are well-meaning but not useful. During a recurrence, it is far easier to call upon a strategy formed in collaboration rather than to scramble to put one together.

Obviously, there will be many situations in which the patient is *already* pregnant and symptomatic. Sometimes, when all else fails and the psychiatric condition threatens the health of mother and fetus, medication becomes unavoidable.

◆ As with any patient, a reassuring, compassionate manner should not preempt the patient's right to know the potential risks and benefits. We approach medicating a pregnant woman as a procedure that warrants informed consent. This requires that the psychiatrist be knowledgeable about the existing data and their limitations. *Unfortunately, controlled studies of the teratogenicity of psychotropics in human beings do not exist.*

◆ We insist that consent be written for medicolegal reasons. Whenever possible, we request the expectant father's consent as well.

◆ As often as is appropriate, we try to provide *written* information to the pregnant couple. This allows them to study, discuss, and integrate it. Frequently, the anxiety about taking any medication during pregnancy interferes with the ability to process what is heard; written patient education materials are often appreciated.

One of the most organized sources of data on psychotropics in pregnancy is the handbook by Briggs et al.[13] Although by no means authoritative, it is a periodically revised sourcebook for reviewing this literature. We have tabulated some of the data relevant to psychotropics in Appendix M ("Effects of Psychotropics During Pregnancy"). *This tabulation is intended as a quick guide, not as a substitute for consulting the primary sources.*

Some notes on the data's limitations:

◆ To repeat, there are no controlled studies of the teratogenicity of psychotropics in human beings.

◆ Most analyses are *retrospective* rather than prospective. Even when data are drawn from collaborative studies assaying thousands of mother-infant pairs, correlational versus causal associations remain entangled. This methodology has implications for whether results are interpreted as "highly likely" or "probably coincidental."

◆ Beware of conclusions based on limited numbers of subjects.

◆ Agents that are teratogenic in one animal species are not necessarily teratogenic in another.

◆ Most data are uncorrected for a medication's relative usage frequency:

  • For example, Briggs et al.[13] assign imipramine (Tofranil) to risk category D, while amoxapine (Asendin) earns risk category C (see Appendix M for an explanation of these categories). Does this reflect amoxapine's truly superior teratogenic profile? Or does amoxapine's infrequent use produce fewer documented side effects than imipramine and thus the appearance of greater safety?

Choosing a medication for a pregnant patient requires a conceptual shift away from selections based on superior efficacy and toward remaining with what has been "tried and true" for the fetus. For example, the high specificity and excellent side-effect profile of the new SSRIs (e.g., fluoxetine [Prozac], sertraline [Zoloft], paroxetine [Paxil]) must be counterbalanced by the greater accumulated experience with the TCAs.

A medication's morphological teratogenicity is only one consideration; others include behavioral teratogenicity, toxicity (fetal or neonatal), and withdrawal (fetal or neonatal). Lack of maternal toxicity does not predict fetal toxicity. Several factors determine the teratogenic risks of a drug:[154]

◆ Exposure to the drug during organogenesis:
  • Central nervous system (CNS): gestational days 10–25
  • Limb development: days 24–26
  • Cardiovascular system: days 20–40
◆ Dosage
◆ Regularity of use
◆ Interaction with other environmental factors, such as other drugs, alcohol, tobacco, and other toxins
◆ Genetic constitution of the fetus

Every clinician must define his or her own approach to medicating pregnant patients. Ovulation detector kits (sold over the counter in pharmacies) may improve chances for quicker conception, reducing the medication-free interval for women who opt to discontinue psychotropic medications while trying to become pregnant.

Anxiolytics and Sedatives

Benzodiazepines

The use of benzodiazepines in pregnancy remains controversial, mainly because of contradictory findings that have both linked diazepam—the prototypical benzodiazepine—to and absolved it from an association with congenital defects. This literature has been burdened and confounded by retrospective methodology. In the 1970s, an association was found between in utero exposure to diazepam and increased rates of oral clefts,[1,125,128,129] with estimates of a 4:1 relative risk that mothers of babies with cleft lip and/or cleft palate had used first-trimester diazepam compared with mothers of infants with other birth defects.[125] However, despite the retrospective methodology, the risk was still relatively small—only 4%—in comparison with the 2% overall risk of birth defects.[125] Furthermore, this association was not corroborated by subsequent studies.[32,123,135] Concurrent substance abuse has further confounded research into benzodiazepine teratogenesis.

One of the most compelling studies was in Sweden by Laegreid et al.,[80] who in 1989 described dysmorphic features, growth retardation, and CNS defects in eight infants exposed to either diazepam ($\geq$ 30 mg/day) or oxazepam ($\geq$ 75 mg/day) throughout gestation. The mothers had been screened for substance abuse and had regular prenatal care.

◆ The mean birth weight of the infants was 1.2 standard deviations below the Swedish average, with only one child weighing above the mean. Six of the newborns had low Apgar scores (mainly due to apnea), five needed resuscitation, all were hypotonic at birth, and all had neonatal drug withdrawal with episodes of opisthotonos and convulsions. Seven of the eight infants lacked rooting and sucking reflexes, causing feeding difficulties. Most of them had craniofacial defects, such as low nasal bridge, uptilted nose, slanted eyes, and epicanthic folds. One infant with severe psychomotor retardation died of sudden infant death syndrome at 11 weeks. Six other children had varying degrees of mental retardation, some with severely disturbed visual perception and all with gross motor disability. Other possible etiologies were ruled out by extensive special examinations; the only common factor among the eight cases was maternal benzodiazepine consumption.

These findings reinforced earlier apprehensions about the safety of diazepam and other benzodiazepines in pregnancy. However, Laegreid et al.'s[80] cases were collected for study "after the fact," chosen because of the same disease stigmata, rather than prospectively evaluated. This retrospective methodology is fraught with its own risk—namely, positioning two potentially independent events as causally linked. Reassuringly, subsequent research published in 1992 by the same group[79] *failed* to confirm teratogenesis in benzodiazepine-exposed infants; sedation and withdrawal were the main side effects seen in these babies.

Additional reassuring findings emerged from a 1992 chart survey by Bergman and co-workers[12] of 104,000 women who delivered babies between 1980 and 1983.

◆ In this survey, about 2,000 women were prescribed benzodiazepines while pregnant (averaging 34 total pills or 10–150 mg of diazepam equivalents daily). Eighty took medication during the second trimester, with 40 of these exposed to benzodiazepines *throughout* pregnancy. Women with heavy benzodiazepine use had many concomitant psychiatric and medical problems, including drug abuse. Among these 80 pregnancies, there were 3 intrauterine deaths, and 2 infants with congenital abnormalities died as newborns. Twelve newborns went through drug withdrawal, with 7 possibly related to benzodiazepines. Of the 64 babies who survived, 6 had teratogenic abnormalities but none had mental retardation, oral clefts, or other features that had been reported by Laegreid and associates.[80] Bergman et al.[12] proposed that the relatively high rate of overall teratogenesis was more likely due to alcohol or other substance use than to benzodiazepine use.

In his 1993 survey, Gelenberg[41] concluded,

> Most infants born to mothers who have presumably taken high doses of benzodiazepines throughout their pregnancies are born without overt consequences . . . The best assessment at present is that *benzodiazepines probably have little if any teratogenic potential*. Of course, most of us prefer to avoid exposing a developing fetus to any unnecessary drugs, but in many instances, pharmacological intervention is less hazardous than the consequences of untreated psychiatric disorders. (pp. 2–3)

High-dose ($\geq$ 30 mg) or extended diazepam ingestion during labor and delivery may produce floppy infant syndrome and withdrawal.[13]

Data on the individual benzodiazepines follow:

◆ **Oxazepam (Serax):** This medication is an active metabolite of diazepam. As mentioned, it was implicated as causing teratogenic effects in one study,[80] but not in subsequent research.[79]

- **Lorazepam (Ativan) and alprazolam (Xanax):** The teratogenic potential of the newer anxiolytics, such as lorazepam and alprazolam, has not been definitively established,[9] but as of 1994, there were no reports of congenital abnormalities with either.[13] Preliminary findings with alprazolam show no pattern of serious adverse events when it is administered in the first trimester (in two small samples, $n = 236$[130] and $n = 542$[144]) or throughout pregnancy ($n = 10$).[37]

- **Clonazepam (Klonopin):** As of 1994, no reports linking clonazepam with congenital defects had been published.[13] Cohen et al.[20] have expressed a preference for clonazepam because its longer duration of action allows smoother tapering with little of the rebound associated with shorter-acting medications.

- **Temazepam (Restoril) and diphenhydramine (Benadryl):** Temazepam is rated X, contraindicated during pregnancy. Diphenhydramine (rated C), when combined with temazepam, may be particularly toxic in pregnancy. One mother had taken diphenhydramine 50 mg for mild itching of the skin and, about 1.3 hours later, took 30 mg of temazepam for sleep.[68] Three hours later she awoke with violent intrauterine fetal movements, which lasted several minutes and then abruptly stopped. A stillborn infant was delivered about 4 hours later, demonstrating no gross or microscopic anomalies on autopsy. In pregnant rabbits, neither drug alone caused fetal mortality, but when combined, 51 (81%) of 63 fetuses were stillborn or died shortly after birth.[68] The mechanism for this interaction is unknown.

- **Triazolam (Halcion):** The manufacturer considers this medication to be *contraindicated* during pregnancy, even though there are no data that support an association with congenital defects.[13]

Barbiturates

Barbiturates have been reported to cause growth retardation, skeletal abnormalities, cleft palate, and respiratory depression due to their accumulation at up to 75% of maternal blood levels.[50] They also are capable of producing withdrawal reactions and cross-tolerance in newborns. They are never preferred to benzodiazepines as anxiolytics in pregnant women.

Antidepressants

Tricyclic Antidepressants

The teratogenic potential of TCAs has been less controversial than that for the benzodiazepines. There has been little definitive evidence of their teratogenicity; most experts consider the tricyclics tried, true, and safe in pregnancy.[20,22,63,77,88]

- Although occasional early reports linked the tricyclics with congenital defects, such as limb anomalies, most of the evidence suggests relative safety during pregnancy.[13] However, these medications are classified in risk category D:[13] "There is positive evidence of human fetal risk, but the benefits may be acceptable despite the risk (e.g., if the drug is needed in a life-threatening situation, or for a serious disease for which safer drugs cannot be used or are ineffective)" (p. xx). Despite this admonition, tricyclics have been used safely in modified doses, with informed consent, plasma concentration monitoring, and in collaboration with an obstetrician.[163]

Some still argue, however, that tricyclics should be restricted to the second or third trimester, and then be given only if absolutely necessary.[61] L. S. Cohen (personal communication, March 1992) has commented,

> The literature suggesting increased rates of limb reduction abnormalities in the setting of in utero exposure to tricyclics is extremely weak and anecdotal. This has been followed by a large series of patients followed during pregnancy, some of whom had tricyclic exposure. These data do not support the association, . . . and use of tricyclic antidepressants during pregnancy has become the treatment of choice for many women with recurrent affective disorder who demonstrate a need for antidepressant pharmacotherapy before, during, and after pregnancy.

It remains for the individual clinician to judge the level of acceptable risk for an individual patient.

Note: The progressive physiological changes of pregnancy require dose *increases;* pregnancy reduces protein-binding capacity, enhances hepatic metabolism, causes progesterone-induced decline in gastrointestinal motility (reducing absorption), and increases the volume of distribution.[35,76] Wisner and colleagues[174] showed that required tricyclic doses increased during the second half of pregnancy; during the final trimester, the mean required dose was 1.6 times that needed during the nonpregnant state.

If clinically feasible, decrease the tricyclic dosage before delivery to lessen the risk of neonatal withdrawal. If a severe neonatal withdrawal syndrome develops, the infant can be given a low dose of antidepressant and gradually tapered off the drug[88] (see section on Neonatal Toxicity).

Nortriptyline and desipramine care the preferred tricyclics for pregnant patients because of their low anticholinergicity and availability of serum monitoring.[20,38,134]

Newer Antidepressants

Fluoxetine. A prospective study on 128 pregnant women showed no increase in congenital anomalies after first-trimester fluoxetine (Prozac) use.[109] There was a nonsignificant increased risk for miscarriage on fluoxetine, however. There are no studies yet on the long-term effects of in utero exposure to fluoxetine or other SSRIs. Fluoxetine has proven quite effective for postpartum depression.[124] However, fluoxetine has been associated with neonatal toxicity,[143] with reversible CNS irritability and increased heart and respiratory rates.

Newer SSRIs. There are no human studies yet available on the newer SSRIs in pregnancy.

Bupropion. In a 1985–1992 surveillance study, three newborns exposed to first-trimester bupropion (Wellbutrin) were without major birth defects.[13] Obviously, these numbers are too small to draw any conclusions about bupropion's safety.

Monoamine Oxidase Inhibitors

First-trimester monoamine oxidase inhibitor (MAOI) exposure has been associated with an increased risk of malformations.[13,62] So little is known about the use of MAOIs in pregnancy that some have recommended against such use.[156]

Electroconvulsive Therapy

ECT has been safely used to treat psychotic depression[119,120,170] and mania,[81] where aggressive intervention was crucial to the well-being of mother and unborn child. ECT may be safer to the first-trimester fetus than long-term pharmacotherapy, but controlled studies are lacking.[119] In general, recent case reports support ECT for all three trimesters of pregnancy.[4] The teratogenic risk of barbiturate anesthesia is not well understood, but brief exposure is unlikely to be a problem.[4] Developmental follow-up of children who were exposed in utero to ECT has revealed no abnormalities.[39,65,142] It is possible to continue breast feeding during ECT.[154] It does not increase the incidence of premature labor in normal pregnancies.

The American Psychiatric Association's[4] recommendations for safely administering ECT during pregnancy follow:

- A complete physical and pelvic examination
- An obstetrician on the treatment team
- Fetal monitoring when gestational age is beyond 10 weeks
- Intubation for advanced pregnancy because of the increased risk of gastric reflux and subsequent aspiration

In two comprehensive 1994 reviews of ECT during pregnancy, Miller[89] and Walker and Swartz[162] formulated additional guidelines:

Before the Procedure:

- Perform a pelvic examination, looking for vaginal bleeding and/or cervical dilatation.
- Discontinue nonessential anticholinergic medication, to avoid excessive delay in gastric emptying. (Pregnancy prolongs gastric emptying time.)
- Check for contractions prior to ECT via uterine tocodynamometry.
- Hydrate intravenously with lactated Ringer's or normal saline solution.
- Give 30 ml of 0.3M sodium citrate (a nonparticulate antacid) by mouth about 15–20 minutes before anesthesia. (This minimizes the risk of pneumonitis secondary to gastric regurgitation and pulmonary aspiration during ECT.)
- Diminish the risk of aspiration by applying pressure on the cricoid cartilage while the patient is anesthetized.
- Test for pseudocholinesterase activity with a succinylcholine substrate.

During the Procedure:

- If the woman is more than 20 weeks pregnant, place a pillow or rolled-up sheet under her **right** hip to displace the uterus to the **left.**
- Add external fetal cardiac monitoring. If fetal heart rate slows, consider increasing O_2 and further displacing the uterus to the left.

♦ Intubate if the pregnancy is beyond the first trimester.
♦ Avoid excessive hyperventilation.

After the Procedure:

♦ Recheck for uterine contractions with tocody-namometry. Observe the mother in the labor and delivery suite if contractions are recurrent. Give tocolytic therapy (which inhibits contractions) when indicated.
♦ Recheck for vaginal bleeding.
♦ Examine a nonstress test after each treatment. "Nonreactive" tests should be followed up with a contraction stress test.
♦ Obtain weekly Doppler imaging of the umbilical artery for gestations after the 25th week if uteroplacental insufficiency is suspected.

Use ECT with caution in *high-risk* pregnancy, such as premature labor, incompetent cervix, multiple pregnancy, hydramnios, antepartum hemorrhage, maternal hypertension including preeclampsia, maternal diabetes, renal disease, RH isoimmunization, and maternal cardiac disease.[99] Successful ECT can be performed in high-risk pregnancy if special precautions are taken.[170]

Miscellaneous Treatments

Sleep deprivation. Partial sleep deprivation improved Hamilton Rating Scale for Depression[53b] scores in three women with postpartum psychotic depression.[157] Patients became either transiently manic or hypomanic. After recovery sleep, each subject was less manic but required further treatment with mood-stabilizing agents.

Light therapy. Light therapy may be potentially useful, but we could locate no studies on its use in pregnancy.[127]

Conclusions

In her excellent 1994 review, Miller[88] concluded:

> Antidepressant agents of choice during pregnancy are desipramine and nortriptyline, due to the comparative wealth of data about them, the ability to monitor serum levels, and a favorable side-effect profile. Fluoxetine is a reasonable alternative if tricyclic agents are less effective or less well tolerated by a given patient, or if the patient is already taking fluoxetine. (p. 72)

For women unwilling to undertake even this level of risk, we recommend ECT.

Neonatal Toxicity

Medications have sequelae other than structural defects. Because psychoactive drugs and metabolites pass freely through the placenta to the fetus, whose blood-brain barrier is relatively open in early gestation, neonatal toxicity can result.[45,93]

♦ For example, Misri and Sivertz[92] reported that eight of nine infants whose mothers were on tricyclic drugs at delivery showed withdrawal symptoms, including *irritability, transient cyanosis, hypotonia, poor sucking, and tachypnea.* Infants born to mothers on more than 150 mg of tricyclics per day showed jaundice and severe withdrawal symptoms, perhaps due to the relative immaturity of the neonatal liver. All symptoms resolved in 3–6 days. Infants born to mothers whose tricyclics had been discontinued 4–7 days prior to delivery showed *negligible withdrawal symptoms.*
♦ These "tricyclic babies" exposed to TCAs in utero had normal developmental parameters at 3-year follow-up, including motor skills and behavioral development.
♦ Of concern is one report[116] of fetal tachyarrhythmias with the highly anticholinergic tricyclic dothiepin. The authors warned that other tricyclics may lead to similar adverse effects in the fetus and newborn.
♦ Neonatal toxicity similar to that with other tricyclics has been reported for clomipramine (Anafranil).[131]
♦ Toxicity in a neonate has been described with fluoxetine,[143] with CNS irritability and increased heart and respiratory rates. Fortunately, there were no sequelae.

The secondary amines (nortriptyline [Pamelor/Aventyl] or desipramine [Norpramin]) are the tricyclics of choice[20] because they allow for plasma monitoring and produce fewer maternal and neonatal anticholinergic effects such as urinary retention or bowel obstruction.[38,134]

Ideally, reduce tricyclics before delivery to minimize neonatal withdrawal. However, weigh the risk of the mother's psychiatric relapse against the benefits of avoiding neonatal withdrawal. If withdrawal symptoms are severe, the infant can be given a low dose of antidepressant and then gradually tapered off the medication.[88]

Breast Feeding

Medication after delivery has been shown to reduce postpartum major depression.[174a] Antidepressants are secreted into the breast milk at different concentrations and with variable neonatal effects. Approximately 10% of the maternal TCA concentration crosses to the milk.[92] The impact of these trace amounts on the infant are controversial.

◆ One study found no detectable levels of desipramine or its metabolite 2-hydroxydesipramine in a breast-feeding infant whose mother was ingesting 300 mg/day, even though it was estimated that the infant was consuming 1/100 of the maternal dose (6 mg/kg).[145]

◆ Other studies found no detectable serum levels in nursing infants of mothers taking amitriptyline[6,12a] or clomipramine.[173]

◆ None of seven breast-feeding infants whose mothers were taking nortriptyline had detectable levels of nortriptyline, but two of four infants developed low concentrations of 10-hydroxynortriptyline.[172] No immediate adverse effects were observed.

◆ Fluoxetine and its metabolite norfluoxetine were found in breast milk at one-quarter to one-fifth the serum concentration.[66]

◆ A few studies on newer antidepressants and breast feeding have begun to appear.[3a]

Adverse consequences are rare, but do occur:

◆ An 8-week-old nursing infant's respiratory depression seemed to correlate with the mother's desmethyl metabolite of doxepin after her dose had been raised from 10 to 75 mg/day; doxepin itself was undetectable in the child's serum.[84]

◆ Fluoxetine was found to be above adult therapeutic levels in a 3-week-old baby of a nursing mother who was taking 20 mg/day.[82] The baby suffered colic (constant crying, sleep disturbance, frequent vomiting, watery stools) while breast feeding, which resolved when switched to a bottle. It could not be determined if other constituents of the breast milk caused the colic.

The decision concerning breast feeding is a complicated one, especially since safe exposure levels to any agent are difficult to establish for an infant. The available information does not warrant absolute recommendations. For women on tricyclics still wishing to breast-feed, the baby's serum tricyclic levels assist in making an informed choice.[88] However, Misri and Sivertz[92] have commented,

Some authors suggest that since the amount of TCAs found in breast milk are very small, there is no risk to the infant, and the mother can be allowed to continue to breast-feed. Other authors believe that, regardless of the amount of drug in the breast milk, there may be long-term effects on the infant, because of possible effects on the neurotransmitter system [and the developing brain] . . . [B]rain concentrations can be ten to thirty times greater than serum concentrations. (p. 169)

Bader and Newman[6] have suggested that there may be unidentified risks of TCAs in the neonate because of accumulation, slow or absent detoxification, enzyme induction, and limited drug excretion.

To further complicate matters, when mothers with a history of unipolar depression insist on medication-free breast feeding, they increase their risk of relapse and hospitalization.[92] Misri and Sivertz[92] have taken the following position:

It is our goal to treat all patients on an outpatient basis to avoid disruption of the family, foster bonding between mother and infant, prevent the psychosocial problems associated with hospitalization for a psychiatric disorder, and to minimize health care costs. From this perspective, it would seem preferable to treat clinically depressed nursing mothers with TCAs (either with or without continuation of breast feeding), rather than to risk an exacerbation of symptoms necessitating maternal-infant separation for inpatient treatment, and ultimately resulting in discontinuation of breast feeding, and treatment with TCAs. Based on the growing information that it is safe to breast-feed during treatment with TCA, we have adopted an attitude of informed and cautious encouragement. (p. 169, italics added)

Note, however, that the American Academy of Pediatrics classifies most antidepressants as "drugs whose effects on the nursing infant is unknown but may be of concern" (p. xx).[13] For benzodiazepines, the risks of infant weight loss, neonatal flaccidity, and respiratory depression are scattered throughout the literature.[13] Breast feeding on tricyclics should be avoided for infants who are preterm, or who have cardiac or neurological problems. Patients who require unusually high doses of tricyclics or complex drug regimens should probably not breast-feed at all.

⚜ SUMMARY

1. The goal of psychiatric management is to minimize risk to the fetus and mother.

2. Routinely inquire about oral contraceptives in depressed women of childbearing age, and hormone replacement therapy in menopausal patients. Consider switching to a preparation containing less progestin.

3. The postpartum blues are loosely defined and of ambiguous etiology. They may lie along a continuum with affective illness or be a nonspecific response to a psychobiological stressor. Premenstrual dysphoria, prior episodes of depression, or depression during the pregnancy predispose to the blues. Demographics, physiological variables, obstetric factors, and stressful life events are inconsistently related to risk. The blues are usually transitory and rarely require treatment.

4. Postpartum major depression may be misattributed to situational stress or to "raging hormones." Although the risk of suicide during the first year after childbirth is lower than that for the general female population, major depression before, during, or after pregnancy is never benign. There are adverse effects on both mother and infant.

5. Pregnancy provides no meaningful protection from panic attacks. Pharmacological intervention is reserved for those women at risk for becoming seriously disabled.

6. Psychopharmacological strategies are summarized in Appendix N ("Guidelines for Using Psychotropics During Pregnancy").

7. Diazepam (Valium) and oxazepam (Serax) have been linked inconsistently with congenital defects, raising concerns about other benzodiazepines. To date, however, the benzodiazepines clonazepam (Klonopin), lorazepam (Ativan), and alprazolam (Xanax) have no teratogenic past. Triazolam (Halcion), and temazepam (Restoril) with diphenhydramine (Benadryl) have been rated "absolutely contraindicated" in pregnancy.

8. The teratogenicity of the tricyclic antidepressants (TCAs) has been less controversial than that of the benzodiazepines. Among the TCAs, desipramine (Norpramin) and nortriptyline (Pamelor, Aventyl)

are preferred. We know of only one study of first-trimester fluoxetine in which it was found safe and effective. Adverse effects in nursing infants have been reported only rarely, but there are no controlled studies or long-term data.

9. The physiological changes of pregnancy require progressive dose increases in order to maintain steady serum levels. If clinically feasible, the medication should be reduced before delivery to minimize neonatal withdrawal or toxicity.

10. Electroconvulsive therapy (ECT) has a good therapeutic track record in pregnant patients.

⚜ REFERENCES

1. Aarskog D: Association between maternal intake of diazepam and oral clefts (letter). Lancet 2:921, 1975

2. Adams P, Rose D, Folkard J, et al: Effect of pyridoxine on depression associated with oral contraceptives. Lancet 1:897–904, 1973

3. Albright A: Postpartum depression: an overview. Journal of Counseling and Development 71:316–320, 1993

3a. Altshuler L, Burt V, McMullen M, et al: Breastfeeding and sertraline: a 24-hour analysis. J Clin Psychiatry 56:243–245, 1995

3b. American Psychiatric Association: Diagnostic and Statistical Manual of Mental Disorders, 3rd Edition. Washington, DC, American Psychiatric Association, 1980

3c. American Psychiatric Association: Diagnostic and Statistical Manual of Mental Disorders, 4th Edition. Washington, DC, American Psychiatric Association, 1994

4. American Psychiatric Association: The Practice of Electroconvulsive Therapy: Recommendations for Treatment, Training, and Privileging (A Task Force Report of the American Psychiatric Association). Washington, DC, American Psychiatric Association, 1990

5. Appleby L: Suicide during pregnancy and in the first postnatal year. BMJ 302:137–140, 1991

6. Bader T, Newman K: Amitriptyline in human breast milk and the nursing infant's serum. Am J Psychiatry 137:855–856, 1980

7. Ballinger C, Buckley D, Naylor G, et al: Emotional disturbance following childbirth: clinical findings and urinary excretion of cyclic AMP. Psychol Med 36:293–300, 1979

8. Ballinger C, Kay D, Naylor G, et al: Some biochemical findings during pregnancy and after delivery in relation to mood change. Psychol Med 12:549–556, 1982

9. Barry W, St. Clair S: Exposure to benzodiazepines in utero (letter). Lancet 1:1436–1437, 1987

10. Beck CT: The lived experience of postpartum depression: a phenomenological study. Nurs Res 41:166–170, 1992

11. Benjamin J, Benjamin M: Panic disorder and pregnancy (letter). J Clin Psychiatry 56:36, 1995

12. Bergman U, Rosa F, Baum C, et al: Effects of exposure to benzodiazepine during fetal life. Lancet 340:694–696, 1992

12a. Breyer-Pfaff U, Nell K, Entenmann A, et al: Secretion of amitriptyline and metabolites into breast milk (letter). Am J Psychiatry 152:812–813, 1995

13. Briggs G, Freeman R, Yaffe S: Drugs in Pregnancy and Lactation, 4th Edition. Baltimore, MD, Williams & Wilkins, 1994

14. Campbell S, Cohn J, Flanagan C, et al: Course and correlates of postpartum depression during the transition to parenthood. Development and Psychopathology 4:29–47, 1992

15. Carroll B, Steiner M: The psychobiology of premenstrual dysphoria. Psychoneuroendocrinology 3:171–180, 1978

16. Coble P, Reynolds C, Kupfer D, et al: Childbearing in women with and without a history of affective disorder, I: psychiatric symptomatology. Compr Psychiatry 35:205–214, 1994

17. Coble P, Reynolds C, Kupfer D, et al: Childbearing in women with and without a history of affective disorder, II: electroencephalographic sleep. Compr Psychiatry 35:215–224, 1994

18. Cogill S, Caplan H, Alexandra H, et al: Impact of maternal depression on cognitive development of young children. BMJ 292:1165–1166, 1986

19. Cohen L, Heller V, Kelley K: Course of panic disorder in 24 pregnant women. Paper presented at the 142nd annual meeting of the American Psychiatric Association. San Francisco, CA, May 6–12, 1989

20. Cohen L, Heller V, Rosenbaum J: Treatment guidelines for psychotropic drug use in pregnancy. Psychosomatics 30:25–33, 1989

21. Cohen L, Rosenbaum J, Heller V: Panic attack–associated placental abruption: a case report. J Clin Psychiatry 50:266–267, 1989

22. Cohen L, Rosenbaum J, Heller V: Psychotropic drug use in pregnancy, in The Practitioner's Guide to Psychoactive Drugs, 3rd Edition. Edited by Gelenberg A, Bassuk E, Schoonover S. New York, Plenum Medical Book, 1991, pp 389–405

23. Cohen L, Sichel D, Dimmock J, et al: Impact of pregnancy on panic disorder: a case series. J Clin Psychiatry 55:284–288, 1994

24. Cohen L, Sichel D, Dimmock J, et al: Postpartum course in women with preexisting panic disorder. J Clin Psychiatry 55:289–292, 1994

25. Condon J, Watson T: The maternity blues: exploration of a psychological hypothesis. Acta Psychiatr Scand 76:164–171, 1987

26. Cowley D, Roy-Byrne P: Panic disorder during pregnancy. Journal of Psychosomatic Obstetrics and Gynaecology 10:193–210, 1989

27. Cox J, Connor Y, Kendell R: Prospective study of the psychiatric disorders of childbirth. Br J Psychiatry 140:111–117, 1982

28. Cox J, Holden J, Sagovsky R: Detection of postnatal depression. Development of the 10-item Edinburgh Postnatal Depression Scale. Br J Psychiatry 150:782–786, 1987

29. Cox J, Murray D, Chapman G: A controlled study of the onset, duration, and prevalence of postnatal depression. Br J Psychiatry 163:27–31, 1993

30. Cullberg J: Mood changes and menstrual symptoms with different gestagen/estrogen combinations: a double blind comparison with placebo. Acta Psychiatr Scand Suppl 236:1–86, 1972

31. Cutrona C: Causal attributions and perinatal depression. J Abnorm Psychol 92:161–172, 1983

32. Czeizel A, Lendvay A: In utero exposure to benzodiazepines (letter). Lancet 1:628, 1987

33. Davidson J: Post partum mood changes in Jamaican women; a description and discussion on its significance. Br J Psychiatry 121:659–663, 1972

34. Dean C, Williams R, Brockington I: Is puerperal psychosis the same as bipolar manic-depressive disorder? a family study. Psychol Med 19:637–647, 1989

35. Eadie M, Lander C, Tyrer J: Plasma drug monitoring in pregnancy. Clin Pharmacokinet 2:427–436, 1977

36. Edwards D, Porter S, Stein G: A pilot study of postnatal depression following caesarean section using two retrospective self-rating instruments. J Psychosom Res 38:111–117, 1994

37. Edwards J, Inman W, Pearce G, et al: Prescription-event monitoring of 10,895 patients treated with alprazolam. Br J Psychiatry 158:387–392, 1991

38. Falterman L, Richardson D: Small left colon syndrome associated with maternal ingestion of psychotropics. J Pediatr 97:300–310, 1980

39. Forssman H: Follow-up of sixteen children whose mothers were given electroconvulsive therapy during gestation. Acta Psychiatr Neurol Scand 30:437–441, 1955

39a. Frautschi S, Cerulli A, Maine D: Suicide during pregnancy and its neglect as a component of maternal mortality. Int J Gynaecol Obstet 47:275–284, 1994

40. Gard P, Handley S, Parsons A, et al: A multivariate investigation of postpartum mood disturbances. Br J Psychiatry 148:567–575, 1986

41. Gelenberg A: Benzodiazepines: not teratogenic? Biological Therapies in Psychiatry Newsletter 16:2–3, 1993

42. George A, Sandler M: Endocrine and biochemical studies in puerperal mental disorders, in Motherhood and Mental Illness 2: Causes and Consequences. Edited by Kumar R, Brockington I. London, Wright, 1988, pp 78–112

43. George A, Wilson K: Monoamine oxidase activity and the puerperal blues syndrome. J Psychosom Res 25:409–413, 1981

44. George D, Ladenheim J, Nutt D: Effect of pregnancy on panic attacks. Am J Psychiatry 144:1078–1079, 1987

45. Gingserg J: The placenta and psychotropic drugs (report of meeting: Psychotropic Drugs in Pregnancy, Infancy, Childhood). Br J Psychiatry 132:200–201, 1978

46. Gitlin M, Pasnau R: Psychiatric syndromes linked to reproductive function in women: a review of current knowledge. Am J Psychiatry 146:1413–1422, 1989

47. Glick I, Bennett S: Psychiatric complications of progesterone and oral contraceptives. J Clin Psychopharmacol 1:350–367, 1982

48. Glover V: Do biochemical factors play a part in postnatal depression? Prog Neuropsychopharmacol Biol Psychiatry 16:605–615, 1992

49. Glover V, Liddle P, Taylor A, et al: Mild hypomania (the highs) can be a feature of the first postpartum week: association with later depression. Br J Psychiatry 164:517–521, 1994

50. Goldberg H, DiMascio A: Psychotropic drugs in pregnancy, in Psychopharmacology: A Generation of Progress. Edited by Lipton M, DiMascio A, Killam K. New York, Raven, 1978, pp 1047–1055

51. Goldman L: The use of hypnosis in obstetrics. Psychiatr Med 10:53–67, 1992

52. Gotlib I, Whiffen V, Wallace P, et al: Prospective investigation of postpartum depression: factors involved in onset and recovery. J Abnorm Psychol 100:122–132, 1991

53. Grant E, Pryse-Davies J: Effects of oral contraceptives on endometrial monoamine oxidase and phosphates. BMJ 3:777–780, 1968

53a. Green M: Diagnosis, management, and implications of maternal depression for children and pediatricians. Curr Opin Pediatr 6:525–529, 1994

53b. Hamilton M: A rating scale for depression. J Neurol Neurosurg Psychiatry 23:56–62, 1960

54. Handley S, Dunn T, Waldron G, et al: Tryptophan, cortisol and puerperal mood. Br J Psychiatry 136:498–508, 1980

55. Hannah P, Adams D, Glover V, et al: Abnormal platelet 5-hydroxytryptamine uptake and imipramine binding in postnatal dysphoria. J Psychiatr Res 26:69–75, 1992

56. Hannah P, Adams D, Lee A, et al: Links between early postpartum mood and post-natal depression. Br J Psychiatry 160:777–780, 1992

57. Harris B: Prospective trial of L-tryptophan in maternity blues. Br J Psychiatry 137:233–235, 1980

58. Harris B: A hormonal component to postnatal depression. Br J Psychiatry 163:403–405, 1993

59. Harris B, Fung H, Johns S, et al: Transient postpartum thyroid dysfunction and postnatal depression. J Affect Disord 17:243–249, 1989

60. Harris B, Lovett L, Newcombe R, et al: Maternity blues and major endocrine changes: Cardiff puerperal mood and hormone study II. BMJ 308:949–953, 1994

61. Hauser L: Pregnancy and psychotropic drugs. Hosp Community Psychiatry 36:817–818, 1985

61a. Hay D, Kumar R: Interpreting the effects of mothers' postnatal depression on children's intelligence: a critique and re-analysis. Child Psychiatry Hum Dev 25:165–181, 1995

62. Heinonen O, Slone D, Shapiro S: Birth Defects and Drugs in Pregnancy. Littleton, MA, PSG, 1977

63. Idanpaan-Heikkila J, Saxen L: Possible teratogenicity of imipramine-chloropyramine. Lancet 2:282–284, 1973

64. Iles S, Gath D, Kennerly H: Maternity blues, II: a comparison between post-operative women and post-natal women. Br J Psychiatry 155:363–366, 1989

65. Impastato D, Gabriel A, Landaro H: Electric and insulin shock therapy during pregnancy. J Nerv Ment Dis 25:542–546, 1964

66. Isenberg K: Excretion of fluoxetine in human breast milk (letter). J Clin Psychiatry 51:169, 1990

67. Jarrahi-Zadeh A, Kane F, Van der Castle R, et al: Emotional and cognitive changes in pregnancy and the early puerperium. Br J Psychiatry 115:797–805, 1969

68. Kargas G, Kargas S, Bruyere HJ, et al: Perinatal mortality due to interaction of diphenhydramine and temazepam (letter). N Engl J Med 313:1417–1418, 1985

69. Kelly A, Deakin B: Postnatal depression and antenatal morbidity (letter). Br J Psychiatry 161:579–581, 1992

70. Kendell R: Suicide in pregnancy and the puerperium. BMJ 302:126–127, 1991

71. Kendell R, Mackenzie W, West C, et al: Day to day changes after childbirth: further data. Br J Psychiatry 145:620–625, 1984

72. Kendell R, μguire R, Conner Y, et al: Mood changes in the first three weeks after childbirth. J Affect Disord 3:317–326, 1981

73. Kennerly H, Gath D: Maternity blues, I: detection and measurement by questionnaire. Br J Psychiatry 155:356–362, 1989

74. Kennerly H, Gath D: Maternity blues, III: associations with obstetric, psychological and psychiatric factors. Br J Psychiatry 155:367–373, 1989

75. Klein D: Commentary: pregnancy and panic disorder. J Clin Psychiatry 55:293–294, 1994

76. Knott C, Reynolds F: Therapeutic drug monitoring in pregnancy. Clin Pharmacokinet 19:425–433, 1990

77. Kuenssberg E, Knox J: Imipramine in pregnancy. BMJ 2:292, 1972

77a. Kumar R: Postnatal mental illness: a transcultural perspective. Soc Psychiatry Psychiatr Epidemiol 29:250–264, 1994

77b. Kumar R, Marks M, Platz C, et al: Clinical survey of a psychiatric mother and baby unit: characteristics of 100 consecutive admissions. J Affect Disord 33:11–22, 1995

78. Kumar R, Robson K: A prospective study of emotional disorders in childbearing women. Br J Psychiatry 144:35–47, 1984

79. Laegreid L, Hagberg G, Lundberg A: The effect of benzodiazepines on the fetus and the newborn. Neuropediatrics 23:18–23, 1992

80. Laegreid L, Olegard R, Wahlstrom J, et al: Teratogenic effects of benzodiazepine use during pregnancy. J Pediatr 114:126–131, 1989

81. LaGrone D: ECT in secondary mania, pregnancy, and sickle cell anemia. Convulsive Therapy 6:176–180, 1990

82. Lester B, et al: Possible association between fluoxetine hydrochloride and colic in an infant. J Am Acad Child Adolesc Psychiatry 32:1253–1255, 1993

83. Levy V: The maternity blues in post-partum and post-operative women. Br J Psychiatry 151:368–372, 1987

84. Matheson I, Pande H, Alertsen A: Respiratory depression caused by N-desmethyldoxepin in breast milk (letter). Lancet 2:1124, 1985

85. McIntosh J: Postpartum depression: women's help-seeking behaviour and perceptions of cause. J Adv Nurs 18:178–184, 1993

86. Metz A, Sichel D, Goff D: Postpartum panic disorder. J Clin Psychiatry 49:278–279, 1988

87. Metz A, Stump K, Cowen P, et al: Changes in platelet alpha-2 adrenoreceptor binding postpartum: possible relation to maternity blues. Lancet 1:495–498, 1983

88. Miller L: Psychiatric medication during pregnancy: understanding and minimizing risks. Psychiatric Annals 24:69–75, 1994

89. Miller L: Use of electroconvulsive therapy during pregnancy. Hosp Community Psychiatry 45:444–450, 1994

90. Millis J, Kornblith P: Fragile beginnings: identification and treatment of postpartum disorders. Health Soc Work 17:192–199, 1992

91. Mishell D: The pharmacologic and metabolic effects of oral contraceptives. Int J Fertil 34 (suppl):21–26, 1989

92. Misri S, Sivertz K: Tricyclic drugs in pregnancy and lactation: a preliminary report. Int J Psychiatry Med 21:157–171, 1991

92a. Montgomery S, sberg M: A new depression scale designed to be sensitive to change. Br J Psychiatry 134:382–389, 1979

93. Moya F, Thornbike V: Passage of drugs across the placenta. Am J Obstet Gynecol 84:1778–1798, 1962

94. Murad F, Kuret J: Estrogens and progestins, in Goodman and Gilman's The Pharmacological Basis of Therapeutics, 8th Edition. Edited by Gilman A, Rall T, Nies A, et al. New York, Pergamon, 1990, pp 1384–1412

94a. Murray D, Cox J, Chapman G, et al: Childbirth: Life event or start of a long-term difficulty? further data from the Stoke-on-Trent controlled study of postnatal depression. Br J Psychiatry 166:595–600, 1995

95. Murray L: The impact of postnatal depression on infant development. J Child Psychol Psychiatry 33:543–561, 1992

96. Neziroglu F, Anemone R, Yaryura T: Onset of obsessive-compulsive disorder in pregnancy. Am J Psychiatry 149:947–950, 1992

97. Northcott C, Stein M: Panic disorder in pregnancy. J Clin Psychiatry 55:539–542, 1994

98. Nott P, Franklin M, Armitage C, et al: Hormonal changes and mood in the puerperium. Br J Psychiatry 128:379–383, 1976

99. Nurnberg H: An overview of somatic treatment of psychosis during pregnancy and postpartum. Gen Hosp Psychiatry 11:328–338, 1989

100. O'Hara M: Social support, life events and depression during pregnancy and the puerperium. Arch Gen Psychiatry 43:569–573, 1986

101. O'Hara M: Post-partum "blues," depression, and psychosis: a review. Journal of Psychosomatic Obstetrics and Gynaecology 7:205–227, 1987

102. O'Hara M, Neunaber D, Zekoski E: Prospective study of postpartum depression: prevalence, course, and predictive factors. J Abnorm Psychol 93:158–171, 1984

103. O'Hara M, Rehm L, Campbell S: Predicting depressive symptomatology. J Abnorm Psychol 91:457–461, 1982

104. O'Hara M, Schlechte J, Lewis D, et al: Controlled prospective study of postpartum mood disorders: Psychological, environmental, and hormonal variables. J Abnorm Psychol 100:63–73, 1991

105. O'Hara M, Schlechte J, Lewis D, et al: Prospective study of postpartum blues. Biologic and psychosocial factors. Arch Gen Psychiatry 48:801–806, 1991

106. O'Hara M, Zekoski E: Postpartum depression: a comprehensive review, in Motherhood and Mental Illness. Edited by Kumar R, Brockington I. London, Butterworth, 1988, pp 17–63

107. O'Hara M, Zekoski E, Philipps L, et al: A controlled prospective study of postpartum mood disorders. J Abnorm Psychol 99:3–15, 1990

108. Parry B, Rush A: Oral contraceptives and depressive symptomatology: biologic mechanisms. Compr Psychiatry 20:347–358, 1979

109. Pastuszak A, Schick-Boschetto B, Zuber C, et al: Pregnancy outcome following first-trimester exposure to fluoxetine (Prozac). JAMA 269:2246–2248, 1993

110. Paykel E, Emms E, Fletcher J, et al: Life events and social support in puerperal depression. Br J Psychiatry 136:336–346, 1980

111. Petersen J: Obstetrics and gynecology, in Psychiatric Care of the Medical Patient. Edited by Stoudemire A, Fogel B. New York, Oxford University Press, 1993, pp 637–656

112. Philipps L, O'Hara M: Prospective study of postpartum depression: 4½-year follow-up of women and children. J Abnorm Psychol 100:151–155, 1991

113. Pitt B: "Atypical" depression following childbirth. Br J Psychiatry 114:1325–1335, 1968

114. Pitt B: "Maternity blues." Br J Psychiatry 122:431–433, 1973

114a. Pons G, Rey E, Matheson I: Excretion of psychoactive drugs into breast milk: pharmacokinetic principles and recommendations. Clin Pharmacokinet 27:270–289, 1994

115. Pop V, de Rooy H, Vader H, et al: Postpartum thyroid dysfunction and depression in an unselected population (letter). N Engl J Med 324:1815–1816, 1991

116. Prentice A, Brown R: Fetal tachyarrhythmia and maternal antidepressant treatment (letter). BMJ 298:190, 1989

117. Protheroe C: Puerperal psychoses: a long-term study 1927–1961. Br J Psychiatry 115:9–30, 1969

118. Raphael B, Martinek N: Social contexts affecting women's well-being in pregnancy and postpartum (comment). Med J Aust 161:463–464, 1994

118a. Raskin A, Schulterbrandt J, Reatig N, et al: Differential response to chlorpromazine, imipramine and placebo: a study of subgroups of hospitalized depressed patients. Arch Gen Psychiatry 23:164–173, 1970

119. Remick R, Maurice W: ECT in pregnancy (letter). Am J Psychiatry 135:761–762, 1978

120. Repke J, Berger N: Electroconvulsive therapy in pregnancy. Obstet Gynecol 63 (suppl):39–40, 1984

121. Robinson L, Walker J, Anderson D: Cognitive-behavioural treatment of panic disorder during pregnancy and lactation. Can J Psychiatry 37:623–626, 1992

122. Rose D, Strong R, Adams P, et al: Experimental vitamin B6 deficiency and the effect of estrogen containing oral contraceptives on tryptophan metabolism and vitamin B6 requirements. Clin Sci 42:465–477, 1972

123. Rosenberg L, Mitchell A, Parsells J, et al: Lack of relation of oral clefts to diazepam use during pregnancy. N Engl J Med 309:1282–1285, 1983

124. Roy A, Cole K, Goldman Z, et al: Fluoxetine treatment of postpartum depression (letter). Am J Psychiatry 150:273, 1993

125. Safra M, Oakley G: Association between cleft lip with or without cleft palate and prenatal exposure to diazepam. Lancet 2:478–540, 1975

126. Saks B, Frank J, Lowe T, et al: Depressed mood during pregnancy and the puerperium: clinical recognition and implications for clinical practice. Am J Psychiatry 142:728–731, 1985

127. Sandyk R: Postpartum psychosis and the pineal gland. Int J Neurosci 62:101–105, 1992

128. Saxen I: Association between oral clefts and drugs taken during pregnancy. Int J Epidemiol 4:37–44, 1975

129. Saxen I, Saxen L: Association between maternal intake of diazepam and oral clefts (letter). Lancet 2:498, 1975

130. Schick-Boschetto B, Zuber C: Alprazolam exposure during early human pregnancy (abstract 26). Teratology 45:460, 1992

131. Schimmell M, Katz E, Shaag Y, et al: Toxic neonatal effects following maternal clomipramine therapy. Clinical Toxicology 29:479–484, 1991

132. Schopf J, Bryois C, Jonquiere M, et al: A family hereditary study of postpartum "psychoses." Eur Arch Psychiatry Neurol Sci 235:164–170, 1985

133. Schweitzer R, Logan G, Strassberg D: The relationship between marital intimacy and postnatal depression. Australian Journal of Marriage and Family 13:19–23, 1992

133a. Seguin L, Potvin L, St-Denis M, et al: Chronic stressors, social support, and depression during pregnancy. Obstet Gynecol 85:583–589, 1995

134. Shearer W, Schreiner R, Marshall R: Urinary retention in a neonate secondary to maternal ingestion of nortriptyline. J Pediatr 81:570–572, 1972

135. Shiono P, Mills J: Oral clefts and diazepam use during pregnancy (letter). N Engl J Med 311:919–920, 1984

136. Sholomskas D, Wickamaratne P, Dogolo L, et al: Postpartum onset of panic disorder: a coincidental event? J Clin Psychiatry 54:476–480, 1993

137. Sholomskas D, Wickamaratne P, Woods S, et al: Panic disorder and pregnancy (letter, reply). J Clin Psychiatry 56:36, 1995

138. Shoupe D, Mishell D: Norplant: Subdermal implant system for long-term contraception. Am J Obstet Gynecol 160:1286–1292, 1989

139. Sichel D, Cohen L, Rosenbaum J, et al: Postpartum onset of obsessive-compulsive disorder. Psychosomatics 34:277–279, 1993

140. Slap G: Oral contraceptives and depression. J Adolesc Health Care 2:53–64, 1981

141. Small R, Astbury J, Brown S, et al: Depression after childbirth: does social context matter? Med J Aust 161:473–477, 1994

142. Sobel D: Fetal damage due to ECT, insulin coma, chlorpromazine, and reserpine. Arch Gen Psychiatry 2:606–610, 1960

143. Spencer M: Fluoxetine hydrochloride (Prozac) toxicity in a neonate. Pediatrics 92:721–722, 1993

143a. Spitzer R, Endicott J, Robins E: Research Diagnostic Criteria: rationale and reliability. Arch Gen Psychiatry 35:773–782, 1978

144. St. Clair S, Schirmer R: First-trimester exposure to alprazolam. Obstet Gynecol 80:843–846, 1992

145. Stancer H, Reed K: Desipramine and 2-hydroxydesipramine in human breast milk and the nursing infant's serum. Am J Psychiatry 143:1597–1600, 1986

146. Stein A, Gath D, Bucher J, et al: The relationship between post-natal depression and mother-child interaction. Br J Psychiatry 158:46–52, 1991

147. Stein D, Hollander E, Simeon D, et al: Pregnancy and obsessive-compulsive disorder (letter). Am J Psychiatry 150:1131–1132, 1993

148. Stein G: The pattern of mental change and body weight change in the first post-partum week. J Psychosom Res 24:165–171, 1980

149. Stein G, Marsh A, Morton J: Mental symptoms, weight changes, and electrolyte excretion in the first post partum week. J Psychosom Res 25:395–408, 1981

150. Stewart D: Prophylactic lithium in postpartum affective psychosis. J Nerv Ment Dis 176:485–489, 1988

151. Stewart D: Thyroid function and postpartum depression (letter). Am J Psychiatry 148:816, 1991

152. Stewart D, Addison A, Robinson G, et al: Thyroid function in psychosis following childbirth. Am J Psychiatry 145:1579–1581, 1988

152a. Stewart D: Schizophrenia and pregnancy. Can Fam Physician 30:1537–1542, 1984

153. Stewart D, Klompenhouwer J, Kendell R, et al: Prophylactic lithium in puerperal psychosis: the experience of three centres. Br J Psychiatry 158:393–397, 1991

154. Stewart D, Robinson G: Psychotropic drugs and electroconvulsive therapy during pregnancy and lactation, in Psychological Aspects of Women's Health Care: The Interface Between Psychiatry and Obstetrics and Gynecology. Edited by Stewart D, Stotland N. Washington, DC, American Psychiatric Press, 1993, pp 71–95

155. Stewart D, Stotland N (eds): Psychological Aspects of Women's Health Care: The Interface Between Psychiatry and Obstetrics and Gynecology. Washington, DC, American Psychiatric Press, 1993

156. Stotland N, Smith T: Psychiatric consultation to obstetrics and gynecology: systems and syndromes, in American Psychiatric Press Review of Psychiatry, Vol 9. Edited by Tasman A, Goldfinger SM, Kaufmann C. Washington, DC, American Psychiatric Press, 1990, pp 537–563

157. Strouse T, Szuba M, Baxter L: Response to sleep deprivation in three women with postpartum psychosis. J Clin Psychiatry 53:204–206, 1992

158. Stuart S: Treatment of postpartum depression with interpersonal psychotherapy (letter). Arch Gen Psychiatry 52:75–76, 1994

159. Susman V, Katz J: Weaning and depression: another postpartum complication. Am J Psychiatry 145:498–501, 1988

160. Villeponteaux V, Lydiard R, Laraia M, et al: The effects of pregnancy on preexisting panic disorder. J Clin Psychiatry 53:201–203, 1992

161. Wagner K, Berenson A: Norplant-associated major depression and panic disorder. J Clin Psychiatry 55:478–480, 1994

162. Walker R, Swartz C: Electroconvulsive therapy during high-risk pregnancy. Gen Hosp Psychiatry 16:348–353, 1994

163. Ware M, DeVane C: Imipramine treatment of panic disorder during pregnancy. J Clin Psychiatry 51:482–484, 1990

164. Warnes H, Fitzpatrick C: Oral contraceptives and depression. Psychosomatics 20:187–194, 1979

165. Watson J, Elliott S, Rugg A, et al: Psychiatric disorder in pregnancy and the first postnatal year. Br J Psychiatry 144:453–462, 1984

166. Webster M, Thompson J, Mitchell E, et al: Postnatal depression in a community cohort. Aust N Z J Psychiatry 28:42–49, 1994

167. Weissman M, Slaby A: Oral contraceptives and psychiatric disturbance: evidence from research. Br J Psychiatry 123:513–518, 1973

168. Whalley L, Roberts D, Wentzel J, et al: Genetic factors in puerperal affective psychoses. Acta Psychiatr Scand 65:180–193, 1982

169. Wilkie G, Shapiro C: Sleep deprivation and the postnatal blues. J Psychosom Res 36:309–316, 1992

170. Wise M, Ward S, Townsend-Parchman W, et al: Case report of ECT during high-risk pregnancy. Am J Psychiatry 141:99–101, 1984

171. Wisner K, Peindl K, Hanusa B: Symptomatology of affective and psychotic illnesses related to childbearing. J Affect Disord 30:77–87, 1994

172. Wisner K, Perel J: Serum nortriptyline levels in nursing mothers and their infants. Am J Psychiatry 148:1234–1236, 1991

173. Wisner K, Perel J, Foglia J: Serum clomipramine and metabolite levels in four nursing mother-infant pairs. J Clin Psychiatry 56:17–20, 1995

174. Wisner K, Perel J, Wheeler S: Tricyclic dose requirements across pregnancy. Am J Psychiatry 150:1541–1542, 1993

174a. Wisner K, Wheeler S: Prevention of recurrent postpartum major depression. Hosp Community Psychiatry 45:1191–1196, 1994

175. Yalom I, Lunde D, Moos R, et al: "Postpartum blues" syndrome: a description and related variables. Arch Gen Psychiatry 18:16–27, 1968

175a. Zelkowitz P, Milet T: Screening for postpartum depression in a community sample. Can J Psychiatry 40:80–86, 1995

176. Zuckerman B, Amaro H, Bauchner H, et al: Depressive symptoms during pregnancy: relationship to poor health behaviors. Am J Obstet Gynecol 160:1107–1111, 1989

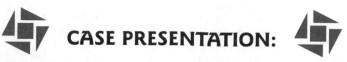

CASE PRESENTATION:
Ms. Sawyer: The Psychotic, Bipolar Pregnant Patient

Ms. Sawyer is an attractive 25-year-old aspiring singer who has been marginally followed in the local clinic for 3 years. She had her first manic episode at age 22, when she was hospitalized with flight of ideas, euphoria, and hyperactivity. At that time, she had the delusion that she was the double of the singer Madonna, because Marilyn Monroe's voice followed her everywhere telling her to dye her hair blond. The police had brought her in after she had created a disturbance at a local record store by attempting to stage her own concert, trailed by several homeless men. There was no history of substance abuse. Family history was negative for psychiatric illness. Past medical history was negative.

The patient had responded well to a combination of thiothixene (Navane) 5 mg po bid and lithium 300 mg qid with levels of approximately 1.0 mEq/ml. She was discharged home, where she lived with a succession of boy-friends. She managed to support herself with waitressing jobs, which changed about every 6 months. She was able to book occasional singing gigs at local bars.

Compliance with lithium was an ongoing struggle between Ms. Sawyer and her therapists at the clinic. She managed, however, to remain out of the hospital. She was lost to follow-up until 10 months later, when the obstetrics resident called because Ms. Sawyer was again psychotic after having delivered a healthy baby girl 1 week earlier. She did not know who the father of the baby was. She was brought in by police from a local record store, where she was singing the Madonna song "Like a Virgin" in a loud voice, draped only in a white bedsheet. In the emergency room she was euphoric, hyperactive, with flight of ideas. She reported that she was "talking to the voice of the Virgin Mary" because she has had a baby, "like Madonna's madonna."

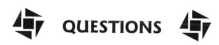 QUESTIONS

Choose all that apply.

1. What is the approximate incidence of postpartum psychosis in the general population?
   a. 1 in 100
   b. 1 in 1,000
   c. 1 in 10,000
   d. 1 in 100,000

2. What is true regarding the onset of psychosis associated with pregnancy?
   a. Most episodes begin before the third week postpartum.
   b. Most episodes begin between weeks 3 and 12 of pregnancy.
   c. Most episodes begin after the twelfth week postpartum.
   d. There is no definable pattern of onset.

3. Following uncomplicated childbirth, the increased risk of psychiatric hospitalization persists for up to
   a. 2 weeks
   b. 2 months
   c. 12 months
   d. 2 years
   e. It is no greater than that for nonpregnant women.

4. How does Ms. Sawyer's presentation compare with that of other postpartum psychotic syndromes?
   a. She is unusual, in that the majority of postpartum disorders requiring hospitalization are schizophreniform rather than affective.
   b. She is fairly typical, in that the majority of postpartum disorders requiring hospitalization are affective in nature rather than schizophreniform.
   c. Paranoid psychotic syndromes account for the majority of psychiatric syndromes following childbirth.

d. Bipolar disorder confers a higher risk for postpartum psychosis than does unipolar disorder.

e. The risk of homicidal activity is no greater for Ms. Sawyer than for someone whose psychosis is unassociated with pregnancy.

5. What are accurate statements about risk factors for postpartum psychosis?

   a. Ms. Sawyer's social or environmental stressors are unlikely to play a role in generating the condition.

   b. Her lower social class correlates with higher risk.

   c. There is no correlation with maternal age.

   d. Parity does not correlate with the risk of developing postpartum psychosis.

   e. Schizophrenic patients are at no greater risk for decompensating after delivery than the population at large.

6. What characterizes affective episodes associated with pregnancy and childbirth (compared with those unassociated with pregnancy)?

   a. They have a higher rate of psychosis.

   b. They are more likely to be accompanied by confusion.

   c. They more often occur during pregnancy than after childbirth.

   d. They confer no greater risk of subsequent affective episodes as long as the woman does not become pregnant.

7. The risk of puerperal psychosis for a woman with a history of affective disorder . . .

   a. Is about double that for a woman with no affective history.

   b. Is over a hundred times greater than for a woman with no affective history.

   c. Is no greater than for anyone else, provided that thyroid function tests and blood estrogen levels remain normal.

   d. Stays high for up to 6–9 months, then drops back to whatever was her nonpregnant baseline.

8. Which of the following is arranged in the correct *descending* order for the risk of hospital admissions for bipolar affective illness?

   a. Postpartum month 1 > Postpartum month 3 > Postpartum year 2 > Antepartum

   b. Antepartum > Postpartum month 1 > Postpartum month 3 > Postpartum year 2

   c. Postpartum month 1 > Postpartum month 3 > Antepartum > Postpartum year 2

   d. Postpartum month 3 > Postpartum month 1 > Postpartum year 2 > Antepartum

9. On the psychiatry service, Ms. Sawyer preaches "the word of the Lord" to the other patients, while actively hallucinating. She retains some reality testing about her infant and is concerned that her parents take good care of the child. Her parents are extremely upset about her condition, and ask how this could have happened. Which of the following are true?

   a. Shifts in estrogen and progesterone have been shown to precipitate postpartum psychosis.

   b. Studies suggest a high genetic loading for general psychiatric disorders in postpartum psychotic patients, but not specifically for pregnancy-related psychiatric disorders.

   c. If Ms. Sawyer had no previous psychiatric history, the risk of future affective episodes would drop back to the risk in the general population.

   d. All of the above.

10. What factors correlate with illness severity in pregnant, chronically mentally ill women?

   a. Low neonatal Apgar scores

   b. Lower neonatal birth weights

   c. More neonatal prematurity

   d. Poor maternal compliance with prenatal follow-up

   e. All of the above

11. If Ms. Sawyer could be carefully followed upon discharge, which of the following would be true?

   a. Experts would agree that Ms. Sawyer's lithium should be discontinued prior to planned conception.

   b. Postpartum affective syndromes tend to have good prognoses, while puerperal schizophrenic illness has the same generally poor prognosis as schizophrenia unassociated with pregnancy.

   c. There would be consensus that valproic acid or carbamazepine would be less *cardiotoxic* to the fetus than lithium.

   d. Most practitioners would use valproic acid or carbamazepine instead of lithium, if first-trimester antimanic agents were required.

12. Ms. Sawyer is discharged home and does well until she is once again lost to follow-up. She reappears in the emergency room, about 1 year later, this time 10 weeks pregnant, and again hallucinating, delusional, and with irritable mood. Her lithium level is zero. She is alert and fully oriented, but cannot concentrate and refuses cogni-

tive testing, claiming that the examiner is a "priest of the devil." She again does not know who the father of her baby is. Physical exam and labs are pending. What characterizes the differential diagnosis at this point?

   a. This clinical picture is consistent with one of the end-organ side effects of *chronic* lithium exposure, even though her present level is zero and acute toxicity is ruled out.

   b. Her presentation is congruent with lupus erythematosus, except for the age at onset.

   c. Within the spectrum of thyroid disease, *hyper*thyroidism, but not *hypo*thyroidism, could present in this way.

   d. Although she is at risk for human immunodeficiency virus (HIV), manic syndromes are not a presenting feature of HIV infection without other systemic signs.

13. The medical workup, including labs, is completely normal. What are the treatment guidelines to apply to a psychotic pregnant patient like Ms. Sawyer?

   a. Phenothiazines have been associated with substantially high rates of fetal malformations.

   b. Electroconvulsive therapy (ECT) is unlikely to be effective for postpartum mania.

   c. Clonazepam (Klonopin) should not be combined with neuroleptics during pregnancy, as it worsens confusion and increases neuroleptic requirements.

   d. High-potency neuroleptics are recommended over low-potency agents during pregnancy.

14. Pregnant psychotic patients should not be given prophylactic anticholinergic or antiparkinsonian agents, but sometimes such drugs become necessary. Although there are no data suggesting which is the safest agent, which agents should be avoided because of possible teratogenicity?

   a. Amantadine (Symmetrel)
   b. Atenolol (Tenormin)
   c. Benztropine (Cogentin)
   d. Bromocriptine (Parlodel)
   e. Diphenhydramine (Benadryl)
   f. Propranolol (Inderal)
   g. Trihexyphenidyl (Artane)

15. Ms. Sawyer responds partially to clonazepam (Klonopin) 0.5 mg bid and haloperidol (Haldol) 2 mg tid. She becomes assaultive toward another patient, whom she is convinced is part of the satanic plot to undo her "virgin divinity." The euphoric mood persists. If Ms. Sawyer became violent and required physical restraint, what instructions should be given to the nurses?

   a. She should be placed supine.
   b. She should be positioned on her right side.
   c. She should be positioned on her left side.
   d. Her position should be changed frequently.

16. Fetuses of mothers placed on carbamazepine (Tegretol) should undergo screening specifically for . . .
   a. Alpha-fetoprotein.
   b. Ceruloplasmin.
   c. Congenital heart disease.
   d. Fragile X syndrome.
   e. None of the above.

17. Fetuses of mothers placed on lithium should undergo screening specifically for . . .
   a. Alpha-fetoprotein.
   b. Ceruloplasmin.
   c. Congenital heart disease.
   d. Fragile X syndrome.
   e. None of the above.

18. Fetuses of mothers placed on valproic acid (Depakene) should undergo screening specifically for . . .
   a. Alpha-fetoprotein.
   b. Ceruloplasmin.
   c. Congenital heart disease.
   d. Fragile X syndrome.
   e. None of the above.

19. If you could have managed Ms. Sawyer before her second pregnancy, which of the following strategies would have won consensus approval from the experts?

   a. Counsel the patient that lithium at *any* time during pregnancy confers an *equally* high risk of congenital deformities, varying according to trimester.

   b. Discontinue lithium at least 2 months before attempted conception.

   c. Advise her that, based on current knowledge, there is no evidence of higher physical or mental abnormalities in developing children who were exposed to lithium in utero but were normal at birth (i.e., did not have Ebstein's anomaly).

   d. None of the above.

20. Ms. Sawyer has been counseled that in utero exposure to lithium may increase the incidence of Ebstein's anomaly. What features are associated with Ebstein's anomaly?

   a. Tricuspid insufficiency
   b. Mitral stenosis
   c. Transposition of the great vessels
   d. Cleft palate
   e. Mental retardation

21. Ms. Sawyer responds quickly to ECT and low-dose neuroleptics. She requires antimanic prophylaxis, but you decide at week 11 to wait a bit longer before beginning lithium, keeping the patient hospitalized. What are the current data on lithium's effects on the developing heart?

    a. Data increasingly support a high frequency of Ebstein's anomaly for children whose mothers took lithium during the first trimester.

    b. Studies of children with Ebstein's anomaly have retrospectively shown a significant rate of in utero lithium exposure.

    c. Based on currently available data, the risk of bearing a baby with Ebstein's anomaly is greater for a woman on lithium than for women in the general population.

    d. The frequency of congenital malformations for children exposed to lithium in utero has been confirmed at about 10% (compared with a malformation frequency of 2% in the general population).

22. Which pharmacokinetic changes occur during pregnancy?

    a. If the patient becomes preeclamptic, an increase in lithium dose would compensate for the expanded volume of distribution.

    b. In the last months of pregnancy, glomerular filtration rate (GFR) *rises*, predisposing to subtherapeutic lithium levels and heightened risk of manic relapse.

    c. At the time of delivery, GFR *rises*, predisposing to subtherapeutic lithium levels and heightened risk of manic relapse.

    d. None of the above.

23. Early into her second trimester, Ms Sawyer is discharged home in the care of her parents on lithium 300 mg bid (level: 1.0 mEq/ml). She is compliant with outpatient psychiatric and obstetrical follow-up. She asks if she will remain on this lithium dose throughout. She hopes it will not make her baby "sick" when it is born. She wants to have natural childbirth this time and asks if she will be able to breast-feed. You respond:

    a. Neonatal lithium toxicity can be avoided as long as maternal blood levels remain in the therapeutic range.

    b. The syndrome of neonatal lithium toxicity resembles that of the adult.

    c. Most of the toxic effects of lithium in the newborn are self-limiting.

    d. The American Academy of Pediatrics considers lithium to be contraindicated during breast feeding.

24. The few studies on prophylactic lithium in women at high risk for postpartum psychosis . . .

    a. Have been inconclusive.

    b. Show minimal effectiveness in women who are *asymptomatic* immediately after delivery.

    c. Show substantial reductions in postpartum psychiatric morbidity.

    d. Indicate that prophylaxis must begin by week 34 in order to be effective.

⬧ Answers

1.	Answer: b (p. 328)	13.	Answer: d (pp. 331–332)
2.	Answer: a (p. 328)	14.	Answer: a, c, e, g (p. 332)
3.	Answer: d (p. 328)	15.	Answer: c, d (pp. 330–331)
4.	Answer: b (p. 328)	16.	Answer: a (pp. 334–335)
5.	Answer: a, c, d (p. 329)	17.	Answer: c (p. 334)
6.	Answer: a, b (p. 328)	18.	Answer: a (p. 335)
7.	Answer: b (p. 329)	19.	Answer: c (pp. 332–334)
8.	Answer: a (p. 328)	20.	Answer: a (p. 333)
9.	Answer: b (p. 329)	21.	Answer: c (pp. 333–334)
10.	Answer: e (p. 330)	22.	Answer: b (p. 334)
11.	Answer: b, c (pp. 329, 333)	23.	Answer: c, d (p. 336)
12.	Answer: a (p. 330)	24.	Answer: c (p. 335)

⚐ POSTPARTUM PSYCHOSIS

Methodological Problems

The criteria for postpartum psychosis have been vague, with early studies calling many different postpartum states "postpartum psychosis": major depression with psychotic features, bipolar disorder with manic episode, schizophrenia, schizophreniform disorder, and brief reactive psychosis. Even more confusing are the variable definitions of the postpartum period—anywhere from 2 to 3 weeks[20] to 6 months after delivery.[95] Hospital admission records often are the only source of epidemiological data, but they frequently lack diagnostic specifics (e.g., psychotic depression versus schizophrenia). This complicates evaluating the literature in a clinically meaningful way.

◆ If onset is within 4 weeks after delivery of a child, DSM-IV[3] adds a "postpartum onset" specifier to the condition (including major depressive, manic, or mixed episode of *major depressive disorder; bipolar I or II disorder;* or *brief psychotic disorder*).

◆ DSM-IV also allows the diagnosis of *psychotic disorder not otherwise specified* for "postpartum psychosis that does not meet criteria for mood disorder with psychotic features, brief psychotic disorder, psychotic disorder due to a general medical condition, or substance-induced psychotic disorder" (p. 315).

A brief survey of the largely pre–DSM-IV literature follows.

Features

Postpartum psychosis occurs infrequently: 1–2 [cases?] per 1,000 births (0.1%–0.2%).[75,76] Knowing the patterns of onset and relapse can be clinically useful: the majority of severe postpartum illnesses begin *before the third week after delivery.*[54,75] Many of these patients will be symptomatic during pregnancy.

◆ The risk varies according to time from delivery: *Postpartum month 1 > Postpartum month 3 > Postpartum year 2 > Antepartum.*[54,72,75,85]

◆ Psychiatric admissions among recently pregnant patients were found to be higher by a factor of 6.0 in the first postpartum month and higher by a factor of 3.8 in the first 3 months postpartum compared with antepartum rates.[75] These risk factors rose even higher (21.7 and 12.7, respectively) when only ICD-9[174a] psychoses were included (roughly equivalent to DSM-III-R[2a] affective disorders and schizophrenia, excluding dysthymia).[54] Similarly, Kastrup and co-workers[72,85] found that the frequency of hospital admissions specifically due to bipolar affective illness was lowest *during* pregnancy, climbed highest in the first month postpartum, then dropped during months 2–12 postpartum, but still remained high (three-fourths, 8, and 2 times the antepartum reference frequency, respectively).

◆ The higher risk of hospitalization continues *for up to 2 years postpartum.*[54,75]

◆ Most postpartum psychiatric syndromes requiring hospitalization are *affective,* with depressive disorders accounting for approximately 60% of these patients.[17,40,73,75,138]

◆ Puerperal affective episodes are accompanied by a *higher rate of confusion and Schneiderian first-rank symptoms* (i.e., auditory hallucinations, experiences of influence, experiences of alienation, thought broadcasting[83]) compared with affective episodes that are unrelated to pregnancy and the postpartum period.[17,41,68,73,114a,154] Although Wisner et al.[173] did not confirm more Schneiderian symptoms in their sample, they did note more bizarre behavior and unusual psychotic symptoms (e.g., tactile, olfactory, and visual hallucinations) compared with psychosis unassociated with pregnancy.

◆ The etiology for the delirium-like quality of postpartum psychosis remains unknown. Wisner et al.[173] have speculated that the extreme interference in circadian rhythms and normal sleep associated with childbirth may account for this.

◆ Of most concern is that *homicidal ideation* occurs in postpartum psychosis. Of the three psychotic women in Wisner et al.'s[173] sample, two attempted to harm their babies. (One poured lighter fluid over the baby and was restrained by a relative as she was about to strike a match; the second mother attempted to stab her baby and herself.) This finding dovetails with Resnick's[126] assessment that *the most dangerous period for child victims of mothers committing filicide was the first 6 months of life.*

Risk Factors

A number of factors are associated with a higher risk for postpartum psychosis.[19]

- **Psychiatric history:** The best-documented risk factor is a history of psychiatric illness:[15,75,97,123] the risk of puerperal psychosis for a woman with a history of affective disorder[15,75,123] is 20%–25%—about 200 times higher than for a woman with no psychiatric history (1–2 cases in 1,000 births, or 0.1%–0.2%). *Bipolar* disorder confers more risk than unipolar disorder for postpartum affective syndromes.[2,75,159]

- **Family history:** Studies suggest a high genetic loading for psychiatric disorders in patients with postpartum psychosis,[37] but not specifically for pregnancy-related psychiatric disorders.[42,120,138b,154]

- **Demographics:** No obvious association with social class or culture has been found.[18,65,80a,108,116] There are conflicting results regarding marital status, with some finding no association[40,77,116,120] and others reporting a higher rate of postpartum psychosis in unwed mothers.[65,76,77,115,160] Unmarried status and psychiatric admission (within 1 month of childbirth) significantly correlated in a recent study; 19% of these women were unmarried, compared with only 10% of unwed mothers in the general population.[75] The unmarried rate in patients with psychosis was also higher than the general population, but this did not reach statistical significance. The relevance of these findings is unclear; they may reflect the general epidemiology of psychosis rather than be specific to puerperal psychiatric illness.

- **Obstetric factors:** Unlike postpartum blues, postpartum psychosis is most common among women who are having their first child,[20,74] with the rate among primiparae being approximately double that of multiparae.[74] There is no obvious association with maternal age.[76,120,160]

- **Stressful life events:** Present studies indicate that social and environmental stresses do not significantly contribute to the genesis of puerperal psychosis.[18,47,92,93]

- **Early versus late onset:** One prospective study of postpartum psychosis differentiated between early (within 3 weeks of delivery) and later onset (within 3 weeks to 6 months of delivery).[95] Several trends suggested demographic and psychiatric differences between the two groups, but these differences were not statistically significant and sample size was small ($n = 16$ early, $n = 9$ late). Early-onset cases were more often characterized by primiparity and younger age at the time of delivery and first psychiatric illness. Women with later-onset psychosis were more often of lower social class, not married (despite their generally increased age and parity), and psychiatrically symptomatic during the 6 months before the index pregnancy. The early-versus-late distinction so far has not been corroborated.[138a]

- **Physiological correlates:** As mentioned, biological findings in puerperal psychiatric syndromes are inconclusive.[96a] Postdexamethasone cortisol levels have been significantly elevated in some studies,[117,147] with evidence of blunted thyroid-stimulating hormone (TSH) response.[117] However, high rates of cortisol nonsuppression have been also found 3–5 days postpartum in women *without* psychiatric illness,[58,147] reverting to baseline when retested 5–24 weeks postpartum.[147]

Prognosis

Woman who suffer pregnancy-related psychotic episodes often want to know their risk for recurrence if they do (or do not) become pregnant again. *Unfortunately, puerperal psychotic illness predisposes to **additional** psychotic episodes unrelated to pregnancy, even in patients without prior psychiatric history.*[8,13,94,118,128,154] The risk of future affective illness also stays higher for these women than for the general population—with or without additional pregnancies.[40,138]

One 25-year follow-up study tracked 82 patients who had been treated for postpartum illness.[40] The diagnostic groups were unipolar depression (52%), bipolar disorder (18%), schizophrenia (16%), "abnormal personality with depression" (8%), "organic disorder" (2%), and "obsessional state with depression" and paranoid disorder (1% each). There were several notable trends:

- The overall prognosis was good, except for schizophrenic illness, which resulted in chronic disability in 50% of patients and deterioration with further childbirth.

- Although clinical lore has it that schizophreniform illness precipitated by an acute stressor augurs a good prognosis, this is not true for schizophreniform presentations associated with pregnancy.[40] *The risk of nonpuerperal recurrence for schizophrenic illness was 100% (versus 43% for recurrent unipolar depression and 66% for recurrent bipolar disorder).*

- Varying according to diagnosis, the risk of developing another postpartum illness ranged from 1 in 3 to 1 in 5 pregnancies.

- The incidence of suicide was 5%.
- The incidence of infanticide was 4%.

Differential Diagnosis

Always rule out medical etiologies for abnormal mental status in pregnancy. Although Ms. Sawyer's clinical picture is consistent with recurrent bipolar illness, a number of other specific conditions should be eliminated. *A primary psychiatric diagnosis should be one of exclusion in pregnant patients—even for those with a psychiatric history.*

- **Human immunodeficiency virus (HIV) infection** should be suspected in a patient with psychosis if the patient has any of the risk factors for HIV infection; Ms. Sawyer's chaotic series of sexual partners places her at high risk. Manic symptoms specifically have been reported as the presenting feature of acquired immunodeficiency syndrome (AIDS) in the absence of systemic signs.[21,39,49,52,78,137] Furthermore, a recent study found that pregnant women were significantly less likely to practice safer sex (i.e., use condoms) than nonpregnant women—even when their sexual partners were intravenous drug users.[43]
- **Systemic lupus erythematosus** (SLE) has a peak incidence in women of childbearing age and may present with prominent psychosis but few medical symptoms. It may be precipitated by pregnancy,[67a] with onset especially during the first 6 weeks postpartum.[59] SLE easily imitates pregnancy-associated psychiatric illnesses. Antinuclear antibodies (ANA) and erythrocyte sedimentation rates (ESR) are important screening tests for this condition.
- **Thyroid disease:** The occurrence of psychiatric symptoms associated with hyperthyroid disease is well recognized, but hypothyroidism (*myxedema*) is an often-overlooked cause of psychosis. *Hypothyroidism can be a complication of **chronic** lithium therapy in bipolar patients like Ms. Sawyer.* "Myxedema madness"[9] may be the first harbinger of hypothyroidism, even without other stigmata of thyroid disease.[66] Although its psychiatric presentations are heterogeneous, paranoid psychosis is said to be most characteristic,[87] usually with features of delirium. Even without obvious clouding of consciousness, there is usually some cognitive impairment, particularly of recent memory.[87]
- **Miscellaneous**
  - The **Fregoli syndrome**, a rare delusional misidentification syndrome similar to Capgras' syndrome, has been associated with postpartum psychosis. In this condition, the patient develops the delusion that a stranger is really a person familiar to them, even though this stranger bears no physical resemblance to that person. Four patients have been reported who developed the Fregoli syndrome postpartum within 14 days of delivery.[112] No medical cause was found. Nosologically, one patient was classified as bipolar, another schizoaffective, and two as having unspecified "functional" psychosis.
  - Postpartum **Capgras' syndrome** has also been described.[34]

Pregnancy and the Chronically Mentally Ill

As mentioned, schizophrenic patients have a much higher risk of decompensating both during and after pregnancy.[33,96,120] There also appears to be a relationship between obstetric complications and chronic mental illness. Low Apgar scores, lower birth weights, and more prematurity have correlated with the chronicity and severity of the mother's mental disturbance.[135,178] Psychotic patients may be unreliable about prenatal care, such as in complying with medical recommendations.[79] Chronically mentally ill pregnant women are less likely to keep prenatal care appointments than are nonpsychiatric pregnant control subjects and "mildly" mentally ill pregnant women.[175] Even in recent studies, maternal social incompetence and the diagnosis of schizophrenia were significant predictors of poorer prenatal care and more complicated births.[56,102,103] The misperceptions and bizarre behavior of women with chronic mental illness interfered with their making use of available services.[102] Genetic risk factors also influence outcome in these women.

Long-term inpatient management of pregnant psychotic patients results in better perinatal care and outcome.[24,105,109,110,152] Miller and colleagues[104] have urged that involuntary hospitalization be considered a priority when other less restrictive options have been unsuccessful. Unfortunately, there are few guidelines to assist clinicians in assessing current or future risk of harm to an infant as a consequence of maternal mental illness, particularly schizophrenia.[80b,104a]

The Violent Pregnant Patient

Sometimes it becomes impossible to manage a psychotic pregnant patient with medications alone and she must be physically restrained. However, it is dangerous to restrain second- and third-trimester patients in the supine (face up) position; compression of the aorta and vena cava by the gravid uterus may obstruct the venous return to the heart and produce the supine hypotensive syndrome.[13a]

◆ When necessary, a patient requiring restraint should be placed on her *left* side (i.e., raising the right hip so that the uterus is displaced to the left).[146]

◆ Frequent positional changes will prevent partial inferior vena cava obstruction and dependent edema.

Physical restraint may lessen the need for chemical restraint, potentially minimizing the exposure of the fetus to psychotropic medication.[24,101] Raskin et al.[122] have argued, however, that

> although restraints themselves can be readily removed, their adverse psychological consequences may be long lasting . . . Administering antipsychotic medication may, in [some] instances, be less traumatic and alleviate delusions sufficiently to build a working relationship, while restraints may intensify paranoia. (p. 1760)

Once again, there is no formula for intervention, and clinicians must tailor their management to the needs of the individual.

⚡ PSYCHOPHARMACOLOGY IN PREGNANCY, PART II

Electroconvulsive Therapy

As mentioned, ECT has been safely used in pregnancy to treat psychotic depression[73a,124,125,172] and secondary mania.[82] As comprehensively reviewed by Mukherjee et al.,[106] ECT does have proven efficacy in the acute treatment of mania and is a treatment option for the severely manic pregnant patient.[32,168] Although there are no prospective, controlled studies comparing complications from ECT with those from other treatments in pregnancy, ECT is considered to be generally safe. (See discussion in the first part of this chapter on Ms. Wright.)

Neuroleptics

Indications in Pregnancy

The goal of pharmacological management in pregnancy is to reduce symptoms with the lowest dose and number of agents. Consider the following indications for neuroleptics during pregnancy:[110]

◆ Gross inability to care for oneself or to cooperate with prenatal care.

◆ Impairment of reality testing, inducing potential danger to self or others.

◆ Disorganized thought, behavior, and perception unresponsive to supportive intervention, up to and including hospitalization.

See also Appendix M ("Effects of Psychotropics During Pregnancy").

Teratogenicity

Neuroleptics are ideally avoided during the first trimester but are preferred to lithium in the first-trimester patient.[91] Their relative teratogenicity has become somewhat controversial, however.

◆ Extensive experience has accrued with the phenothiazines, especially chlorpromazine (Thorazine), which has long been used for the hyperemesis of pregnancy. (Haloperidol has also been used extensively for the treatment of hyperemesis.[164]) Early research showed that phenothiazines were not strong organ or behavioral teratogens—at least in antiemetic doses.[4,11,16,80,98,133,149,151] Although there were occasional early reports of problems associated with these drugs,[111,133,166] most of the data were inconclusive and anecdotal.

These reassuring results, however, were challenged by two studies. The first, a comprehensive prospective study,[133] was conducted in 1977 by the French National Institute of Health and Medical Research, which surveyed more than 12,000 pregnancies. Of concern were 189 births of unequivocal, nonchromosomally based malformations and a significant increase in malformed infants for women who had taken phenothiazines during the first 3 months after the last menstrual period.

A second paper in 1984 by Edlund and Craig[48] reanalyzed the data of the California Child Health and Development Project (1959–1966),[98] which had shown no increase in congenital anomalies after phenothiazine exposure in more than 19,000 births.

◆ Edlund and Craig[48] showed a trend for increased abnormalities linked to phenothiazine exposure after 4 weeks, with the most critical period being from gestational weeks 6–10.

The infants of subjects medicated early (1–4 weeks after conception) showed no significant congenital disorders. *This study suggested that there may exist a specific toxic window for phenothiazines.* Moreover, Edlund and Craig[48] pointed out that many studies may have minimized potential adverse effects by using nonpsychotic subjects who ingested small antiemetic or anxiolytic amounts of phenothiazines rather than the larger antipsychotic dosages. (Note, too, that children of psychotic women have a higher risk of fetal abnormality independent of drug exposure.[152a,155,175])

What, then, is the clinician to use? Cohen and colleagues at the Massachusetts General Hospital Perinatal Psychiatry Clinical Research program advise medicating with the high-potency neuroleptics (L. S. Cohen, personal communication, March 1992). Stewart and Robinson[155] agree (see also Appendix M). Neuroleptics are not recommended for breast-feeding mothers.[118a]

To date, few data exist on the use of clozapine (Clozaril) during pregnancy.[12,84,167] No adverse sequelae have been reported in the newborns of mothers who took the drug. Clozapine was not included in the 1994 edition of Briggs et al.[16]

Medications for Neuroleptic Side Effects

There are few available data on agents used to treat extrapyramidal side effects (EPS) and neuroleptic malignant syndrome:

- **Benztropine** (Cogentin) and **trihexyphenidyl** (Artane): In 1977, the Collaborative Perinatal Project found a significant increase of minor malformations in infants exposed prenatally to anticholinergic medications.[60] These concerns remained for both agents in the 1994 edition of Briggs et al.[16] In addition, potential adverse anticholinergic side effects in the fetus and neonate include functional intestinal obstruction, tachycardia, and urinary retention.[99]
- **Diphenhydramine** (Benadryl) has been associated with major and minor congenital anomalies, including oral clefts.[60,136] Briggs et al.[16] have stated that conclusions are not possible about diphenhydramine's teratogenicity, as the data are confounded by exposure to other drugs. An interaction between diphenhydramine and temazepam (Restoril) resulted in violent intrauterine fetal movements and the subsequent birth of a stillborn infant.[71] Moreover, there may be an association between antihistamine exposure in the last 2 weeks of pregnancy and retrolental fibroplasia in premature infants.
- **Amantadine** (Symmetrel) has been implicated as a human teratogen,[36,107] mainly relative to cardiovascular defects. It was also anecdotally associated with complications such as miscarriage, hydatidiform mole, preeclampsia, and first-trimester bleeding in a series of four cases.[55] Briggs et al.[16] have argued, however, that the number of exposures is too small to draw definitive conclusions about this medication.
- Beta-adrenergic blocking agents, such as **propranolol** (Inderal) and **atenolol** (Tenormin), have not been linked with increased congenital anomalies or other complications.[121,131] Pregnancy does enhance propranolol's effect on slowing maternal heart rate,[132] however.
- First-trimester **bromocriptine** (Parlodel) has shown no evidence of increased teratogenicity or miscarriage.[16,161] Little is known about the effects of **dantrolene** (Dantrium) during pregnancy.

Miller[100] has proposed the following guidelines for managing EPS during pregnancy:

1. Avoid prophylactic treatment with anticholinergic or antiparkinsonian agents.
2. Monitor electrolytes, particularly calcium (pregnant women are at risk for inadequate calcium intake), since hypocalcemia may predispose to acute dystonic reactions from neuroleptics.[81]
3. When severe dystonic or parkinsonian side effects do occur, try switching to a lower-potency neuroleptic at the lowest effective dose.
4. There are no data suggesting which agents are the safest during pregnancy, except that amantadine (Symmetrel) should be avoided if possible.
5. Significant akathisia during pregnancy can be safely treated with propranolol (Inderal) or atenolol (Tenormin). (Normal pregnancy can induce a state of motor restlessness that may resemble drug-induced akathisia.)
6. If a pregnant woman develops neuroleptic malignant syndrome, bromocriptine can be safely used in conjunction with supportive measures.

Adjuvant Clonazepam

Clonazepam (Klonopin) has some antimanic activity,[25,26] low teratogenic potential,[16,156] and when used as an adjuvant may reduce the total required dose of neuroleptics.[26,27,134]

Lithium: When? Why? How?

Before Conception

Everyone agrees that lithium is best avoided during pregnancy, but sometimes antimanic prophylaxis spares the need for more medication later on. As mentioned, ovulation detector kits (sold over the counter in pharmacies) may hasten planned conception for women who opt to discontinue psychotropics while trying to become pregnant. As usual, recommendations vary:

◆ The number of prior affective episodes correlates with future risk of relapse. Cohen et al.[32] advise discontinuing lithium one menstrual period *before* attempted conception in patients with a history of a single manic episode or only rare episodes.

◆ For more fragile patients, Cohen (personal communication, March 1992) and colleagues recommend that lithium be discontinued only *after* pregnancy is documented.[31] They argue that since conception may take several months, this approach minimizes the lithium-free period, thus lowering the risk of recurrence of affective disorder. Also, in the setting of early pregnancy (i.e., after one missed menstrual period, or at approximately 2 weeks postconception) the window of lithium exposure is small. They cite evidence that nonspecific toxic insults to the conceptus during this period result in either complete repair (and a normal pregnancy) or a nonviable blighted ovum (and spontaneous abortion).[44]

◆ Markovitz and Calabrese[91] disagree; they insist that even a 2-week lithium exposure by the conceptus is unacceptable. These authors point out that the "all or nothing," blight-or-repair phenomenon has never been documented for lithium and remains hypothetical. They recommend using alternatives to lithium, such as valproic acid (see below).

◆ Schou[140] feels that women of fertile age should use contraception while taking lithium, and that lithium should be discontinued 1–2 months before planned conception[141] or stopped after pregnancy occurs.[140] If the woman's history suggests a high likelihood of bipolar relapse, he advises resuming lithium after the first trimester, when organogenesis has been largely completed.[140]

During Pregnancy

When neuroleptics fail to control mania, which antimanic agent is the best choice? By far the most clinical experience is with lithium, which freely crosses the placenta, equilibrating between maternal and cord serum.[142] First-trimester lithium was implicated as causing cardiovascular defects in the 1970s by the Lithium Baby Register project. (The cardiovascular system is formed during the third through ninth week after conception.[50]) This was a joint Danish, American, and Canadian study that pooled information about 225 babies who had been exposed to lithium in utero.[144,145,171]

◆ Of these children, 11% ($n = 25$) had malformations at birth—compared with the malformation frequency of 2% in the general population; 8% ($n = 18$) of the 225 babies had malformations involving the heart and vessels, with 3% ($n = 6$) having the rare Ebstein's anomaly. The latter occurs in the general population only once in about 20,000 births (0.005%).[53,63]

◆ **Ebstein's malformation** is characterized by downward displacement of the tricuspid valve into the right ventricle, due to anomalous attachment of the tricuspid leaflets.[51] The tricuspid valve tissue is dysplastic. Although the clinical manifestations are variable, patients may come to medical attention because of progressive cyanosis from right-to-left atrial shunting, symptoms due to tricuspid regurgitation and right ventricular dysfunction, or paroxysmal atrial tachyarrhythmias.[51] The degree of right ventricular impairment depends on the magnitude of the tricuspid valve regurgitation and the extent to which the right ventricular inflow is "atrialized." Most patients survive at least to the third decade. Surgical approaches have included prosthetic replacement of the tricuspid valve.[51] Mental retardation and cleft palate are not features of Ebstein's anomaly.

Several subsequent investigations have *failed* to confirm a greater risk of congenital heart malformations with first-trimester lithium exposure:

◆ In 1982, data registers of women with manic-depressive illness and infants with congenital malformations were linked.[70] A higher but *nonsignificant* incidence of malformations was found in infants exposed to lithium ($N = 59$; $n = 7$ malformations; $n = 4$ heart defects) compared with those exposed either to other drugs or to no drugs at all ($N = 118$; $n = 4$ malformations; $n = 2$ heart defects). No infant had Ebstein's anomaly. Note, however, the limitations of small sample size.

◆ In 1989, another study of 50 children exposed to lithium in utero revealed no cardiovascular malformations.[38] Again, note the small sample size.

◆ In 1990, a different cohort of 59 children with Ebstein's anomaly retrospectively showed that none had been exposed to lithium in utero.[177]

In 1992, Jacobson and associates[63] conducted a prospective study of first-trimester fetal lithium exposure. The subjects were 148 women (ages 15–40) who had taken first-trimester lithium (as early as 3 weeks) matched with 148 lithium-free pregnant control subjects. The case subjects were taking lithium 50–2,400 mg daily for "major affective disorders."

◆ There was no difference between the lithium-treated mothers and the control subjects in total number of live births, frequency of major anomalies, spontaneous or therapeutic abortions, ectopic pregnancies, or prematurity.

◆ In the lithium group, one case of Ebstein's anomaly was diagnosed at 16 weeks gestation, leading the mother to terminate her pregnancy.

Comment.   The authors[63] interpreted their data as further challenging the lithium–Ebstein's anomaly link, concordant with others who have concluded that at most there is a *weak* association between the two.[69,140,169] There is another possible interpretation, however: 1 case of Ebstein's anomaly in 148 patients approximates a rate of 0.68%—or about 135 times the estimated rate in the general population of 1 in 20,000 (0.005%).[53] Nonetheless, we agree that these are fairly good odds—better, certainly, than the original data (3%) reported by the Baby Register Project or the likely risk of bipolar relapse. These inferences were recently supported by a 1994 review[29a,30] of existing research, which concluded that *patients should be informed that the risk of major malformations with first-trimester lithium is somewhat greater than that of the general population*—on the order of 4%–12% as compared with 2%–4% in untreated comparison groups.[29a]

We concur with Gelenberg,[53] who has written,

> For a woman with a serious bipolar disorder well controlled with lithium, [the possibility of Ebstein's anomaly] pales in comparison with the likelihood of experiencing a severe mood episode, which would threaten the life of the mother, the well-being of the fetus, the security of the mother-infant bond postpartum, and the long-term course of the mother's mood disorder. (pp. 1–2)

Summary.   As warned, readers looking for certitude will not find it here. To summarize:

1. Patients who have been exposed to lithium prior to week 12 should have fetal cardiac ultrasound at weeks 18–20.
2. High-potency neuroleptics are preferred, but should be deferred if possible until the second trimester, substituting aggressive environmental management

(e.g., hospitalization, one-to-one nursing) to maintain safety.
3. ECT remains a viable option.
4. Although there are less-cardiotoxic alternatives to lithium, they are not without their problems (see below).
5. *The goal of pharmacological management is to minimize risk to the fetus, not necessarily to achieve prepregnancy symptom control for the mother.* This means tolerating substantial psychiatric symptomatology without definitive pharmacological intervention—at least through the first trimester. This can be taxing for the clinician, trying for the psychiatric staff, and most of all, terrifying for the exhausted patient and family. Frequent staff and family meetings help maintain a "team approach" while minimizing divisiveness, splitting, and acting out; it is disturbing to watch a pregnant, manic patient for 12 long weeks and "do" what feels like "nothing."

Pregnancy pharmacokinetics and lithium.   For pregnant patients on lithium, adjust the dose according to changes in GFR, which varies throughout pregnancy. A rough guideline follows:

◆ **Last months of pregnancy:** ↑ GFR, ↓ lithium levels: Therefore, ↑ lithium dose to maintain serum levels.[14,143]
◆ **As delivery approaches:** ↓ GFR, ↑ lithium levels: Therefore, to avoid toxicity, ↓ lithium dose by 30%–50%[29] or discontinue lithium[140] 2–3 days before the expected delivery date. This also lowers lithium concentrations and diminishes the risk of toxicity in the newborn.
◆ **For preeclampsia:** The sodium-restricted diet may produce toxicity: ↓ sodium intake, ↑ sodium and lithium reabsorption, ↑ lithium levels.[45] Therefore, to avoid toxicity, ↓ lithium.

Lithium alternatives.   Both carbamazepine (Tegretol) and valproic acid (Depakene) have been recommended as alternatives to first-trimester lithium because they are less cardiotoxic to the fetus. They are not, however, without problems:

◆ **Carbamazepine** has teratogenic activity (i.e., developmental delay, fingernail hypoplasia, minor craniofacial defects).[23,28,32,67,170] Of even greater concern was the discovery in 1991[130] that it confers a 1% risk of neural tube defects such as spina bifida—about 13.7 times the expected rate.[6,61,62,86,88,113,129] It is now clearly recommended that an alpha-fetoprotein analysis of amniotic fluid be conducted to rule out this possibility.[86] Unlike lithium, however, carbamazepine is considered by the American Academy of Pediatrics to be compatible with breast feeding.[35]

◆ **Valproic acid** in the first trimester has been implicated in causing spina bifida in 1%–2% of infants.[127] Markovitz and Calabrese[91] note that spina bifida can be detected at 20 weeks gestation with alpha-fetoprotein analysis and ultrasonography. These authors recommend valproic acid management for manic patients who fail neuroleptic management and would be willing to consider a therapeutic abortion at 20 weeks.[91] Furthermore, they argue that valproic acid is less cumbersome than lithium and does not require the same careful attention to fluid and electrolyte alterations.[22]

   • These recommendations must be tempered, however, by findings that in utero exposure to valproic acid produces other problems not necessarily detectable before birth. For example, deformities of the head, face, digits, and urogenital tract; intrauterine growth retardation; and fetal or newborn distress constitute the *fetal valproic syndrome.*[7,46,64,86,165,177]

   • Unlike lithium, valproic acid is considered by the American Academy of Pediatrics to be compatible with breast feeding.[35]

◆ The calcium channel blocker **verapamil** (Calan) was safely used during pregnancy in three manic women[57] and has not been linked with congenital defects,[16] but more extensive data are lacking. The American Academy of Pediatrics considers it to be compatible with breast feeding.[35]

While considering the pros and cons of each management strategy, never underestimate the emotional impact of a second-trimester abortion—however therapeutic—on an already vulnerable patient who has wanted the pregnancy.

After Childbirth

Be sure to follow high-risk patients closely in the first *2–4 weeks* postpartum.[54] Early warning signs of relapse should signal immediate intervention. Opinion varies, however, about the merits of prophylactic lithium for bipolar patients who are *asymptomatic* after delivery but remain at high risk for postpartum psychosis.[1,68,114,123,150,158]

Recently, Stewart et al.[154] identified 21 women at high risk for postpartum psychosis according to family affective history, personal bipolar history, and previous "puerperal psychosis" (most commonly bipolar I and major

depressive disorder, but also with schizoaffective disorder and unspecified "functional" psychosis). These women were given prophylactic lithium carbonate either late in the third trimester (week 34) or immediately after delivery. (The rationale for initiating lithium prophylaxis at week 34 was to achieve a therapeutic serum lithium level by postpartum days 3–4, when the risk of psychosis is particularly high.)

◆ Nineteen women remained nonpsychotic while on lithium.

◆ Three had mild, brief periods of confusion, insomnia, fatigue, or depression that were treated with lorazepam, and which the authors speculated may have been attenuated forms of puerperal illness.

◆ Only two women (10%) on prophylactic lithium suffered a recurrence of their puerperal psychiatric illness. One woman had a major depression without psychotic features that started 6 days after delivery and required a 13-day hospitalization. This illness was milder than her previous episode, which had prominent psychotic features and required an 8-week admission. The second woman, who had taken lithium throughout her pregnancy, still experienced recurrent puerperal psychosis on postpartum day 8. She was hospitalized for 4 months and underwent ECT.

◆ Seventeen women took lithium for at least 6 months. Three stopped the medication after 4–6 months and remained euthymic. One discontinued the lithium and suffered a psychotic relapse at 3 months postpartum.

◆ Of concern was an unexplained stillbirth in one patient who had received lithium at week 34.

This report[154] corroborates the findings of several other studies[10,153,163] that postdelivery lithium protects against recurrent puerperal psychosis in high-risk women.

◆ *However, the authors advise against lithium prophylaxis in asymptomatic* **pregnant** *patients, even late in the third trimester.*[154]

◆ The emergence of symptoms immediately after delivery for a patient resuming lithium does not always signal the need for more lithium; it may also indicate a delay in achieving steady state while the GFR is reequilibrating. Be cautious about overly brisk dose increases.

Clearly, these recommendations are based on relatively few subjects, and are intended to serve as guidelines only.

Neonatal lithium toxicity. The serum half-life of lithium in newborns is prolonged, averaging 68–96 hours, as compared with the adult's 10–20 hours.[89] Lithium levels that are therapeutic in the mother may be toxic in the neonate; neonatal levels of 1.0 mEq/ml have been associated with cyanotic states, bradycardia, impaired respiratory function, and "floppy babies."[5] The picture of lithium toxicity in newborns is different from that in adults. Most of these toxic effects are self-limiting, disappearing in 1–2 weeks as lithium is eliminated by the kidneys.[16] Although these effects are considered reversible, data on long-term effects are lacking.[174]

◆ For example, fetal red blood cell choline levels (the metabolic precursor to acetylcholine) are elevated during maternal therapy with lithium.[90] The clinical significance of this effect is unknown, but it may be related to the teratogenicity of lithium due to its effect on cellular lithium transport.[90]

Van Gent and Verhoeven[162] have recommended that the newborn exposed to lithium be observed in the neonatal ward to monitor for lithium toxicity.

Breast feeding. Nursing infants' blood lithium concentrations are 10%–50% of the mothers',[144,157] with infant serum levels approximately equal to those of the breast milk.[16] There is only one report of an adverse effect on a breast-feeding infant during the course of the child's common cold, with restlessness, muscle twitches, and serum lithium level in the baby of 1.4 mmol/L.[148] Cessation of breast feeding led to complete recovery.

Schou[140] has stressed that the psychological and physical benefits of breast feeding must be weighed against the risks, and each case considered individually to help the mother make her own choice. The American Academy of Pediatrics, however, considers lithium to be *contraindicated* during breast feeding because of the potential for lithium-induced toxicity in the nursing infant.[35] (Perhaps this is due to newborns' vulnerability to dehydration, which heightens their risk for lithium toxicity.) As mentioned, carbamazepine (Tegretol), valproic acid (Depakene), and verapamil (Calan) are considered compatible with breast feeding[35] and may be viable options for mothers who require antimanic prophylaxis and also desire to nurse.

Lithium children. We know of only one follow-up study on the effects of lithium on later childhood development. Schou[139,140] conducted a questionnaire follow-up study on 60 "lithium children," age 5 years or older,

who had shown no malformations at birth. Their siblings, who had no prenatal exposure to lithium, served as the control group (n = 57). Physical and mental abnormalities were no higher among the lithium children. This study was limited by small sample size, the young age of the subjects, and the dependence on mothers' assessments rather than objective examinations.

⚜ SUMMARY

1. Postpartum psychosis is an infrequent but serious condition. Always rule out medical conditions such as human immunodeficiency virus (HIV) infection, systemic lupus erythematosus (SLE), or thyroid disease.

2. The majority of severe postpartum illnesses occur within the first month after delivery. Most syndromes are affective in nature, with depression most prominent. Puerperal affective episodes show a higher rate of confusion and Schneiderian first-rank symptoms (i.e., auditory hallucinations, experiences of influence, experiences of alienation, thought broadcasting), compared with affective episodes that are unrelated to pregnancy and the postpartum period.

3. A woman with an affective history has a risk of postpartum psychosis that is about 200 times higher than that for someone with no psychiatric history. Preexisting bipolar disorder confers a higher risk than unipolar disorder for postpartum psychosis, which is most common among women having their first child. There is no obvious association with maternal age, demographics, or stressful life events. The physiological correlates remain unclear.

4. The prognosis for pregnancy-related schizophreniform illness is poor; there is a high likelihood of an enduring schizophrenic course. Moreover, women with pregnancy-related affective psychoses are at risk for recurrent psychotic episodes unrelated to pregnancy.

5. Schizophrenic women have a much higher risk of psychotic recurrence both during and after pregnancy. They also have a higher rate of obstetric complications. Inpatient management of pregnant psychotic patients has been associated with better perinatal care and outcome.

6. The violent pregnant patient should be restrained on her *left* side, with frequent positional changes. Judicious physical restraint may lessen the need for chemical restraint.

7. ECT has been safely used in the treatment of mania, depression, and psychosis in pregnancy.

8. The relative teratogenicity of the phenothiazines versus the high-potency agents is controversial. Experts in the field now advise using the high-potency neuroleptic haloperidol.

9. Avoid prophylactic treatment with anticholinergic or antiparkinsonian agents. Monitor electrolytes, particularly calcium (pregnant women are at high risk for inadequate calcium intake), since hypocalcemia may predispose to neuroleptic-induced dystonic reactions. There are no data suggesting which anti–extrapyramidal side effects (EPS) medications are the safest during pregnancy, except that amantadine (Symmetrel) should be avoided if possible. Significant akathisia can be safely treated with propranolol (Inderal) or atenolol (Tenormin). (Remember that normal pregnancy can induce a state of motor restlessness that may resemble drug-induced akathisia.) If a pregnant woman develops neuroleptic malignant syndrome, bromocriptine (Parlodel) can be used with supportive measures.

10. Recommendations are conflicting about when to stop lithium for brittle bipolar patients who become pregnant. Everyone agrees that first-trimester medications should be avoided if possible, and that hospitalization is a safe alternative.

11. The main hazard of first-trimester lithium is congenital heart disease (Ebstein's malformation), but the chance of this anomaly is much lower than the risk of manic relapse. Women exposed to lithium prior to week 12 should have fetal cardiac ultrasound at weeks 18–20. In the third trimester, the increased glomerular filtration rate (GFR) requires increased lithium doses to maintain serum levels. As delivery approaches, declining GFR requires reduced lithium to avoid maternal and newborn toxicity. Prophylactic lithium after delivery minimizes psychiatric morbidity in high-risk patients. Despite its advocates in the psychiatric literature, breast feeding on lithium is considered contraindicated by the American Academy of Pediatrics. Carbamazepine (Tegretol), valproic acid (Depakene), and verapamil (Calan) are considered to be compatible with breast feeding and may present viable options for nursing mothers who require antimanic prophylaxis.

12. Antimanic alternatives to lithium, such as carbamazepine and valproic acid, are less cardiotoxic but more neurotoxic to the fetus. Alpha-fetoprotein analysis and ultrasonography should be done at week 20 to screen for spina bifida.

REFERENCES

1. Abou-Saleh M, Coppen A: Puerperal affective disorders and response to lithium (letter). Br J Psychiatry 142:539, 1983
2. Akiskal H, Walker P, Puzantian V, et al: Bipolar outcome in the course of depressive illness: phenomenologic, familiar, and pharmacologic predictors. J Affect Disord 5:115–128, 1983
2a. American Psychiatric Association: Diagnostic and Statistical Manual of Mental Disorders, 3rd Edition, Revised. Washington, DC, American Psychiatric Association, 1987
3. American Psychiatric Association: Diagnostic and Statistical Manual of Mental Disorders, 4th Edition. Washington, DC, American Psychiatric Association, 1994
4. Ananth J: Congenital malformations with psychopharmacologic agents. Compr Psychiatry 16:437–445, 1975
5. Ananth J: Side effects on fetus and infant of psychotropic drug use during pregnancy. Pharmacopsychiatry 11:246–260, 1976
6. Anonymous: Teratogenesis with carbamazepine. Lancet 337:1316–1317, 1991
7. Ardinger H, Atkin J, Blackston R, et al: Verification of the fetal valproate syndrome phenotype. Am J Med Genet 29:171–185, 1988
8. Arentsen K: Postpartum psychoses, with particular reference to the prognosis. Dan Med Bull 15:97–100, 1968
9. Asher R: Myxoedematous madness. BMJ 2:555–562, 1949
10. Austin M: Puerperal affective psychosis: is there a case for lithium prophylaxis? Br J Psychiatry 161:692–694, 1992
11. Ayd FJ: Children born of mothers treated with chlorpromazine during pregnancy. Clin Med 71:1758–1763, 1964
12. Barnas C, Bergant A, Hummer M, et al: Clozapine concentrations in maternal and fetal plasma, amniotic fluid, and breast milk (letter). Am J Psychiatry 151:945, 1994
13. Benvenuti P, Cabras P, Servi P, et al: Puerperal psychoses: a clinical case study with follow-up. J Affect Disord 26:25–30, 1992
13a. Blumenfeld M, Gabbe S: Placental abruption, in Gynecology and Obstetrics. Edited by Sciarra J. Philadelphia, PA, JB Lippincott, 1989, pp 1–18
14. Boobis A, Lewis P: Pharmacokinetics in pregnancy, in Clinical Pharmacology in Obstetrics. Edited by Lewis PP. Boston, MA, PSG Publishers, 1983, pp 5–16
15. Bratfos O, Haug J: Puerperal mental disorders in manic-depressive females. Acta Psychiatr Scand 42:285–294, 1966
16. Briggs G, Freeman R, Yaffe S: Drugs in Pregnancy and Lactation, 4th Edition. Baltimore, MD, Williams & Wilkins, 1994
17. Brockington I, Cernyk K, Schofield E, et al: Puerperal psychosis: phenomenon and diagnosis. Arch Gen Psychiatry 38:829–833, 1981
18. Brockington I, Martin C, Brown G, et al: Stress and puerperal psychosis. Br J Psychiatry 157:331–334, 1990

19. Brockington I, Meakin C: Clinical clues to the aetiology of puerperal psychosis. Prog Neuropsychopharmacol Biol Psychiatry 18:417–429, 1994

20. Brockington I, Winokur G, Dean C: Puerperal psychosis, in Motherhood and Mental Illness. Edited by Brockington I, Kumar R. London, Academic Press, 1982, pp 37–69

21. Buhrich N, Cooper D, Freed E: HIV infection associated with symptoms indistinguishable from functional psychosis. Br J Psychiatry 152:649–653, 1988

22. Calabrese J, Gulledge A: Psychotropics during pregnancy and lactation: a review. Psychosomatics 26:413–426, 1985

23. Calabrese J, Gulledge A: Carbamazepine, clonazepam use during pregnancy (letter). Psychosomatics 27:464, 1986

24. Chang S, Renshaw D: Psychosis and pregnancy. Compr Ther 12:36–41, 1986

25. Chouinard G: Antimanic effects of clonazepam. Psychosomatics 26 (suppl):7–11, 1985

26. Chouinard G, Annable L, Turnier L, et al: A double-blind randomized clinical trial of rapid tranquilization with i.m. clonazepam and i.m. haloperidol in agitated psychotic patients with manic symptoms. Can J Psychiatry 38 (suppl):S114–S121, 1993

27. Cohen B, Lipinski JJ: Treatment of acute psychosis with non-neuroleptic agents. Psychosomatics 27 (suppl 1):7–16, 1986

28. Cohen LS: Pregnancy in the bipolar patient. Biological Therapies in Psychiatry 11:42–44, 1988

29. Cohen L: Personal communication, March 1992

29a. Cohen L, Friedman J, Jefferson J, et al: A reevaluation of risk of in utero exposure to lithium. JAMA 271:146–150, 1994

30. Cohen L, Friedman J, Jefferson J, et al: The risk of in utero exposure to lithium (letter; reply). JAMA 271:1828–1829, 1994

31. Cohen L, Heller V: On the use of anticonvulsants for manic depression during pregnancy (letter). Psychosomatics 31:462, 1990

32. Cohen L, Heller V, Rosenbaum J: Treatment guidelines for psychotropic drug use in pregnancy. Psychosomatics 30:25–33, 1989

33. Cohler B, Gallant D, Grunebaum H, et al: Pregnancy and birth complications among mentally ill and well mothers and their children. Soc Biol 22:269–278, 1975

34. Cohn C, Rosenblatt S, Faillace L, et al: Capgras' syndrome presenting as post partum psychosis. South Med J 70:942, 1977

35. Committee on Drugs, American Academy of Pediatrics: Transfer of drugs and other chemicals into human milk. Pediatrics 93:137–150, 1994

36. Coulson A: Amantadine and teratogenesis (letter). Lancet 2:1044, 1975

37. Craddock N, Brockington I, Mant R, et al: Bipolar affective puerperal psychosis associated with consanguinity. Br J Psychiatry 164:359–364, 1994

38. Cunniff C, Sahn D, Reed K, et al: Pregnancy outcome in women treated with lithium. Teratology 39:447–448, 1989

39. Dauncey K: Mania in early stages of AIDS. Br J Psychiatry 152:716–717, 1988

40. Davidson J, Robertson E: A follow-up study of postpartum illness, 1946–1978. Acta Psychiatr Scand 71:451–457, 1985

41. Dean C, Kendell R: The symptomatology of puerperal illnesses. Br J Psychiatry 139:128–133, 1981

42. Dean C, Williams R, Brockington I: Is puerperal psychosis the same as bipolar manic-depressive disorder? a family study. Psychol Med 19:637–647, 1989

43. Deren S, Beardsley M, Davis R, et al: HIV risk factors among pregnant and nonpregnant high-risk women in New York City. J Drug Educ 23:57–66, 1993

44. Dicke J: Teratology: principles and practice. Med Clin North Am 73:567–581, 1989

45. Dickson L, Miller W, Hyatt M: Pregnancy complicated by acute mania and preeclampsia. Psychosomatics 33:221–224, 1992

46. DiLiberti J, Farndon P, Dennis N, et al: The fetal valproate syndrome. Am J Med Genet 19:473–481, 1984

47. Dowlatshahi D, Paykel E: Life events and social stress in puerperal psychoses: absence of effect. Psychol Med 20:655–662, 1990

48. Edlund M, Craig T: Antipsychotic drug use and birth defects: an epidemiologic reassessment. Compr Psychiatry 25:32–37, 1984

49. El-Mallakh R: Mania and paranoid psychosis in AIDS (letter). Psychosomatics 32:362, 1991

50. Friedman W: Congenital heart disease, in Harrison's Principles of Internal Medicine, 11th Edition. Edited by Braunwald E, Isselbacher K, Petersdorf R, et al. New York, McGraw-Hill, 1987, pp 983–951

51. Friedman W, Child J: Congenital heart disease in the adult, in Harrison's Principles of Internal Medicine, 13th Edition. Edited by Isselbacher K, Braunwald E, Wilson J, et al. New York, McGraw-Hill, Health Professions Division, 1994, pp 1037–1046

52. Gabel R, Barnar N, Norko M, et al: AIDS presenting as mania. Compr Psychiatry 27:251–254, 1986

53. Gelenberg A: Lithium teratogenesis revisited. Biological Therapies in Psychiatry Newsletter 15:1–2, 1992

54. Gitlin M, Pasnau R: Psychiatric syndromes linked to reproductive function in women: a review of current knowledge. Am J Psychiatry 146:1413–1422, 1989

55. Golbe L: Parkinson's disease and pregnancy. Neurology 37:1245–1249, 1987

56. Goodman S, Emory E: Perinatal complications in births to low socioeconomic status schizophrenic and depressed women. J Abnorm Psychol 101:225–229, 1992

57. Goodnick P: Verapamil prophylaxis in pregnant women with bipolar disorder (letter). Am J Psychiatry 150:1560, 1993

58. Greenwood J, Parker G: The dexamethasone suppression test in the puerperium. Aust N Z J Psychiatry 18:282–284, 1984

59. Hahn B: Systemic lupus erythematosus, in Harrison's Principles of Internal Medicine, 12th Edition. Edited by Wilson J, Braunwald E, Isselbacher K, et al. New York, McGraw-Hill, Health Professions Division, 1991, pp 1432–1437

60. Heinonen O, Slone D, Shapiro S: Birth Defects and Drugs in Pregnancy. Littleton, MA, PSG, 1977

61. Hesdorffer D, Hauser W: Spina bifida in infants of women taking carbamazepine (letter). N Engl J Med 325:664, 1991

62. Hughes R: Spina bifida in infants of women taking carbamazepine (letter). N Engl J Med 325:664, 1991

63. Jacobson S, Jones K, Johnson K, et al: Prospective multicentre study of pregnancy outcome after lithium exposure during the first trimester. Lancet 339:530–533, 1992

64. Jager-Roman E, Deichi A, Jakob S, et al: Fetal growth, major malformations, and minor anomalies in infants born to women receiving valproic acid. J Pediatr 108:997–1004, 1986

65. Jansson B: Psychic insufficiencies associated with childbearing. Acta Psychiatr Scand Suppl 172:7–168, 1963

66. Jefferson J, Marshall J: Neuropsychiatric Features of Medical Disorders. New York, Plenum Medical Book, 1981

67. Jones K, Lacro R, Johnson K, et al: Pattern of malformations in the children of women treated with carbamazepine during pregnancy. N Engl J Med 320:1661–1666, 1989

67a. Jones W: Autoimmune disease and pregnancy. Aust N Z J Obstet Gynaecol 34:251–258, 1994

68. Kadrmas A, Winokur G, Crowe R: Postpartum mania. Br J Psychiatry 135:551–554, 1979

69. Källén B: Comments on "Teratogen update: lithium" (letter). Teratology 38:597, 1988

70. Källén B, Tandberg A: Lithium and pregnancy: a cohort study on manic-depressive women. Acta Psychiatr Scand 68:134–139, 1982

71. Kargas G, Kargas S, Bruyere HJ, et al: Perinatal mortality due to interaction of diphenhydramine and temazepam (letter). N Engl J Med 313:1417–1418, 1985

72. Kastrup M, Lier L, Rafaelsen O: Psychiatric illness in relation to pregnancy and childbirth, I: methodologic considerations. Nordisk Psykiatrisk Tidsskrift 43:531–534, 1989

73. Katona C: Puerperal mental illness: comparisons with non-puerperal controls. Br J Psychiatry 141:447–452, 1982

73a. Kellner C, Beale M, Prtichett J: The risk of in utero exposure to lithium (letter). JAMA 271:1828, 1994

74. Kendell R: Emotional and physical factors in the genesis of puerperal mental disorders. J Psychosom Res 29:3–11, 1985

75. Kendell R, Chalmers J, Platz C: Epidemiology of puerperal psychoses. Br J Psychiatry 150:662–673, 1987

76. Kendell R, Rennie D, Clarke J, et al: The social and obstetric correlates of psychiatric admission in the puerperium. Psychol Med 1:341–350, 1981

77. Kendell R, Wainwright S, Hailey A, et al: The influence of childbirth on psychiatric morbidity. Psychol Med 11:342–350, 1976

78. Kieburtz K, Zettelmaier A, Ketonen L, et al: Manic syndrome in AIDS. Am J Psychiatry 148:1068–1070, 1991

79. Krener P, Simmons M, Hansen R, et al: Effect of pregnancy on psychosis: life circumstances and psychiatric symptoms. Int J Psychiatry Med 19:65–84, 1989

80. Kris E: Children of mothers maintained on pharmacotherapy during pregnancy and postpartum. Current Therapeutic Research 31:690–695, 1965

80a. Kumar R: Postnatal mental illness: a transcultural perspective. Soc Psychiatry Psychiatr Epidemiol 29:250–264, 1994

80b. Kumar R, Marks M, Platz C, et al: Clinical survey of a psychiatric mother and baby unit: characteristics of 100 consecutive admissions. J Affect Disord 33:11–22, 1995

81. Kuny S, Binswanger U: Neuroleptic-induced extrapyramidal symptoms and serum calcium levels: results of a pilot study. Pharmacopsychiatry 21:67–70, 1989

82. LaGrone D: ECT in secondary mania, pregnancy, and sickle cell anemia. Convulsive Therapy 6:176–180, 1990

83. Leon R, Bowden C, Faber R: Diagnosis and psychiatry: examination of the psychiatric patient, in Comprehensive Textbook of Psychiatry, 5th Edition. Edited by Kaplan H, Sadock B. Baltimore, MD, Williams & Wilkins, 1989, pp 449–462

84. Lieberman J, Safferman A: Clinical profile of clozapine adverse reactions and agranulocytosis, in Clozapine in Treatment-Resistant Schizophrenia. Edited by Lapierre Y, Jones B. London, Royal Society of Medicine, 1992, pp 3–14

85. Lier L, Kastrup M, Rafaelsen O: Psychiatric illness in relation to pregnancy and childbirth, II: diagnostic profiles, psychosocial and perinatal aspects. Nordisk Psykiatrisk Tidsskrift 43:535–542, 1989

86. Lindhout D, Omtzigt J: Teratogenic effects of antiepileptic drugs: implications for the management of epilepsy in women of childbearing age. Epilepsia 35 (suppl 4):S19–S28, 1994

87. Lishman W: Organic Psychiatry, 2nd Edition. Oxford, UK, Blackwell Scientific, 1987

88. Little B, Santos-Ramos R, Newell J, et al: Megadose carbamazepine during the period of neural tube closure. Obstet Gynecol 82:705–708, 1993

89. Mackay A, Loose R, Glen A: Labour on lithium. BMJ 1:878, 1976

90. Mallinger A, Hanin I, Stumpf R, et al: Lithium treatment during pregnancy: a case study of erythrocyte choline content and lithium transport. J Clin Psychiatry 44:381–384, 1983

91. Markovitz P, Calabrese J: On the use of anticonvulsants for manic depression during pregnancy (letter). Psychosomatics 31:463–464, 1990

92. Marks M, Wieck A, Checkley S, et al: Life stress and postpartum psychosis: a preliminary report. Br J Psychiatry Suppl 10:45–49, 1991

93. Martin C, Brown G, Goldberg D, et al: Psycho-social stress and puerperal depression. J Affect Disord 16:283–293, 1989

94. McGorry P, Connell S: The nosology and prognosis of puerperal psychosis: a review. Compr Psychiatry 31:515–534, 1990

95. McNeil T: A prospective study of postpartum psychoses in a high-risk group, II: relationships to demographic and psychiatric history characteristics. Acta Psychiatr Scand 75:35–43, 1987

96. McNeil T, Kaij L: Women with nonorganic psychosis: pregnancy's effect on mental health during pregnancy. Acta Psychiatr Scand 70:140–148, 1984

96a. Meakin C, Brockington I, Lynch S, et al: Dopamine supersensitivity and hormonal status in puerperal psychosis. Br J Psychiatry 166:73–79, 1995

97. Meltzer E, Kumar R: Puerperal mental illness, clinical features and classification: a study of 142 mother-and-baby admissions. Br J Psychiatry 147:647–654, 1985

98. Milkovich L, Van den Berg B: An evaluation of the teratogenicity of certain antinauseant drugs. Am J Obstet Gynecol 125:244–248, 1976

99. Miller L: Clinical strategies for the use of psychotropic drugs during pregnancy. Psychiatr Med 9:275–298, 1991

100. Miller L: Psychiatric medication during pregnancy: understanding and minimizing risks. Psychiatric Annals 24:69–75, 1994

101. Miller W, Resnick M: Restraining the violent pregnant patient (letter). Am J Psychiatry 148:269, 1991

102. Miller W, Resnick M, Williams M, et al: The pregnant psychiatric inpatient: a missed opportunity. Gen Hosp Psychiatry 12:373–378, 1990

103. Miller WJ, Bloom J, Resnick M: Chronic mental illnesses and perinatal outcome. Gen Hosp Psychiatry 14:171–176, 1992

104. Miller WJ, Bloom J, Resnick M: Prenatal care for pregnant chronic mentally ill patients. Hosp Comm Psychiatry 43:942–943, 1992

104a. Mowbray C, Oyserman D, Zemencuk J, et al: Motherhood for women with serious mental illness: pregnancy, childbirth, and the postpartum period. Am J Orthopsychiatry 65:21–38, 1995

105. Mugtader S, Hamann M, Molnar G: Management of psychotic pregnant patients in a medical-psychiatric unit. Psychosomatics 27:31–33, 1986

106. Mukherjee S, Sackeim H, Schnur D: Electroconvulsive therapy of acute manic episodes: a review of 50 years' experience. Am J Psychiatry 151:169–176, 1994

107. Nora J, Nora A, Way G: Cardiovascular maldevelopment associated with maternal exposure to amantadine (letter). Lancet 2:607, 1975

108. Nott P: Psychiatric illness following childbirth in Southampton: a case register study. Psychol Med 12:557–561, 1982

109. Nurnberg G, Prudic J: Guidelines for treatment of psychosis during pregnancy. Hosp Community Psychiatry 35:67–71, 1984

110. Nurnberg H: An overview of somatic treatment of psychosis during pregnancy and postpartum. Gen Hosp Psychiatry 11:328–338, 1989

111. O'Leary J, O'Leary J: Nonthalidomide ectromelia. Obstet Gynecol 23:17–20, 1964

112. O'Sullivan D, Dean C: The Fregoli syndrome and puerperal psychosis. Br J Psychiatry 159:274–277, 1991

113. Oakeshott P, Hunt G: Carbamazepine and spina bifida (letter). BMJ 303:651, 1991

114. Oates M: The treatment of psychiatric disorders in pregnancy and the puerperium. Clin Obstet Gynecol 13:385–395, 1986

114a. Oosthuizen P, Russouw H, Roberts M: Is puerperal psychosis bipolar mood disorder? a phenomenological comparison. Compr Psychiatry 36:77–81, 1995

115. Paffenbarger R: Epidemiological aspects of mental illness associated with childbearing, in Motherhood and Mental Illness. Edited by Brockington I, Kumar R. London, Academic Press, 1982, pp 19–36

116. Paffenbarger RJ: The picture puzzle of the postpartum psychoses. Journal of Chronic Diseases 13:161–173, 1961

117. Paykel E, del Campo A, White W, et al: Neuroendocrine challenge studies in puerperal psychoses: dexamethasone suppression and TRH stimulation. Br J Psychiatry 159:262–266, 1991

118. Platz C, Kendell R: A matched-control follow-up and family study of "puerperal psychosis." Br J Psychiatry 153:90–94, 1988

119. Pons G, Rey E, Matheson I: Excretion of psychoactive drugs into breast milk: pharmacokinetic principles and recommendations. Clin Pharmacokinet 27:270–289, 1994

120. Protheroe C: Puerperal psychoses: a long-term study, 1927–1961. Br J Psychiatry 115:9–30, 1969

121. Pruyn S, Phelan J, Buchanan G: Long-term propranolol therapy in pregnancy: maternal and fetal outcome. Am J Obstet Gynecol 135:485–489, 1979

122. Raskin V, Dresner N, Miller L: Risks of restraints versus psychotropic medication for pregnant patients (letter). Am J Psychiatry 148:1760–1761, 1991

123. Reich T, Winokur G: Postpartum psychoses in patients with manic depressive disease. J Nerv Ment Dis 151:60–68, 1970

124. Remick R, Maurice W: ECT in pregnancy (letter). Am J Psychiatry 135:761–762, 1978

125. Repke J, Berger N: Electroconvulsive therapy in pregnancy. Obstet Gynecol 63 (suppl):39–40, 1984

126. Resnick P: Child murder by parents: a psychiatric review of filicide. Am J Psychol 126:73–82, 1969

127. Robert E, Giubaud P: Maternal valproic acid and congenital neural tube defects (letter). Lancet 2:937, 1982

128. Rohde A, Marneros A: Postpartum psychoses: onset and long-term course. Psychopathology 26:203–209, 1993

129. Rosa F: Spina bifida in infants of women taking carbamazepine (letter). N Engl J Med 325:664–665, 1991

130. Rosa F: Spina bifida in infants of women treated with carbamazepine during pregnancy. N Engl J Med 324:674–677, 1991

131. Rubin P: Beta-blockers in pregnancy. N Engl J Med 305:1323–1326, 1981

132. Rubin P, Butters L, McCabe R, et al: The influence of pregnancy on drug action: concentration-effect modelling with propranolol. Clin Sci 73:47–52, 1987

133. Rumeau-Rouquette C, Goujard J, Huel G: Possible teratogenic effects of phenothiazines in human beings. Teratology 15:57–64, 1977

134. Salzman C, Green A, Rodriguez-Villa R, et al: Benzodiazepines combined with neuroleptics for management of severe disruptive behavior. Psychosomatics 27:17–21, 1986

135. Sameroff A, Zax M: Perinatal characteristics in the offspring of schizophrenic women. J Nerv Ment Dis 157:191–199, 1973

136. Saxen I: Cleft palate and maternal diphenhydramine intake. Lancet 1:407–408, 1974

137. Schmidt U, Miller D: Two cases of hypomania in AIDS. Br J Psychiatry 152:839–842, 1988

138. Schopf J, Bryois C, Jonquiere M, et al: On the nosology of severe psychiatric postpartum disorders: results of a catamnestic investigation. Eur Arch Psychiatry Neurol Sci 234:54–63, 1984

138a. Schopf J, Rust B: Follow-up and family study of postpartum psychoses, II: early versus late onset postpartum psychoses. Eur Arch Psychiatry Clin Neurosci 244:135–137, 1994

138b. Schopf J, Rust B: Follow-up and family study of postpartum psychoses, III: characteristics of psychoses occurring exclusively in relation to childbirth. Eur Arch Psychiatry Clin Neurosci 244:138–140, 1994

139. Schou M: What happened later to the lithium babies: a follow-up study of children born without malformations. Acta Psychiatr Scand 54:193–197, 1976

140. Schou M: Lithium treatment during pregnancy, delivery, and lactation: an update. J Clin Psychiatry 51:410–413, 1990

141. Schou M: Lithium use and pregnancy (letter). J Clin Psychiatry 52:279, 1991

142. Schou M, Amdisen A: Lithium and placenta (letter). Am J Obstet Gynecol 122:541, 1975

143. Schou M, Amdisen A, Steenstrup O: Lithium and pregnancy, II: hazards to women given lithium during pregnancy and lactation. BMJ 2:137–138, 1973

144. Schou M, Goldfield M, Weinstein M, et al: Lithium and pregnancy, I: report from the register of lithium babies. BMJ 2:135–136, 1973

145. Schou M, Weinstein M: Problems of maintenance treatment during pregnancy, delivery, and lactation. Agressologie 21A:7–9, 1980

146. Shnider S, Levinson G (eds): Anesthesia for Obstetrics, 2nd Edition. Baltimore, MD, Williams & Wilkins, 1987

147. Singh B, Gilhotra M, Smith R, et al: Postpartum psychoses and the dexamethasone suppression test. J Affect Disord 11:173–177, 1986

148. Skausig O, Schou M: Diegivning under lithium—behandling. Ugeskr Laeger 139:400–401, 1977

149. Slone D, Siskind V, Heinonen O, et al: Antenatal exposure to the phenothiazines in relation to congenital malformations, perinatal mortality rate, birth weight, and intelligence quotient score. Am J Obstet Gynecol 128:486–488, 1977

150. Sneddon J, Kerry R: Puerperal psychosis (letter). Br J Psychiatry 136:520, 1980

151. Sobel D: Fetal damage due to ECT, insulin coma, chlorpromazine, and reserpine. Arch Gen Psychiatry 2:606–610, 1960

152. Spielvogel A, Wile J: Treatment of the psychotic pregnant patient. Psychosomatics 27:487–492, 1986

153. Stewart D: Prophylactic lithium in postpartum affective psychosis. J Nerv Ment Dis 176:485–489, 1988

154. Stewart D, Klompenhouwer J, Kendell R, et al: Prophylactic lithium in puerperal psychosis: the experience of three centres. Br J Psychiatry 158:393–397, 1991

155. Stewart D, Robinson G: Psychotropic drugs and electroconvulsive therapy during pregnancy and lactation, in Psychological Aspects of Women's Health Care: The Interface Between Psychiatry and Obstetrics and Gynecology. Edited by Stewart D, Stotland N. Washington, DC, American Psychiatric Press, 1993, pp 71–95

156. Sullivan F, McElhatton P: A comparison of the teratogenic activity of the antiepileptic drugs carbamazepine, clonazepam, ethosuximide, phenobarbital, phenytoin, and pyrimidone in mice. Toxicol Appl Pharmacol 40:365–378, 1977

157. Sykes P, Quarrie J, Alexander F: Lithium carbonate and breastfeeding. BMJ 4:1299, 1976

158. Targum S, Davenport Y, Webster M: Postpartum mania in bipolar manic-depressive patients withdrawn from lithium carbonate. J Nerv Ment Dis 167:572–574, 1979

159. Targum S, Gershon E: Pregnancy, genetic counseling and the major psychiatric disorders, in Genetic Diseases in Pregnancy: Maternal Effects and Fetal Outcome. Edited by Schulman J, Simpson J. New York, Academic Press, 1981, pp 413–438

160. Tetlow C: Psychoses of childbearing. Journal of Mental Science 101:629–639, 1955

161. Turkalj I, Braun P, Krupp P: Surveillance of bromocriptine in pregnancy. JAMA 247:1589–1591, 1982

162. van Gent E, Verhoeven W: Bipolar illness, lithium prophylaxis, and pregnancy. Pharmacopsychiatry 25:187–191, 1992

163. Van Hulst A, Klompenhouwer J: The role of prophylactic lithium in prevention of recurrence of puerperal psychosis, in Proceedings of the 9th International Congress of Psychosomatic Obstetrics and Gynecology: The Free Woman: Women's Health in the 1990s. Edited by Van Hall E, Everaerd W. Carnforth, Lanes, UK, Parthenon, 1989, pp 417–423

164. Van Waes A, Van de Velde E: Safety evaluation of haloperidol in the treatment of hyperemesis gravidarum. J Clin Pharmacol 9:224–227, 1969

165. Verloes A, Frikiche A, Gremillet C, et al: Proximal phocomelia and radial aplasia in fetal valproic syndrome. Eur J Pediatr 149:266–267, 1990

166. Vince D: Congenital malformations following phenothiazine administration during pregnancy. Can Med Assoc J 100:223, 1969

167. Waldman M, Safferman A: Pregnancy and clozapine (letter). Am J Psychiatry 150:168–169, 1993

168. Walker R: ECT and twin pregnancy. Convulsive Therapy 8:131–136, 1992

169. Warnaky J: Teratogen update: lithium. Teratology 38:593–596, 1988

170. Waters C, Belai Y, Gott P, et al: Outcomes of pregnancy associated with antiepileptic drugs. Arch Neurol 51:250–253, 1994

171. Weinstein M: Lithium treatment of women during pregnancy and the post-delivery period, in Handbook of Lithium Therapy. Edited by Johnson F. Lancaster, UK, MTP Press, 1980, pp 421–429

172. Wise M, Ward S, Townsend-Parchman W, et al: Case report of ECT during high-risk pregnancy. Am J Psychiatry 141:99–101, 1984

173. Wisner K, Peindl K, Hanusa B: Symptomatology of affective and psychotic illnesses related to childbearing. J Affect Disord 30:77–87, 1994

174. Woody J, London W, Wilbanks G: Lithium toxicity in a newborn. Pediatrics 47:94–96, 1971

174a. World Health Organization: Manual of the International Statistical Classification of Diseases, Injuries, and Causes of Death, 9th Revision. Geneva, Switzerland, WHO, 1977

175. Wrede G, Mednick S, Huttunen M, et al: Pregnancy and delivery complications in the births of an unselected series of Finnish children with schizophrenic mothers. Acta Psychiatr Scand 62:369–381, 1980

176. Ylagan L, Budorick N: Radial ray aplasia in utero: a prenatal finding associated with valproic acid exposure. J Ultrasound Med 13:408–411, 1994

177. Zalzstein E, Koren G, Einarson T, et al: A case-control study of the association between first trimester exposure to lithium and Ebstein's anomaly. Am J Cardiol 65:817–818, 1990

178. Zax M, Sameroff A, Babigian H: Birth outcomes in the offspring of mentally disordered women. Am J Orthopsychiatry 47:218–230, 1977

The Gynecology/Oncology Patient

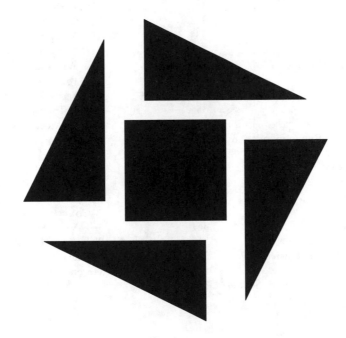

CHAPTER 9

CONTENTS

- Introduction to Chapter 9 345
- Case Presentation: Mrs. Reid (Part I): Menopause,
  Chronic Pelvic Pain, and Hysterectomy 346
- Questions 346
- Answers 349
- Discussion 350
  - ◆ Menopause 350
    - Overview 350
    - Menopause and Psychiatric Morbidity 350
      - Hormone Studies 353
    - Symptoms and Estrogen Deficiency: Facts
      and Fiction 3353
      - Kupperman Menopausal Index 353
      - Sexuality 354
      - Sleep 355
    - Hormone Replacement Therapy 355
      - Psychological Functioning 355
      - Insomnia 355
    - Psychodynamics 355
      - Comment: Menopause and Psychoanalysis . . 356
    - Summary and Treatment Recommendations . 357
  - ◆ Chronic Pelvic Pain 358
    - Incidence and Definition 358
    - Treatment 359
    - Conclusions 360
  - ◆ Hysterectomy 360
    - Psychiatric Sequelae 361
      - Effects on Sexuality 362
      - Abdominal Versus Vaginal Hysterectomy . . . 362
      - Oophorectomy 362
      - Risk Factors for Adverse Psychiatric Sequelae 363

- Conclusions 363
  - ◆ References 364
- Case Presentation: Mrs. Reid (Part II):
  Breast Cancer 370
- Questions 370
- Answers 372
- Discussion 373
  - ◆ Breast Cancer 373
    - Uncertainty About Treatment 373
    - Patient Issues in Medical Decision Making . . 373
    - Psychological Variables in Coping 374
    - Comparison With Other Illnesses 375
    - Treatment 375
      - Mastectomy Versus Limited Resection 375
      - Breast Reconstruction 376
      - Adjuvant Chemotherapy 377
      - Posttreatment Adjustment Reactions 377
      - Sexual Side Effects of Breast Cancer
        Treatments 377
    - Cancer Morbidity, Mortality, and the Psyche . 378
      - Methodological Problems 379
      - Coping Styles 379
      - Impact of Psychosocial Treatment on
        Disease Progression 379
    - Prognosis, Psychotherapy, and
      Countertransference 381
      - Some Practical Guidelines for Psychotherapy . 381
  - ◆ "Physician, Heal Thyself" 383
  - ◆ Summary 384
  - ◆ References 385

As mentioned in the introduction to Chapter 8, we have selectively focused on the medical-psychiatric issues in women's health. The volume by Stewart et al.[155] integrates many of the psychosocial issues that we only skim here.

As always, use the questions as you find helpful.

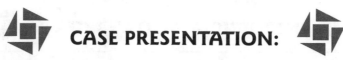

CASE PRESENTATION:

Mrs. Reid (Part I): Menopause, Chronic Pelvic Pain, and Hysterectomy

Mrs. Reid is a 53-year-old woman who is referred to you by her gynecologist for "postmenopausal depression." Mrs. Reid has been her patient for many years and was doing well until about 1 year ago, when she began experiencing hot flashes and irregular periods. Her menses have since ceased entirely, without obvious sequelae. On her most recent routine visit, she had become tearful when her doctor asked her how work was going. Mrs. Reid had responded, "Everything is fine there, but I'm having a hard time coping." The patient could offer no specific precipitant for her distress, prompting the gynecologist's concern regarding menopause-associated depression and the psychiatric referral.

Mrs. Reid had been in psychotherapy in her early 20s when she was undergoing a workup for unexplained chronic pelvic pain. She has no history of substance abuse and has never been on psychotropic medication. There is no history of postpartum or premenstrual depression. She has never been on oral contraceptives. Prior sexual functioning had been satisfactory. She has worked for 25 years as a schoolteacher, is married, and has two grown children. There was no family history of psychiatric illness or substance abuse.

Mental status exam reveals a dark-haired, sportily dressed woman who appears thoughtful and is easy to engage. Her speech is measured, but goal-directed, coherent, and logical. Affect is full. Mood is sad. There is no suicidal ideation. Her thought content centers on concerns about her job and how it is affecting her psychologically. There are no hallucinations or delusions. She is alert and fully oriented. Higher cognitive functions are tested individually and are entirely intact. Capacity for insight and judgment are assessed as above average.

 QUESTIONS

Choose all that apply.

1. Mrs. Reid said the most difficult thing about menopause was that she never knew when she was going to get a hot flash, which was embarrassing, especially when she was teaching. Her periods had been heavy and painful for many years, "a real nuisance." She denied any other symptoms, except relief that "it was all over." Mrs. Reid acknowledged being upset since her boss recently failed to promote her to assistant principal. She regretted not having furthered her own education as a younger woman. In retrospect, she would have liked to have pursued a doctorate in comparative literature and taught at the college level, but stated, "Few women went that far when I was young. You became a teacher because that was the thing that women did." Which of the following is/are true?

   a. Most of the psychiatric literature supports the gynecologist's impression that menopause is a time of high risk for psychiatric disorder.

   b. Estrogen deficiency has been implicated for the symptoms listed in the Kupperman menopausal index (vasomotor symptoms, paresthesias, insomnia, nervousness, melancholia, vertigo, weakness, arthralgia and myalgia, headaches, palpitations, and formication).

   c. The view that menopause has a deleterious effect on mental health was based on studies that were methodologically flawed.

   d. Vasomotor symptoms and vaginal dryness have been convincingly related to hormonal (rather than psychological) menopausal changes.

2. When queried about her feelings concerning her career, Mrs. Reid stated that she felt regret, not guilt. "This was a different kind of 'doing something wrong'!" Her pride in her work with learning-disabled children often lessened her sense of dissatisfaction with her job. One child had done particularly well on standardized testing

the week before, which cheered her and was quite heartening. She treasured the small bouquet of flowers the child brought her. Her marriage was at times "rocky," since her husband did not seem to understand her regrets. Mrs. Reid does admit to diminished sexual interest, and states that intercourse with her husband has become painful in the past 2 years. Her appetite for food "has never been good." She experiences difficulty sleeping, awakening frequently in the middle of the night. Which are true?

    a. Kraepelin's original distinction between involutional melancholia and other types of affective illness has not been substantiated.

    b. No direct temporal relationship between menopause and the onset of mental illness has been confirmed.

    c. Involutional melancholic and manic-depressive patients were found to have *equivalent* risks of affective disorder in first-degree relatives.

    d. There are few data to substantiate the notion that sexual interest declines in women after the menopause, especially when contrasted with men of comparable age.

    e. Mrs. Reid's vegetative symptoms are the prodrome of an affective syndrome.

3. The term *climacteric* . . .
    a. Is synonymous with menopause.
    b. Is synonymous with perimenopause.
    c. Is the transition period from reproductive to non-reproductive status.
    d. Refers to the first amenorrheic period.

4. The hormonal changes of menopause include . . .
    a. Decline in the production of estradiol, which is the main form of ovarian estrogen.
    b. Decline in follicle-stimulating hormone (FSH).
    c. Increase in FSH.
    d. Decline in luteinizing hormone (LH).

5. The most reliable marker of menopause is thought to be . . .
    a. Self-report of at least 1 year of amenorrhea.
    b. High FSH levels with amenorrhea.
    c. Low estrogen levels with amenorrhea.
    d. Irregular menstrual cycles and age above 50 years.

6. The gynecologist is surprised that you do not recommend medication, and is concerned that Mrs. Reid is "not telling you everything." Her impression is that menopausal women like Mrs. Reid have a high incidence of

nervousness, "blues," and irritability secondary to hormonal changes. She seems satisfied, however, that you will be monitoring Mrs. Reid closely in weekly psychotherapy, and wants to be informed if her psychiatric status changes. All of the following are true except . . .

    a. One would expect to see nonspecific complaints of "nerves," irritability, and headache peak at the time of menopause.

    b. Mrs. Reid might be at greater risk for psychiatric symptoms if she were still menstruating, and therefore presumably immediately premenopausal.

    c. Research has substantiated that nonpsychiatric complaints, such as hot flashes and sweats, sharply increase at menopause and are not merely artifactual.

    d. Nonspecific somatic and psychological complaints were found to be more common in women under 45 years of age than in those over 45.

7. Methodological pitfalls in the menopause research have included all of the following except . . .
    a. Reliance on clinic samples
    b. Use of general population surveys
    c. Definitions of menopause based on age
    d. Exclusive focus on melancholia and depression

8. Over the next 6 months, Mrs. Reid's insight about her own background and past choices continues to expand, but she still complains of occasional hot flashes, low sexual interest, dyspareunia, and middle insomnia. She denies dysphoric symptoms and states that her mood has improved since she has been in psychotherapy. She doesn't understand, then, why she is still symptomatic. Her gynecologist recommends estrogen replacement therapy, but Mrs. Reid is opposed to the idea of taking medication. How do you help guide her?

    a. Dyspareunia related to vaginal atrophy responds well to estrogen therapy.

    b. Antidepressants are effective in relieving both depression and hot flashes associated with menopause.

    c. Menopausal-related insomnia responds well to estrogen replacement therapy.

    d. Exogenous estrogens have proven efficacy for improving libido.

9. The most commonly occurring neuropsychiatric side effect of hormone replacement therapy involves progestin-induced . . .
    a. Psychosis.
    b. Mania.

  c. Depression.

  d. Anxiety.

10. Sherwin and colleagues[138,141–146] have pioneered the relationship between affect and sex hormones. Their findings have included which of the following?

  a. In two prospective studies of women who had undergone oophorectomy, depression scores covaried inversely with circulating levels of estradiol.

  b. In two prospective studies of women who had undergone oophorectomy, depression scores covaried inversely with circulating levels of testosterone.

  c. Increased feelings of well-being on estrogens are most apparent in severely depressed women.

  d. The symptoms of estrogen deficiency are usually less severe in women who have undergone surgical (versus natural) menopause.

11. The hormone replacement regimen that was shown to increase the sexual desire, sexual arousal, and frequency of sexual fantasies of surgically menopausal women included the addition of . . .

  a. Testosterone.

  b. LH.

  c. FSH.

  d. Estriol.

12. It is clinically difficult to distinguish psychogenic desire disorders from . . .

  a. Female androgen deficiency syndrome.

  b. Overreplacement of estrogen.

  c. Thyrotoxicosis.

  d. Estrogen deficiency.

13. Estrogen's mood-enhancing effects have been postulated to be mediated by . . .

  a. Effects on monoamine oxidase activity.

  b. Effects on tryptophan.

  c. Effects on cortisol.

  d. Placebo effects.

  e. None of the above.

14. What is likely to be the impact of preexisting attitudes about women's experience of the menopause?

  a. In general, neutral feelings about the cessation of menses become more negative as women actually experience menopause.

  b. In general, neutral feelings about the cessation of menses become more positive as women actually experience menopause.

  c. Women who expected some beneficial effect had lower levels of depression during menopause.

  d. The psychological experience of menopause tends to be independent of women's preexisting expectations.

15. Mrs. Reid begins to respond to estrogen, administered in patches, with no adverse side effects. She tells you more about her previous psychiatric history. She had been in therapy briefly in her early 20s when repeated medical tests for chronic pelvic pain of 2 years' duration, including laparoscopy, proved negative. She felt as though "people thought I was crazy. I thought maybe they were right . . . it was all in my head." The pain subsided completely after the birth of her second child, with no clear etiology. What has been discovered in the research on chronic pelvic pain?

  a. The onset of pelvic pain usually correlates with psychological precipitants.

  b. A significantly higher incidence of stressful life events distinguishes chronic pelvic pain patients without a physical etiology from nonpain control subjects.

  c. The majority of patients with the abdominal pelvic pain syndrome are not clinically depressed or anxious.

  d. There is consensus that most patients with chronic pelvic pain have normal findings on laparoscopy.

  e. A history of early childhood family disruptions distinguishes chronic pelvic pain patients from control subjects.

16. Several recent studies have explored the correlation between chronic pelvic pain and childhood sexual abuse. What have been the preliminary conclusions?

  a. A significantly higher incidence of childhood sexual abuse has been confirmed in chronic pain patients.

  b. Findings of a higher incidence of sexual abuse disappeared when control groups were used as comparison.

  c. Women with chronic pelvic pain have higher scores on measures of dissociation.

  d. Patients with histories of childhood sexual abuse and chronic pain are more likely to respond to pharmacological therapy alone than are patients without abuse histories.

17. What treatments have been effective for chronic pelvic pain?

  a. Cognitive interventions

  b. Behavioral interventions

  c. Stress analysis

d. None of the above; chronic pelvic pain tends to be resistant to interventions other than analgesics.

18. Mrs. Reid's vaginal itching and dryness improve with the estrogen. The hot flashes also disappear. Slowly, she and her husband resume regular intercourse, which makes her feel "as if I'm part of the world again." However, she begins to experience pelvic pain upon deep thrusting during intercourse. Workup reveals two large pelvic masses consistent with fibroids. The gynecologist hopes to avoid surgery but suspects that hysterectomy may be required in the near future, which greatly upsets the patient. Once again, the gynecologist is concerned about depression, since she feels that there is a strong association between hysterectomy and psychiatric morbidity. Which statements are true?
   a. Psychological distress increases after hysterectomy in the majority of study patients.
   b. No consistent relationship between hysterectomy and psychiatric illness has emerged from the literature.
   c. Research has confirmed a high incidence of psychological morbidity in women who are about to undergo hysterectomy.
   d. Research has confirmed a high incidence of psychological morbidity in women who have already had a hysterectomy.

19. Factors that seem predictive of psychiatric morbidity associated with hysterectomy include . . .
   a. Age.
   b. Social class.
   c. Prior psychiatric history.
   d. Type of gynecological pathology.
   e. Preoperative mental status.

20. *Menorrhagia* refers to . . .
   a. Excessively profuse menstruation.
   b. Painful menstruation.
   c. Cessation of menstruation.
   d. Painful intercourse.

21. Mrs. Reid is extremely anxious about the anticipated surgery. While many associations to her flawed sense of femininity are brought up, there are several practical concerns. She has never experienced general anesthesia before, and wonders what it will be like to be "totally out." She is concerned about yet another deterioration in her sexual life and worries that she will become clinically depressed after the surgery. What are some of the data that guide you in helping Mrs. Reid prepare for surgery?
   a. The majority of women experience a decline in sexual functioning posthysterectomy.
   b. Preoperative psychiatric disorder has emerged as a strong risk factor for postoperative psychiatric disorder.
   c. Combined hysterectomy and bilateral salpingo-oophorectomy are associated with a higher incidence of psychiatric disorders than simple hysterectomy.
   d. None of the above.

Answers

1.	Answer: c, d (pp. 350–351, 353)	12.	Answer: a (p. 354)
2.	Answer: a, b, c (pp. 350–351, 354)	13.	Answer: a, b (p. 353)
3.	Answer: b, c (p. 351)	14.	Answer: b, c (p. 356)
4.	Answer: a, c (p. 351)	15.	Answer: c (pp. 358–359)
5.	Answer: b (p. 351)	16.	Answer: a, c (p. 359)
6.	Answer: a (p. 351)	17.	Answer: a, b, c (pp. 359–360)
7.	Answer: b (p. 350)	18.	Answer: b, c (pp. 361–362)
8.	Answer: a, c (p. 355)	19.	Answer: c, e (p. 361)
9.	Answer: c (p. 355)	20.	Answer: a (p. 358)
10.	Answer: a, b (p. 353)	21.	Answer: b (pp. 362–363)
11.	Answer: a (p. 354)		

◈ MENOPAUSE

Overview

Wading through the research on menopause and psychiatric morbidity is daunting. At first, the confusion seems to stem from reviews that have overly condensed details from the original studies, thereby obscuring them; consulting the original studies, however, reveals minutiae and methodological problems that appear to defy conclusions. Nonetheless, it is encouraging that there is a trend to depathologize menopause, statistically debunking old Jekyll-Hyde stereotypes of the menopausal woman as "oppressed by fears of impending evils . . . with a melancholy of her own, compounded of many simples, extracted from many objects."[31] (See also the fascinating essay by Marilyn Maxwell[97] on portrayals of menopausal women in literature.)

Most of the early studies used tenuous definitions of menopause, yet their conclusions live on, stamped as established fact. We found the 1991 paper by Schmidt and Rubinow[134] to be the most cogent, comprehensive, and critical guide to this literature. Papers by Ballinger[10] and by Gise and Weston[58] also directed our reading. Here we will present an overview of the trends as applicable to clinical situations arising on a consultation-liaison service. The ambitious reader is referred to the originals.

Finally, note that Mrs. Reid's gynecologist is female. Misassumptions about menopause and female psychology are by no means linked to the Y chromosome. When a patient focuses *exclusively* on the male gender of a physician who has upset her, however realistically, he may have become an object of transference—that is, there may be displacement of feelings about other significant men in her life. Be careful of colluding in therapy with a reverse-sexist, "this is what men are like" stance. Such a posture may represent a form of resistance that blocks further exploration of other issues (self-esteem, sexuality, etc.). (The psychodynamics of men's views of menopausal women has been explored in an interesting essay by Phillips.[119])

Menopause and Psychiatric Morbidity

Many patients present gynecological symptoms without being sick gynecologically. Their illness represents a psychic conflict sailing under a gynecological flag.[129]

While Rogers's[129] statement poetically captures the psychosomatic determinants of certain gynecological complaints, it fails to depict most menopausal women, whose physical symptoms are usually medical, not psychological, in etiology. Menopause has accrued many medical, psychological, and cultural meanings, but the gynecological and psychiatric literatures have become quite discrepant. For example, some gynecological textbooks still insist that psychiatric symptoms (e.g., depression, lack of confidence, poor concentration) are attributable to estrogen deficiency.

◆ *However, the impression that menopause is a time of high risk for psychiatric disorder has not been consistently supported by subsequent psychiatric research.*

Several methodological problems with the early menopause literature are worthy of note:

◆ Much of the early research was based on clinic attendees, who are not representative of the population at large. Conclusions about the association between the "menopausal years" and psychiatric illness based on clinic samples have not been upheld in general population surveys.[3a,7,54,60,72] Attendance at clinics is determined by a complex interaction of personal, economic, social, and cultural factors that can skew the data derived from them. Referral bias, sociocultural issues, and personality factors may influence who winds up in the clinic waiting room rather than the gynecologist's office.

◆ Gynecology clinic attendees have been shown to have 1) increased rates of psychiatric disturbance compared with the general population;[26] 2) higher scores on the General Health Questionnaire,[58a] indicating significant emotional disturbance;[9] 3) greater likelihood of previous psychiatric contact;[9] and 4) less demonstrable physical illness accounting for their clinic visit.[103] Menorrhagia and pelvic pain appeared to be the most common complaints.

◆ Criteria for establishing menopausal status have varied. Most studies have failed to obtain adequate biological evidence of ovarian dysfunction in their "menopausal" subjects.

◆ A reliable endpoint for the "menopausal period" has been lacking. For example, a mood disorder occurring

10 years after menopause cannot meaningfully be considered as menopause related.[134]

◆ Affective symptoms have not been distinguished from affective syndromes.

The World Health Organization[126] has defined *menopause* as the permanent cessation of menstruation resulting from loss of ovarian activity, and the *climacteric* or *perimenopause* as the transition period from reproductive to nonreproductive status (i.e., the period immediately before menopause and at least the first year afterward). During the climacteric and menopause, there is a decline in production of estradiol, which is the main form of ovarian estrogen. This markedly increases FSH and, to a lesser extent, LH.

◆ FSH levels that are consistently elevated (> 25 IU/L), combined with a 6-month history of menstrual cycle irregularity, constitute biological evidence of the climacteric.[134]

◆ FSH levels that are greater than 40 IU/L, coupled with a 6-month history of amenorrhea, also reasonably define menopause.[134]

Research has used markers of menopause other than hormone levels, such as absolute age, onset of irregular menstrual cycles, and patient self-reports of at least 1 year of amenorrhea.

◆ Samples that are selected by age, for example, are unlikely to be homogeneous, with age ranges from 41 to 59 years. (The mean age of menopause is thought to be roughly 50–51 years.[163])

◆ Studies that use the 1-year amenorrhea criterion may be confounded by retrospective reporting bias and possible misattribution (e.g., menstrual irregularity also occurs in women who are not yet menopausal); uterine bleeding may occur in postmenopausal women.

◆ Not even hormone levels are completely reliable. For example, in one study,[113] 3 of 12 amenorrheic patients were found to have serum estradiol/estrone ratios within the *pre*menopausal range, even though FSH levels were in the *post*menopausal range (> 40 IU/L). This finding suggested that there was residual ovarian estrogen production and only partial ovarian failure.

A surge of papers in the past 30–40 years have challenged the notion of menopause as psychotoxic:

◆ A 1957 study of 54 consecutive female first admissions to a psychiatric hospital between the ages of 40 and 55 years uncovered no direct temporal relationship between the onset of mental illness and the menopause.[160]

◆ Hopkinson[68] in 1964 compared patients who had their first depressive illness before and after the age of 50 years. They were similar, except that agitation (thought to be particularly characteristic of involutional melancholia) was more common in the early-onset group.

◆ Nonspecific complaints of "nerves," irritability, and headache were more common in women *under* 45 years of age than those over 45.[46]

◆ Several studies of women over 45 who were immediately premenopausal (i.e., assumed to be still menstruating) showed a higher frequency of psychiatric symptoms ("mental imbalance," fatigue, depression, and irritability) than in subjects who were already postmenopausal.[24,46,72,154] Predictably, nonpsychiatric complaints, like hot flashes and sweats, *did* increase sharply at age-defined menopause.

◆ Postmenopausal women unequivocally reported more hot flashes, joint pain, and sleep difficulties than perimenopausal women. However, several studies showed that physical discomfort did not always correspond with psychological distress;[62,95,96,98] many women perceived *lower* levels of stress in their daily lives after menopause.[96]

Kraepelin's concept of *involutional melancholia*,[82] as distinct from other types of affective illness, has not been substantiated on the basis of diagnostic features,[78,152] premorbid personality,[152] etiology,[152] clinical course,[152] or response to electroconvulsive therapy (ECT).[78] Involutional melancholia was included in DSM-I[1] and DSM-II,[1a] but deleted from DSM-III.[1b] Some additional evidence arguing against the validity of involutional melancholia as a distinct entity follows:[134]

◆ Patients with menopause-related major depressive episodes have no unique clinical pattern or history of previous depressive episodes.

◆ The risk of suicide or psychiatric hospitalization is not consistently increased during the menopausal period.

◆ There appears to be no increased prevalence of depression during menopause.

◆ The risk of affective disorder in first-degree relatives of involutional melancholic versus manic-depressive patients does not differ.

Two 1970s studies[175,177] by distinguished researchers set the stage for viewing involutional melancholia as "myth." However, their conclusions were convincingly challenged by a recent critical review.[134] In the first study, Weissman[175] examined a sample of 422 consecutive female outpatients admitted with major (nonbipolar) depression. Only an age criterion was used for defining menopausal status: the premenopausal group (< 45 years of age, n = 347), the menopausal group (45–55 years of age, n = 58), and the presumed postmenopausal group (> 56 years of age, n = 17). No significant differences were found in symptom patterns or number of previous depressive episodes. Weissman concluded that there was insufficient evidence for involutional-onset depression to stand as a distinct entity.

◆ Upon subsequent evaluation of these data, however, Schmidt and Rubinow[134] were struck by the substantial risk for developing a depressive episode in the postmenopausal group—65% of the postmenopausal depressed group had no previous history of depression (i.e., they experienced their first depressive episode late in life, in the postmenopausal period).

◆ A substantial proportion of women first become psychiatrically distressed postmenopausally, reminiscent of the "involutional" description. Again, the age criterion of menopause limits the conclusions that can be drawn either way.

In the second study, Winokur[177] examined a sample of 71 consecutively admitted women with admission diagnoses of affective disorder. Twenty-eight patients were defined as menopausal on the basis of a 3-year history of amenorrhea. He compared the risk of hospitalization for a depressive episode in these 28 patients with the overall risk of developing an affective syndrome in the total sample of 71 women (age range 20–80 years). No significant differences were found, prompting the following conclusions: 1) menopause was not supported as precipitating an episode of affective disorder; 2) affective disorders were not more likely to occur during menopause; and 3) the study of menopause-associated depression was unlikely to promote further understanding of affective disorder. Winokur also found no association between the menopausal years and admissions for depression or attempted suicide.[177,178]

Schmidt and Rubinow[134] have taken issue with these conclusions:

◆ Winokur *used different severity criteria* for the diagnosis of depression during menopause than for depressions that were not menopause related.

◆ The reasoning for this methodology was circular: because of the high symptom frequency of depression (38%) and nervousness (75%) in his menopausal patients, more stringent diagnostic criteria (e.g., need for hospitalization) were needed to qualify for the depressive diagnosis in the menopausal patients.

◆ Moreover, Winokur stated that since the symptoms reported during menopause were "similar to those which patients suffering from affective disorder complain of" (p. 93),[177] the addition of the hospitalization criterion was necessary.

Schmidt and Rubinow[134] have stated,

> Given the high frequency of reports of menopause-related affective symptoms in this group, it seems unwarranted to conclude that there is "little value in looking specifically at the menopausal state for clues to the etiology of ordinary affective disorder."[177] Additionally, even if the menopause-related symptoms were phenomenologically distinct from major affective disorder, the affective symptoms occurring so frequently during menopause require further explanation. (p. 846)

They argue that the current data do *not* convincingly refute a menopause-related affective syndrome. Furthermore, they cite evidence from two studies[23,153] that reported that involutional versus early-onset depression was associated with less family history of depression:

> Thus, while menopausal major depression does not appear phenomenologically distinct, . . . *other forms of affective disorder* may be associated with this period. In fact, many of the original reports described a clinical picture during menopause that was more consistent with neurasthenia or atypical depression. *The presupposition that menopause-related affective syndromes, if they exist, will be manifested by melancholia may have interfered with the identification and characterization of other affective syndromes (e.g., atypical depression) occurring at this time . . . .*[134] (p. 846, italics added)

The relationship between affective symptoms and menopause remains controversial. Earlier studies are severely limited by imprecise definitions of menopause and other problems in methodology. We summarize some of the hormonal research next.

Hormone Studies

Sherwin and colleagues[138,141–146] have taken a more quantitative approach by investigating affective changes as a function of sex hormone levels.

◆ In two prospective studies of women who had undergone oophorectomy ("surgical menopause"), depression scores covaried inversely with levels of both estradiol and testosterone.[138,143]

◆ When a placebo was substituted for estrogen in these surgically menopausal women, depression scores increased.

These results indicate a positive association between mood and sex hormone levels in healthy, nondepressed women. Note that women who have undergone surgical menopause usually experience more severe symptoms of estrogen deficiency, due to the abrupt change in their hormonal environment.[140]

Affective responses to exogenous estrogen were investigated in postmenopausal women whose pretreatment depression differed in intensity on the Beck Depression Inventory.[13a,135] Conjugated estrogens (Premarin) enhanced the mood of euthymic women but not those who were depressed.

Estrogen could hypothetically affect mood in several ways:[140]

◆ Regularly cycling depressed women have higher levels of plasma monoamine oxidase (MAO) activity than do nondepressed women.[81] It has been shown that exogenous estrogen decreases MAO activity in the amygdala and hypothalamus of rats,[89] thereby hypothetically maintaining higher serotonin levels in the brain.

◆ Significant negative correlations have been found between depression scores and free plasma tryptophan in women who have undergone oophorectomy; mood and free tryptophan levels have been enhanced after treatment with exogenous estrogen.[5] Estrogen displaces tryptophan, which is the serotonin precursor, from its binding sites to plasma albumin in vitro and in vivo.[4] This would allow more free tryptophan to be available to the brain, where it could be metabolized to serotonin.

◆ A prospective study of surgically menopausal women found increased density of tritiated imipramine bind-

ing sites on platelets coincident with higher estradiol levels and lower depression scores.[146] To the extent that estrogen increases serotonin's concentrations or its time in the synapse, estrogen would enhance mood.[140]

Comment. These studies refute the notion of the menopausal woman as a melancholic "madwoman of Shalott," and have practical implications: Beware of assuming that menopausal patients' expressions of negative self-image or defective femininity are "age appropriate." Colluding with such attitudes fosters stereotypes, which should be challenged in psychotherapy. It would be equally spurious, however, to relegate subtler menopause-associated symptomatology to the status of myth; premenstrual dysphoric disorder has just been rescued from that fate. A critical review of the available research shows that conclusions about the "nonexistence" of menopause-related mood syndromes are premature. The literature has suffered from selective interpretation of data, lack of methodological precision, and failure to investigate syndromes other than major depressive disorder. Prospective, longitudinal studies of biologically confirmed menopause are needed before definitive conclusions can be drawn about the psychiatric consequences of this phase of life.

Symptoms and Estrogen Deficiency: Facts and Fiction

Kupperman Menopausal Index

The Kupperman menopausal index[84] is based on 11 items: vasomotor symptoms (hot flashes and cold sweats), paresthesias, insomnia, nervousness, melancholia, vertigo, weakness, arthralgia and myalgia, headaches, palpitations, and formication. It does not distinguish among possible etiologies, although gynecological authors have long attributed all of these symptoms to the hazards of estrogen deficiency. Utian and Serr[166] found that the symptoms that were most likely to be estrogen related fell into two groups:

◆ An early-onset group: hot flashes, sweats, and atrophic vaginitis
◆ A late-onset group: osteoporosis

The other Kupperman symptoms were *independent* of estrogen deficiency, and clustered according to sociocultural or psychosocial factors. It is generally accepted that only vasomotor symptoms and vaginal dryness—*not* psychological symptoms—are convincingly related to the hormonal changes of menopause.[179]

The vasomotor phenomena of hot flashes and cold sweats are estimated to persist for 1 year in 65% of postmenopausal women, and for 5 years in about 20%.[20] Moreover, there are certain vegetative complaints occurring with estrogen deficiency that may mistakenly be attributed to primary psychiatric illness. We discuss them below.

Sexuality

Sexual complaints center on *dyspareunia,* which is often related to vaginal atrophy, and *vaginitis,* which also results from estrogen deficiency. More ambiguous is the finding of postmenopausal diminished sexual drive. Suggestions that there would be an increase in sexual drive after menopause (e.g., because of freedom from pregnancy fears[93]) have not been supported by research. All studies have indicated quite the contrary—namely, a drop in sexual interest.

Here are a few of the more important findings:

◆ Hallstrom[61] showed a significant decline in postmenopausal sexual interest that was independent of increasing age. Decline in sexual interest did significantly correlate with low social class, the symptom of depression, and a poor marital relationship, especially one in which the husband was experienced as unsupportive.

◆ Osborn et al.[112] confirmed the increase in sexual dysfunction with age in a community survey of women aged 35–59 years. Sexual dysfunction was found in 33%, consisting mainly of reduced sexual interest, vaginal dryness, infrequent orgasm, and dyspareunia. However, rather than assuming that menopause was the sole culprit, the authors looked at other potential etiologies. They found that there was no association of sexual dysfunction with menopausal symptoms per se, such as flashes and sweats, vaginal dryness, and cessation of menstrual periods. In contrast, sexual dysfunction *was* significantly positively associated with psychiatric disorder, "neuroticism," and marital disharmony.

◆ Exogenous estrogen fails to increase sexual desire or libido commensurate with improvements in atrophic vaginitis, dyspareunia, and vaginal lubrication.[100,101,104]

◆ Sherwin and colleagues[143–145] have demonstrated that *the addition of **testosterone**,* which is normally produced by the ovaries, to an estrogen replacement regimen *increased sexual desire, sexual arousal, and the frequency of sexual fantasies* in the women who re-

ceived this treatment compared with those treated with estrogen alone. These findings are consistent with those of other investigators who used subcutaneous pellets containing estradiol and testosterone.[25,28]

◆ Kaplan and Owett[75] evaluated the sexual functioning of 11 women, ages 40–57 years, who developed androgen (testosterone) deficiency after medical or surgical treatments. They found that testosterone deficiency in these women produced a marked decrease in libido and sexual responsiveness. They concluded that the *female androgen deficiency syndrome* is often clinically indistinguishable from psychogenic desire disorders (see also p. 378).

These results are interesting in light of studies showing that men and women age differently relative to sexual desire:

◆ Priest and Crisp[121] found that 25% of women in their early 40s indicated a decline in their sexual interest; this figure increased to 75% of women in their early 60s. The change was more marked in women than in men of comparable age.

◆ Pfeiffer and colleagues[118] reported that a high percentage (51%) of older women (ages 61–65) acknowledged absent sexual interest; in this regard they differed significantly from their younger (ages 46–50) counterparts (7%) and were in marked contrast with male subjects (whose decline in sexual interest was 0% for ages 46–50, and only 11% for ages 61–65).

These data suggest that female libido undergoes a significant diminution with advancing age, becoming increasingly discrepant from that of males.

Several papers provide useful reviews on sexuality and menopause.[6,40,128,131]

Comment. Obviously, factors other than hormones influence sexual functioning throughout life. Previous sexual functioning, personality, cultural factors, personal illness, and the quality of the marital relationship influence female sexuality. It is important to take an adequate sexual history. Sometimes there may be countertransferential reluctance to discuss sexuality, especially when the patient is older than oneself. It is also often startling for beginning therapists when older patients develop maternal and paternal transferences to them, regardless of their relative youth. Awareness of one's own, often subliminal, reactions to the patient's sexuality help maintain therapeutic effectiveness.

Sleep

Perimenopausal sleep difficulties occur *independently* of psychiatric conditions; estrogen deficiency produces difficulty falling asleep and staying asleep.[8,161,162] In addition, sleep may be disrupted because of hot flashes, which occur more frequently at night.[140] Estrogen replacement therapy is often helpful (see below).

Hormone Replacement Therapy

Hormone replacement therapy with estrogen eliminates hot flashes, helps prevent osteoporosis, and may reduce the risk of coronary disease.[149] Dyspareunia related to vaginal atrophy also responds well to this treatment. *Diminished libido, however, does not directly improve with estrogen replacement therapy,*[12,159] but responds better to testosterone.[143-145]

Psychological Functioning

While the physiological benefits of estrogen replacement therapy have been well established, the mood benefit is more ambiguous. Results have been variable:

◆ Estradiol was significantly more effective than progestin, combination estradiol-progestin, or placebo in improving sexual functioning, depression, fatigue, anxiety, irritability, and insomnia in a large study.[39]

◆ One review concluded that estrogen replacement did improve psychological functioning, but that progestins should be minimized because of possible adverse effects.[38] (Progestin is added because of the epidemiological association between unopposed estrogen and endometrial cancer.) Unfortunately, progestin-induced *depression* is a complication.[67,139]

◆ In contrast, others discovered a large placebo effect of estrogen on psychological state,[32] failing to corroborate any direct therapeutic effect specifically on psychological symptoms.[55,158,162,165]

Nonetheless, many early menopausal psychological symptoms correlate with vasomotor symptoms, which clearly respond to hormone replacement therapy.[54,94] One woman with no prior psychiatric history described the experience of these vasomotor changes:

> . . . like opening an oven, and having a hot blast come at you, all at once, but from within your own body. You feel like you're suffocating and turning red as a beet. If there is no relief in sight, such as opening a window or door for cool air, you can only sit absolutely still, waiting for the blast to pass. It is so sudden, so unpredictable, that there is no time to adjust socially or to compensate for one's momentary loss of concentration. Even though objectively no one else might notice, it feels as if one's most private bodily functions are on public display. It's a feeling of one's body being foreign and out of control.

The psychological relief afforded by eliminating hot flashes and improving vaginal dryness should come as no surprise.[27,164] *However, hormone replacement therapy is no substitute for antidepressant medications for affective illness.* Antidepressants are effective in this population for improving mood, irritability, headache, and insomnia.[49,80,176] Hot flashes, on the other hand, have been found to be resistant to antidepressant treatment and to respond preferentially to hormone replacement.

As always, be sure to rule out medical disorders in patients who present with new psychological complaints or cognitive changes. When complaints are related to the hormone therapy rather than to a primary psychiatric disorder, discuss with the gynecologist modifying the estrogen-to-progestin ratio (i.e., decreasing the progestin) or changing to another pattern of administration (e.g., sequential hormone replacement versus continuous combination therapy).

Note also that estrogen replacement therapy has been anecdotally associated with panic attacks.[37,120]

Insomnia

The effects of estrogen on insomnia have been encouraging, with several double-blind studies showing improvement over placebo.[27,161,162] Some feel that estrogens improve sleep quality independently of their effect on disruptive vasomotor symptoms,[27,133] but not everyone agrees.[142] Ballinger[10] has gone so far as to state that estrogen replacement should be encouraged for patients with new-onset insomnia during the menopausal years, particularly if they also experience marked vasomotor symptoms. Despite some debate, there is consensus that estrogen is appropriate for insomnia only when the sleep disturbance is not secondary to a psychiatric condition such as depression.

Psychodynamics

In contrast to childbirth, preparation for the menopause has been a neglected area.[70] Phase-appropriate introspection about certain life choices does not solely result from hormonal changes, nor does it invariably warrant pharmacological intervention. For example, Avis and McKinlay[3] examined women's attitudes toward menopause in a randomly sampled, prospective study ($N = 2,565$, ages 45–55).

- They found that the majority of women reported *relief* or neutral feelings about the cessation of menses; feelings became more positive with time.
- Negative attitudes toward menopause were related to general symptom reporting and depression.
- Preexisting negative attitudes correlated with subsequent symptom reporting during menopause.

Personal characteristics,[39a] especially prior depression,[2] are more related to the so-called menopause syndrome than to menopause itself.

> Women for whom menopause is problematic have varied reactions. Those who have not had children may become depressed when they experience a resurgence of regret that their children no longer exist, even within the realm of possibility. Women with children whose roles as mothers have been singularly invested may also become depressed because of the loss of capacity. Fears about health and body integrity may reappear at this time of physical and hormonal shifts. Minor physical changes may trigger ancient panics about the mysteries of the body. Narcissistic concerns about aging heighten. Women worry that their sexual appeal and responsiveness will diminish. For some women at menopause, it feels as though life is over when the biological clock has stopped.[73] (p. 133)

Several papers[10,11,19,22,30a,76] detail the impact of cultural, social, and family issues on mental health in menopausal women (e.g., children leaving home, reevaluation of personal role and future goals). Datan[36] discussed the relationship between culture and psychological well-being in women at midlife. Attitudes of women from five Israeli subcultures were compared: Israel-born Moslem Arabs, and immigrant Jews born in North Africa, Persia, Turkey, and Central Europe. She writes,

> To the researchers' complete astonishment, women across the five cultures unanimously welcomed menopause and the cessation of fertility, despite great differences in childbearing history and . . . attitude toward size of their families. Two-thirds of the modern European women expressed regret that their families were so small . . . but, when asked whether they regretted their lost fertility or the loss of the chance to bear additional children, they, along with women in other cultures, emphatically declared that they were pleased to be finished with the business of childbearing and childrearing.[36] (p. 126)

The anthropologist Flint[48] has observed that in cultures where women's status and privileges increase at menopause, menopausal symptoms are minimal. In contrast, according to Gise and Weston,[58]

> North American society is youth-oriented with negative stereotypes of aging women that may promote symptoms at menopause. Menopausal symptoms are increased in women of lower socioeconomic status, especially those with low self-satisfaction and low self-esteem.[169] Women who have focused their psychological investment on childrearing to the exclusion of other interests seem to be at increased risk. (p. 273)

The effects of menopause have often been confused with the impact of negative life events that may coincide with this period, such as the loss of a spouse, difficulties with teenage or young-adult children, or the assumption of a caregiving role with elderly parents or in-laws.[58] Bowles[19] has also explored the impact of sociocultural beliefs on forming the attitudes toward menopause.

Comment: Menopause and Psychoanalysis

The views of menopause attributed to psychoanalytic theory are sometimes dismissed by reducing them to the kind of "quotable quotes" that make feminists wince, such as Benedek's[15] "symbolic castration" of menopause (1950) or the "mortification of menopause" theory of Helene Deutsch (1944)[42]—as though nothing different had been said by psychoanalysts since. This stereotyping perpetuates yet another myth of menopause; 50-year-old papers do not represent a current body of knowledge. An antianalytic bias deflects investigation from psychodynamic research and relegates psychoanalytic contributions to the status of the Dead Sea Scrolls. Given the ambiguity of the findings of biological research, no field of inquiry should be summarily dismissed—the clinician faced with a troubled patient needs all the help he or she can get.

Harris[63] critically reviews three psychoanalytical positions on menopause: 1) the traditional Freudian model, which was dominant from the beginning of the century until midcentury, when it became modified by 2) ego psychology and subsequently by 3) object relations theory. There is also a growing literature on the psychodynamics of middle age.[1c,29,43,50,59,69,79,87,99,105,111,137,167,168,170] The psychoanalyst Kalinich[73] has captured the current developmental, psychodynamic view of menopause. We quote her at length:

> Menopause wraps up a portion of a woman's life into a discrete package: its closure is clear; the ovarian cycle is finished; the womb is quiet once and for all. As a marker in a woman's life, it is so clearly defined that it can bring with it psychological hazards. For most women, however, menopause is basically uneventful. The "change" is experienced quietly and privately, with considerable nostalgia. Even if the menstrual periods were difficult, annoying or painful, their regular return provided a certain comfort and security. Women can miss this. And menopause, like retirement, does stand as a concrete reminder of the relative imminence of death. A certain kind of productivity is a thing of the past; most of life has been lived . . . As a child the thought that life began at forty seemed ludicrous to me . . . But now, having myself crossed into the middle years, when the simple facts of passing time are less easily denied, I must say that [it] . . . makes more sense to me. The pleasure in feeling a certain consolidation of all the hard-won gains of youth makes me comprehend the point. In certain ways, one really does "arrive" at a destination, or a destiny, that has been prepared by the steps taken in the early years. In that sense, life really does begin. Menopausal or not, with or without children, the middle years are special ones. And the biological clock . . . because it stops, helps preserve the middle years for living. It preserves them for being in time rather than for passing it . . . It insists that we exist in some way other than the way we did

> when we were young. In that way it readies us for old age by demanding that we actually live a bit before we are translated from this life. In a culture that privileges youth, this notion of aging is an important one for a therapist or an analyst to grasp. With it he or she will be able to help patients to hear in each tick of the clock the timbre of the music to come rather than the echo of notes already played.[73] (pp. 133–134)

Summary and Treatment Recommendations

1. Menopause is a time of enormous physiological and psychological complexity. The clinician must be wary of assumptions about what a menopausal woman should or should not feel. As damaging as the myth of melancholic menopause is the neglect of psychiatric signs because they were unexpected. There appears to be a subgroup of patients vulnerable to psychiatric distress during the climacteric and menopause. Psychiatric *symptoms* must be distinguished from *syndromal* states. In addition, menopausal somatic symptoms may induce behavioral or affective reactions that can be diagnostically confusing. For example, some women with severe daytime hot flashes report social avoidance similar to that observed in agoraphobic or social-phobic patients.[134] Failure to inquire about somatic symptoms might lead to the misdiagnosis of a primary anxiety disorder.

2. Both affective and relevant somatic symptoms (e.g., hot flashes, vaginal dryness) should be monitored. Endocrinological measures of FSH, LH, and estradiol are the most reliable way to assess menopause.

3. The literature has emphasized major depressive disorder at the expense of investigating other types of symptoms. Clinical evaluation should include a thorough history and mental status examination, screening for a range of psychiatric symptomatology, not only major depressive disorder.

4. Patients with natural menopause who present with depression and signs of estrogen deficiency should be given a trial of hormone replacement therapy unless there are contraindications (e.g., a history of breast cancer).[134]

5. Sometimes moderate to severe mood symptoms are accompanied by only minimal symptoms of estrogen deficiency. In these cases, the decision of hormone replacement versus antidepressant therapy depends

on factors such as past personal or family affective history and possible contraindications to exogenous estrogen.[134]

6. Patients experiencing surgically or medically induced menopause may pose special problems. These patients are usually younger, and the impact of their medical condition (e.g., cancer) is more complicated. Estrogen deficiency symptoms are usually more severe, due to the abruptness of the hormonal changes. Before prescribing psychotropics, remember that inadequate estrogen replacement or sequential hormone replacement (as opposed to continuous combination therapy) can precipitate mood changes. Recommend adjusting these medications first.

7. Intervention should optimally include the following components: providing balanced information about the menopause to women and their families; discussing attitudes and examining pessimistic beliefs; health promotion sessions focusing on diet, exercise, and smoking; stress management sessions; and group discussion of personal, health, and social issues faced by women during midlife.[70]

8. As with any life event, the context of a woman's individual psychodynamics frames her personal reactions to menopause. Exploring the impact of aging on self-esteem and life goals is very meaningful for patients who are making the transition to this next phase of life.

⬡ CHRONIC PELVIC PAIN

Incidence and Definition

Some definitions:

◆ **Menorrhagia:** *Excessively* profuse or prolonged menstruation
◆ **Menorrhalgia** (also termed *dysmenorrhea*): Painful menstruation
◆ **Dyspareunia:** Painful sexual intercourse
◆ **Chronic pelvic pain:** Pain of greater than 6 months' duration

Chronic pelvic pain has been called one of the most perplexing problems facing the gynecologist.[90] Approximately 25% of noncontraceptive gynecological visits involve some kind of pain complaint, and about 50% of laparoscopies are performed to evaluate pain.[124] While pain-inducing conditions such as dysmenorrhea and ectopic pregnancy do respond to pharmacological and surgical treatments, many types of pain are chronic and respond poorly or not at all.

Chronic pelvic pain patients are a heterogeneous population characterized by a spectrum of biological and psychological factors.

◆ For example, it is not possible to meaningfully predict laparoscopic findings in chronic pelvic pain patients: normal pelvic organs are found in as few as 17% to as many as 90%.[83,86,123,130,136]

Even more confusingly, although the pain location often correlates with lesion location, the perception of pain intensity demonstrates *no direct relationship* to the amount of tissue pathology.[47,157]

Many early studies found higher levels of psychopathology in pain patients compared with control subjects,[30,114,123,125,130] paving the way for assumptions of a psychiatric etiology for pain without documentable physical pathology. Tightened methodology, however, has challenged these assumptions. For example, Hodgkiss and Watson[66] found that laparoscopy-positive and -negative chronic pelvic pain patients *did not differ* on measures of psychiatric morbidity or illness behavior, although both groups tended to be more depressed than nonpain control subjects.

In a 1989 study by Slocumb et al.,[148] 41 gynecological patients with the abdominal pelvic pain syndrome were matched with control subjects, who were nonpain patients attending the gynecology clinic for other complaints. (The abdominal pelvic pain syndrome is diagnosed in about 78% of pain clinic patients.[147] It is defined as pain in one or more of the soft tissues in the paracervical area, vaginal cuff, abdominal wall, vaginal wall, and over the sacrum. The pain often occurs during coitus, menses, ovulation, and upon bladder or bowel distention.) All patients either had no evidence of pelvic disease or showed other systemic signs. The pain patients had already tried a variety of treatments, which had been ineffective, including medications (antibiotics, oral contraceptives, and analgesics), laparoscopy, hysterectomy, and laparotomy. Patients were administered the Hopkins Symptom Checklist[41a] and the Symptom Questionnaire.[76a,77a] Not surprisingly, the chronic pain patients were self-rated as

◆ Significantly more anxious, depressed, and hostile than control subjects.
◆ Having more nonpelvic somatic symptoms than control subjects.

The pertinent negatives of this study, however, ran counter to the common clinical assumptions about chronic pain patients:

◆ *The majority of the chronic pain patients (56%) rated themselves within the normal range on all scales.*
◆ Stressful life events did *not* significantly differ between the two groups, corroborating the findings of another study that failed to correlate the onset of pain with psychological precipitants.[56]
◆ *No significant differences* in early home life (e.g., bereavement, family disruptions) were found between the two groups. This contradicts other studies that have found that childhood bereavement is associated with adulthood somatization.[17,45,77]

These negative findings are cautions against stereotypes. However, there is growing evidence of a *subgroup* of chronic pelvic pain patients who are especially vulnerable to psychiatric distress:

◆ Several investigators have reported that patients with chronic pelvic pain are significantly more likely to have a history of sexual and physical abuse[21,116,122,171,172] and to use dissociation as a coping mechanism.[172]

These data are reminders to avoid default psychiatric diagnoses when medical etiologies are obscure, and to evaluate each pain patient without preconceptions of what you will find.

Treatment

Delivering appropriate medical care often poses a dilemma. Clearly, avoiding unnecessary surgical procedures has priority. However,

> Clinicians should not be misled by the presence of pathologic personality traits or neurotic features in chronic pain patients. Often physicians tend to disregard the validity of patients' pain reports if a strong "characterologic overlay" is present.[16] (p. 296)

Team collaboration and a nonjudgmental approach are crucial. Note that the two conditions most often associated with chronic pelvic pain—endometriosis and adhesions—are often difficult to detect by noninvasive means, including techniques such as magnetic resonance imaging (MRI); *only laparoscopy* makes the definitive

diagnosis.[151] Laparoscopy also permits the treatment of certain conditions, such as adhesions.[150]

Pearce and colleagues[115] investigated the results of a prospective randomized, controlled trial of two different psychological interventions in the treatment of chronic pelvic pain. The subjects were 78 women with chronic pelvic pain of at least 6 months' duration and without obvious laparoscopic pathology who were assigned to a pain analysis, stress analysis, or minimal-intervention group. All were told that their pain was due to abnormalities in pelvic blood flow. The stress analysis group members were trained in identifying and implementing alternative cognitive and behavioral responses in stressful situations, as well as being taught relaxation strategies. Women in the pain analysis group focused on monitoring events occurring before and after pain, participated in graded exercise, and received reinforcement of "well behaviors." Compared with subjects in the minimal-intervention control group, women in both the stress analysis and the pain analysis groups reported significantly lower pain intensity ratings at 6-month follow-up.

Multidisciplinary pain management approaches were significantly effective in two recent studies. Kames et al.[74] implemented a 6- to 8-week interdisciplinary program for 16 chronic pain patients that included both somatic and behavioral therapies.

◆ Acupuncture and psychological therapy (stress management, relaxation, hypnosis, sex education, and cognitive therapy) were used in all patients. Tricyclic antidepressants were given to approximately 50% of the patients. Narcotics were reduced until they were eliminated, and nonsteroidal antiinflammatory drugs were used in about one-third of patients. A small percentage also received trigger-point injections.
◆ Participants showed a dramatic decrease in pain levels after treatment compared with waiting-list control subjects. Anxiety and depression also decreased and psychosocial functioning improved, including return to work, increased social activities, and improved sexual activity.

Peters et al.[116] randomly assigned 106 chronic pelvic pain patients to either a standard-approach or an integrated-approach group. In the standard-approach group, physical causes of pelvic pain were excluded first and diagnostic laparoscopy was routinely performed. If no somatic cause was found, other causes such as psychological disturbances became the focus. In the second group, an integrated approach was started from the beginning, with equal attention to somatic, psychological, dietary, environmental, and physiotherapeutic factors. Laparoscopy was not routinely performed in this group. Both groups were similar in patient characteristics and pain severity.

◆ The integrated-approach group showed significantly greater improvement in pain, disturbance of daily activities, and associated pain symptoms at 1-year follow-up.
◆ Laparoscopy played no important role in relieving pain.
◆ However, it was not possible to determine which specific components of the treatment were most effective.

Note that women with chronic pelvic pain and childhood sexual abuse histories are likely to require multimodal treatment strategies, incorporating behavioral and insight-oriented psychotherapies with pharmacotherapy, as has been emphasized by Walker and colleagues.[172] Chronic pelvic pain patients with histories of childhood sexual abuse may not be compliant with antidepressant treatment.[173] In addition, one study found that pharmacotherapy tended to be less effective for these patients than for pain patients without abuse histories.

Patients with chronic pelvic pain are often unwilling to consider their symptoms as other than somatically based. Steege and Stout[151] have suggested framing this association in a way that is already acceptable to most people: that psychological factors such as worry, muscle tension, or depression worsen their pain. This strategy helps to establish the rapport needed for exploring psychological, behavioral, and cognitive patterns that exacerbate the pain symptoms. The goal of treatment is to develop strategies for interrupting these patterns. Steege and Stout[151] have the patient record pain ratings throughout the day, and then tailor treatment interventions that include

◆ Relaxation training directed at reducing muscle tension.
◆ Stress analysis to identify difficult life areas.
◆ Assertiveness training to teach skills for dealing with people or circumstances directly, rather than letting the pain complaints "speak" for the patient.
◆ Cognitive interventions directed at specific emotional responses to pain that may secondarily increase anxiety, depression, and perceived pain.

Steege and Stout[151] note,

Psychological approaches may also involve spouses or families to assist in defining a val-

ued role in the family despite some possible limitations in previous activities. Changes in sexual activity often accompany pelvic pain, and specific education and counseling may be required to allow the patient to return to a level of comfort. Sexual counseling suggestions often include information about adequate physiological arousal, changes in sexual positions, and instruction in vaginal relaxation exercises to treat a conditioned vaginismus response. As a trusting therapeutic relationship is established and coping skills are developed, some women may be receptive to pursuing psychotherapeutic approaches that are inclusive of broader issues related to unresolved emotional issues from past experiences. (p. 262)

Tricyclic antidepressants often lessen pain occurring in the presence of affective illness,[18,88,174] as well as in its absence.[16,35,57,173] The newer serotonergic agents are also being tried.[151]

Conclusions

Current research on chronic pain patients remains inconclusive, but clearly reveals distressed people—regardless of pathology. It is unequivocal that anxiety and depression magnify pain perception, and that pain is less tolerable for patients with emotional difficulties. However, psychological distress is as easily a *consequence* of persistent pain as the cause of it. Slocumb and colleagues[148] have recommended that patients *not* be told that psychological factors are the main *cause* of their pain, given our inadequate knowledge concerning causation.

✦ HYSTERECTOMY

Hysterectomy has been the most frequently performed major operation in the United States.[108] Unfortunately, the loss of the uterus is sometimes trivialized by physicians of both genders, at times treated as though it were the excision of a vestigial organ like the appendix, especially if the woman already has children. Reactions that are perceived as untoward may be misattributed to endogenous depression (or worse, designated "hysterical"), and may spur well-meaning referral to a psychiatrist, often specifically for medication. A woman's experience of her uterus depends in part on biology, but more importantly on her individual and cultural conceptions of femininity. The uterus can be seen as a childbearing organ; an excretory organ; a sexual organ; a regulator of bodily processes; a reservoir of strength; and a maintainer of youth or attractiveness.[44] Reactions to its loss, as with any medical procedure, must be understood within the individual woman's psychological framework.

However, as therapeutically noxious as trivializing hysterectomy is assuming that it inevitably bodes psychological ill.

◆ Before the early 1970s, many studies in Great Britain and the United States reported high rates of posthysterectomy psychiatric morbidity compared with other surgical procedures.

◆ This led to the assumption that hysterectomy was *causally* related to psychiatric disorder. This view has persisted despite the demonstration[132] that these studies had significant methodological flaws: reliance on retrospective rather than prospective data; use of nonstandardized psychological assessment instruments; failure to control for other procedures (e.g., oophorectomy); failure to distinguish the cause for hysterectomy (i.e., benign or malignant lesions); sample size differences; and flawed methods of data collection.

Gath et al.[51,54a] have provided a helpful review of the early literature and subsequent research on hysterectomy.

Psychiatric Sequelae

The alleged psychotoxicity of hysterectomy was challenged by two prospective studies that showed a high incidence of psychological morbidity in women *who were about to undergo* elective hysterectomy.[52,53,91,92,132] Martin et al.[91,92] in the United States and Gath et al.[52,53] in Great Britain prospectively compared pre- and posthysterectomy psychiatric functioning using structured psychiatric interviews and psychological rating scales. They found that psychiatric distress *declined* after hysterectomy. Several findings were of note:

◆ Both investigations reported a high prevalence of *preoperative* psychiatric illness (57%–58%). Depression was the most common diagnosis.

◆ Posthysterectomy psychological outcome differed in timing, but not in trend. The United Kingdom patients showed a marked *diminution* in psychiatric morbidity, from 58% preoperatively to 29% at 18-month follow-up.[53] This was similar to the significant posthysterectomy psychiatric improvement found in another prospective British study.[33] The American sub-

jects were also less symptomatic at 1-year follow-up, but the decline was not as dramatic.[91,92]

◆ Age, marital status, number of children, social class, and types of gynecological pathology *did not predict* posthysterectomy reactions. The strongest predictors of postoperative psychiatric morbidity were
  • Previous psychiatric history
  • Preoperative mental state

◆ Of clinical relevance, the American investigators detected an unexpected and inordinately high incidence of Briquet's syndrome (27% versus the expected 1%–2%).[91,92] (Briquet's syndrome was not specifically mentioned in the British sample.) Not surprisingly, these patients continued to be symptomatic after surgery. The authors suggest careful preoperative screening for these patients, who are at risk for having an unnecessary hysterectomy based on psychiatric distress rather than on gynecological illness.

Another project prospectively investigated psychological outcome in 60 women ages 30–55 years undergoing hysterectomy for benign conditions.[132] Assessments occurred within 2 weeks of the operation, after 4 months, and at 14 months.

◆ There was a high prevalence of preoperative psychological morbidity (55%), which *declined* after surgery (31.7%).

◆ The main risk factors for poor psychological outcome were previous scores on mental health measures and a personality inventory.

◆ The authors concluded that there was no evidence that hysterectomy led to greater psychological distress.

These findings are very similar to those of Gath et al.[53] and to the nonsignificant trends found by Martin's group.[91]

Lalinec-Michaud and colleagues[85] compared patients having hysterectomies, other pelvic surgery, or cholecystectomy. There were no differences among groups in depressive symptomatology, and all appeared to do well postsurgically, although a significant number of subjects dropped out during the follow-up period. The authors emphasized that although women undergoing hysterectomy do have anxiety and depressive symptoms, such symptoms are no more common than in control subjects and tend to remit postsurgically.

Youngs and Wise[180] have written,

> For the majority of patients, menses are perceived as a necessary experience. Even among

patients in whom menstruation has been painful and troublesome, many view the menstrual period as a valuable and important function . . . [Some] patients . . . report lessening of sexual desire, diminished ability to respond sexually, diminished sexual attractiveness, and concern over husband's possible infidelity. Specific concerns relate to "defective sexual equipment" or belief that hysterectomy was punishment for sexual misdeeds. (p. 257)

Comment.   While hysterectomy itself does not invariably induce psychiatric morbidity, and may *improve* quality of life, never underestimate the symbolic meanings of any medical illness or surgical procedure.

◆ Steer carefully between the twin risks of trivializing hysterectomy and colluding with the patient's catastrophic interpretation of it.

◆ It is therapeutically nihilistic to agree with a hysterectomy patient's view that a degraded sense of self and femininity is now her fate.

◆ Exploring the meanings of her lost uterus relative to her preexisting conflicts and fantasies helps the patient rework its meanings.

◆ Of course, an insight-oriented therapy is not always feasible or appropriate. Many patients respond better to cognitive approaches that challenge misassumptions in a more directive way.

Technical differences aside, all good psychotherapies have in common that they beckon the patient to consider that her interpretation of a real event is not inescapable; they offer the hope of other meanings, and in doing so, the promise that the pain can heal.

Effects on Sexuality

The adverse sexual effects of hysterectomy have been reported to be as high as 37%[41,102] and as low as 6%.[71] A recent study showed deterioration in sexual adjustment after hysterectomy.[107] However, while the procedure has adverse sexual effect in some patients, this is by no means universal.

◆ Many women show improved sexual functioning after hysterectomy.[33,52,53,65,91]

◆ Many reports indicate that patients resume their level of preoperative sexual functioning by between 2 and 4 months posthysterectomy.[33,52,53,59a,64]

◆ The best predictive factors for sexual functioning after surgery have been defined as presurgical coital frequency, cyclicity of arousability, frequency of desire, and frequency of orgasm.[63a,64]

Not surprisingly, preoperative orgasmic functioning and attitudes toward the sexual partner also influence postoperative sexual functioning.[64]

In their scholarly review of the psychological aspects of gynecological surgery, Oates and Gath[110] caution against biased interpretations of hysterectomy data:

The findings of some studies that over a third of women experienced a deterioration in their sexual life, together with the widespread equation of hysterectomy with castration and belief on the part of the public that hysterectomy affects sexual life, have led to the assumption that hysterectomy has a negative impact on sexual functioning in a significant number of women. Few, if any, of these studies were prospective and most used very variable and nonstandardized ways of assessing sexual functioning. The negative interpretation of their results is misleading. *The results of most of these studies, even the earliest ones, could be interpreted in an alternative and more positive way as showing that in the majority of women studied, hysterectomy led to either no change or an improvement in sexual functioning.* Almost all studies show that the women whose sexual functioning deteriorated were outnumbered by those women whose sexual functioning improved [or remained the same]. (pp. 733–734, italics added)

Abdominal Versus Vaginal Hysterectomy

Gath and colleagues[51–53] found no evidence for a differential psychological effect of abdominal versus vaginal hysterectomy—although women appreciate no scar. There are insufficient data in the literature to draw definitive conclusions.

Oophorectomy

Oates and Gath[110] reviewed the psychiatric morbidity after hysterectomy alone compared with hysterectomy and oophorectomy. Several reports showed that oophorectomy did not significantly contribute to posthysterectomy psychiatric disorders, including psychosexual dysfunction,[52,53,102] whether or not replacement hormones were provided.[13,52,91,127]

◆ These findings are perplexing; clearly, if oophorectomy leads to estrogen deficiency with vasomotor symptoms, vaginal atrophy, and diminished lubrication, untreated oophorectomy patients would be expected to do more poorly. Moreover, women with surgical menopause experience more severe symptoms of estrogen deficiency, due to the abrupt change of their hormonal environment.[140] (Refer to the work of Sherwin and colleagues[138,139,142-146] on surgical menopause and hormone therapy, which was summarized above.)

Oophorectomy has been associated with body-image changes.[14]

Risk Factors for Adverse Psychiatric Sequelae

There are several risk factors for adverse psychiatric sequelae:

◆ Regardless of methodology or controversy, preoperative psychiatric disorder remains a strong risk factor for postoperative psychiatric problems. Previous depression greatly increases the risk of depression afterward.

◆ A majority of patients receiving psychiatric treatment after hysterectomy were likely to have received similar treatment before the operation.[91]

◆ The patient's preoperative mental state affects outcome[52] even in the absence of a psychiatric history: patients who received a psychiatric diagnosis before the operation were also more likely to receive one postoperatively.[91]

◆ The gynecological diagnosis will influence the medical prognosis, and therefore the psychiatric outcome (e.g., endometriosis, fibroids, and cancer have different medical courses and psychological outcomes).

The effects of age, marital status and satisfaction, parity, and social class influence psychiatric outcome, but not consistently, except for younger women who have not had children or completed their families. For these patients, lost fertility may be wrenching, as profound a grief as the loss of a loved person. Helping the patient to mourn and to move on to changed expectations are important goals of therapy.

Conclusions

To suffer with heavy vaginal bleeding, painful intercourse, long-lasting dysmenorrhea, or chronic pain erodes the spirit; it is no wonder that women who have endured these conditions become depressed or psychiatrically symptomatic. Psychiatric evaluation of prospective hysterectomy candidates should include screening for somatoform disorder, as there exists a subgroup with somatoform rather than somatic illness that undergoes hysterectomy. However, the majority seek hysterectomy as a treatment that brings symptomatic relief.

◆ A recent study[106] confirmed that relief of heavy bleeding and pain was the major advantage of hysterectomy; close to one-third of the subjects reported that there was no disadvantage to the procedure at all.

◆ Preoperative mental status and mood, as well as a previous psychiatric history, have more closely correlated with postsurgical outcome than have generalizations about hysterectomy itself.

Explore the patient's understanding of the purpose, indications, and expected results of the procedure. If surgery is elective and the patient would benefit from psychotherapy or psychotropic drugs, the hysterectomy should be postponed if possible.[117] Petersen[117] has proposed the following outline for approaching psychiatric evaluation before or after hysterectomy:

◆ What is the meaning of the hysterectomy for the patient?

◆ Did she want more children?

◆ Is she concerned about an altered sense of femininity?

◆ Is she worried about a change in her sexual responsiveness?

◆ What do her partner and family think about the procedure?

◆ What previous reactions to stress has she had, and what was helpful for coping with them?

◆ What support systems are available to her?

◆ Are there other situational stresses affecting the patient that indicate that surgery should be postponed?

That the uterus is rich in psychosexual meanings makes its loss particularly poignant for most women. There are fears of lost femininity, desirability as a woman, and youth; grief over lost fertility; and resentment toward the medical profession, which is often perceived as trivializing the procedure.[109,156] The early retrospective studies appear to have made an interpretative mistake: they concluded that hysterectomy was the single causative factor for anguish, rather than a difficult step toward a cure that, like many medical treatments, leaves some of its sufferers exhausted and sometimes ambivalent.

⚜ REFERENCES

1. American Psychiatric Association: Diagnostic and Statistical Manual: Mental Disorders. Washington, DC, American Psychiatric Association, 1952

1a. American Psychiatric Association: Diagnostic and Statistical Manual of Mental Disorders, 2nd Edition. Washington, DC, American Psychiatric Association, 1968

1b. American Psychiatric Association: Diagnostic and Statistical Manual of Mental Disorders, 3rd Edition. Washington, DC, American Psychiatric Association, 1980

1c. Auchincloss E, Michels R: The impact of middle age on ambitions and ideals, in The Middle Years: New Psychoanalytic Perspectives. Edited by Oldham J, Liebert R. New Haven, CT, Yale University Press, 1989, pp 40–57

2. Avis N, Brambilla D, McKinlay S, et al: A longitudinal analysis of the association between menopause and depression: results from the Massachusetts Women's Health Study. Annals of Epidemiology 4:214–220, 1994

3. Avis N, McKinlay S: A longitudinal analysis of women's attitudes toward the menopause: results from the Massachusetts Women's Health Study. Maturitas 13:65–79, 1991

3a. Avis N, McKinlay S: The Massachusetts Women's Health Study: an epidemiologic investigation of the menopause. J Am Med Wom Assoc 50:45–49, 63, 1995

4. Aylward M: Plasma tryptophan levels and mental depression in post-menopausal subjects: effects of oral piperazine-oestrone sulphate. International Research Communications System (IRCS) Journal of Medical Science 1:30–34, 1973

5. Aylward M: Estrogens, plasma tryptophan levels in perimenopausal patients, in The Management of the Menopause and Post-Menopausal Years. Edited by Campbell S. Baltimore, MD, University Park Press, 1976, pp 135–147

6. Bachmann G: Sexual function in the perimenopause. Obstet Gynecol Clin North Am 20:379–389, 1993

7. Ballinger C: Psychiatric morbidity and the menopause: screening of general population sample. BMJ 3:344–346, 1975

8. Ballinger C: Subjective sleep disturbance at the menopause. J Psychosom Res 20:509–513, 1976

9. Ballinger C: Psychiatric morbidity and the menopause: survey of a gynaecological outpatient clinic. Br J Psychiatry 131:83–89, 1977

10. Ballinger C: Psychiatric aspects of the menopause. Br J Psychiatry 156:773–787, 1990

11. Ballinger C, Smith A, Hobbs P: Factors associated with psychiatric morbidity in women—a general practice survey. Acta Psychiatr Scand 71:272–280, 1985

12. Bancroft J: Hormones and sexual behavior. Psychol Med 7:553–556, 1977

13. Barker M: Psychiatric illness after hysterectomy. BMJ 2:91–95, 1968

13a. Beck A: Depression Inventory. Philadelphia, PA, Philadelphia Center for Cognitive Therapy, 1978

14. Bellerose S, Binik Y: Body image and sexuality in oophorectomized women. Arch Sex Behav 22:435–459, 1993

15. Benedek T: Climacterium: a developmental phase. Psychoanal Q 11:19–26, 1950

16. Beresin E: Imipramine in the treatment of chronic pelvic pain. Psychosomatics 27:294–296, 1986

17. Birchnell J: Early parent death and the clinical scales of the MMPI. Br J Psychiatry 132:574–579, 1978

18. Blumer D, Heilbronn M: Antidepressant treatment for chronic pain: treatment outcome of 1,000 patients with the pain-prone disorder. Psychiatric Annals 14:796–800, 1984

19. Bowles C: The menopausal experience: sociocultural influences and theoretical models, in The Meanings of Menopause: Historical, Medical and Clinical Perspectives. Edited by Formanek R. Hillsdale, NJ, Analytic Press, 1990, pp 157–175

20. Brenner P: The menopausal syndrome. Obstet Gynecol 72 (suppl):6–11, 1988

21. Briere J, Runtz M: Symptomatology associated with childhood sexual victimization in a nonclinical adult sample. Child Abuse Negl 12:51–59, 1988

22. Brown G, Harris T: Social Origins of Depression. London, Tavistock, 1978

23. Brown R, Sweeney J, Loutsch E, et al: Involutional melancholia revisited. Am J Psychiatry 141:24–28, 1984

24. Bungay G, Vessey M, McPherson C: Study of symptoms in middle life with special reference to the menopause. BMJ 2:181–183, 1980

25. Burger H, Hailes J, Menelaus M, et al: The management of persistent menopausal symptoms with oestradiol-testosterone implants: clinical, lipids and hormonal results. Maturitas 6:351–358, 1984

26. Byrne P: Psychiatric morbidity in a gynaecology clinic: an epidemiological survey. Br J Psychiatry 144:28–34, 1984

27. Campbell S: Double blind psychometric studies on the effects of natural estrogens on post-menopausal women, in Management of Menopause and Post-Menopausal Years. Edited by Campbell S. Lancester, UK, MTP Press, 1976, pp 149–158

28. Cardozo L, Gibb D, Tuck S, et al: The effects of subcutaneous hormone implants during the climacteric. Maturitas 5:177–184, 1984

29. Carney J, Cohler B: Developmental continuities and adjustment in adulthood: social relations, morale, and the transformation from middle to late life, in The Course of Life, Vol 6: Late Adulthood. Edited by Pollock G, Greenspan S. Madison, CT, International Universities Press, 1993, pp 199–226

30. Castelnuovo-Tedesco P, Krout B: Psychosomatic aspects of chronic pelvic pain. Psychiatr Med 1:109–126, 1970

30a. Chirawatkul S, Manderson L: Perceptions of menopause in northeast Thailand: contested meaning and practice. Soc Sci Med 39:1545–1554, 1994

31. Conklin W: Some neuroses of the menopause. Transactions of the American Association of Obstetrics and Gynecology 2:301–311, 1889

32. Coope J, Thomson J, Poller L: Effects of "natural oestrogen" replacement therapy on menopausal symptoms and blood clotting. BMJ 4:139–143, 1975

33. Coppen A, Bishop M, Beard R, et al: Hysterectomy, hormones and behaviour: a prospective study. Lancet 1:126–128, 1981

34. Corney R, Crowther M, Everett H, et al: Psychosexual dysfunction in women with gynaecological cancer following radical pelvic surgery. Br J Obstet Gynaecol 100:73–78, 1993

35. Couch J, Hassanein R: Amitriptyline in migraine prophylaxis. Arch Neurol 36:695–699, 1979

36. Datan N: Aging into transitions. Cross-cultural perspectives on women at midlife, in The Meanings of Menopause: Historical, Medical and Clinical Perspectives. Edited by Formanek R. Hillsdale, NJ, Analytic Press, 1990, pp 117–131

37. Dembert M, Dinneen M, Opsahl M, et al: Estrogen-induced panic disorder (letter). Am J Psychiatry 151:1246, 1994

38. Dennerstein L: Psychologic and sexual effects, in Menopause: Psychology and Pharmacology. Edited by Mishell D. Chicago, IL, Year Book Medical, 1987, pp 225–234

39. Dennerstein L, Burrows G, Hyman G: Hormone therapy and affect. Maturitas 1:247–259, 1979

39a. Dennerstein L, Smith A, Morse C: Psychological well-being, mid-life and the menopause. Maturitas 20:1–11, 1994

40. Dennerstein L, Smith A, Morse C, et al: Sexuality and the menopause. Journal of Psychosomatic Obstetrics and Gynecology 15:59–66, 1994

41. Dennerstein L, Wood C, Burrows G: Sexual response following hysterectomy and oophorectomy. Obstet Gynecol 49:92–96, 1977

41a. Derogatis L, Lipman R, Rickels K, et al: The Hopkins Symptom Checklist (HSCL): a self-report symptom inventory. Behav Sci 19:1–15, 1974

42. Deutsch H: The Psychology of Women. New York, Grune & Stratton, 1944

43. Dewald P: Adult phases of the life cycle, in The Course of Life, Vol 6: Late Adulthood. Edited by Pollock G, Greenspan S. Madison, CT, International Universities Press, 1993, pp 129–152

44. Drellich M, Bieber I: The psychological importance of the uterus and its functions. J Nerv Ment Dis 126:322–336, 1958

45. Duncan C, Taylor H: A psychosomatic study of pelvic congestion. Am J Obstet Gynecol 64:1–12, 1952

46. Dunnell K, Cartwright A: Medicine Takers, Prescribers and Hoarders. Boston, MA, Routledge & Kegan Paul, 1972

47. Fedele L, Parazzini F, Bianchi S, et al: Stage and localization of pelvic endometriosis and pain. Fertil Steril 53:155–158, 1990

48. Flint M: The menopause: reward or punishment? Psychosomatics 16:161–173, 1975

49. Foldes J: Psychosomatic approach to the menopausal syndrome, in Psychosomatic Medicine in Obstetrics and Gynecology. Edited by Morris N. Basel, Switzerland, Karger, 1972, pp 517–621

50. Formanek R (ed): The Meanings of Menopause: Historical, Medical and Clinical Perspectives. Hillsdale, NJ, Analytic Press, 1990

51. Gath D, Cooper P: Psychiatric aspects of hysterectomy and female sterilization, in Recent Advances in Clinical Psychiatry, Vol 4. Edited by Granville-Grossman K. London, Churchill, 1982, pp 75–100

52. Gath D, Cooper P, Bond A, et al: Hysterectomy and psychiatric disorder, II: demographic, psychiatric and physical factors in relation to psychiatric outcome. Br J Psychiatry 140:343–350, 1982

53. Gath D, Cooper P, Day A, et al: Hysterectomy and psychiatric disorder, I: levels of psychiatric morbidity before and after hysterectomy. Br J Psychiatry 140:335–342, 1982

54. Gath D, Osborn M, Bungay G, et al: Psychiatric disorder and gynaecological symptoms in middle aged women: a community survey. BMJ 294:213–218, 1987

54a. Gath D, Rose N, Bond A, et al: Hysterectomy and psychiatric disorder: are the levels of psychiatric morbidity falling? Psychol Med 25:277–284, 1995

55. George G, Utian W, Beumont P: Effect of exogenous estrogens on minor psychiatric symptoms in postmenopausal women. S Afr Med J 47:2387–2388, 1973

56. Gidro-Frank L, Gordon T, Taylor H: Pelvic pain and female identity. Am J Obstet Gynecol 79:1184–1202, 1960

57. Gingras M: A clinical trial of Tofranil in rheumatic pain in general practice. J Int Med Res 4:41–49, 1976

58. Gise L, Weston S: Reproductive endocrinology, in Medical Psychiatric Practice, Vol 2. Edited by Stoudemire A, Fogel B. Washington, DC, American Psychiatric Press, 1993, pp 237–300

58a. Goldberg D: The Detection of Psychiatric Illness by Questionnaire. Oxford, UK, Oxford University Press, 1972

59. Gould R: Transformational tasks in adulthood, in The Course of Life, Vol 6: Late Adulthood. Edited by Pollock G, Greenspan S. Madison, CT, International Universities Press, 1993, pp 23–68

59a. Graig G, Jackson P: Sexual life after vaginal hysterectomy (letter). BMJ 3:97, 1975

60. Hallstrom T: Mental Disorder and Sexuality in the Climacteric. Gothenburg, Sweden, Scandinavian University Books, 1973

61. Hallstrom T: Sexuality in the climacteric. Clin Obstet Gynecol 4:227–239, 1977

62. Hallstrom T, Samuelsson S: Mental health in the climacteric: The longitudinal study of women in Gothenburg. Acta Obstet Gynecol Scand Suppl 130:13–18, 1985

63. Harris H: A critical view of three psychoanalytical positions on menopause, in The Meanings of Menopause: Historical, Medical and Clinical Perspectives. Edited by Formanek R. Hillsdale, NJ, Analytic Press, 1990, pp 65–76

63a. Helstrom L: Sexuality after hysterectomy: a model based on quantitative and qualitative analysis of 104 women before and after subtotal hysterectomy. J Psychosom Obstet Gynaecol 15:219–229, 1994

64. Helstrom L, Lundberg P, Sorbom D, et al: Sexuality after hysterectomy: a factor analysis of women's sexual lives before and after subtotal hysterectomy. Obstet Gynecol 81:357–362, 1993

65. Helstrom L, Weiner E, Sorbom D, et al: Predictive value of psychiatric history, genital pain and menstrual symptoms for sexuality after hysterectomy. Acta Obstet Gynecol Scand 73:575–580, 1994

66. Hodgkiss AD, Watson JP: Psychiatric morbidity and illness behaviour in women with chronic pelvic pain. J Psychosom Res 38:3–9, 1994

67. Holst J, Backstrom T, Hammerback S, et al: Progestogen addition during oestrogen replacement therapy—effects on vasomotor symptoms and mood. Maturitas 11:13–20, 1989

68. Hopkinson G: A genetic study of affective illness in patients over 50. Br J Psychiatry 110:244–254, 1964

69. Horowitz M: The developmental and structural viewpoints: on the fate of unconscious fantasies in middle life, in The Middle Years: New Psychoanalytic Perspectives. Edited by Oldham J, Liebert R. New Haven, CT, Yale University Press, 1989, pp 7–16

70. Hunter M: Predictors of menopausal symptoms: psychosocial aspects. Baillieres Clin Endocrinol Metab 7:33–45, 1993

71. Jackson P: Sexual adjustment to hysterectomy and the benefits of a pamphlet for patients. N Z Med J 90:471–472, 1979

72. Jaszmann L, Van Lith N, Zaat J: The perimenopausal symptoms: the statistical analysis of a survey. Medical Gynaecology and Sociology 4:268–277, 1969

73. Kalinich L: The biological clock, in The Middle Years: New Psychoanalytic Perspectives. Edited by Oldham J, Liebert R. New Haven, CT, Yale University Press, 1989, pp 123–134

74. Kames L, Rapkin A, Naliboff B, et al: Effectiveness of an interdisciplinary pain management program for the treatment of chronic pelvic pain. Pain 41:41–46, 1990

75. Kaplan H, Owett T: The female androgen deficiency syndrome. J Sex Marital Ther 19:3–24, 1993

76. Kaufert P, Gilbert P, Tate R: The Manitoba Project: a re-examination of the link between menopause and depression. Maturitas 14:143–155, 1992

76a. Kellner R: Abridged Manual of the Symptom Questionnaire. Albuquerque, NM, University of New Mexico, 1976

77. Kellner R: Somatization and Hypochondriasis. New York, Praeger-Greenwood, 1986

77a. Kellner R: A symptom questionnaire. J Clin Psychiatry 48:268–274, 1987

78. Kendell R: The Classification of Depressive Illness (Maudsley monograph 18). London, Oxford University Press, 1968

79. Kernberg O: The interaction of middle age and character pathology: treatment implications, in The Middle Years: New Psychoanalytic Perspectives. Edited by Oldham J, Liebert R. New Haven, CT, Yale University Press, 1989, pp 209–223

80. Kerr M: Amitriptyline in emotional states at the menopause. N Z Med J 72:243–245, 1970

81. Klaiber E, Broverman D, Vogel W, et al: Effects of estrogen therapy on plasma MAO activity and EEG driving responses of depressed women. Am J Psychiatry 128:1492–1498, 1972

82. Kraepelin E: Lecture I—introduction: melancholia, in Lectures on Clinical Psychiatry. Edited by Johnston T. New York, Bailliere, Tindall & Cox, 1906

83. Kresch A, Steifer D, Sach L, et al: Laparoscopy in 100 women with chronic pelvic pain. Obstet Gynecol 64:672–674, 1984

84. Kupperman H, Wetchler B, Blatt M: Contemporary therapy of the menopausal syndrome. JAMA 171:1627–1637, 1959

85. Lalinec-Michaud M, Engelsmann F, Marino J: Depression after hysterectomy: a comparative study. Psychosomatics 29:307–314, 1988

86. Levitan Z, Eibschitz I, De Vries K, et al: The value of laparoscopy in women with chronic pelvic pain and a "normal pelvis." Int J Gynaecol Obstet 23:71–74, 1985

87. Lieberman M: A reexamination of adult life crises: spousal loss in mid- and late life, in The Course of Life, Vol 6: Late Adulthood. Edited by Pollock G, Greenspan S. Madison, CT, International Universities Press, 1993, pp 69–110

88. Lindsay P, Wyckoff M: The depression-pain syndrome and its response to antidepressants. Psychosomatics 22:571–577, 1981

89. Luine V, Khylchevskaya R, McEwen B: Effect of gonadal steroids on activities of monoamine oxidase and choline acetylase in rat brain. Brain Res 86:293–306, 1975

90. Lundberg W, Wall J, Mathers J: Laparoscopy in evaluation of pelvic pain. Am J Obstet Gynecol 42:872–876, 1973

91. Martin R, Roberts W, Clayton P: Psychiatric status after hysterectomy: One year prospective follow-up. JAMA 244:350–353, 1980

92. Martin R, Roberts W, Clayton P, et al: Psychiatric illness and non-cancer hysterectomy. Diseases of the Nervous System 38:974–980, 1977

93. Masters V, Johnson V: Human Sexual Response. Boston, MA, Little, Brown, 1966

94. Matthews K: Myths and realities of the menopause. Psychosom Med 54:1–9, 1992

95. Matthews K, Bromberger J, Egeland G: Behavioral antecedents and consequences of the menopause, in The Menopause. Edited by Korenman S. Norwell, MA, Serono Symposia, 1990, pp 1–15

96. Matthews K, Wing R, Kuller L, et al: Influences of natural menopause on psychological characteristics and symptoms of middle-aged healthy women. J Consult Clin Psychol 58:345–351, 1990

97. Maxwell M: Portraits of menopausal women in selected works of English and American literature, in The Meanings of Menopause: Historical, Medical and Clinical Perspectives. Edited by Formanek R. Hillsdale, NJ, Analytic Press, 1990, pp 255–279

98. McKinlay J, McKinlay S, Brambilla D, et al: Health status and utilization behavior associated with menopause. Am J Epidemiol 125:110–121, 1987

99. Modell A: Object relations theory: psychic aliveness in the middle years, in The Middle Years: New Psychoanalytic Perspectives. Edited by Oldham J, Liebert R. New Haven, CT, Yale University Press, 1989, pp 17–26

100. Montgomery J, Studd J: Psychological and sexual aspects of the menopause. Br J Hosp Med 45:300–302, 1991

101. Morrell M, Dixon J, Carter S, et al: The influence of age and cycling status on sexual arousability in women. Am J Obstet Gynecol 148:166–174, 1984

102. Munday R, Cox L: Hysterectomy for benign lesions. Med J Aust 17:759–763, 1967

103. Munro A: Psychiatric illness in gynaecological outpatients: a preliminary study. Br J Psychiatry 115:807–809, 1969

104. Myers L, Morokoff P: Physiological and subjective sexual arousal in pre- and postmenopausal women taking replacement therapy. Psychophysiology 23:283–290, 1986

105. Nadelson C: Issues in the analyses of single women in their thirties and forties, in The Middle Years: New Psychoanalytic Perspectives. Edited by Oldham J, Liebert R. New Haven, CT, Yale University Press, 1989, pp 105–122

106. Nathorst-Boos J, Fuchs T, von Schoultz B: Consumer's attitude to hysterectomy: the experience of 678 women. Acta Obstet Gynecol Scand 71:230–234, 1992

107. Nathorst-Boos J, von Schoultz B: Psychological reactions and sexual life after hysterectomy with and without oophorectomy. Gynecol Obstet Invest 34:97–101, 1992

108. National Center for Health Statistics: Detailed diagnosis and surgical procedures for patients discharged from short stay hospitals: United States, 1983 (Vital and Health Statistics Series 13, No. 82). Washington, DC, US Government Printing Office, 1985

109. Notman M: Emotional impact of gynecological surgery, in Psychological Experience of Surgery. Edited by Blacher R. New York, Wiley, 1987, pp 99–115

110. Oates M, Gath D: Psychological aspects of gynaecological surgery. Baillieres Clin Obstet Gynaecol 3:687–749, 1989

111. Ornstein P: Self Psychology: the fate of the nuclear self in the middle years, in The Middle Years: New Psychoanalytic Perspectives. Edited by Oldham J, Liebert R. New Haven, CT, Yale University Press, 1989, pp 27–39

112. Osborn M, Hawton K, Gath D: Sexual dysfunction among middle aged women in the community. BMJ 296:959–962, 1988

113. Padwick M, Endacott J, Whitehead M: Efficacy, acceptability, and metabolic effects of transdermal estradiol in the management of postmenopausal women. Am J Obstet Gynecol 152:1085–1091, 1985

114. Pasnau R, Soldinger S, Andersen B: Pelvic pain, in Psychological Disorders in Obstetrics and Gynecology. Edited by Priest R. London, Butterworth, 1985, pp 49–69

115. Pearce S, Matthews A, Beard R: A controlled trial of psychological approaches to the management of pelvic pain in women. Paper presented at the 8th annual scientific sessions of the Society of Behavioral Medicine, Washington, DC, March 1987

116. Peters A, van Horst E, Jellis B, et al: A randomized clinical trial to compare two different approaches in women with chronic pelvic pain. Obstet Gynecol 77:740–744, 1991

117. Petersen J: Obstetrics and gynecology, in Psychiatric Care of the Medical Patient. Edited by Stoudemire A, Fogel B. New York, Oxford University Press, 1993, pp 637–656

118. Pfeiffer E, Verwoerdt A, Davis G: Sexual behavior in middle life. Am J Psychiatry 128:1262–1267, 1972

119. Phillips S: Reflections of self and other: men's views of menopausal women, in The Meanings of Menopause: Historical, Medical and Clinical Perspectives. Edited by Formanek R. Hillsdale, NJ, Analytic Press, 1990, pp 281–295

120. Price W, Heil D: Estrogen-induced panic attacks. Psychosomatics 29:433–435, 1988

121. Priest R, Crisp A: The menopause and its relationship with reported somatic experiences, in Psychosomatic Medicine in Obstetrics and Gynecology. Edited by Morris N. Basel, Switzerland, Karger, 1972, pp 605–607

122. Rapkin A, Kames L, Darke L, et al: History of physical and sexual abuse in women with chronic pelvic pain. Obstet Gynecol 76:92–96, 1990

123. Renaer M: Chronic pelvic pain without obvious pathology in women. Eur J Obstet Gynecol 10:415–463, 1980

124. Renaer M: Chronic Pelvic Pain in Women. Berlin, Springer-Verlag, 1981

125. Renaer M, Vertommen H, Nijs P, et al: Psychological aspects of chronic pelvic pain in women. Am J Obstet Gynecol 134:75–80, 1979

126. Research on the Menopause: WHO Technical Report Series 670. Geneva, Switzerland, World Health Organization, 1981

127. Richards D: A post-hysterectomy syndrome. Lancet 2:983–985, 1974

128. Riley A: Sexuality and the menopause. Sexual and Marital Therapy 6:135–146, 1991

129. Rogers F: Emotional factors in gynecology. Am J Obstet Gynecol 59:321–327, 1950

130. Rosenthal R, Ling F, Rosenthal T, et al: Chronic pelvic pain: psychological features and laparoscopic findings. Psychosomatics 25:833–841, 1984

131. Roughan P, Kaiser F, Morley J: Sexuality and the older woman. Clin Geriatr Med 9:87–106, 1993

132. Ryan M, Dennerstein L, Pepperell R: Psychological aspects of hysterectomy. Br J Psychiatry 154:516–522, 1989

133. Schiff I, Regenstein Q, Schinfeld J, et al: Interactions of oestrogens and the hours of sleep on cortisol, FSH, LH, and prolactin in hypogonadal women. Maturitas 2:179–183, 1980

134. Schmidt P, Rubinow D: Menopause-related affective disorders: a justification for further study. Am J Psychiatry 148:844–852, 1991

135. Schneider M, Brotherton P, Hailes J: The effect of exogenous oestrogens on depression in menopausal women. Med J Aust 2:162–163, 1977

136. Semchyshyn S, Strickler R: Laparoscopy—is it replacing clinical acumen? Obstet Gynecol 48:615–618, 1976

137. Shanok R: Towards an inclusive adult developmental theory: epigenesis reconsidered, in The Course of Life, Vol 6: Late Adulthood. Edited by Pollock G, Greenspan S. Madison, CT, International Universities Press, 1993, pp 243–260

138. Sherwin B: Affective changes with estrogen and androgen replacement therapy in surgically menopausal women. J Affect Disord 14:177–187, 1988

139. Sherwin B: The impact of different doses of estrogen and progestin on mood and sexual behavior in postmenopausal women. J Clin Endocrinol Metab 72:336–343, 1991

140. Sherwin B: Menopause: myths and realities, in Psychological Aspects of Women's Health Care: The Interface Between Psychiatry and Obstetrics and Gynecology. Edited by Stewart D, Stotland N. Washington, DC, American Psychiatric Press, 1993, pp 227–248

141. Sherwin B: Sex hormones and psychological functioning in postmenopausal women. Exp Gerontol 29:423–430, 1994

142. Sherwin B, Gelfand M: Effects of parenteral administration of estrogen and androgen on plasma hormone levels and hot flushes in the surgical menopause. Am J Obstet Gynecol 148:552–557, 1984

143. Sherwin B, Gelfand M: Sex steroids and affect in the surgical menopause: a double-blind cross-over study. Psychoneuroendocrinology 10:325–335, 1985

144. Sherwin B, Gelfand M: The role of androgen in the maintenance of sexual functioning in oophorectomized women. Psychosom Med 49:397–409, 1987

145. Sherwin B, Gelfand M, Brender W: Androgen enhances sexual motivation in females: a prospective, cross-over study of sex steroid administration in the surgical menopause. Psychosom Med 47:339–351, 1985

146. Sherwin B, Suranyi-Cadotte B: Up-regulatory effect of estrogen on platelet ³H-imipramine binding sites in surgically menopausal women. Biol Psychiatry 28:339–348, 1990

147. Slocumb J: Neurological factors in chronic pelvic pain: trigger points and the abdominal pelvic pain syndrome. Am J Obstet Gynecol 149:536–543, 1984

148. Slocumb J, Kellner R, Rosenfeld R, et al: Anxiety and depression in patients with the abdominal pelvic pain syndrome. Gen Hosp Psychiatry 11:48–53, 1989

149. Speroff L: Menopause and hormone replacement therapy. Clin Geriatr Med 9:33–55, 1993

150. Steege J, Stout A: Resolution of chronic pelvic pain following laparoscopic adhesiolysis. Am J Obstet Gynecol 165:278–283, 1991

151. Steege J, Stout A: Chronic gynecologic pain, in Psychological Aspects of Women's Health Care: The Interface Between Psychiatry and Obstetrics and Gynecology. Edited by Stewart D, Stotland N. Washington, DC, American Psychiatric Press, 1993, pp 249–266

152. Stenback A: On involutional and middle-age depression. Acta Psychiatr Scand 39 (suppl 169):14–32, 1963

153. Stenstedt A: Involutional melancholia. Acta Psychiatrica et Neurologica Scandinavica 34 (suppl 127), 1959

154. Stewart D, Boydell K, Derzko C, et al: Psychologic distress during the menopausal years in women attending a menopause clinic. Int J Psychiatry Med 22:213–220, 1992

155. Stewart D, Stotland N (eds): Psychological Aspects of Women's Health Care: The Interface Between Psychiatry and Obstetrics and Gynecology. Washington, DC, American Psychiatric Press, 1993

156. Stotland N, Smith T: Psychiatric consultation to obstetrics and gynecology: systems and syndromes, in American Psychiatric Press Review of Psychiatry, Vol 9. Edited by Tasman A, Goldfinger SM, Kaufmann C. Washington, DC, American Psychiatric Press, 1990, pp 537–563

157. Stout A, Steege J, Dodson W, et al: Relationship of laparoscopic findings to self-report of pelvic pain. Am J Obstet Gynecol 164:73–79, 1991

158. Strickler R, Borth R, Cecutti A, et al: The use of estrogen replacement in the climacteric syndrome. Psychol Med 7:531–639, 1977

159. Studd J, Collins W, Chakravarti S, et al: Oestradiol and testosterone implants in the treatment of psychosexual problems in the postmenopausal woman. Br J Psychiatry 84:314–315, 1977

160. Tait A, Harper J, McClatchey W: Psychiatric illness in involutional women, I: clinical aspects. J Ment Sci 103:132–145, 1957

161. Thomson J, Oswald I: Effect of estrogen on the sleep, mood, and anxiety of menopausal women. BMJ 2:1317–1319, 1977

162. Thomson J, Oswald I: Hormones and sleep. Curr Med Res Opin 4 (suppl 3):67–72, 1977

163. Treolar A: Menstrual cyclicity and the pre-menopause. Maturitas 3:249–264, 1981

164. Utian W: The mental tonic effect of estrogens administered to oophorectomized females. S Afr Med J 46:1079–1082, 1972

165. Utian W: The true clinical features of post-menopause and oophorectomy and their response to estrogen therapy. S Afr Med J 46:732–737, 1972

166. Utian W, Serr D: The climacteric syndrome, in Consensus on Menopause Research. Edited by Van Keep P, Greenblatt R, Albeaux-Fernet M. Lancaster, UK, MTP Press, 1976, pp 1–4

167. Vaillant G: The evolution of defense mechanisms during the middle years, in The Middle Years: New Psychoanalytic Perspectives. Edited by Oldham J, Liebert R. New Haven, CT, Yale University Press, 1989, pp 58–72

168. Vaillant G, Koury S: Late midlife development, in The Course of Life, Vol 6: Late Adulthood. Edited by Pollock G, Greenspan S. Madison, CT, International Universities Press, 1993, pp 1–22

169. vanKeep P, Kellerhals J: The impact of socio-cultural factors on symptom formation. Psychother Psychosom 23:251–263, 1974

170. Viederman M: Middle life as a period of mutative change, in The Middle Years: New Psychoanalytic Perspectives. Edited by Oldham J, Liebert R. New Haven, CT, Yale University Press, 1989, pp 224–239

171. Walker E, Katon W, Harrop-Griffiths J, et al: Relationship of chronic pelvic pain to psychiatric diagnoses and childhood sexual abuse. Am J Psychiatry 145:75–80, 1988

172. Walker E, Katon W, Neraas K, et al: Dissociation in women with chronic pelvic pain. Am J Psychiatry 149:534–537, 1992

173. Walker E, Roy-Byrne P, Katon W, et al: An open trial of nortriptyline in women with chronic pelvic pain. Int J Psychiatry Med 21:245–252, 1991

174. Ward N, Bloom V, Friedel R: The effectiveness of tricyclic antidepressants in the treatment of coexisting pain and depression. Pain 7:331–341, 1979

175. Weissman M: The myth of involutional melancholia. JAMA 242:742–746, 1979

176. Wheatley D: The use of psychotropic drugs in the female climacteric, in Psychosomatic Medicine in Obstetrics and Gynecology. Edited by Morris N. Basel, Switzerland, Karger, 1972, pp 612–616

177. Winokur G: Depression in the menopause. Am J Psychiatry 130:92–93, 1973

178. Winokur G, Cadoret R: The irrelevance of the menopause to depressive illness, in Topics in Psychoendocrinology. Edited by Sachar E. New York, Grune & Stratton, 1975, pp 59–66

179. World Health Organization: Research on the menopause: report of a WHO scientific group (Technical Report Series 670). Geneva, Switzerland, WHO, 1981

180. Youngs D, Wise T: Psychological sequelae of elective gynecologic surgery, in Psychosomatic Obstetrics and Gynecology. Edited by Youngs D, Ehrhardt A. New York, Appleton-Century-Crofts, 1980, pp 255–264

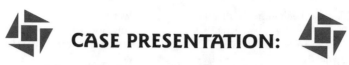

CASE PRESENTATION:

Mrs. Reid (Part II): Breast Cancer

Mrs. Reid (whom we described earlier in this chapter) recuperates rapidly from her hysterectomy. She continues to work on self-esteem issues and terminates therapy after 2 years of treatment. She returns several years later, at the age of 57, when mammography reveals a lesion consistent with breast cancer. She requests help in coping with her anxiety about her diagnosis and the upcoming workup.

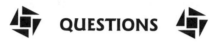

QUESTIONS

Choose all that apply.

1. What medical-system stressors is Mrs. Reid more likely to face today compared with women 20 years ago?
   a. Full disclosure of survival prognosis is usually emphasized over reassurance about the future.
   b. Treatment options now stress the importance of tolerating radical breast surgery in order to eradicate the cancer, rather than breast-conserving approaches.
   c. There is greater uncertainty about what constitutes optimal treatment.
   d. There is less autonomy about specific treatment decisions.

2. In assessing Mrs. Reid's adaptation to this newest life stress, which of the following are *false*?
   a. Prior psychiatric disorder predisposes to less-favorable psychological outcome postsurgically.
   b. Coping styles characterized by a confrontational, "tackling" stance result in less emotional distress in the early rehabilitative stages after mastectomy than do more passive coping styles.
   c. The majority of men cope well in response to a mate's mastectomy.
   d. Partners who view the mastectomy scar early have a poorer psychological outcome.

3. Breast cancer patients with better prognoses are those who are . . .
   a. Older and postmenopausal at onset.
   b. Younger and premenopausal at onset.

   c. Estrogen-receptor positive.
   d. Estrogen-receptor negative.

4. With increased use of mammography, many women are being diagnosed with early breast cancer. These patients often seek referral specifically to a psychiatrist, at least initially, believing that psychiatrists' medical background qualifies them more than other mental health professionals to make medical-psychological recommendations. It is important for the psychiatric consultant to have an idea of the patient's prognosis, as this knowledge will inform therapeutic technique and strategy. Which choice best estimates the 5-year survival time for primary breast cancer patients who present with a large tumor diameter (greater than 5 cm) and positive axillary nodes?
   a. Only about 20% survive 5 years.
   b. Less than half survive 5 years.
   c. Two-thirds will make it 5 years.
   d. Over 95% survive 5 years.

5. Which choice best approximates average 5-year survival time for primary breast cancer patients who have a tumor diameter less than 2 cm and negative axillary nodes?
   a. Only about 20% survive 5 years.
   b. Less than half survive 5 years.
   c. Two-thirds will make it 5 years.
   d. Over 95% survive 5 years.

6. The median survival time of women with metastatic breast cancer is
   a. 6 months.
   b. 1 year.

c. 2 years.

d. 3 years.

7. Mrs. Reid must decide whether to have a mastectomy or limited resection ("lumpectomy") followed by radiation. She is confused about which method offers the best chance of survival. Her husband accompanies her to her visit with you. Mr. Reid wants to know the likelihood that his wife will emerge from this experience without "severe psychological damage." Which of the following are important data to consider in helping the Reids with this issue?

a. Women without prior psychiatric history undergoing mastectomy for stage I and II breast cancer showed a significantly greater incidence of psychiatric sequelae, such as suicidal ideation, when compared with women having cholecystectomy, those having biopsy for benign breast disease, or healthy control subjects.

b. Women who were well-adjusted premastectomy, and whose disease is at an early stage, can expect at 1 year to have a quality of life *equivalent* to unaffected peers.

c. Studies have demonstrated significantly better psychological adaptation for women choosing limited breast resection over mastectomy.

d. Only a small cohort of patients now chooses mastectomy over limited resection and radiation.

8. Mrs. Reid opts for mastectomy. She is found to have stage I (node negative) disease. She is enormously relieved after the surgery, denies depression or anxiety, and speaks about having reconstruction. Which of the following are true statements concerning recent findings about the psychological response to breast reconstruction?

a. Breast reconstruction has been associated with a better outlook on life, but general and social *daily functioning* are usually unaffected.

b. Only a minority of patients have realistic expectations of breast reconstruction and are not disappointed with the results.

c. Most patients report seeking reconstruction in order to please their husband or significant other.

d. Reconstructed patients report enhanced sexual satisfaction.

e. Patients who sought reconstructive surgery to improve the relationship with their partner were more likely to have had a history of impaired interpersonal relations.

9. Psychological response to breast reconstruction has been found to be dependent on . . .

a. Age.

b. Social class.

c. The surgeon's estimate of the success of outcome.

d. None of the above.

10. During his wife's hospitalization, Mr. Reid requests a meeting with you to discuss her care. Mrs. Reid gives consent. He wants to know what to expect next, given the good news about negative lymph nodes and the way that she has psychologically "breezed through" her treatment so far. Which is/are true?

a. Mrs. Reid is likely to avoid the stress of adjuvant chemotherapy, since is it rarely recommended for stage I disease.

b. Patients are less likely to require psychological intervention as their oncological treatment approaches termination, especially if they have successfully navigated the surgery.

c. Weight *gain* is a side effect of adjuvant chemotherapy.

d. Tamoxifen frequently causes depression.

11. Clinical experience with the sexual dysfunction associated with breast cancer has shown . . .

a. Mastectomy per se has no adverse physical effect on the female sexual response cycle.

b. Most sexual problems of the mastectomy patient who has completed chemotherapy are the result of the male partner's reaction to the missing breast.

c. Most experts in the field urge *early* return to sexual activity.

d. Tamoxifen is one of the few oncological agents that spares sexual functioning.

e. In the absence of affective illness, diminished libido is most likely to be from psychological rather than physiological causes.

12. Likely factors in the sexual dysfunction of breast cancer patients include . . .

a. Physiological impairment of the excitement phase of sexual response

b. Diminished testosterone (androgen)

c. Atrophy of the vaginal mucosa

d. Diminished clitoral sensation

e. All of the above

13. Mrs. Reid returns to your office very concerned about how she can best improve her prognosis. Some of her friends tell her that she should "get her anger out," because repressed anger can retrigger the cancer. Others

caution that she should try to avoid depression as much as possible and "laugh her way to health." They give her stacks of books on the subject, acquired from local bookstores. She feels she is coping well on her own, but doesn't feel like laughing. She's in a quandary. Is she jeopardizing a cure? Should she return to regular psychotherapy? Can her state of mind influence her illness? Can psychotherapy improve her prognosis? How do you respond?

a. Studies have shown that cancer morbidity and mortality do correlate with psychological factors.

b. Studies have shown no correlation between cancer morbidity or mortality and psychological factors.

c. There are no studies indicating improved *survival time* when patients are randomized to standard oncological care plus intensive psychosocial treatment and compared with control groups receiving standard oncological care alone.

d. Psychotherapeutic interventions that are the least stressful for patients emphasize "visualizing" the cancer illness (e.g., visualizing white cells ferociously attacking cancer cells).

e. A recent survey of attitudes about the effect of psychological factors on cancer revealed that the majority of respondents (consisting of oncology caregivers and university students) believed that stress and coping style were *not* contributing *causes* of cancer.

f. Both a and b are correct.

🔁 Answers

1. Answer: a, c (pp. 373–374)
2. Answer: d (pp. 374–375)
3. Answer: a, c (p. 381)
4. Answer: b (p. 381)
5. Answer: d (p. 381)
6. Answer: c (p. 381)
7. Answer: b (pp. 375–376)
8. Answer: d, e (pp. 376–377)
9. Answer: d (pp. 376–377)
10. Answer: c (p. 377)
11. Answer: a, c (pp. 377–378)
12. Answer: e (p. 378)
13. Answer: f (pp. 378–381)

◄⁊ BREAST CANCER

The psychiatrist who works with women facing breast cancer soon discovers that the issues are not limited to self-esteem, femininity, and sexuality. Changes in the medical system and philosophy of treating breast cancer greatly impinge on a woman's psychological adaptation to her disease and its treatment. Rowland and Holland[87] have pointed out that as breast cancer became recognized as a systemic rather than local disease, the premise underpinning radical breast cancer surgery shifted. Treatment is now aimed at achieving the maximum disease-free survival with *breast-conserving treatments* that provide best cosmesis but do not compromise cure. Recognition that radical or modified radical mastectomy do not prevent micrometastases has led to newer approaches using breast-conserving methods combined with irradiation. Comparable survival rates have been achieved, although follow-up periods are not yet as long as with the older methodologies. The early psychosocial research on radical mastectomy is no longer as clinically relevant in light of these changes, but the reader interested in a historical survey can consult several good reviews.[47,61,67]

Here we highlight the more pressing consultation-liaison issues that come up with breast cancer. Additional reviews will round out the reader's understanding of this important area.[1,34,87]

Uncertainty About Treatment

Despite the less-mutilating procedures, patients today face greater uncertainty and differing opinions about what constitutes optimal therapy.[96] Gone are the days when the path to treatment lay direct and unambiguous, however disfiguring. Survival statistics are readily available in the lay press, a response to the demand for greater patient autonomy and full disclosure. These statistics are frightening, at best. Rowland and Holland[87] have commented,

> The result of these changes is a vastly altered sociocultural climate for women dealing with breast cancer [as compared with 15–20 years ago] . . . The emotional problems are different today, but equally compelling. Although fears about breast loss and threat to body im-

> age and sexual function have decreased with the introduction of breast-conserving treatment techniques, fears and anxieties about having made the right treatment choice and about the likelihood of survival have increased. A change that is integral to the initial emotional burden [of breast cancer] today is the patient's increased level of participation in primary treatment decisions. (p. 189)

Although many women experience their enhanced participation as positive, others feel overwhelmed as they are forced to share therapeutic and prognostic uncertainty. The "bad old days" of medical paternalism and inevitably mutilating surgery are gone—but so, too, is the reassuring illusion of the omnipotent physician. Patients must now be actively involved with treatment decisions, often aware that no "best" treatment exists.[22] As one patient described,

> I feel like I'm walking a tightrope, having to make life-and-death decisions for myself with little education or experience, during the most stressful period of my life. There is no certainty about which is the best thing to do. This is even more upsetting than the idea of losing my breast.

Patient Issues in Medical Decision Making

Previous experiences, personal data, demographic characteristics, and factors relating to family, friends, and physician all influence how patients make decisions regarding their treatment.[42,107] Many are too shocked at the time of diagnosis to register details about their illness.[76] Some patients assume a less active stance toward decision making, preferring to rely on their physician for guidance.[22,80] Certainly anxiety and information overload can interfere.[92]

The verbal interaction with the doctor greatly influences what happens later. *In one study, the primary factor in a patient's acceptance of an outlined treatment was trust in the physician.*[80] Shapiro and colleagues[94] evaluated the effect of various physician facial expressions on patient recall.

- Forty women at risk for breast cancer viewed videotapes of an oncologist presenting mammogram results looking either worried or unworried.
- Although the mammogram results and the oncologist were the same in both presentations, women receiving results from the "worried" physician recalled significantly less information, perceived the clinical situation as significantly more serious, reported significantly higher levels of state anxiety, and had significantly higher pulse rates.

Predictably, nuances in communication and facial expression are not top priority for the surgeon or oncologist. Often the consulting psychiatrist assists the patient in processing the information and her feelings about the way she has received it. A thoughtless remark or casual comment, seemingly innocuous to the medical person who makes it, can induce a tailspin of panic and despair in the patient. Psychiatric intervention can mitigate untoward psychological reactions while assisting informed decision making and medical compliance.

Rowland and Holland[87] have delineated four typical response types and suggested useful interventions for each:

Response Type 1: "You decide for me, Doctor."

- **Patient:** Accustomed to accepting the authority and decisions of the physician. May be—or prefer to remain—less well informed about treatment options.
- **Strategy:** A physician who outlines options but accepts a strong role in decision making will be most helpful for a patient like this. Such a patient will do poorly with a statement like "Come back in a week and let me know your decision," which may be frightening because it is interpreted as the doctor's not knowing what to do.

Response Type 2: "I demand that you do the . . . procedure."

- **Patient:** More medically sophisticated; has consulted all available resources and obtained all relevant materials. May have already made a decision.
- **Strategy:** This patient must be treated as a full participant in the decision process and may benefit from written materials to supplement her own research. It is important to listen and respond to the patient's many questions. Failure to include her may result in an adversarial stance toward the physician.

Response Type 3: "I can't decide."

- **Patient:** Overwhelmed by the knowledge of the breast lump, with its threat to life or an intact body. Finds the medical options too painful to consider.
- **Strategy:** This type of patient is often referred for psychiatric consultation. It may be helpful to postpone the surgery and review possible treatments in a safe, secure setting. Asking "How would you respond to that?" as the patient is verbally guided through each treatment option may be effective in reducing anxiety and exploring their ramifications. Usually, certain aspects of a treatment emerge as more acceptable to the patient, and cancer therapy can then proceed.

Response Type 4: "Given the options, your recommendations, and my preferences, I choose . . . "

- **Patient:** Mature, anxious, but able to engage in constructive discussion with the physician about treatment.
- **Strategy:** With a patient like this, discussion of relevant facts, accompanied by written material, regarding all facets of the treatment usually leads to a decision.

Psychological Variables in Coping

A woman's phase of life greatly affects her adjustment to breast cancer and its treatment. Young, single women are particularly vulnerable to breast cancer's psychological assaults on self-esteem and hope.[6a,72a,91a] On the other hand, older women more often are experiencing additional losses or illnesses. There is no easy time to have breast cancer.[69a]

Coping styles influence adaptation:

- Prior psychiatric illness predisposes to poor adaptation. When subjects with preexisting psychiatric disorder were eliminated from a study of adaptation to breast cancer, no serious psychopathological sequelae were found in the year after mastectomy.[6]
- Poor adaptation has been associated with previous unsatisfactory or negative sexual experiences, overly intense emotional investment in breasts, body image problems,[91] and a high number of stressful life events before diagnosis.[63]
- Prior experiences with breast cancer in friends or other family members may also increase vulnerability for problems.[58a,110] Cultural factors are also relevant.[82a]

- A confrontational, "tackling" stance is thought to be optimal; women who use avoidance and capitulation have been found to be more emotionally distressed in the early rehabilitative stages after mastectomy.[78]
- Patients who have a sense of control over events and who take an active role in rehabilitation tend to adjust better than those with a helpless outlook.[60]
- A tendency to suppress emotional reactions (such as anger, helplessness, and a fatalistic attitude) toward cancer correlates with greater psychological morbidity.[28,109]
- Preexisting pessimism about one's life magnifies the risk for adverse psychological reactions.[9]

Positive coping behavior can be learned or enhanced, and if implemented, has been shown to improve health outcomes.[24,26]

The response from significant people in the patient's life is potent. Patients may be particularly pained by relatives' withdrawal or avoidance of them. Families should be included in psychiatric interventions, and are often themselves in significant distress.[44,117] Wellisch and colleagues[111] studied men's adjustment to breast cancer:

- Although most men managed well overall in response to their partner's mastectomy, a subgroup remained distressed postsurgically.[73,111]
- Men who gave least support to their partners had significant psychiatric problems, particularly substance abuse, a history of infidelity or abuse, an inability to tolerate the patient's increased dependency needs, or a chronic pattern of poor communication.
- Active participation, visiting after the operation, seeing the scar early, assisting with dressing changes, and resuming sexual relations early were associated with more psychologically comfortable outcomes.

Self-help organizations, such as Reach to Recovery[85,113] and SHARE, provide peer visitors and support to patients undergoing various procedures, including reconstruction. A number of institutions sponsor programs that combine peer and professional support in group counseling.[11,31]

Comparison With Other Illnesses

Expectably, in a large prospective study, breast cancer patients had more psychological distress than women having cholecystectomy, those having biopsy for benign breast disease, or healthy control subjects.[6] Notably, however, there were not significantly more psychiatric sequelae,

such as suicidal ideation. *Women who were well-adjusted premastectomy, and whose disease was at an early stage, could expect to have a quality of life at 1 year equivalent to that of unaffected peers.* Not surprisingly, women with stage II disease who received adjuvant chemotherapy were more distressed throughout the year and at 12 months. Predictors of poorer outcome were additional illness, expectation of poor support from others, and *a tendency to perceive life events as less under one's own control.*[79]

- Note that this study was conducted before women with stage I disease were routinely given chemotherapy. Times are very different now; chemotherapy adds to the distress of treatment, regardless of stage.

Treatment

Mastectomy Versus Limited Resection

Limited resection ("lumpectomy") has advantages over radical mastectomy relative to[5,32,58,74,83,89,103]

- Self-image
- Self-consciousness
- Sexual function

However, some have reported less-than-expected emotional benefit relative to more-mutilating surgery.[35,118] Differences between treatment groups apparently *diminish over time,*[75] and women choosing breast-conserving procedures experience *as much* psychological discomfort (about issues other than body image) as those undergoing radical mastectomy.[4,21,59,90]

It may seem surprising that many women (51%) still chose mastectomy over limited resection.[115] There may be fears about recurrence and cancer residua, suspicion about a "newer" procedure, and worries about having compromised survival for the sake of saving the breast. Lasry and Margolese[57] studied fear of recurrence in patients undergoing mastectomy versus breast-conserving surgery.

- Fear of recurrence was more related to the number of surgical interventions than to the type of surgery (lumpectomy versus mastectomy).
- Expectably, patients with multiple operations reported a greater fear of cancer recurrence and a more impaired body image.
- Patients who underwent radical mastectomy had no less fear of recurrence, nor did lumpectomy patients express more fear of cancer than their mastectomy counterparts.

Some patients are so relieved to be spared mastectomy that the strain of lumpectomy may take them by surprise. The 6 weeks of daily radiation therapy is a major intrusion on life and psyche, with potential complications such as cardiac toxicity (with left–chest wall radiation) and the risk of contralateral breast cancer. Moreover, while preserving the breast has important psychological advantages, many women underestimate the psychic toll of watching the irradiated breast lose normal sensitivity and consistency. Delayed reactions to the trauma of their illness occur in the lumpectomy group,[87] becoming more apparent with daily visits for radiation therapy and heightened by the accompanying fatigue. Moreover, Levy et al.[59] found that patients choosing breast-conservation surgery rated themselves as having less energy and receiving less emotional support than those choosing modified radical mastectomies. Schain et al.[89] have written,

> Mastectomy per se is not the sole culprit in posttreatment emotional morbidity. The "treatment is to blame" hypothesis can finally be dismissed as a . . . simplistic explanation for psychological sequelae experienced by mastectomy [and lumpectomy] patients. (p. 1227)

Psychosocial support may be different for patients receiving breast-conserving procedures compared with mastectomy. Spiegel[99] has speculated:

> Perhaps what is particularly stressful about mastectomy . . . the removal of the breast and the obvious disfigurement it produces . . . has an unintended positive consequence. Perhaps it elicits more nurturance and support from spouses and partners, who cannot so easily put the disease out of their minds . . . Perhaps the damage inflicted by the loss of a breast is made up for by the enhanced comfort and support . . . the reordering of what is important in a relationship . . . that comes from the daily, inescapable, and visible evidence of the threat the cancer poses to the couple and the family. (pp. 347–348)

The view that "it is 'just' a lumpectomy" allows friends and families to deny the impact on themselves and their loved one. Certainly, these data highlight the value of helping a woman choose the treatment that *seems right for her,* within the parameters of medical advice. Support-

ing her decision as an active, effective strategy in eradicating cancer promotes compliance and enhanced quality of life. Prospective studies are needed to further assess the relative psychological outcome for women choosing breast-conserving procedures over mastectomy.

Breast Reconstruction

Long-term and prospective data on the impact of breast reconstruction have begun to accrue, and influence the choice of mastectomy versus lumpectomy. Advances in surgical techniques have led to fewer complications and better outcomes. Moreover, tissue-sparing methods have made surgical reconstruction more feasible.

Rowland et al.[88] assessed 83 women undergoing reconstructive surgery with respect to surgical and psychological status. Evaluations were at the time of consultation for breast reconstruction and were repeated 2 months or more after surgery.

- The most frequently cited reasons for seeking surgery were to be rid of the prosthesis, to "feel whole again," and to restore breast symmetry and decrease self-consciousness about appearance.
- Most women sought surgery for reasons of their own; 60% reported that their husband or significant other was neutral or even opposed to reconstruction, despite having been supportive (85%) after mastectomy.
- Results were overwhelmingly positive: 83% were satisfied, 12% were dissatisfied, and 5% were neutral.
- Response to reconstruction was found to be independent of a woman's age, her social class, or her surgeon's estimate of the success of outcome.
- There was improvement in general daily functioning and in social roles, and a decrease in psychiatric symptoms.
- Women were rated as more comfortable with their sexuality. Although the frequency of sex did not increase, sexual satisfaction was enhanced and more closely approximated premastectomy levels.
- In most cases, women felt the surgery had met or exceeded their expectations. However, those who had anticipated that surgery would improve sexual relations and/or relations with their partner were at risk for disappointment postreconstruction. These patients were more likely to have had a history of impaired interpersonal relations predating their mastectomy. They also reported greater loss of role and social function postmastectomy, and significantly more symptomatology on a standard checklist.

◆ Women of all age groups sought out breast reconstruction, lending "support to the contention that attractiveness is not primarily a concern of younger women and that older women may react as strongly as younger women to breast loss" (p. 248).[88]

The medical issues concerning immediate versus delayed reconstruction are controversial, but the evidence argues in favor of early reconstruction in minimizing the psychosocial trauma experienced by mastectomy patients.[7,16,66,72,104,112] However, some clinicians anecdotally report that immediate reconstruction may interfere with mourning the cancer diagnosis and loss of a breast.[87]

Adjuvant Chemotherapy

Adjuvant chemotherapy is increasingly recommended for stage I (node negative) disease since the discovery of improved survival (by almost 10%).[13] Chemotherapy is stressful, and patients benefit from active support. Not surprisingly, depression is more common in patients receiving adjuvant chemotherapy than in those undergoing radiotherapy alone.[51] Weight gain is a less well known but distressing side effect of adjuvant chemotherapy, reported in 50% of patients (who gained more than 10 pounds).[52] It occurs independently of treatment regimen, estrogen receptor status, age, or menopausal status. It adds one more cosmetic insult to the injury of hair loss and should be considered when choosing an antidepressant. The mechanism is unknown.[17]

Tamoxifen is an antiestrogen medication administered to postmenopausal women with lymph node involvement and to those with positive estrogen receptor tumors. It has few adverse neuropsychiatric side effects, although its antiestrogen effects can be upsetting.[87] There is one report of tamoxifen-associated reduction in tricyclic antidepressant levels.[53a]

Posttreatment Adjustment Reactions

Intense psychological reactions often peak as treatment ends.[87] We have observed this repeatedly. Patients may be less aware of their emotional reactions throughout the information-gathering phase, surgery, and immediate postoperative period. The emotional pain often hits with a shock later. The frequent visits to the physician and clinic, initially terrifying but gradually part of the patient's "routine," can be difficult to relinquish.[87] Fears about recurrence often reach their height as treatment terminates.[49] Holland[46] has written,

The staff often assumes that patients feel relief upon reaching the end of a lengthy, onerous treatment regimen. [There are] data that suggest quite the contrary: women were significantly more depressed and angry at the end of their treatment and were also anxious about termination, with its consequences of the loss of the comfortable relationship with the staff, the loss of the close monitoring, and the [feeling of] increased vulnerability to their disease. (p. 140)

Although most patients "count down" to the end of treatments, it is frightening to surrender "*doing* something to cure the cancer." This is often the time that patients need help in the difficult readaptation to normal life, while maintaining vigilant hope.

Sexual Side Effects of Breast Cancer Treatments

As important as knowing the latest psychopharmacological treatments is knowing how to screen for psychosexual dysfunction. Several papers review the treatment of sexual dysfunction in the medical setting.[1a,2,20,93] Clinicians should be able to discuss sexuality in a way that combines concern, warmth, and a relaxed professional demeanor. In her review of sexual dysfunction in cancer patients, Auchincloss[2] advises that a cool, extremely "professional" stance does little to set an anxious patient at ease, whereas an overly familiar or joking style is inappropriate.

Simply asking about sexual function is reassuring to many patients. It conveys that the topic is acceptable, that concerns can be freely raised . . . , and that problems can be discussed and treated.[2] (p. 397)

The sexual side effects of breast cancer treatment are often ignored. Kaplan[55] has written,

This important aspect of cancer has been largely neglected by researchers, oncologists, and surgeons, as well as by mental health specialists. This is unfortunate, because a diagnosis of breast cancer and mastectomy typically create a condition of emotional vulnerability. Women with breast cancer are often more afraid of losing their husbands or lovers, or, if single, of not being able to attract new partners, than they are about the possibility of facing a cruel and untimely death. To make things worse, adjuvant chemotherapy and hormone treatments, which represent a promising new advance in breast cancer management, often impair female sexuality on a physical basis. The potential threat to her sexuality can be a major source of stress for the recovering cancer patient. But unfortunately, most women face this difficult issue alone because it is a rare doctor, nurse, or social worker who will bring up the subject of sex during the postsurgical care of their patients, while women themselves are often reluctant to voice their concerns because they feel embarrassed and guilty to be thinking about sex when they "should be grateful" for being alive. (pp. 3–4)

Several observations from this helpful paper follow:

◆ Mastectomy itself does not physiologically inhibit female sexual response, but psychologically may induce sexual avoidance because the woman anticipates rejection by her partner.

Happily, such concerns are largely unfounded. The great majority of husbands and lovers, provided of course that they were attracted to their partners before surgery, and that she continues to be sexually responsive, do *not* lose sexual interest nor do they develop potency problems. In most cases, men "tune out" their partner's missing breast(s), and focus instead on the pleasurable erotic stimulation of lovemaking.[55] (p. 5)

◆ Most experts urge *early* return to sexual activity in order to prevent sexual avoidance; once established, it is difficult to reverse. Effective conjoint sex therapy and individual counseling methods may bring relief.[2,48,114]
◆ The antiestrogen tamoxifen is much less toxic than chemotherapy, but has been associated with vaginal soreness, drying, and shrinking, as well as diminished libido.
◆ The physiological effects of chemotherapy, such as fatigue, depression, nausea, vomiting, hair loss, and weight gain, may exacerbate preexisting sexual and self-esteem problems.
◆ Destruction of ovarian functioning is desirable in the treatment of estrogen-sensitive cancers, because it reduces estrogen production. Drugs like adriamy-

cin, cyclophosphamide, and phenylalanine mustard (L-PAM) impair fertility, menstruation, and sexual functioning by interfering with the production of estrogen and testosterone.

◆ Induction of premature menopause impairs all three phases of female sexual response—desire, excitement, and orgasm.

• Estrogen deficiency impairs the female excitement phase, which is mediated by perivaginal vasodilatation that causes the vagina to lubricate and swell during arousal. Atrophy of the vaginal mucosa results in painful intercourse, secondarily inhibiting libido.

• *Female libido and orgasm depend on testosterone,* which is also secreted by the ovaries. The chief feature of female testosterone deficiency *(female androgen deficiency syndrome)* is the global loss of sexual desire and diminished sexual pleasure and fantasy.

• The sudden loss of ovarian androgens that occurs after surgical or chemical menopause is often more profound than in natural menopause, in which the ovaries continue to secrete some androgens for many years.

The resulting physical unresponsiveness and difficulty achieving orgasms

can be a real "turnoff" for [the woman's] partner. A partner's arousal is a powerful aphrodisiac for most men. Conversely, her lack of responsiveness can be disturbing, and this can precipitate a cycle of performance anxiety and impotence that eventually damages a couple's relationship much more than the surgical removal of the breast(s).[55] (p. 8)

Kaplan advises hormone testing for breast cancer patients with nonsituational sexual complaints, especially those with diminished libido, orgasmic dysfunction, and diminished clitoral sensation. Levels of testosterone 20 ng/ml or below are suggestive of female androgen deficiency syndrome. Kaplan and her group have been exploring testosterone replacement therapy, finding good response and few adverse side effects.[55,56]

Cancer Morbidity, Mortality, and the Psyche

The mind's effect on bodily health needs little advocacy. For example, an interesting study surveyed oncology caregivers' and university students' beliefs about psychological influences in cancer.[19] Overall, the majority agreed strongly that psychological factors influenced physical health and the course of cancer, *including its curability*. Many also believed that stress and coping style were contributing *causes of cancer*. Both groups rated psychological interventions as being very helpful *physically* to persons with cancer, with most respondents desiring such approaches if they themselves were to develop cancer.

Consultation-liaison psychiatrists are often asked about the correlation between psychological factors and the risks for cancer morbidity and mortality. There are both positive and negative results in the literature: some studies have found that risk correlates with psychological factors[81,84,95] while others have not.[3,10,15,43,54,119] Some of the available evidence—and its methodological limitations—follow.

Methodological Problems

In their detailed recent survey, Mulder et al.[71] summarized several problems in researching psychosocial factors and breast cancer:

◆ Variability in psychological self-report questionnaires
◆ Heterogeneous cancer diagnoses
◆ Differing intervals of psychosocial assessments from time of diagnosis
◆ Inclusion of patients at different stages of the disease
◆ Differences in statistical methods
◆ Failure to control for clinicopathological factors
◆ Potentially confounding behavioral factors, such as compliance with medical treatment, physical exercise, dietary intake, smoking, and alcohol and drug abuse

In addition, diagnosing depression in patients with cancer is often challenging,[65] complicated by neurovegetative symptoms that often obscure the diagnosis.

Coping Styles

Although methodology limits the validity of some study results, the trends regarding coping and disease outcome are worth mentioning:

◆ In 1975, Greer and Morris[38] found that women with malignancies at breast biopsy had more difficulty expressing anger than those with benign lesions. The mood assessment occurred *before* the patients knew the biopsy results.
◆ A 1979 study by Derogatis et al.[18] reported that patients rated by the medical staff as *less* cooperative lived significantly longer (although the long-surviv-

ing group had significantly less radiotherapy before the study and may have been less ill).

◆ A prospective study of nonmetastatic breast cancer (n = 62) by Greer, Pettingale, and Morris[39,40,82] reported that patients' psychological responses to cancer were significantly related to disease outcome 5, 10, and 15 years later. Patients who responded with a fighting spirit or denial (positive avoidance) were significantly more likely to be alive and free of recurrence than were patients with fatalistic or helpless responses. Psychological response was not related to clinical stage, measures of tumor load, histological grade, or mammographic appearance.
◆ Repressive coping styles were found in many breast cancer patients,[36] with extroversion and social activity predictive of longer survival.[45] Unlike findings in earlier studies, low levels of anger predicted better outcome.
◆ Another study found that severe stress from adverse life events was significantly associated with an increased risk of breast cancer relapse.[84]
◆ Those melanoma patients who self-reported more psychosocial distress had faster disease progression.[105]
◆ A less favorable prognosis was found in malignant melanoma patients who were relatively cooperative but unassertive.[106]

Among the negative studies, Cassileth et al.[10] found that psychosocial factors did not predict cancer progression. Zonderman et al.[119] reported no relationship between depression and cancer mortality. Barraclough et al.[3] found no contribution of psychosocial stress or depression to relapse of breast cancer.

Many people—with or without a medical diagnosis—fear the "toxicity" of acknowledging negative or angry feelings. Right now, the effects of coping on cancer remain ambiguous.[53] Nonetheless, we encourage that verbalizing such feelings is beneficial—inducing relief, not relapse—and that any psychological strategy that improves comfort and well-being promotes good health.

Impact of Psychosocial Treatment on Disease Progression

Several investigations have explored the impact of psychosocial treatment on disease progression. Results have varied:

◆ Psychotherapy significantly reduced a variety of somatic and psychological symptoms in cancer patients, whose nausea and vomiting also diminished.[30]

◆ Patients randomized to receive group support treatment and somatic (chemotherapy or radiation) treatment were found to live longer than patients who received somatic treatment alone.[41]

◆ Linn et al.[62] and Morgenstern et al.[70] could demonstrate no effect of psychosocial treatment on survival from an individual counseling program with end-stage mixed-type cancer patients and a group support program with mixed-stage breast cancer patients, respectively.

◆ Gellert et al.[33] similarly found that an adjunctive psychosocial support program showed no favorable impact on survival time in breast cancer patients followed over 10 years. The support program consisted of weekly cancer peer support and family therapy, individual counseling, and use of positive mental imagery.

One of the most publicized studies has been by Spiegel, Bloom, and colleagues.[100–102] These investigators used a randomized, prospective psychosocial support trial for metastatic breast cancer patients. Eighty-six women were assigned randomly to either routine oncological care or a year of weekly support groups. The patients in the latter group experienced less mood disturbance, fewer phobic responses, and less pain than the control group. Most importantly, *the patients randomized to psychosocial treatment lived almost twice as long as control subjects* (average: 18.9 months versus 36.6 months, respectively). The difference was statistically significant, and no baseline differences could account for the observed differences in survival time. Spiegel[97] has written,

> This was the first time that we had undertaken a study absolutely convinced that the outcome would show no difference between intervention and control samples. We were thus doubly surprised to find a substantial difference. This study provides convincing evidence that patients randomized to intensive psychosocial treatment live longer, that something happens that slows the progression of the illness . . . Furthermore, it must be emphasized that at no time did we convey to the patients, nor did we believe ourselves, that the intervention would have any effect on longevity. Thus, there was no placebo component to the survival time. (pp. 363–364)

Mulder, Spiegel, and colleagues[71] later speculated that the patients in the intervention group may have been more compliant with medical treatment, or may have stimulated each other in good health behaviors, such as physical exercise or eating well. Undetected preexisting differences between the intervention and control groups may also have existed regarding medical status and psychosocial variables, including coping styles, social support, and stressful life events. This study remains to be replicated.

Most recently, Fawzy et al.[26] evaluated recurrence and survival for 68 patients with malignant melanoma who had participated in a 6-week structured psychiatric group intervention 5–6 years earlier,[23,24,27] shortly after their diagnosis and initial surgical treatment. These investigators used a randomized, controlled experimental study design.

◆ For control patients, there was a trend for recurrence and a (statistically significant) higher death rate than for experimental patients (13/34 versus 7/34, and 10/34 versus 3/34, respectively).

◆ Male gender and greater lesion depth ("Breslow depth") predicted higher rates of recurrence and lower survival.

◆ Only Breslow depth and psychiatric treatment were significant; even after adjusting for Breslow depth, the treatment effect remained significant.

◆ Baseline affective distress and baseline coping were significant psychobehavioral predictors of recurrence and survival.

◆ Interestingly, *higher* levels of baseline distress predicted lower rates of recurrence and death; the authors speculated that distress might spark illness awareness and behavioral motivation rather than being a negative factor.

◆ Baseline coping and enhanced active-behavioral coping over time also predicted lower rates of recurrence and death.

◆ *Positive coping could be learned or enhanced, and if implemented, improved health outcomes.*

The authors detailed the clinical implications of their findings:

◆ Patients with high distress and poor baseline coping need interventions aimed at enhancing their resources and improving their coping behavior.

◆ Patients with high distress and good coping should be encouraged and supported.

◆ Patients who minimize the threat of cancer, presenting with low baseline distress and coping, appear to be at greatest medical risk. "The theme for interventions in this subgroup should be, 'Don't minimize, mobilize!' " (p. 688).[26] Interventions must focus on helping such individuals understand the realistic threat and motivating them to mobilize their resources.

Fawzy et al.[26] concluded that psychiatric interventions that enhance coping and reduce distress appear to benefit survival; such interventions are not, however, proposed as an alternative treatment for cancer. These authors recently performed a critical review of other psychosocial interventions available for cancer patients.[25]

Comment.   Many cancer patients come to treatment having heard about these findings and wanting to know more. More research is required before making definitive conclusions regarding the psychosocial support–cancer survival relationship.[58b,71a,86a,108] On the other hand, quality-of-life improvements with psychosocial interventions, including groups,[11,31] are undisputed. That psychological health might benefit the body is usually encouraging for people; it is something that they can "do" to help themselves. We never challenge the patient who derives hope from the more optimistic study results. We have found it necessary, however, to work vigorously with the frequent corollaries to this belief—namely, that acknowledging painful feelings is "bad for one's health" and that medical complications are the result of the "wrong attitude."

Prognosis, Psychotherapy, and Countertransference

Good consultation-liaison psychiatrists are an acknowledged blessing to any medical service, but probably nowhere is our presence more welcome than on an oncology service. Certain facts, such as 5-year survival, have practical importance for formulating a psychotherapeutic strategy and help distinguish realistic fears about prognosis from panicky fantasies:

◆ Estrogen receptor–positive patients and older, postmenopausal women with breast cancer have better overall survival than younger, premenopausal receptor-negative patients.[50]

◆ Five-year survival for primary breast cancer varies from approximately **45%** (tumor diameters > 5 cm with positive axillary nodes) to **96.3%** (tumors < 2 cm without nodal involvement).[8,12,86]

◆ Median survival time of metastatic breast cancer is approximately **2 years,**[71] but this ranges from a few months to three decades.[29,77]

Some Practical Guidelines for Psychotherapy

One of our goals in psychotherapy is to demystify cancer, reducing it from the fantasied "monster" disease to an illness that is admittedly dangerous, like many others, but potentially curable or at least manageable.

◆ Sometimes it is possible to illustrate this by semantic distancing, such as referring to cancer as the "C-word" or "the Big C." When respectfully and not flippantly delivered, this strategy often brings a smile of self-recognition, creating some psychological distance for exploring how terrifying fantasies about cancer may be at odds with the facts.

◆ When *reasonable and realistic* after treatment is completed, the patient with good prognosis is encouraged to consider herself as having "had" breast cancer (past tense). This strategy seeks to limit self-identifying as a "cancer patient" indefinitely. The ongoing medical surveillance is framed as an active step toward maintaining *health*, rather than the cancer-patient role.

◆ For more advanced disease, deemphasize cure and instead stress chronicity (i.e., reframe the goal as learning to live with cancer as a chronic illness). Analogies to other chronic illnesses (such as chronic heart disease or diabetes, depending on the personal or family history of the patient)—which, though also incurable, are manageable—are often reassuring. These other illnesses rarely have the same mythic proportions of cancer and thus lend perspective to the terrifying fantasies about cancer. We never mislead the patient about the facts; it is the fantasies that we seek to challenge, as these add to the misery and fear.

◆ For frightened, metastatically ill patients who are not ready to explore issues about death, highlighting the broad range of survival statistics or acknowledging that the doctors "don't always know," sometimes allows the patient enough hope to make the most of the "here and now."

◆ **Never** make statements implying that the patient "is a better/stronger/saner person" for having cancer (unless, of course, such descriptions come from her). Amazingly, many patients hear this from family and friends, who apparently are at a loss for what else to say. We recommend empathy with the viewpoint that statements like these, while well-intentioned, are infuriating; they distance the speaker from the patient's pain and fear, which makes the patient feel more isolated and terribly alone.

Expect some psychological regression during periodic oncological checkups, even for patients with limited disease and good prognosis. When appropriate, challenge the view that the patient is a "walking time bomb." Instead, repeatedly emphasize that she is taking aggressive action to ensure continued health, detecting problems before they progress—like patients with any other serious illness.

◆   As with all psychotherapeutic strategies, proper timing, dose, and tact are important in effecting this cognitive shift while still remaining empathic to the ongoing terror about a recurrence.

Many an anxious patient tries to use her psychotherapy to discuss specific survival statistics rather than her feelings. Try to redirect these specifics to the oncologist, and focus on exploring with the patient her feelings about what she has learned. As mentioned, many cancer patients—regardless of education or sophistication—often imagine that there are toxic effects of sharing painful emotions.

> "Don't cry," one patient's husband said, "you'll make the cancer spread." Although this statement reflects his intolerance of the emotional discomfort that comes from sharing fear and sadness and also reflects the ill-begotten and mistaken belief that expression of emotion leads to dissemination of cancer, it points out that there are factors in family life that may facilitate or inhibit shared coping.[99] (p. 347)

One patient experienced her cancer as just punishment for prior misdeeds within her family.[116] Both of her sisters had been previously diagnosed with more advanced breast cancer. Her guilt about having a better prognosis than her sisters' related to preexisting survivor guilt about their abusive father, who had spared her, his favorite. Compliance with her medical care improved as she explored aspects of her painful past, all the while fearful that discussing upsetting feelings would activate the cancer.

Remember, inadvertent slips or even unique wording can panic a patient.

◆   For example, a graduate student found a 2-cm breast lump during the course of a 3-year psychotherapy. She had sailed through her lumpectomy and chemotherapy without incident. A very logical and practical person, she coped by "taking charge" and "staying organized." The radiation oncologist at their first meeting unthinkingly mused aloud that the one positive lymph node had been located in an "atypical" place. Despite reassurances that this had no impact on prognosis, the patient became frantic, stating "I don't want to be 'interesting' and I'm sick of being 'atypical.' " There ensued weeks of nightmares about death, an inability to concentrate on her studies, and ruminations about survival statistics.

Clearly, the meanings of the oncologist's comments were psychologically loaded by the patient's preexisting fears and fantasies. One cannot protect a patient from the many personalities that become involved in oncological treatment. Our approach is to tailor a hybrid therapy, borrowing strategies from insight-oriented, cognitive, and supportive psychotherapies: we persist in examining hidden meanings and fantasies derived from the past, reframing thoughts that maintain negative feelings in the here and now, and reinforcing adaptive defenses.[14,23,24,26,37,68,69,98] Medications are added when appropriate.

◆   The graduate student gained insight that "atypical" contained associations to feeling defective since adolescence relative to her attractive older sisters. This extended to other women who had body types that she idealized. She had felt she could compete with other women only with her breasts, which had been the sole "perfect" part of her; they, too, had "let her down." A brief course of temazepam (Restoril, 15 mg) restored sleep. In addition to the exploratory work, reinforcing her "stay logical" defensive style helped her find a different radiation oncologist whose approach was more upbeat and reassuring. The patient was supported in her desire to learn yoga, and encouraged to "get centered again" and "stay organized."

Oncology patients often ask about interventions that emphasize "visualizing" (e.g., visualizing white cells ferociously attacking cancer cells) or "laughing the cancer away." This approach may be helpful for some patients but—beware!—may seem silly or burdensome for others. There is no easy treatment in oncology, including this one.

◆   Patients often feel defensive and guilty when they "can't relate" to this kind of inspirational approach, especially when championed by well-meaning but insistent relatives and friends, desperate to be of help.

◆ *Medical setbacks may be misattributed to the patient's inadequate motivation to get well*—a transgression that costs not only survival, but saddles an already beleaguered patient with feelings of guilt and inadequacy. Since everyone brings to her illness preexisting conflicts wrought from a lifetime of living, *this approach may reinforce the idea that expressing negative feelings is dangerous.*

As mentioned, your knowledge of the illness course and prognosis has important implications for technique: selecting techniques that rely on an unstructured unfolding of unconscious fantasies may be helpful in the long run, but can potentially outsurvive the patient; choosing a short-term approach for no other reason than "the patient has cancer" reduces treatment strategy to diagnostic stereotype. Either extreme deprives the patient of appropriate treatment and may signal countertransference issues:

◆ For example, embarking on a psychodynamic treatment that requires a long-term commitment may reflect the psychiatrist's denial of the disease's lethality, the patient's mortality, and what both stir up personally. (See the case report by Mayer[64] on the analysis of a dying patient.)

◆ Similarly, a short-term approach that disintegrates into "hit and run" may signal avoidance, a countertransference escape from the unconscious issues elicited by the patient, consciously rationalized as therapeutic expediency.

⚜ "PHYSICIAN, HEAL THYSELF"

This wise admonishment seems a fitting conclusion to this final chapter. Oncological psychiatry, like most of consultation-liaison psychiatry, is not for the fainthearted. It constantly challenges the fine balance of emotional responsiveness and neutrality that is the hallmark of the effective physician. Consultation psychiatry sometimes feels like a M.A.S.H.–unit siege on the psyche, especially on an oncology service. A sense of humor and camaraderie with fellow staff help maintain perspective.

◆ Some final words on "neutrality." It is often confused with "impassivity," which is an allegedly "analytic" stance.

◆ In lay terms, impassivity is more accurately termed *coldness*. A physician's emotional coldness may reflect defensive distancing, consciously rationalized as "technique"; it is *poison* to working with seriously ill

patients. Medical patients are already struggling with anxiety about abandonment and separation; they may pick up the clinician's inaccessibility, and accurately conclude that the contact will not be helpful.

◆ Unfortunately, this attitude may be generalized to all psychiatrists, and make future psychiatric intervention more difficult.

◆ *"Neutrality" does not mean being emotionally "neutered."*

◆ See Appendix P ("Practical Suggestions for Bedside Manner in the General Hospital Setting").

Following through to the end of any medical illness assaults one's own psyche, as well as the patient's, with realistically terrifying issues. Clinicians must be alert to becoming psychologically symptomatic themselves. This is an authentic occupational hazard; clues are feeling "stuck" at one of two poles:

◆ Feeling helplessly overwhelmed as a physician by the inexorability of the patient's illness, or

◆ Being fixed in sterile hyperintellectualization that drains emotional responsiveness from patients, friends, and family.

Both extremes feel foreign and are very uncomfortable. They may be more consciously accessible as perceptions of "burnout": forgetting appointments, having trouble making time for a patient, dreaming repeatedly or ruminating about the patient's situation, and so forth. We strongly recommend that the clinician be open to supervision with an experienced peer or a more senior colleague.

◆ Regular collaboration with another psychiatric colleague, even at the bedside, helps to reestablish the appropriate balance between clinical distance and emotional accessibility.

◆ *Moreover, personal psychiatric consultation may be helpful and bring relief!*

The latter is an often much-resisted option. Although unlikely to refuse personal consultation with an internist for persistent fever and cough, many of us paradoxically resist availing ourselves of the psychiatric resources that we so ardently provide for our patients. The prospect of obtaining or refusing personal psychiatric treatment brings us face to face with our own hidden prejudices about what it means to see a psychiatrist.

The immediate goal of supervision or personal psychiatric intervention should be to highlight and remedy areas of countertransference interference. This strategy allows the psychiatrist more flexibility in making good therapeutic decisions and staying emotionally available to a besieged patient. Consulting competently and with compassion in the medical setting, especially under fire and often against all odds, returns a deeply rewarding, gratifying experience.

⚛ SUMMARY

1. Changes in the medical system and philosophy of treating breast cancer greatly impinge on a woman's psychological adaptation to her disease and its treatment. Treatment is now aimed at achieving the maximum disease-free survival with breast-conserving treatments that provide the best cosmesis but do not compromise cure. The recognition that radical and modified radical mastectomy do not prevent micrometastases has led to newer approaches using breast-conserving methods combined with irradiation. Comparable survival rates have been achieved, although follow-up periods are not yet as long as those with the older methodologies.

2. Despite the less mutilating procedures, patients today face greater uncertainty and differing opinions about what constitutes optimal therapy. Survival statistics are readily available in the lay press—a response to the demand for greater patient autonomy and full disclosure. These statistics are frightening. While many patients will experience their enhanced participation as positive, others feel overwhelmed as they are forced to share therapeutic and prognostic uncertainty.

3. Previous experiences, personal data, demographic characteristics, and factors relating to family, friends, and physician all influence how patients make decisions regarding their treatment. The verbal interaction with the doctor greatly influences what happens later. Predictably, nuances in communication and facial expression are not top priority for the surgeon or oncologist. Often, the consulting psychiatrist assists the patient in processing the information and her feelings about the way she has received it. A thoughtless remark or casual comment, seemingly innocuous to the medical professional who makes it, can induce a tailspin of panic and despair in the patient. Psychiatric intervention can mitigate untoward psychological reactions while assisting informed decision-making and medical compliance.

4. A woman's phase of life greatly affects her adjustment to breast cancer and its treatment. Young, single women are particularly vulnerable to breast can-

cer's psychological assaults on self-esteem and hope. On the other hand, older women more often are experiencing additional losses or illnesses. There is no easy time to have breast cancer.

5. Coping styles influence adaptation. Prior psychiatric illness predisposes to poor adaptation. When subjects with preexisting psychiatric disorder were eliminated from a study of adaptation to breast cancer, no serious psychopathological sequelae were found in the year after mastectomy. Poor adaptation has been associated with previous unsatisfactory or negative sexual experiences, overly intense emotional investment in breasts, body image problems, and a high number of stressful life events before diagnosis. Prior experiences with breast cancer in friends or other family members may also increase vulnerability to problems. A confrontational, "tackling stance" is thought to be optimal; women who use avoidance and capitulation have been found to be more emotionally distressed in the early rehabilitative stages after mastectomy. Patients who have a sense of control over events and who take an active role in rehabilitation tend to adjust better than those with a helpless outlook.

6. Limited resection ("lumpectomy") has advantages over radical mastectomy relative to self-image, self-consciousness, and sexual function. However, some have reported less-than-expected emotional benefit for lumpectomy as opposed to more mutilating surgery. Differences between treatment groups apparently diminish over time, and women choosing breast-conserving procedures experience as much psychological discomfort (about issues other than body image) as those undergoing radical mastectomy. While preservation of the breast has important psychological advantages, many women underestimate the psychic toll of watching the irradiated breast lose normal sensitivity and consistency. Delayed reactions to the trauma of the illness occur in the lumpectomy group, becoming more apparent with daily visits for radiation therapy and heightened by the accompanying fatigue. Moreover, some researchers found that patients choosing breast-conservation surgery rated themselves as having less energy and receiving less emotional support than those choosing modified radical mastectomies.

7. For most women, breast reconstruction meets or exceeds their expectations. However, those who had anticipated that surgery would improve sexual relations and/or relations with their partner were at risk for disappointment postreconstruction. These pa-

tients were more likely to have had a history of impaired interpersonal relations predating their mastectomy. They also reported greater loss of role and social function postmastectomy and significantly more symptomatology on a standard checklist.

8. Adjuvant chemotherapy is increasingly recommended for Stage I (node negative) disease since the discovery of improved survival (by almost 10%). Chemotherapy is stressful, and patients benefit from active support. Tamoxifen is an antiestrogen medication administered to postmenopausal women with lymph node involvement and to those with positive estrogen receptor tumors. It has few adverse neuropsychiatric side effects, although its antiestrogen effects can be upsetting.

9. *Intense psychological reactions often peak as treatment ends.* Patients may be less aware of their emotional reactions throughout the information gathering, surgery, and immediate postoperative period. The emotional pain often hits with a shock later. The frequent visits to the physician and clinic, initially terrifying but gradually part of the patient's "routine," can be difficult to relinquish. Fears about recurrence often reach their height as treatment terminates.

10. The sexual side effects of breast cancer treatment are often ignored. Although mastectomy itself does not physiologically inhibit female sexual response, it may induce sexual avoidance because the woman anticipates rejection by her partner. In addition, breast cancer treatment affects sexual physiology. Destruction of ovarian functioning is desirable in the treatment of estrogen-sensitive cancers because it reduces estrogen production. Induction of premature menopause impairs all three phases of female sexual response—desire, excitement, and orgasm. Atrophy of the vaginal mucosa results in painful intercourse, secondarily inhibiting libido. Reduction of ovarian testosterone can result in the *female androgen deficiency syndrome*, characterized by a global loss of sexual desire and diminished sexual pleasure and fantasy.

11. Psychiatrists are often asked about the correlation between psychological factors and the risks for cancer morbidity and mortality. There are both positive and negative results in the literature: some studies have found that risk correlates with psychological factors and others have not. There are several methodological problems in this research, which are reviewed in the text. Many cancer patients come to treatment having heard about these findings and wanting to know more. More research is required before making definitive conclusions regarding the psy-

chosocial support–cancer survival relationship. On the other hand, quality-of-life improvements with psychosocial interventions are undisputed. That psychological health might benefit the body is usually encouraging for people; it is something they can "do" to help themselves. Never challenge the patient who derives hope from the more optimistic study results. However, work vigorously with the frequent corollaries to this belief—namely, that acknowledging painful feelings is "bad for one's health" and that medical complications are the result of the "wrong attitude."

12. Review the psychotherapeutic techniques for demystifying cancer. One goal is to reduce cancer from the fantasied "monster" disease to an illness that is admittedly dangerous, like many others, but potentially curable or at least manageable. Certain facts, such as 5-year survival, have practical importance for formulating a psychotherapeutic strategy and help distinguish realistic fears about prognosis from panicky fantasies. Selecting techniques that rely on an unstructured unfolding of unconscious fantasies may be helpful in the long run, but can potentially outsurvive the patient; choosing a short-term approach for no other reason than that "the patient has cancer" reduces treatment strategy to diagnostic stereotype. Either extreme deprives the patient of appropriate treatment and may signal countertransference issues.

13. Oncologic psychiatry, like most of consultation-liaison psychiatry, constantly challenges the fine balance of emotional responsiveness and neutrality that is the hallmark of the effective physician. Following through to the end of any medical illness assaults the clinician's own psyche, as well as the patient's, with realistically terrifying issues. Clinicians must be alert to becoming psychologically symptomatic themselves. This is an authentic occupational hazard; warning signs include feeling "stuck" at one of two poles—feeling helplessly overwhelmed by the inexorability of the patient's illness, or being fixed in sterile hyperintellectualization that drains emotional responsiveness from patients, friends, and family. Try to remain open to supervision with an experienced peer or a more senior colleague.

❧ REFERENCES

1. Andersen B, Doyle-Mirzadeh S: Breast disorders and breast cancer, in Psychological Aspects of Women's Health Care: The Interface Between Psychiatry and Obstetrics and Gynecology. Edited by Stewart D, Stotland N. Washington, DC, American Psychiatric Press, 1993, pp 425–446

1a. Anonymous: The importance of sexual rehabilitation after breast cancer treatment. Oncology 8:15–16, 1994

2. Auchincloss S: Sexual dysfunction in cancer patients: issues in evaluation and treatment, in Handbook of Psychooncology. Edited by Holland J, Rowland J. New York, Oxford University Press, 1990, pp 383–413

3. Barraclough J, Pinder P, Cruddas M, et al: Life events and breast cancer prognosis. BMJ 304:1078–1081, 1992

4. Bartelink H, van Dam F, van Dongen J: Psychological effects of breast conserving therapy in comparison with radical mastectomy. Int J Radiat Oncol Biol Phys 11:381–385, 1985

5. Blichert T: Breast-conserving therapy for mammary carcinoma: psychosocial aspects, indications and limitations. Ann Med 24:445–451, 1992

6. Bloom J, Cook M, Fotopoulis S, et al: Psychological response to mastectomy: a prospective comparison study. Cancer 59:189–196, 1987

6a. Bloom J, Kessler L: Risk and timing of counseling and support interventions for younger women with breast cancer. Monographs—National Cancer Institute 16:199n206, 1994

7. Brown H: Patient issues in breast reconstruction. Cancer 68:1167–1169, 1991

8. Carter C, Allen C, Henson D: Relation of tumor size, lymph node status and survival in 24,740 breast cancer cases. Cancer 63:181–187, 1989

9. Carver C, Pozo-Kaderman C, Harris S, et al: Optimism versus pessimism predicts the quality of women's adjustment to early stage breast cancer. Cancer 73:1213–1220, 1994

10. Cassileth B, Lusk E, Miller D, et al: Psychosocial correlates of survival in advanced malignant disease? N Engl J Med 312:1551–1555, 1985

11. Cella D, Sarafian B, Snider P, et al: Evaluation of a community-based cancer support group. Psycho-Oncology 2:123–132, 1993

12. Chevallier B, Heintzmann M, Mosseri V, et al: Prognostic value of estrogen and progesterone receptors in operable breast cancer. Cancer 62:2517–2524, 1988

13. Clinical Alert: National Cancer Institute. May 16, 1988

14. Cocker K, Bell D, Kidman A: Cognitive behaviour therapy with advanced breast cancer patients: a brief report of a pilot study. Psycho-Oncology 3:233–237, 1994

15. Dattore P, Shontz F, Coyne L: Premorbid personality differentiation of cancer and noncancer groups: a test of the hypothesis of cancer proneness. J Consult Clin Psychol 48:388–394, 1980

16. Dean C, Chetty U, Forrest A: Effects of immediate breast reconstruction on psychosocial morbidity after mastectomy. Lancet 1:459–462, 1983

17. Demark-Wahnefried W, Winer E, Rimer B: Why women gain weight with adjuvant chemotherapy for breast cancer. J Clin Oncol 11:1418–1429, 1993

18. Derogatis L, Abeloff M, Melisaratos N: Psychosocial coping mechanisms and survival time in metastatic breast cancer. JAMA 242:1504–1508, 1979

19. Doan B, Gray R, Davis C: Belief in psychological effects on cancer. Psycho-Oncology 2:139–150, 1993

20. Fagan P, Schmidt CJ: Sexual dysfunction in the medically ill, in Psychiatric Care of the Medical Patient. Edited by Stoudemire A, Fogel B. New York, Oxford University Press, 1993, pp 307–322

21. Fallowfield L, Baum M, Maguire G: Effects of breast conservation on psychological morbidity associated with diagnosis and treatment of early breast cancer. BMJ 293:1331–1334, 1986

22. Fallowfield L, Hall A, Maguire P, et al: Psychological effects of being offered choice of surgery for breast cancer. BMJ 309:448, 1994

23. Fawzy F, Cousins N, Fawzy N, et al: A structured psychiatric intervention for cancer patients, I: changes over time in methods of coping and affective disturbance. Arch Gen Psychiatry 47:720–725, 1990

24. Fawzy F, Fawzy N: A structured psychoeducational intervention for cancer patients. Gen Hosp Psychiatry 16:149–192, 1994

25. Fawzy F, Fawzy N, Arndt L, et al: Critical review of psychosocial interventions in cancer care. Arch Gen Psychiatry 52:100–113, 1995

26. Fawzy F, Fawzy N, Hyun C, et al: Malignant melanoma: effects of an early structured psychiatric intervention, coping, and affective state on recurrence and survival 6 years later. Arch Gen Psychiatry 50:681–689, 1993

27. Fawzy F, Kemeny M, Fawzy N, et al: A structured psychiatric intervention for cancer patients, II: changes over time in immunological measures. Arch Gen Psychiatry 47:729–735, 1990

28. Ferrero J, Barreto M, Toledo M: Mental adjustment to cancer and quality of life in breast cancer patients: an exploratory study. Psycho-Oncology 3:223–232, 1994

29. Fey M, Brunner K, Sonntag R: Prognostic factors in metastatic breast cancer. Cancer Clinical Trials 4:237–247, 1981

30. Forester B, Kornfield D, Fleiss J: Psychotherapy during radiotherapy: effects on emotional and physical distress. Am J Psychiatry 142:22–27, 1985

31. Forester B, Kornfield D, Fleiss J, et al: Group psychotherapy during radiotherapy: effects on emotional and physical distress. Am J Psychiatry 150:1700–1706, 1993

32. Ganz P, Schag C, Polinsky M, et al: Rehabilitation needs and breast cancer: the first month after primary therapy. Breast Cancer Res Treat 10:243–253, 1987

33. Gellert G, Maxwell R, Siegel B: Survival of breast cancer patients receiving adjunctive psychosocial support therapy: a 10-year follow-up study. J Clin Oncol 11:66–69, 1993

34. Glanz K, Lerman C: Psychosocial impact of breast cancer: a critical review. Ann Behav Med 14:204–212, 1992

35. Goldberg J, Scott R, Davidson P, et al: Psychological morbidity in the first year after breast surgery. Eur J Surg Oncol 18:327–331, 1992

36. Goldstein D, Antoni M: The distribution of repressive coping styles among nonmetastatic and metastatic breast cancer patients as compared to noncancer controls. Psychology and Health 3:245–258, 1989

37. Greer S, Moorey S, Baruch J, et al: Adjuvant psychological therapy for patients with cancer. BMJ 301:675–680, 1992

38. Greer S, Morris T: Psychological attributes of women who develop breast cancer: a controlled study. J Psychosom Res 19:147–153, 1975

39. Greer S, Morris T, Pettingale K: Psychological response to breast cancer: effect on outcome. Lancet 2:785–787, 1979

40. Greer S, Morris T, Pettingale K, et al: Psychological response to breast cancer and 15-year outcome (letter). Lancet 335:49–50, 1990

41. Grossarth-Maticek R, Schmidt P, Vetter H, et al: Psychotherapy research in oncology, in Health Care and Human Behavior. Edited by Steptoe A, Matthews A. London, Academic Press, 1984, pp 325–341

42. Hack T, Degner L, Dyck D: Relationship between preferences for decisional control and illness information among women with breast cancer: a quantitative and qualitative analysis. Soc Sci Med 39:279–289, 1994

43. Hahn R, Petitti D: Minnesota Multiphasic Personality Inventory–rated depression and the incidence of breast cancer. Cancer 61:845–848, 1988

44. Hilton B: Issues, problems, and challenges for families coping with breast cancer. Semin Oncol Nurs 9:88–100, 1993

45. Hislop T, Waxler N, Coldman A, et al: The prognostic significance of psychosocial factors in women with breast cancer. Journal of Chronic Diseases 40:729–735, 1987

46. Holland J: Radiotherapy, in Handbook of Psychooncology. Edited by Holland J, Rowland J. New York, Oxford University Press, 1990, pp 134–145

47. Holland J, Mastrovito R: Psychologic adaptation to breast cancer. Cancer 46:1045–1052, 1980

48. Holland J, Rowland J: Psychological reactions to breast cancer and its treatment, in Breast Disease. Edited by Harris J, Hellman S, Henderson I, et al. Philadelphia, PA, JB Lippincott, 1987, pp 632–647

49. Holland J, Rowland J, Lebovits A, et al: Reactions to cancer treatment: assessment of emotional response to adjuvant radiotherapy as a guide to planned interventions. Psychiatr Clin North Am 2:347–358, 1979

50. Host H, Lund E: Age as a prognostic factor in breast cancer. Cancer 57:2217–2222, 1986

51. Hughson A, Cooper A, McArdle C, et al: Psychological impact of adjuvant chemotherapy in the first two years after mastectomy. BMJ 293:1268–1271, 1986

52. Huntington M: Weight gain in patients receiving adjuvant chemotherapy for carcinoma of the breast. Cancer 56:572–574, 1985

53. Hurny C: Coping and survival in early breast cancer: an update. Recent Results Cancer Res 127:211–220, 1993

53a. Jefferson J: Tamoxifen-associated reduction in tricyclic antidepressant levels in blood (letter). J Clin Psychopharm 15:223–224, 1995

54. Kaplan G, Reynolds P: Depression and cancer mortality and morbidity: prospective evidence from the Alameda County Study. J Behav Med 11:1–13, 1988

55. Kaplan H: A neglected issue: the sexual side effects of current treatments for breast cancer. J Sex Marital Ther 18:3–19, 1992

56. Kaplan H, Owett T: The female androgen deficiency syndrome. J Sex Marital Ther 19:3–24, 1993

57. Lasry J, Margolese R: Fear of recurrence, breast-conserving surgery, and the trade-off hypothesis. Cancer 69:2111–2115, 1992

58. Lee M, Love S, Mitchell J, et al: Mastectomy or conservation for early breast cancer: psychological morbidity. Eur J Cancer 28A:1340–1344, 1992

58a. Lerman C, Lustbader E, Rimer B, et al: Effects of individualized breast cancer risk counseling: a randomized trial. J Natl Cancer Inst 87:286–292, 1995

58b. Levenson J, Bemis C: Cancer onset and progression, in Psychological Factors Affecting Medical Conditions. Edited by Stoudemire A. Washington, DC, American Psychiatric Press, 1995, pp 81–97

59. Levy S, Haynes L, Herberman R, et al: Mastectomy versus breast conservation surgery: mental health effects at long-term follow-up. Health Psychol 11:349–354, 1992

60. Levy S, Herberman R, Maluish A, et al: Prognostic risk assessment in primary breast cancer by behavioral and immunological parameters. Health Psychol 4:99–113, 1985

61. Lewis R, Bloom J: Psychosocial adjustment to breast cancer: a review of selected literature. Int J Psychiatry Med 9:1–17, 1978–1979

62. Linn M, Linn B, Harris R: Effects of counseling for late stage cancer patients. Cancer 49:1048–1055, 1982

63. Maunsell E, Brisson J, Deschenes L: Psychological distress after initial treatment of breast cancer: assessment of potential risk factors. Cancer 70:120–125, 1992

64. Mayer E: Some implications for psychoanalytic technique drawn from analysis of a dying patient. Psychoanal Q 63:1–19, 1994

65. McDaniel J, Musselman D, Porter M, et al: Depression in patients with cancer: diagnosis, biology, and treatment. Arch Gen Psychiatry 52:89–99, 1995

66. McKenna R, Greene T, Hang-Fu L, et al: Implications for clinical management in patients with breast cancer: long-term effects of reconstruction surgery. Cancer 68:1182–1183, 1991

67. Meyerowitz B: Psychosocial correlates of breast cancer and its treatment. Psychol Bull 8:108–131, 1980

68. Moorey S, Greer S: Psychological Therapy for Cancer Patients: A New Approach. Oxford, UK, Heinemann Medical Books, 1989

69. Moorey S, Greer S, Watson M, et al: Adjuvant psychological therapy for patients with cancer: outcome at one year. Psycho-Oncology 3:39–46, 1994

69a. Mor V, Malin M, Allen S: Age differences in the psychosocial problems encountered by breast cancer patients. Monogr Natl Cancer Inst 16:191–197, 1994

70. Morgenstern H, Gellert G, Walter S, et al: The impact of a psychosocial support program on survival with breast cancer: the importance of selection bias in program evaluation. Journal of Chronic Diseases 37:273–282, 1984

71. Mulder C, Van der Pompe G, Spiegel D, et al: Do psychosocial factors influence the course of breast cancer? a review of recent literature, methodological problems, and future directions. Psycho-Oncology 1:155–167, 1992

71a. Neuhaus W, Zok C, Gohring U, et al: A prospective study concerning psychological characteristics of patients with breast cancer. Arch Gynecol Obstet 255:201–209, 1994

72. Noone R, Frazier T, Hayward C, et al: Patient acceptance of immediate reconstruction following mastectomy. Plast Reconstr Surg 69:632–640, 1982

72a. Northouse L: Breast cancer in younger women: effects on interpersonal and family relations. Monogr Natl Cancer Inst 16:183–190, 1994

73. Omne-Ponten M, Holmberg L, Bergstrom R, et al: Psychosocial adjustment among husbands of women treated for breast cancer: mastectomy vs breast-conserving surgery. Eur J Cancer 29A:1393–1397, 1993

74. Omne-Ponten M, Holmberg L, Burns T, et al: Determinants of the psychosocial outcome after operation for breast cancer: results of a prospective comparative interview study following mastectomy and breast conservation. Eur J Cancer 28A:1062–1067, 1992

75. Omne-Ponten M, Holmberg L, Sjoden P: Psychosocial adjustment among women with breast cancer stages I and II: six-year follow-up of consecutive patients. J Clin Oncol 12:1778–1782, 1994

76. Paraskevaidis E, Kitchener H, Walker L: Doctor-patient communication and subsequent mental health in women with gynaecological cancer. Psycho-Oncology 2:195–200, 1993

77. Paterson A, Lees A, Hannson J, et al: Impact of chemotherapy on survival in metastatic breast cancer (letter). Lancet 2:312, 1980

78. Penman D: Coping strategies in adaptation to mastectomy. Doctoral dissertation, Yeshiva University, 1979. Diss Abstr Int 40:5825B, 1980

79. Penman D, Bloom J, Fotopoulis S, et al: The impact of mastectomy on self-concept and social function: a combined cross-sectional and longitudinal study with comparison groups. Women Health 11:101–130, 1987

80. Penman D, Holland J, Bahna G, et al: Informed consent for investigational chemotherapy: patients' and physicians' perceptions. J Clin Oncol 2:849–855, 1984

81. Persky V, Kempthorne-Rawson J, Shekelle R: Personality and risk of cancer: 20-year follow-up of the Western Electric study. Psychosom Med 49:435–449, 1987

82. Pettingale K, Morris T, Greer S: Mental attitudes to cancer: an additional prognostic factor (letter). Lancet 1:750, 1985

82a. Powell D: Social and psychological aspects of breast cancer in African-American women. Ann N Y Acad Sci 736:131–139, 1994

83. Pozo C, Carver C, Noriega V, et al: Effects of mastectomy versus lumpectomy on emotional adjustment to breast cancer: a prospective study of the first year postsurgery. J Clin Oncol 10:1292–1298, 1992

84. Ramirez A, Craig T, Watson J, et al: Stress and relapse of breast cancer. BMJ 298:291–293, 1989

84a. Renshaw D: Beacons, breasts, symbols, sex and cancer. Theor Med 15:349–360, 1994

85. Rinehart M: The Reach to Recovery program. Cancer 74 (1 suppl):372–375, 1994

86. Rosen P, Groshen S, Saigo P, et al: Pathological prognostic factors in stage I and stage II breast carcinoma: a study of 644 patients with median follow-up of 18 years. J Clin Oncol 7:1239–1251, 1989

86a. Rowland J: Psycho-oncology and breast cancer: a paradigm for research and intervention. Breast Cancer Res Treat 31:315–324, 1994

87. Rowland J, Holland J: Breast cancer, in Handbook of Psychooncology. Edited by Holland J, Rowland J. New York, Oxford University Press, 1990, pp 188–207

88. Rowland J, Holland J, Chaglassian T, et al: Psychological response to breast reconstruction: expectations for and impact on postmastectomy functioning. Psychosomatics 34:241–250, 1993

89. Schain W, d'Angelo T, Dunn M, et al: Mastectomy versus conservative surgery and radiation therapy: psychosocial consequences. Cancer 73:1221–1228, 1994

90. Schain W, Edwards B, Gorrell C, et al: Psychosocial and physical outcomes of primary breast cancer therapy: mastectomy vs excisional biopsy and irradiation. Breast Cancer Res Treat 3:377–382, 1983

91. Schain W, Wellisch D, Pasnau R, et al: The sooner the better: a study of psychological factors in women undergoing immediate versus delayed breast reconstruction. Am J Psychiatry 142:40–46, 1985

91a. Schover L: Sexuality and body image in younger women with breast cancer. Monogr Natl Cancer Inst 16:177–182, 1994

92. Scott D: Anxiety, critical thinking and information processing during and after breast biopsy. Nurs Res 32:24–29, 1983

93. Segraves R, Segraves K: Female sexual disorders, in Psychological Aspects of Women's Health Care: The Interface Between Psychiatry and Obstetrics and Gynecology. Edited by Stewart D, Stotland N. Washington, DC, American Psychiatric Press, 1993, pp 351–374

94. Shapiro D, Boggs S, Melamed B, et al: The effect of varied physician affect on recall, anxiety, and perceptions in women at risk for breast cancer: an analogue study. Health Psychol 11:61–66, 1992

95. Shekelle R, Raynor W, Ostfeld A, et al: Psychological depression and 17-year risk of death from cancer. Psychosom Med 43:117–125, 1981

96. Sheldon J, Fetting J, Siminoff L: Offering the option of randomized clinical trials to cancer patients who overestimate their prognoses with standard therapies. Cancer Invest 11:57–62, 1993

97. Spiegel D: Can psychotherapy prolong cancer survival? (editorial). Psychosomatics 31:361–366, 1990

98. Spiegel D: Psychological Treatment Manual for Patients With Cancer, 1991 (Available on request from D. Spiegel, M.D., Associate Professor, Department of Psychiatry and Behavioral Medicine, Stanford University School of Medicine, Stanford, CA 94305)

99. Spiegel D: Conserving breasts and relationships (editorial; comment). Health Psychol 11:347–348, 1992

100. Spiegel D, Bloom J: Group therapy and hypnosis reduce metastatic breast carcinoma pain. Psychosom Med 45:333–339, 1983

101. Spiegel D, Bloom J, Kraemer H, et al: Effect of psychosocial treatment on survival of patients with metastatic breast cancer. Lancet 2:888–891, 1989

102. Spiegel D, Bloom J, Yalom I: Group support for patients with metastatic breast cancer. Arch Gen Psychiatry 38:527–533, 1981

103. Steinberg M, Juliano M, Wise L: Psychological outcome of lumpectomy versus mastectomy in the treatment of breast cancer. Am J Psychiatry 142:34–39, 1985

104. Stevens L, McGrath M, Druss R, et al: The psychological impact of immediate breast reconstruction for women with early breast cancer. Plast Reconstr Surg 73:619–628, 1984

105. Temoshok L: Biopsychosocial studies on cutaneous malignant melanoma: psychosocial factors associated with prognostic indicators, progression, psychophysiology, and tumor-host response. Soc Sci Med 20:833–840, 1985

106. Temoshok L, Heller B, Sagebiel R, et al: The relationship of psychosocial factors to prognostic indicators in cutaneous malignant melanoma. J Psychosom Res 29:139–153, 1985

107. Valanis B, Rumpler C: Helping women to choose breast cancer treatment alternatives. Cancer Nurs 8:167–175, 1985

108. Van Der Pompe G, Antoni M, Mulder C, et al: Psychoneuroimmunology and the course of breast cancer—an overview: the impact of psychosocial factors on progression of breast cancer through immune and endocrine mechanisms. Psycho-Oncology 3:271–288, 1994

109. Watson M, Greer S, Rowden L, et al: Relationships between emotional control, adjustment to cancer and depression and anxiety in breast cancer patients. Psychol Med 21:51–57, 1991

110. Wellisch D, Gritz E, Schain W, et al: Psychological functioning of daughters of breast cancer patients, II: characterizing the distressed daughter of the breast cancer patient. Psychosomatics 33:171–179, 1992

111. Wellisch D, Jamison K, Pasnau R: Psychosocial aspects of mastectomy, II: the man's perspective. Am J Psychiatry 135:543–546, 1978

112. Wellisch D, Schain W, Noone B, et al: Psychosocial correlates of immediate versus delayed reconstruction of the breast. Plast Reconstr Surg 76:713–718, 1985

113. Willits M: Role of "Reach to Recovery" in breast cancer. Cancer 74 (7 suppl):2172–2173, 1994

114. Witkin M: Psychosexual counseling of the mastectomy patient. J Sex Marital Ther 4:20–28, 1978

115. Wolberg W, Tanner M, Romsaas E, et al: Factors influencing options in primary breast cancer treatment. J Clin Oncol 5:68–74, 1987

116. Wyszynski A: Managing noncompliance in the "difficult" medical patient: the contributions of insight. Psychother Psychosom 54:181–186, 1990

117. Zahlis E, Shands M: The impact of breast cancer on the partner 18 months after diagnosis. Semin Oncol Nurs 9:83–87, 1993

118. Zevon M, Rounds J, Karr J: Psychological outcomes associated with breast conserving surgery: a meta-analysis. Paper presented at the eighth annual meeting of the Society of Behavioral Medicine, Washington, DC, March 1987

119. Zonderman A, Costa P, McCrae R: Depression as a risk for cancer morbidity and mortality in a nationally representative sample. JAMA 262:1191–1195, 1989

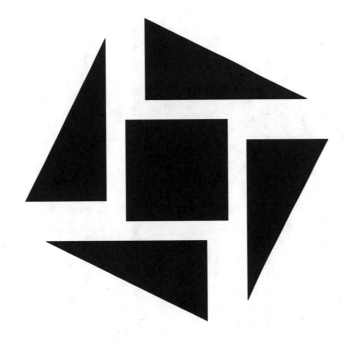

APPENDIXES

Appendix A.   A Consultation-Liaison Guide to DSM-IV

Note.   The code on Axis I usually remains the same regardless of medical etiology, except for dementia; on Axis III give the specific ICD-9-CM code for the medical condition.

	Most prominent symptom			
	Cognitive deficits			
	Delirium	Dementia	Amnestic disorder	Miscellaneous
Mental disorder due to a general medical condition (GMC)	293.0: DELIRIUM DUE TO (GMC) (*Axis I code does not change with GMC*) (e.g., delirium due to alcoholic cirrhosis [hepatic encephalopathy]; delirium due to thiamine deficiency [Wernicke's encephalopathy])	DEMENTIA DUE TO (GMC) 294.1: *fill in GMC; use this code also for:* head trauma, Parkinson's disease, Huntington's disease 294.9: HIV disease 290.1: Pick's disease, Creutzfeldt-Jakob disease	294.0: AMNESTIC DIS-ORDER DUE TO (GMC) (*Axis I code does not change with GMC*) *Specify* if transient or chronic	
Substance-induced (SI) disorders (*specify substance*)	(*SUBSTANCE*)-INTOXICATION DELIRIUM 291.0: Alcohol 292.81: Amphetamine, cannabis, cocaine, hallucinogen, in-halant, opioid, phencyclidine, sedative, hypnotic, anxiolytic 292.81: Other [or unknown] substance (e.g., steroids) (*SUBSTANCE*)-WITHDRAWAL DELIRIUM (*same codes as above*) (e.g., alcohol withdrawal delirium ["DTs"])	(SI) PERSISTING DEMENTIA 291.2: Alcohol 292.82: Inhalant, sedative, hypnotic, anxiolytic 292.82: Other [or unknown] substance	(SI) PERSISTING AMNESTIC DISORDER 291.1: Alcohol 292.83: Sedative, hyp-notic, anxiolytic 292.83: Other [or un-known] substance (e.g., alcohol-induced persisting amnestic disorder due to thiamine deficiency—Korsakoff's syndrome [formerly alcohol amnestic disorder])	SUBSTANCE-RELATED DISORDERS (OTHER) 303.00: Alcohol intoxication 291.8: Alcohol withdrawal (*specify* if with perceptual disturbances) 292.89: (*Substance*) intoxi-cation (*specify* if with perceptual disturbances) (i.e., amphetamine, cannabis, cocaine, hallucinogen, inhalant, opioid, phen-cyclidine)

Other related diagnoses

DELIRIUM DUE TO MULTIPLE ETIOLOGIES
(Use multiple codes based on specific delirium and specific etiologies)
780.09: DELIRIUM NOT OTHERWISE SPECIFIED (NOS)

DEMENTIA OF THE ALZHEIMER'S TYPE
Early onset (≤ age 65)
290.1_ (0: uncomplicated, 1: with delirium, 2: with delusions, 3: with depressed mood)
Late onset (> age 65)
290._ (0: uncomplicated, 3: with delirium, 2: with delusions, 21: with depressed mood)

VASCULAR DEMENTIA (DSM-III-R "multi-infarct dementia")
290.4_ (0: uncomplicated, 1: with delirium, 2: with delusions, 3: with depressed mood)

DEMENTIA DUE TO MULTIPLE ETIOLOGIES
(Use multiple codes based on specific dementias and specific etiologies)

294.8: DEMENTIA NOS

294.8: AMNESTIC DISORDER NOS

294.9: COGNITIVE DISORDER NOS
(e.g., postconcussional disorder, mild neurocognitive disorder)

(continued)

Appendix A.   A Consultation-Liaison Guide to DSM-IV (continued)

	Most prominent symptom			
	Delusions or hallucinations (DSM-III-R: Organic delusional disorder; organic hallucinosis)	Mood disturbance (DSM-III-R: Organic mood disorder)	Anxiety, panic attacks, or compulsions (DSM-III-R: Organic anxiety disorder)	Catatonia (DSM-III-R: Not specified)
Mental disorder due to a general medical condition (GMC)	293.8: PSYCHOTIC DISORDER DUE TO (GMC) 1: with delusions 2: with hallucinations	293.83 MOOD DISORDER DUE TO (GMC) Specify type: with depressive, manic, or mixed features; or with major depressive-like episode	293.83 ANXIETY DISORDER DUE TO (GMC) Specify type: with general-ized anxiety, panic attacks, or obsessive-compulsive symptoms	293.89 CATATONIC DISORDER DUE TO (GMC)
Substance-induced (SI) disorders (specify substance)	(SI) PSYCHOTIC DISORDER (specify: onset during intoxication or withdrawal) ALCOHOL: 291._ (5: with delusions, 3: with halluci-nations [e.g., "alcoholic hallucinosis"]) OTHER: 292.1_ (1: with delusions, 2: with hallucinations) Includes: amphetamine, cannabis, cocaine, hallucinogen, inhalant, opioid, phencyclidine, sedative, hypnotic, anxiolytic, . . . and Other [or unknown] substance (e.g., steroids)	(SI) MOOD DISORDER (specify: onset during intoxication or withdrawal) 291.8: Alcohol 292.84: Amphetamine, cannabis, cocaine, hallucinogen, inhal-ant, opioid, phencyclidine, sedative, hypnotic, anxiolytic 292.84: Other [or unknown] substance (e.g., steroid) Specify type: with depressive, manic, or mixed features	(SI) ANXIETY DISORDER (specify: onset during intoxication or withdrawal) 291.8: Alcohol 292.89: Amphetamine, caffeine, cannabis, cocaine, hallucinogen, inhalant, phencyclidine, sedative, hypnotic, anxiolytic 292.89: Other [or unknown] substance (e.g., steroids) Specify type: with general-ized anxiety, panic attacks, phobic or obsessive-compulsive symptoms	

| Other related diagnoses | 298.9: PSYCHOTIC DISORDER NOS (e.g., postpartum psychosis that does not meet criteria for mood disorder with psychotic features, brief psychotic disorder, psychotic disorder due to a GMC, or substance-induced psychotic disorder | 296.90: MOOD DISORDER NOS 296.__: MOOD DISORDER WITH POSTPARTUM ONSET (*specify*: major depressive, manic, or mixed episode in major depressive disorder, bipolar I disorder, or bipolar II disorder) | 300.00 ANXIETY DISORDER NOS |

(continued)

Appendix A. A Consultation-Liaison Guide to DSM-IV (continued)

Most prominent symptom

	Personality change (DSM-III-R: Organic personality disorder)	Sexual dysfunction (DSM-III-R: Not specified)	Sleep disturbance (DSM-III-R: Not specified)	Miscellaneous
Mental disorder due to a general medical condition (GMC)	310.1: Personality change due to (GMC) *Specify type:* labile, disinhibited, aggressive, apathetic, paranoid, other, combined, unspecified	SEXUAL DYSFUNCTION DUE TO (GMC) **Hypoactive sexual desire disorder** due to (GMC) (625.8: Female/608.89: Male) **Dyspareunia** due to (GMC) (625.0: Female/608.89: Male) 607.84: **Male erectile disorder** due to (GMC) **Other sexual dysfunction** due to (GMC) (625.8: Female/608.89: Male)	780.___ SLEEP DISORDER DUE TO (GMC) .52: Insomnia type .54: Hypersomnia type .59: Parasomnia type .59: Mixed type	293.9: MENTAL DISORDER NOS DUE TO (GMC) (Use when criteria are not met for a specific mental disorder due to a GMC [e.g., dissociative symptoms due to complex partial seizures])
Substance-induced (SI) disorders (*specify substance*)		(SI) SEXUAL DYSFUNCTION (*specify:* onset during intoxication) 291.8: Alcohol 292.89: Amphetamine, cannabis, cocaine, opioid, sedative, hypnotic, anxiolytic 292.89: Other [or unknown] substance (e.g., steroids) *Specify if:* with pain or impaired desire, arousal, or orgasm	(SI) SLEEP DISORDER (*specify:* onset during withdrawal or intoxication) 291.8: Alcohol 292.89: Amphetamine, caffeine, cocaine, opioid, sedative, hypnotic, anxiolytic 292.89: Other [or unknown] substance (e.g., steroids) *Specify type:* insomnia, hypersomnia, parasomnia, mixed	

Other diagnoses

316: PSYCHOLOGICAL FACTORS
AFFECTING MEDICAL CONDITION
Specify:
"Mental disorder . . .
"Psychological symptoms . . .
"Personality traits or coping
  style . . .
"Maladaptive health be-
  haviors . . .
"Stress-related physio-
  logical response . . .
"Other or unspecified
  factors . . .
  . . . affecting (GMC)"

Appendix B–1. Mini–Mental State Examination

Maximum score	Score	
		ORIENTATION
5	( )	What is the (year) (season) (date) (day) (month)?
5	( )	Where are we? (state) (country) (town) (hospital) (floor)
		REGISTRATION
3	( )	Name 3 objects (1 second to say each).
		Then ask the patient all 3 after you have said them. Give 1 point for each correct answer. Then repeat them until patient learns all 3. Count trials and record. Trials _____
		ATTENTION AND CALCULATION
5	( )	Serial 7's; 1 point for each correct. Stop after 5 answers.
		Alternatively, spell "world" backwards. (Score is number of letters in correct order [e.g., dlrow = 5; dlorw = 3].)
		RECALL
3	( )	Ask for the 3 objects repeated above. Give 1 point for each correct.
		LANGUAGE
2	( )	Name a pencil, and a watch.
1	( )	Repeat the following: "No ifs, ands, or buts."
3	( )	Follow a 3-stage command: "Take a paper in your right hand, fold it in half, and put it on the floor."
1	( )	Read and obey the following: "Close your eyes." (Print on blank paper in large letters.)
1	( )	Write a sentence. (Give the patient a blank piece of paper and ask patient to write a sentence for you. Do not dictate it. It must contain a subject and verb, and be sensible. Correct grammar and punctuation are not necessary.)
1	( )	Copy design. (On a clean piece of paper, draw intersecting pentagons, each side about 1 inch, and ask patient to copy the figure exactly as it is. All 10 angles must be present and 2 must intersect to score 1 point. Tremor and rotation are ignored.)
		SENSORIUM
—	—	Estimate the patient's level of sensorium: alert, drowsy, stupor, coma.

Source. Folstein M, Folstein S, McHugh P: "Mini-Mental State," a practical method for grading the cognitive state of patients for the clinician. *J Psychiatr Res* 12:189–198, 1975. Used with permission of the publisher.

Appendix B–2. Statistical Distribution of Trail Making Test Scores by Age

	Score (seconds)									
	Age 20–39		Age 40–49		Age 50–59		Age 60–69		Age 70–79	
	Trails		Trails		Trails		Trails		Trails	
Percentile	A	B	A	B	A	B	A	B	A	B
90	21	45	22	49	25	55	29	64	38	79
75	26	55	28	57	29	75	35	89	54	132
50	32	69	34	78	38	98	48	119	80	196
25*	42	94	45	100	49	135	67	172	105	292
10**	50	129	59	151	67	177	104	282	168	450

Note. *Mildly suggestive of cerebral dysfunction. **Moderately suggestive of cerebral dysfunction.

Source. Adapted from Davies A: The influence of age on Trail Making Test performance. *J Clin Psychol* 24:96–98, 1968; and from Horton AM: Some suggestions regarding the clinical interpretation of the Trail Making Test. *Clin Neuropsychol* 1:20–23, 1979.

Appendix C.   Guide to Treating Delirium With Haloperidol and Lorazepam

Goal

To completely calm the patient; partial control of agitation is not adequate.[5] Try to avoid oversedation.

Caution!

◆ Regularly scheduled high-dose therapy that continues without frequent mental status examinations may lead to overmedicating.
◆ Check vital signs regularly.
◆ Monitor for akathisia mimicking worsening agitation.
◆ Torsade de pointes ventricular arrhythmia has been described with high-dose haloperidol, although rarely, in patients with progressive QT interval widening.[7,12,15,17]
◆ Human immunodeficiency virus (HIV)–infected patients may be more sensitive to extrapyramidal side effects and neuroleptic malignant syndrome.[3,11]

Day 1→Neuroleptization

Initial haloperidol dose:[5]
◆ Mild agitation: 0.5–2.0 mg iv or im
◆ Moderate agitation: 2.0–5.0 mg iv or im
◆ Severe agitation: 5.0–10.0 mg iv or im
Reduce dose for the elderly or for patients with impaired hepatic metabolism; increase dose if the patient has been previously exposed to neuroleptics.[9]

If initial dose is not effective:

Method A:[5]
◆ If a 2-mg dose does not calm the patient after 30 minutes, slowly administer 1 mg of iv lorazepam over 1 minute.
◆ If there is no effect within 5 minutes, repeat dosing in haloperidol units of 5–10 mg, at intervals of 30 minutes.
◆ If patient is still agitated 30 minutes after lorazepam, give another 1–2 mg iv lorazepam.
◆ If still unsuccessful 5 minutes later, give 10 mg haloperidol.
◆ After calm is achieved, recurrence of agitation should signal additional dosing.[5]

Method B:[1,2]
◆ Begin with haloperidol 3 mg iv [or im] + lorazepam 0.5–1.0 mg iv.
◆ Double doses and repeat in 30 minutes if little or no response.
◆ Successive doses can be doubled every 30 minutes until sufficient control is achieved.

Day 2 and Beyond→Titration

◆ Administer the same number of milligrams as required on day 1 over the next 24 hours in divided doses;[16]
◆ Assuming the patient remains calm, reduce the dose thereafter by 50% every 24 hours;[16]
◆ After complete lucidity has been achieved with the resolution of delirium, the patient will probably need small doses of haloperidol only at night (0.5–3.0 mg), given orally.[5]

—or—

◆ Administer half the total dose used for initial neuroleptization in divided doses for initial daily maintenance therapy.
◆ Subsequent daily doses should be gradually tapered as the delirium clears, titrating to behavior.[6]

Notes on Administration

Haloperidol

◆ Empirically recommended potency ratio: 1 mg haloperidol iv or im = 2 mg haloperidol po[5]

◆ May be given safely intramuscularly, by direct intravenous injection,[4] or as an intravenous infusion in 30–50 ml of fluid.[8]

◆ Flush intravenous line with 2 ml normal saline before and after bolus infusion.

◆ Avoid mixing with heparin or phenytoin, which precipitate haloperidol.

◆ Do not use the decanoate form intravenously, as it is prepared in a sesame oil vehicle.[8]

◆ Upper intravenous dosing limit not established. (There are reports of single-bolus doses of 150 mg iv[5] and infusions of as much as 945 mg over a 24-hour period.)[14]

◆ Intravenous haloperidol may be used in patients receiving epinephrine drips, but a pressor other than epinephrine (e.g., norepinephrine) should be used after very large doses to avoid unopposed beta-adrenergic activity.[5]

Lorazepam

◆ Combination ratio: 1 mg lorazepam to 5 mg haloperidol po[10]

◆ May be given orally, intramuscularly, or intravenously by diluting in an equal volume of sterile water, 5% dextrose, or injectable normal saline.[8]

◆ Should be administered at maximum rate of 2 mg/minute.[13]

◆ Up to 240 mg have been given in critically ill cancer patients over a 24-hour period.[1,2]

◆ Manufacturer recommends a maximum single dose of no more than 4 mg iv or im.

References

1. Adams F: Neuropsychiatric evaluation and treatment of delirium in the critically ill cancer patient. Cancer Bull 36:156–60, 1984

2. Adams F, Fernandez F, Andersson B: Emergency pharmacotherapy of delirium in the critically ill cancer patient: intravenous combination drug approach. Psychosomatics 27 (suppl 1):33–37, 1986

3. Breitbart W, Marotta R, Call P: AIDS and neuroleptic malignant syndrome. Lancet 2:1488–1489, 1988

4. Cassem E, Lake C, Boyer W (eds): Psychopharmacology in the ICU, in The Pharmacologic Approach to the Critically Ill Patient, 2nd Edition. Edited by Chernow B. Baltimore, MD, Williams & Wilkins, 1988, pp 491–510

5. Cassem N, Hackett T: The setting of intensive care, in Massachusetts General Hospital Handbook of General Hospital Psychiatry, 3rd Edition. Edited by Cassem N. St. Louis, MO, Mosby Year Book, 1991, pp 373–399

6. Eisendrath S, Link N: Mental changes in the ICU: detection and management. Drug Ther Hosp Ed 8:18–26, 1983

7. Fayer S: Torsade de pointes ventricular tachyarrhythmia associated with haloperidol (letter). J Clin Psychopharmacol 6:375–376, 1986

8. Fish D: Treatment of delirium in the critically ill patient. Clin Pharm 10:456–466, 1991

9. Goldstein M, Haltzman S: Intensive care, in Psychiatric Care of the Medical Patient. Edited by Stoudemire A, Fogel B. New York, Oxford University Press, 1993, pp 241–265

10. Horvath T, Siever L, Mohs R, et al: Organic mental syndromes and disorders, in Comprehensive Textbook of Psychiatry, 5th Edition. Edited by Kaplan H, Sadock B. Baltimore, MD, Williams & Wilkins, 1989, pp 599–641

11. Hriso E, Kuhn T, Masdeu J, et al: Extrapyramidal symptoms due to dopamine-blocking agents in patients with AIDS encephalopathy. Am J Psychiatry 148:1558–1561, 1991

12. Kriwisky M, Perry G, Tarchitsky D, et al: Haloperidol-induced torsade de pointes. Chest 98:482–484, 1990

13. McEvoy G (ed): Central nervous system agents (American Hospital Formulary Service [AHFS] drug information 89). Bethesda, MD, American Society of Hospital Pharmacists, 1989, pp 981–1305

14. Tesar G, Murray G, Cassem N: Use of high-dose intravenous haloperidol in the treatment of agitated cardiac patients. J Clin Psychopharmacol 5:344–347, 1985

15. Wilt J, Minnema A, Johnson R, et al.: Torsade de pointes associated with the use of intravenous haloperidol. Ann Intern Med 119:391–394, 1993

16. Wise M, Rundell J: Concise Guide to Consultation Psychiatry. Washington, DC, American Psychiatric Press, 1988

17. Zee-Cheng C, Mueller C, Seifert C, et al.: Haloperidol and torsade de pointes (letter). Ann Intern Med 102:418, 1985

Appendix D.   Managing Insomnia and Restlessness in Delirium

	Half-life	Insomnia[a]	Restlessness[a]
Triazolam[b]	1.7–3.0 hours	0.25–0.5 mg po hs	—
Chloral hydrate	4–12 hours	500 mg–2 gm po hs	—
Oxazepam	8–12 hours	15–45 mg po hs	15–30 mg po tid-qid
Temazepam	10–20 hours	15–30 mg po hs	15–30 mg po bid-tid
Lorazepam	10–20 hours	2–4 mg po, im, or iv	0.5–3 mg bid-tid (po, im, or iv)

[a]This is the younger adult dosage. Reduce to one-third to one-half for debilitated or geriatric patients.

[b]Although triazolam produces infrequent next-day sedation, fast sleep onset, and good sleep depth, problems include increased day-time anxiety, retrograde amnesia in older people, severe agitation and delirium 30 minutes to 2 hours after routine administration of 0.125–0.25 mg.[2] In addition, rebound insomnia due to its ultrashort elimination half-life commonly occurs in the early morning hours, necessitating a second triazolam dose. For elderly patients, this exceeds the recommended dose of no more than 0.125 mg, further impairing short-term memory and concentration.[3] We feel that these side effects make triazolam a poor choice for delirium.

Source.   Adapted from Liston E: Delirium, in Treatments of Psychiatric Disorders: A Task Force Report of the American Psychiatric Association, Vol 2. Washington, DC, American Psychiatric Association, 1989, pp 804–815.

References

1. Liston E: Delirium, in Treatments of Psychiatric Disorders: A Task Force Report of the American Psychiatric Association, Vol 2. Washington, DC, American Psychiatric Association, 1989, pp 804–815

2. Patterson J: Triazolam syndrome in the elderly. South Med J 80:1425–1426, 1987

3. Regestein Q: Treatment of insomnia in the elderly, in Clinical Geriatric Psychopharmacology, 2nd Edition. Edited by Salzman C. Baltimore, MD, Williams & Wilkins, 1992, pp 235–253

Appendix E. Differential Diagnosis of the Delirious Psychotic Patient With Cirrhosis

	Mental status exam	Relationship to alcohol	Physical exam and symptoms	Psychiatric treatment
Alcohol hallucinosis (W, I, T)	Sensorium intact; prominent auditory hallucinations usually voices, often threatening; may resemble schizophrenia	Usually within 48 hours or less after heavy alcohol ingestion in person with alcohol dependence	—	Haloperidol 2–5 mg po bid for psychotic symptoms
Alcohol withdrawal (uncomplicated) (H, D)	Irritability, anxiety, malaise; transient hallucinations or illusions (poorly formed); depressed mood or irritability	Peak symptoms 24–48 hours after last drink; usually disappear within 5–7 days unless delirium tremens develop	Tremulousness; nausea, vomiting; autonomic hyperactivity; insomnia; headache	Chlordiazepoxide detoxification
Alcohol withdrawal seizures ("rum fits") (R, A, W)	Loss of consciousness; postictal confusion	Peak symptoms 7–38 hours after last drink	Generalized tonic-clonic seizures; urinary incontinence; may be focal signs	Diazepam, chlordiazepoxide detoxification for prevention
Delirium tremens (alcohol withdrawal delirium) (A, L)	Confusion; disorientation; perceptual disturbances, often hallucinatory and threatening	Gradual onset after 2–3 days; peaks 4–5 days after last drink; first episode usually after 5–15 years of heavy drinking	Marked autonomic hyperactivity (tachycardia, sweating); stigmata of delirium	Chlordiazepoxide detoxification; haloperidol for psychotic symptoms of delirium*
Hepatic encephalopathy (delirium due to hepatic insufficiency) (L, I, R, I)	Confusion > psychosis Change in personality as part of delirious prodrome	Onset may be temporally independent of alcohol intake	Pyramidal and extrapyramidal motor signs predominate over sensory; may fluctuate in parallel with psychotic symptoms Postulated > GABA-ergic tone	Avoid medications undergoing oxidative hepatic metabolism Haloperidol for psychotic symptoms;* lorazepam/oxazepam for withdrawal
Wernicke's encephalopathy (U)	Confusion > psychosis Change in personality as part of delirious prodrome	Onset may be temporally independent of alcohol intake	Ophthalmoplegia; cerebellar ataxia; often followed by Korsakoff residua	Thiamine 100 mg iv with MgSO$_4$ 1–2 ml in 50% solution prior to glucose loading
Korsakoff syndrome/psychosis (alcohol-induced persisting amnestic disorder) (M)	Not a true "psychosis"; retrograde and anterograde amnesia; confabulation; frontal lobe symptoms (apathy, inertia, loss of insight)	Not temporally related to alcohol ingestion	Stigmata of alcohol dependence possible; may have Wernicke's encephalopathy history	No effective treatment; institutionalization often needed

Note. *Haloperidol for delirium is discussed in detail in Chapter 2 (Mr. Davis).

Source. Adapted with permission of publisher from Franklin JE, Frances RJ: Alcohol-induced organic mental disorders, in *The American Psychiatric Press Textbook of Neuropsychiatry*, 2nd Edition. Edited by Yudofsky SC, Hales RE. Washington, DC, American Psychiatric Press, 1992, p. 564.

Appendix F   A Mini-Outline of Competency and Informed Consent

Requirements for Competency (adapted from [2,3])

Required criterion	Operational description	Conditions that might interfere
Evidencing a choice or preference	To minimally be able to express a consistent preference or decision for or against something (A person who is unable or unwilling to express a preference presumably lacks the capacity to make a choice.)	Muteness and inability to write, gesture, or signal Catatonia Unintelligibility Pathological ambivalence
Factual understanding	To have the capacity to reason and make judgments To make the decision voluntarily and without coercion by either the patient's family or the staff To understand the illness and its prognosis To understand the risks and benefits of treatment options, including nontreatment	Low IQ Low education Poor attention span Dementia Receptive aphasia (The patient need not possess this level of understanding at the time of admission; he or she need only to be able to receive and retain it in some reasonable form *during the decision-making process*.)
Reasoning	To use the information logically in order to reach a decision	Psychosis Impaired memory Poor information processing Other cognitive deficits
Insight and appreciation	To have a broad level of understanding relative to the implications and significance of the facts To recognize that his or her welfare is at stake pending the outcome of the decision To appreciate that he or she will benefit or suffer from the consequences of the decision To be realistic in his or her decision making	Denial Delusions Suicidal intent Confabulation

Four exceptions to informed consent:[12,30]

1—Emergencies

2—Incompetency

3—Waiver (i.e., when the patient has waived the right to be informed; the clinician should involve family or significant other in the decision process whenever possible)

4—*Therapeutic privilege* (i.e., the physician withholds information because it would be harmful to the patient; rarely invoked) (e.g., disclosure of terminal illness)

Guidelines for Informing a Patient Before a Procedure or Treatment[*]

Before a diagnostic procedure or treatment:

◆ Establish risk/benefit ratios (if known); consider patient's age, concomitant medical conditions, and relevant statistics.

◆ Disclose serious and frequent risks (> 1%) versus benefits of recommended treatment, alternate treatments, no treatment.

◆ Ask if patient desires more information.

◆ Ask patient the meaning of information.

◆ If patient has poor memory, inform repeatedly.

Before a new or experimental procedure or treatment:

◆ Explain rationale.

◆ If drug is not FDA approved, state and explain to patient (consult Institutional Review Board).

◆ If problems exist, consider consultation.

Before discharge, discuss prescribed treatments with patient:

◆ Interactions with other drugs, alcohol.

◆ Occupational risks, danger if driving, etc.

◆ Risks if patient is pregnant or nursing.

◆ What to do in case of missed dose.

Documentation:

◆ What was patient told?

◆ How did patient respond?

◆ If patient was not asked to sign informed consent, why not?

Some Facts

◆ Consent does not exist unless there is competency.[9]

◆ All adults are presumed to be competent,[6] until proven otherwise.

◆ Competency is usually specific and defined in relation to a specified act, e.g., to make a will (testamentary capacity), to testify in court (testimonial capacity), to consent or refuse treatment (decision-making capacity).[23] Being competent to perform one act does not mean that one is necessarily competent to perform another.

◆ "Physicians, psychologists, and others may express their opinions regarding the functioning and the abilities of an individual, *but by no means determine the competency of that individual.* Legal judgments of competency often make use of such input, but other factors such as state laws, legal precedents, and the specific case circumstances are also taken into account. These factors mean that competency is individually determined in each case, and rigid standards cannot be applied across cases as criteria for competency or incompetency."[3, p. 516 (italics added)]

◆ In the consultation-liaison setting, a "competency" determination is more accurately an assessment of a patient's decision-making *capacity*.[6] Requests are most frequently for[7,13,16]

   ❖ Refusing treatment or disposition.

   ❖ Signing out against medical advice.

   ❖ Giving informed consent for a procedure.

◆ Note that there is no uniform legal standard across in the United States for assessing competence to refuse medical treatment[12] (unlike testamentary competency for making a will).

◆ Medical or psychiatric emergencies: neither competency nor consent is required.[30]

◆ Competency and "committability" are different legally and clinically; persons who are "committed" to remain in a treatment facility because of dangerousness to self or others are still legally "competent" to make treatment decisions until they are adjudicated "incompetent" to do so.[6]

◆ Competency is not an all-or-nothing phenomenon[3] and can vary from hour to hour (e.g., during delirium).[30]

◆ The patient need not understand the technical details of the action or its consequences, yet should be able to articulate the key aspects of the action in layman's terms.[14]

Comment.

◆ "Unfortunately—from both risk management and ethical standpoints—treatment staffs rarely, if ever, question a patient's competency when the patient and everyone surrounding the patient is in agreement with the action to be taken."[6, p. 930]

◆ "Consultants are often tempted to meet the needs of their consultees by telling them what they want to hear; nowhere is this more true than in the assessment of a patient's competency to consent to or refuse treatment. This is compounded by the consultant's own temptation, as a physician, to seek out an outcome that is in the best clinical interests of the

[*]Originally from [12]; adapted by [30]; used with permission.

patient. . . . Such temptations must be strongly resisted; the assignment of the consultant is to be objective and focused on the issue at hand, rather than on what the consultant or consultee sees as the best overall outcome. Such isolation of purpose is often difficult. . . . Finally, the consultant must keep in mind that he is that: a consultant whose job it is to advise and not decide. The consultee may choose to disregard an assessment that a patient is incompetent [i.e., lacks capacity] to make treatment decisions and proceed with treatment. It is the treating physician who assumes both the legal and moral liability of his own actions. The consultant can only serve as a guidepost."[23, p. 635]

Practical Advice for Evaluating Capacity[6]

◆ Review the patient's medical history and current medical condition.

◆ Look especially for a history of changes in orientation and cognition.

◆ Perform a thorough clinical interview and mental status, looking for evidence of impaired cognition or a specific psychiatric disorder.

◆ Try to carry out the evaluation as a *dialogue*, rather than a mechanical question and answer session.[6] The ability to form an alliance with the examiner often predicts the patient's ability to engage in a course of treatment,[6] a kind of "interpersonal competency."[5] Encourage the patient to ask questions, and volunteer thoughts or feelings about the particular procedures; this allows a more natural way of assessing thought process and content.

◆ Auerbach and Banja[3] suggest adding to the traditional mental status exam and interview questions that tap

   ❖ Patient's awareness of current deficits, treatments, and expectations.

   ❖ Feelings about current treatments.

   ❖ Patient's understanding about who decides what treatment the patient gets.

   ❖ Patient's plans after discharge—immediate and long term.

   ❖ Patient's handling of hypothetical scenarios:

      ◆ What would you do if you were given $10,000?

      ◆ Patient's version of the treatment scenario.

◆ Also speak with members of the treatment team and, with the patient's permission, family members.

◆ The patient who maintains an effective social facade and verbal prosody can mislead naive observers into inferring higher functioning, especially if the assessment is not performed over time.[3] On the other hand, clinicians who are very familiar with the patient might assume a level of understanding that is not justified.

◆ If the patient refuses to give consent, try to understand the reasons for the refusal, looking for factors that could impair the patient's judgment, such as depression or dementia.

◆ **Note:** Remember that competency is not all or nothing; the patient may have the capacity to make a treatment decision or power of attorney, but not a contract. "Persons who have cognitive deficits—even permanent ones—may still have the capacity to understand the nature and consequences of certain procedures. A person diagnosed as having dementia is not thereby 'incompetent' in the legal or the psychological sense. Each case is context dependent, and the clinician must go through all the above steps with even the most cognitively impaired patients to determine if they may indeed have the capacity to understand the nature and consequences of the particular procedure being proposed for them."[6, p. 930]

◆ *In an emergency, neither competency nor consent is required.*[30]

◆ Prior to the diagnostic procedure or treatment, try to understand the risk/benefit ratio, factoring in data from the treatment team, the patient's age, medical conditions, and other relevant facts.[12,30]

◆ Discuss serious and frequent (> 1%) risks versus benefits of the recommended treatment, alternate treatments, and no treatment.[12,30]

◆ Ask if the patient wants more information and determine if she/he can explain the meaning of the information you have given.[12,30]

◆ Be sure to document what the patient was told, how the patient responded, and, if informed consent was not signed, why not.

Strict Versus Lenient Standards of Competency

Several authors[23,30] have suggested applying Roth et al.'s[22] differential standards of competency, based on the favorability of the risk/benefit outcome for the patient.

◆ Favorable risk/benefit outcome: Use a strict standard if the patient is *refusing* a treatment that has high likelihood of a favorable outcome with relatively low risk (e.g., intravenous antibiotics for an infected toe in a diabetic); use a lenient standard if the patient is *consenting* to such a treatment.

◆ Unfavorable risk/benefit outcome: Use a strict standard if the patient is *consenting to* a treatment that has a high risk for a minimal or unlikely beneficial outcome (e.g., experimental chemotherapy with high toxicity for someone with disseminated cancer); use a lenient standard if the patient is *refusing* such a treatment.

"While some criticize this approach as being too open to manipulation by a paternalistic physician, it accurately reflects professional obligations to ensure that patients make a truly informed decision based upon a rational weighing of the risks and benefits involved. A similar approach was endorsed by the President's Commission for the Study of Ethical Problems in Medicine and Biomedical and Behavioral Research."[23, p. 630]

Grisso and Appelbaum[8a] have recently compared standards for assessing competency.

Documentation

Use phrases such as the following when documenting your findings in the patient's chart:[6]

◆ "The patient appears to have X diagnosis because . . . "
◆ "Treatment will be instituted so that . . . "
◆ "This treatment has the following risks . . . ; nonetheless, the risks are outweighed by the following benefits: . . . "
◆ "The patient has been informed of the above treatment plan, as well as of the following treatment option: . . . "
◆ "As evidenced by the following, the patient has the capacity to give informed consent: . . . "

Modify the scheme accordingly when the patient is giving "informed refusal," or when the patient is found to lack the capacity ("is not competent") to give consent.

The Incompetent Patient

◆ The incompetent patient may require a surrogate decision maker, who is usually the family, a designated family member, or significant other.[12] Until then, the physician makes emergency decisions. Unless there are health care proxy laws in a particular state that automatically empower next of kin or other individuals to give consent for an incapacitated individual, no nonemergency treatment may continue without some type of judicial intervention (e.g., court order; declaration of incompetence and appointment of a guardian).[6]

◆ Ideally, the patient has previously prepared an advance directive while competent, such as a *living will* or *durable power of attorney.*[12,26] (See below.)

Advance Directives

By law, the competent patient always retains the right to make his or her own medical decisions and to contravene or even revoke the advance directive.[20]

◆ The **Living Will** is a document that allows competent individuals ("testators") to leave instructions for future caregivers about what procedures they do or do not wish should they ever lack the capacity to give consent.[6] Limitation: The document usually cannot be applied to nourishment and hydration supports.[20]
◆ The **Durable Power of Attorney for Health Care** goes beyond the living will, granting the right to control all aspects of personal care and medical treatment, including treatment refusal and withdrawal.[20] Unlike the traditional power of attorney, the "durable" version remains valid even when the individual lacks the capacity to make decisions.[6] Legislatures are beginning to address this on a state level (e.g., in 1990, New York recognized the need for this document with the passage of the New York Health Care Proxy Law).

When evaluating someone who plans to execute an advance directive, perform the usual evaluation for "competency" (capacity), exploring the individual's understanding and reasons underlying treatment requests or refusals. Document your clinical impressions in the event that there is dispute about the validity of the directive, or if there is disagreement with the patient's appointed proxy about decision-making capacity.[22a]

Do-Not-Resuscitate (DNR) Orders

◆ Any competent patient has the right to reject or to insist on resuscitative treatment.[18]
◆ **Note:** If a person with a severe psychiatric disorder, such as major depression, refuses resuscitation because death is an "appropriate, deserved" outcome, they are considered to be incompetent. The consultant should recommend that the family seek guardianship.[30]
◆ *Once made by a competent person, the DNR decision can rarely be overruled.*[30] If a competent patient either requests or declines resuscitation and later becomes incompetent, the court (not the family) may be the

only party able to reverse the patient's original decision.[18] (However, some states permit family, significant other, physician, and/or the hospital ethics committee to intervene to resuscitate the patient who has become incompetent, if a chance of recovery exists.)

References

1. Albert H, Kornfeld D: The threat to sign out against medical advice. Ann Intern Med 79:888–891, 1973

2. Appelbaum P, Grisso T: Assessing patients' capacities to consent to treatment. N Engl J Med 319:1635–1638, 1988

3. Auerbach V, Banja J: Competency determinations, in Medical Psychiatric Practice, Vol 2. Edited by Stoudemire A, Fogel B. Washington, DC, American Psychiatric Press, 1993, pp 515–535

4. Brennan T: AIDS and the limits of confidentiality: the physician's duty to warn contacts of seropositive individuals. J Gen Intern Med 4:242–246, 1989

5. Bursztajn H, Hamm R: The clinical utility of utility assessment. Med Decis Making 2:161–165, 1982

6. Deaton R, Colenda C, Bursztajn H: Medical-legal issues, in Psychiatric Care of the Medical Patient. Edited by Stoudemire A, Fogel B. New York, Oxford University Press, 1993, pp 929–938

7. Farnsworth M: Competency evaluations in a general hospital. Psychosomatics 31:60–66, 1990

8. Greco P, Schulman K, Lavizzo-Mourey R, et al: The patient self-determination act and the future of advance directives. Ann Intern Med 115:639–643, 1991

8a. Grisso T, Appelbaum P: Comparison of standards for assessing patients' capacities to make treatment decisions. Am J Psychiatry 152:1033–1037, 1995

9. Groves J, Vaccarino J: Legal aspects of consultation, in Massachusetts General Hospital Handbook of General Hospital Psychiatry, 2nd Edition. Edited by Hackett T, Cassem N. Littleton, MA, PSG Publishing, 1987, pp 591–604

10. Gutheil T, Appelbaum P: Clinical Handbook of Psychiatry and the Law. New York, McGraw-Hill, 1982

11. Gutheil T, Bursztajn H, Brodsky A: Malpractice prevention through the sharing of uncertainty. N Engl J Med 311:49–51, 1984

12. Howe E: Forensic issues in critical care medicine, in Problems in Critical Care. Edited by Wise M. Philadelphia, PA, JB Lippincott, 1988, pp 171–187

13. Katz M, Abbey S, Rydall A, et al: Psychiatric consultation for competency to refuse medical treatment: a retrospective study of patient characteristics and outcome. Psychosomatics 36:33–41, 1995

14. Mahler J, Perry S: Assessing competency in the physically ill: guidelines for psychiatric consultants. Hosp Community Psychiatry 39:856–861, 1988

15. Mahler J, Perry S, Miller F: Psychiatric evaluation of competency in physically ill patients who refuse treatment. Hosp Community Psychiatry 41:1140–1141, 1990

16. Mebane A, Rauch H: When do physicians request competency evaluations? Psychosomatics 31:40–46, 1990

17. Melton G: Ethical and legal issues in AIDS-related practice. Am Psychol 43:941–947, 1988

18. Miles S, Cranford R, Schultz A: The do-not-resuscitate order in a teaching hospital. Ann Intern Med 96:660–664, 1982

19. Myers B, Barrett C: Competency issues in referrals to a consultation liaison service. Psychosomatics 27:782–789, 1986

20. Overman W: Living wills and advance medical treatment directives, in Medical Psychiatric Practice, Vol 2. Edited by Stoudemire A, Fogel B. Washington, DC, American Psychiatric Press, 1993, pp 537–560

21. Overman W, Stoudemire A: Guidelines for legal and financial counseling of Alzheimer's disease patients and their families. Am J Psychiatry 145:1495–1500, 1988

22. Roth L, Meisel A, Lidz C: Tests of competency to consent to treatment. Am J Psychiatry 134:279–284, 1977

22a. Schneiderman L, Teetzel H: Who decides who decides? When disagreement occurs between the physician and the patient's appointed proxy about the patient's decision-making capacity. Arch Intern Med 155:793–796, 1995

23. Shouton R, Groves J, Vaccarino J: Legal aspects of consultation, in Massachusetts General Hospital Handbook of General Hospital Psychiatry, 3rd Edition. Edited by Cassem N. St. Louis, MO, Mosby Year Book, 1991, pp 619–638

24. Siner D: Advance directives in emergency medicine: medical, legal and ethical implications. Ann Emerg Med 18:1364–1369, 1989

25. Spar J, Garb A: Assessing competency to make a will. Am J Psychiatry 149:169–174, 1992

26. Steinbrook R, Lo B: Decision making for incompetent patients by designated proxy. N Engl J Med 310:1598–1601, 1984

27. Strain J, Taintor Z, Gise L: Informed consent: mandating the consultation. Gen Hosp Psychiatry 7:228–233, 1985

28. Wanzer S, Adelstein S, Cranford R: The physician's responsibility toward hopelessly ill patients. N Engl J Med 310:955–959, 1984

29. Weir R, Gostin L: Decisions to abate life-sustaining treatment for nonautonomous patients: ethical standards and legal liability for physicians after Cruzan. JAMA 264:1846–1853, 1990

30. Wise M, Rundell J: A Concise Guide to Consultation Psychiatry, 2nd Edition. Washington, DC, American Psychiatric Press, 1994

Appendix G. Neuropsychiatric Effects of Electrolyte and Acid-Base Imbalance

Type	Causes	Symptoms	Comment
Hyponatremia	Diuretics, antidepressants, lithium, neuroleptics, excessive parenteral fluids, renal disease, inappropriate secretion of antidiuretic hormone, polydipsia, carbamazepine	Early: impaired taste, anorexia, fatigue, headache, muscle cramps, thirst, mild confusion Late: confusion (Na < 115), delirium, convulsions	Mental symptoms are related to the serum sodium level and the rapidity of its fall. Insidious hyponatremia may be tolerated until Na < 100. EEG: loss of alpha activity and irregular discharges of high-amplitude theta waves.
Hypernatremia	Febrile illness with dehydration, diarrhea, CNS lesions, nonketotic hyperosmolar coma, hyperalimentation, severe burns, sodium bicarbonate	Thirst, depression of consciousness (Na > 160) Delirium, lethargy, stupor, coma	Mental symptoms are related to the serum sodium level and the rapidity of its rise. Insidious hypernatremia may be tolerated until Na > 170. EEG: varying degrees of slow-wave activity, but may be normal.
Hypokalemia	Vomiting, diarrhea, diabetic ketoacidosis, laxative addiction, renal tubular acidosis, diuretics	Muscular weakness and cramps, lethargy, apathy, paresthesias, drowsiness, irritability, hyporeflexia	Symptoms appear with K < 3, but vary with the acuteness of onset and the presence/absence of acidosis. ECG changes: T-wave depression, prominent U waves, arrhythmias.
Hyperkalemia	Excessive intake of K-supplementation or K-containing drugs, nonsteroidal anti-inflammatory agents, K-sparing diuretics, renal failure, trauma	Weakness, hyporeflexia, paresthesias, sensory perception deficits, delirium, cardiac arrhythmias	ECG changes: tall T waves, increased PR interval and QRS widening, fatal arrhythmias.
Hypocalcemia	Hypoparathyroidism, sepsis, renal failure, malabsorption syndrome, drugs (e.g., phenytoin)	Delirium, irritability, fatigue, weakness, depression, muscle cramps, tetany, seizures	Rate of onset may determine appearance of symptoms. Delirium is most likely when onset is acute. EEG: progressive slowing of background activity, as well as low-voltage, fast activity, sharp waves, and spikes.

(continued)

Appendix G. Neuropsychiatric Effects of Electrolyte and Acid-Base Imbalance (*continued*)

Type	Causes	Symptoms	Comment
Hypercalcemia	Malignancy, hyperparathyroidism	Early: anorexia, nausea, vomiting, headache, difficulty walking Delirium (may be the presenting feature), lassitude, drowsiness, anxiety, depression, stupor, coma	Confusion tends to correlate with serum Ca levels. Hypercalcemia presents a life-threatening medical emergency. EEG: diffuse slowing of background activity interrupted by high-voltage bursts of delta waves.
Hypomagnesemia	Starvation, malabsorption syndrome, chronic alcoholism, diuretics, severe diarrhea, aldosteronism, severe body fluid loss, diabetic acidosis, hyperthyroidism, acute intermittent porphyria	Depression, apathy, anxiety, weakness, tremor, fasciculations, irritability, tetany, seizures, delirium, hallucinations	Usually occurs in association with other electrolyte abnormalities e.g., hypocalcemia and hypokalemia). Severe hypomagnesemia may be asymptomatic in the absence of other electrolyte abnormalities. Magnesium is essential for normal calcium and potassium metabolism.
Hypermagnesemia	Renal failure; magnesium-containing oral purgatives, antacids, or rectal enemas; adrenal insufficiency	Drowsiness, lethargy, weakness; eventual narcosis and coma	—
Hypophosphatemia	Diabetic ketoacidosis, acute and chronic alcoholism, severe burns, respiratory alkalosis, hyperalimentation, phosphate-binding antacids	Mild: weakness, malaise, ano-rexia bone pain, joint stiffness, intention tremor Severe: irritability, apprehension, muscular weakness, numbness, paresthesias, dysarthria, confusion, obtundation, seizures, coma	Hypophosphatemia is common, usually mild, and without consequence.
Hyperphosphatemia	—	Definite clinical manifestations have have not been attributed to hyperphosphatemia	—

	Causes	Symptoms	Description
Metabolic acidosis	Renal failure, diabetic ketoacidosis, lactic acidosis, intoxications (ammonium chloride, salicylate, methanol), starvation ketosis, alcoholic ketoacidosis, alkali loss (diarrhea, ureteroenterostomy)	Chronic: asymptomatic, or with fatigue and anorexia Severe: hyperventilation, labored breathing (Kussmaul respiration), progressive depression of consciousness, stupor, coma, convulsions	Defined as arterial blood pH < 7.40. Primary respiratory acidosis: occurs with increased P_{CO_2}. Primary metabolic acidosis: involves compensatory hyperventilation and decreased P_{CO_2}. Symptoms usually difficult to separate from those of the underlying disorder. Depressed levels of consciousness tend to correlate with acidotic cerebrospinal fluid.
Metabolic alkalosis	Vomiting, chloride depletion (gastric drainage, diuretic therapy, posthypercapneic alkalosis), hyperadrenocorticism, potassium depletion	Lethargy, confusion at pH > 7.55. Other: irritability, neuromuscular hyperexcitability, muscle weakness, apathy, stupor (Coexisting hypocalcemia or cerebrovascular disease predisposes to disturbances of consciousness during alkalosis) (Hypoventilation secondary to metabolic alkalosis reflects the compensatory need to retain CO_2 and can augment hypoxia and contribute to mental status symptoms)	Defined as arterial blood pH > 7.40. Metabolic alkalosis is the acid-base disturbance most often encountered in the hospital setting. Primary respiratory alkalosis: occurs when CO_2 removal by the lungs exceeds its production in the body, with resulting hypocapnia; may be caused by hyperventilation, mechanical overventilation, pneumonia, or hepatic failure.

Source. Adapted from the following:
1. Jefferson JW, Marshall JR: Neuropsychiatric Features of Medical Disorders. New York, Plenum Medical Book, 1981
2. Lipowski ZJ: Delirium: Acute Confusional States. New York, Oxford University Press, 1990
3. Arieff AI, Griggs RC: Metabolic Brain Dysfunction in Systemic Disorders. Boston, MA, Little, Brown, 1992

Appendix H.   The Use of Psychotropics in Renal Failure

Drug	Route of excretion — Hepatic	Route of excretion — Renal	Half-life in ESRD (hours)	Supplement for dialysis — HD	Supplement for dialysis — CAPD	Adjustment for renal failure[a] (GFR, mL/minute) > 50	10–50	< 10
ANTIDEPRESSANTS								
Note. Tricyclics may cause anticholinergic side effects, urinary retention, orthostatic hypotension, confusion, and excessive sedation.								
Amitriptyline	✓	Renal < 5%	Unchanged	None	None	None	None	None
Amoxapine	✓	—	?	?	?	None	None	None
Bupropion	✓	—	?	?	?	None	None	None
Clomipramine[b]	✓	—	?	?	?	?	?	?
Desipramine	✓	Renal < 5%	?	None	None	None	None	None
Doxepin	✓	—	Increased (to 10–30 hours)	None	None	None	None	None
Fluoxetine	✓	—	Unchanged	?	?	None	None	None
Imipramine	✓	Renal < 5%	?	None	None	None	None	None
Maprotiline	✓	—	?	?	?	None	None	None
Nortriptyline	✓	—	Increased[b] (to 15–66 hours)	None	None	None	None	None
Phenelzine	✓	—	?	?	?	None	None	None
Protriptyline	✓	—	?	None	None	None	None	None
Sertraline[b]	✓	—	?	?	?	?	?	?
Trazodone[b]	✓	—	?	?	?	None	?	?
BARBITURATES								
Note. May cause excessive sedation and increase osteomalacia in ESRD.								
Pentobarbital	✓	—	Unchanged	None	?	None	None	None
Phenobarbital	✓	Renal 30%	Increased (to 117–160 hours)	Dose after dialysis	1/2 normal dose	q8–12h	q8–12h	q12–16h
Secobarbital	✓	—	?	None	None	None	None	None
BENZODIAZEPINES, ANXIOLYTICS, AND HYPNOTICS								
Note. May cause excessive sedation and encephalopathy in ESRD.								
Alprazolam	✓	—	Unchanged	None[b]	?	None	None	None
Buspirone	✓	—	Increased (5.8 hours)	None	?	None	None	None (active metabolite accumulates[b])
Chloral hydrate	✓	—	?	None	?	None	Avoid	Avoid (active metabolite; excessive sedation)

(continued)

Appendix H.   The Use of Psychotropics in Renal Failure *(continued)*

Drug	Route of excretion Hepatic	Route of excretion Renal	Half-life in ESRD (hours)	Supplement for dialysis HD	Supplement for dialysis CAPD	Adjustment for renal failure[a] (GFR, mL/minute) > 50	10–50	< 10
BENZODIAZEPINES, ANXIOLYTICS, AND HYPNOTICS *(continued)*								
Chlorazepate[b]	✓	—	Unchanged	?	?	None	None	None
Chlordiazepoxide	✓	Active metabolite excreted by kidney	Unchanged	None	?	None	None	Decrease to 50%
Clonazepam	✓	—	?	None	?	None	None	None
Diazepam	✓	Active metabolite excreted by kidney	Unchanged	None	?	None	None	None (active metabolite; decreased protein binding, increased volume of distribution in ESRD)
Ethchlorvynol	✓	—	?	None	None	None	Avoid	Avoid (removed by hemoperfusion; excessive sedation; plasma levels rebound after dialysis)
Flurazepam	✓	—	Unchanged	None	?	None	None	None (active metabolite)
Lorazepam	✓	—	Increased (32–70 hours)	None	?	None	None	None
Meprobamate	✓	Renal 10%	Unchanged	None	?	q6h	q9–12h	q12–18h (excessive sedation)
Oxazepam	✓	—	Increased (25–90 hours)	None	?	None	None	None (in ESRD: increased glucuronide metabolite and volume of distribution, decreased protein binding)
Prazepam[b]	✓	—	Unchanged	?	?	None	None	None
Temazepam	✓	—	?	None	None	None	None	None
Triazolam	✓	—	Unchanged	None	None	None	None	None
ANTIPSYCHOTICS								
Note. Phenothiazines may cause anticholinergic side effects, urinary retention, orthostatic hypotension, confusion, and extrapyramidal symptoms.								
Chlorpromazine	✓	—	Unchanged	None	None	None	None	None
Haloperidol	✓	—	?	None	None	None	None	None

(continued)

Appendix H.   The Use of Psychotropics in Renal Failure *(continued)*

Drug	Route of excretion — Hepatic	Route of excretion — Renal	Half-life in ESRD (hours)	Supplement for dialysis — HD	Supplement for dialysis — CAPD	Adjustment for renal failure[a] (GFR, mL/minute) > 50	Adjustment for renal failure[a] (GFR, mL/minute) 10–50	Adjustment for renal failure[a] (GFR, mL/minute) < 10
MISCELLANEOUS AGENTS								
Atenolol[b]	—	> 90% excreted unchanged	Increased (to 15–35 hours)	25–50 mg	None	None	Decrease to 50% q 48h	Decrease to 30%–50% q 96h
Benztropine	✓	—	?	?	?	?	?	?
Carbamazepine	✓	Active metabolite excreted renally	Variable, even in healthy individuals	None	None	None	None	None
Diphenhydramine	✓	Renal < 4%	?	None	None	None[b]	None[b]	None[b]
						(may cause urinary retention)		
Hydroxyzine	✓	Active metabolite excreted renally[b]	?	?	?	None	?	?
Lithium	—	✓	Increased (to 40 hours)	Dose after dialysis	None	None	Decrease to 50%–75% maint.	Decrease to 25%–50% maint.
Propranolol	✓	—	Decreased (1–6 hours)	None	None	None	None	None
Sodium valproate	✓	—	Unchanged	None	None	None	None	None
						(decreased protein binding in uremia)		
Trihexyphenidyl	Unknown[b]	Unknown[b]	?	?	?	?	?	?

Note.   CAPD = chronic ambulatory peritoneal dialysis; ESRD = end-stage renal disease; GFR = glomerular filtration rate; HD = hemodialysis; maint. = maintenance dose; ? = not known.

[a]Adjustment for renal failure:

   Interval Extension Method: Lengthen the intervals between individual doses, keeping the dose size normal.

   Dose Reduction Method: Reduce the size of the individual doses; percentages indicate fraction of normal dose to be used.

[b]Bennett WM, Aronoff GR, Golper TA, et al: *Drug Prescribing in Renal Failure*, 3rd Edition. Philadelphia, PA, American College of Physicians, 1994.

Source.   Adapted with permission from Bennett WM, Aronoff GR, Golper TA, et al: *Drug Prescribing in Renal Failure: Dosing Guidelines for Adults*, 2nd Edition. Philadelphia, PA, American College of Physicians, 1991.

Appendix I. Definitional Criteria for AIDS Dementia Complex (ADC) (HIV-1–Associated Dementia [HAD] Complex) and Cognitive Impairment—American Academy of Neurology AIDS Task Force

---

Probable **(must have *each* of the following)**

1. a. Acquired abnormality in at least two of the following cognitive abilities (present for at least 1 month):
   - attention/concentration
   - speed of processing of information
   - abstraction/reasoning
   - visuospatial skills
   - memory/learning
   - speech/language

   The decline should be verified by reliable history and mental status examination. In all cases, when possible, history should be obtained from an informant, and examination should be supplemented by neuropsychological testing.

   b. Cognitive dysfunction causing impairment of work or activities of daily living

2. At least **one** of the following:

   a. Acquired abnormality in motor function or performance verified by clinical examination (e.g., slowed rapid movements, abnormal gait, limb incoordination, hyperreflexia, hypertonia, or weakness), neuropsychological tests (e.g., fine motor speed, manual dexterity, perceptual motor skills), or both.

   b. Decline in motivation or emotional control or change in social behavior. This may be characterized by any of the following: change in personality with apathy, inertia, irritability, emotional lability, or new onset of impaired judgment, characterized by socially inappropriate behavior or disinhibition.

3. Absence or clouding of consciousness during a period long enough to establish the presence of criterion 1, above.

4. Evidence of another etiology has been sought and ruled out, including active CNS opportunistic infection or malignancy, psychiatric disorders (e.g., depressive disorder), active alcohol or substance use, or substance withdrawal. If another potential etiology (e.g., major depression) is present, it cannot be the cause of the above cognitive, motor, or behavioral symptoms and signs in order to diagnose HAD.

Possible **(must have *one* of the following)**

1. Other potential etiology present (must have **each** of the following):
   a. Same as criteria 1, 2, and 3 in **Probable**
   b. Other potential etiology is present, but the cause of criterion 1 above is uncertain

2. Incomplete clinical evaluation (must have **each** of the following):
   a. Same as criteria 1, 2, and 3 in **Probable**
   b. Etiology cannot be determined (appropriate laboratory or radiologic investigations not performed)

Source. Adapted from: Janssen RS, Cornblath DR, Epstein LG, et al: Nomenclature and research case definitions for neurological manifestations of human immunodeficiency virus type-1 (HIV-1) infection: report of a working group of the American Academy of Neurology AIDS Task Force. *Neurology* 41:778–785, 1991.

Appendix J.   Revised Human Immunodeficiency Virus (HIV) Classification System for Adolescents and Adults (Centers for Disease Control and Prevention 1993)

CD$^+$T-cell categories	Clinical categories		
	A. Asymptomatic, acute (primary) HIV or PGL	B. Symptomatic, not (A) or (C) conditions	C. AIDS-indicator conditions
1. ≤ 500/μl	A1	B1	C1
2. 200–499/μl	A2	B2	C2
3. < 200/μl AIDS-indicator T-cell count	A3	B3	C3

One or more of the conditions listed below place the patient in Category A; conditions listed in Categories B and C must not have occurred:
- PGL (persistent generalized lymphadenopathy)
- Asymptomatic HIV infection
- Acute (primary) HIV infection with accompanying illness or history of acute HIV infection

Symptomatic conditions in an HIV-infected individual that are not included among those listed in Category C and that meet at least one of the following criteria:
(a) The conditions are attributed to HIV infection or are indicative of a defect in cell-mediated immunity.
(b) The conditions are considered to be complicated by HIV infection.

Examples:
- Constitutional symptoms, such as fever or diarrhea > 1 month
- Cervical dysplasia
- Peripheral neuropathy
- Herpes zoster (shingles)

Includes clinical conditions listed in AIDS surveillance case definition. Once a Category C condition has occurred, the person remains in Category C.

Examples:
- HIV encephalopathy/ AIDS dementia complex (ADC)
- HIV wasting syndrome
- *Pneumocystis carinii* pneumonia
- Tuberculosis
- Lymphoma
- Cryptosporidiosis
- Kaposi's sarcoma
- Cytomegalovirus
- Coccidioidomycosis
- Progressive multifocal leukoencephalopathy
- Toxoplasmosis

Note.   AIDS = acquired immunodeficiency syndrome.

Source.   Adapted from Centers for Disease Control: 1993 Revised Classification System for HIV Infection and Expanded Surveillance Case Definition for AIDS Among Adolescents and Adults. *Morbidity and Mortality Weekly Report* 41(RR-17):1–13, 1992.

Appendix K. Management Strategies for the Patient With HIV-Associated Minor Cognitive-Motor Impairment and AIDS Dementia Complex (ADC)

HIV-Associated Minor Cognitive-Motor Impairment—Advice to Patients

1. **Use memory aids** (e.g., write down appointments, important information, or conversations). These reduce the need to ask for help and allow the individual to maintain a sense of control.
2. **Slow down and do one task at a time.** Performing multiple or simultaneous tasks can produce confusion, mistakes, and frustration.
3. **Use verbal monitoring** (i.e., talk aloud as a task is completed). Problem-solving aloud is a form of self-cueing that facilitates concentration and maintains focus.
4. **Keep mentally active in nonstressful ways.** Activities such as Scrabble, cards, checkers, crossword puzzles, jigsaw puzzles, and video games reinforce concentration abilities and keep many impaired individuals stimulated and involved in the world. These activities should be challenging but not overly difficult or frustrating.
5. **Get enough rest and schedule appointments early in the day.** Fatigue can worsen cognitive problems and lead to irritability and angry outbursts.
6. **Avoid stressful situations by planning ahead.** For example, shopping, running errands, or dining can be conducted during off-hours, when stimulation and stress are less.
7. **Learn stress-reduction techniques and relaxation exercises** to reduce tension and anxiety.
8. **Encourage regular exercise. Activities such as walking** can reduce stress and maintain involvement in the world. Motor skills and coordination may be retained longer with regular use. Passive exercise such as massage also may be beneficial.
9. **Self-manage medications as long as possible.** Devices such as watches with an alarm, or automated pill boxes that beep when it is time for the next dose, are helpful.
10. **Give up tasks that have become too difficult** (e.g., balancing a checkbook). Encourage the patient to find assistance. This can be reassuring and lessen anxiety for the patient who may be frightened by the cognitive changes.

The Patient With ADC—Advice to Caregivers

1. **Maintain orientation** cues regarding the date, place, and time, by visibly displaying calendars and clocks. Use an orientation blackboard with the date and the patient's daily schedule, as well as night lights to minimize "sundowning."
2. **Keep the environment and routine consistent.** Sudden changes, such as traveling on vacation, can be extremely disorienting. Familiarity is important in reducing confusion (e.g., furniture, utensils, personal articles should be kept in the same place).
3. **Monitor stimulation;** too much or too little can cause increased confusion, fearfulness, and agitation.
4. **Prepare the patient for change.** Cognitive impairment limits the ability to adjust quickly to change; sudden changes or surprises may increase confusion or cause anxiety.
5. **Avoid challenging demented patients directly,** either by questioning their reasoning for a particular behavior or by trying to convince them of another course of action. Demented patients are unable to appropriately respond to questions because of deficits in reasoning and memory. Confrontation may increase their frustration and confusion.
6. **Redirect or distract** the patient from inappropriate or troublesome behavior (e.g., by calling the patient's name and shifting to a different focus or activity).
7. **Maintain calm when faced with the demented patient's agitation or confusion.** Displays of emotion on the part of caregivers are likely to escalate the patient's agitation.

Source.   Adapted from Boccellari A, Zeifert P: Management of neurobehavioral impairment in HIV-1 infection. *Psychiatric Clinics of North America* 17:183–203, 1994.

Appendix L.   The Questions Patients Ask: A Pretest of Countertransference

Medical patients often ask questions that verge on the existential. Few people—especially those blessed with good health—reflect on these uncomfortable issues before being personally confronted with them. Consider the following questions, not in order to prepare canned answers, but to explore your own "gut responses." Remember, countertransference is never "wrong" or shameful, but creates problems when acted out by the unaware therapist.

The following is an adaptation of an exercise that was originally developed by Winiarski (1991) for therapists working with HIV-infected patients. We have found it to be useful preparation for working with other types of medical patients as well.

1. Why me?

◆ What is your gut response? Be alert to statements that carry value judgments, especially in illnesses like AIDS or lung cancer, where behavior played a role in contracting the illness.

◆ Responses to the "why me?" which imply blame (e.g., "Because you smoked"; "Because you were promiscuous and had anal intercourse"; "Because you shot up drugs") will affect how safe the patient feels within the therapy. These statements are variations of "Because you did not follow the rules." The converse is, "Those who followed the rules did not become infected." Where do you stand on rules and social norms? Are you a rule follower, and uncomfortable with those who are not? Do you become angry with those who flout convention? Do you protect yourself with the fantasy that illness "happens" only to those who invite or "deserve" it?

◆ Explore your own attitudes regarding drug use, especially if you work with HIV-infected patients. Is drug use a symptom of a personality disorder? Is a person responsible for having a personality disorder? Is it environment?

2. Will I die in pain?

◆ This is the one of several questions concerning fears of dying. If you do not know the answer, how willing are you to learn about the medical facts? about pain control?

◆ Have you thought of what you personally fear about dying? about death?

◆ What are your attitudes regarding pain control for medical patients? for medically ill substance abusers? Are you the kind of person who will not take an aspirin and frown at others for "overmedicating?"

◆ People experience pain differently, but can you remain nonjudgmental with the low pain threshold patient? Intravenous drug users, in particular, report low pain thresholds. Yet they are least likely to be treated for pain, because their physicians fear being manipulated. As the psychiatric consultant, how would you negotiate this dilemma?

3. Will I die alone?

4. Will you stay with me until the end?

◆ It's easy to miss the request to the therapist in question 3, which is a subtle version of the more obvious plea in question 4. At one level, the patient may be asking, "Will you abandon me as others have, or as I fear others will?" Or, "Will you be by my bedside, and see me through this journey?"

◆ Think through your responses—practical and emotional—beforehand. Are you willing to visit a deteriorating patient in the hospital? Where do you draw the line relative to the dictates of your schedule? If your August vacation were planned, would you change it if your patient were dying? How would you respond to direct queries such as, "Yes, your schedule is busy, but can't you get to the hospital?" What stops you? What fears of loss and impotence may underlie your inability to "stay until the end" of a terminal illness?

◆ These questions tap how close you can be to your patient, and how much loss you can tolerate. If you find it hard to tolerate loss, do you disparage yourself and, possibly, the patient?

◆ On the other hand, is the "caretaker" in you being manipulated? What lies behind your eagerness to stand by and hold the patient's hand? Is there grandiosity or a rescue fantasy? Beware! Both may render a therapist ineffectual.

◆ Are you overinvolved? Is your overinvolvement a reaction to negative feelings about the patient? What might these be? Would your answer differ depending on the patient's gender or illness? Is it the function of the therapist to be at the bedside?

5. Can you stand to look at me?

◆ What is your honest response? How necessary is it for you to have a patient who appears attractive or normal? What feelings and fears are elicited in you when you imagine being with someone disfigured?

◆ For example, Kaposi's sarcoma lesions may cause severe swelling of arms, legs, and face. Cancer patients often lose their hair and become cachectic. Neurosurgical patients and those with head and neck malignancies often become disfigured.

◆ These are not easy sights for anyone. Psychotherapy, however, is a potentially intimate encounter, posing a special mandate for the therapist to have explored counterreactions in advance.

6. Wouldn't you kill yourself if you were me?

◆ This is one of the most difficult and provocative of questions. *You should be clear regarding your response before you start therapy with a patient.*

◆ Your beliefs in the quality and quantity of life—your despair and optimism—are tapped by this question. Do you believe in the individual's right to commit "rational" suicide? Or do you feel that no suicidal ideation is rational, that it reflects a severe psychiatric disturbance, no matter how thoughtful the client appears?

◆ Would you be willing to collude in the suicide of a terminally ill patient, if you were certain you would not suffer professional or legal repercussions? Or are you convinced that you would intervene to prevent a suicide under any circumstances?

◆ If you would intervene to block a suicide under any circumstances, should you state this at the beginning of therapy? How do you manage the potential reply, "Sure, I'll talk to you about my life, except for my considerations of suicide." How does cutting off the possibility of that discussion limit the effectiveness and relevance of the therapy for the patient?

◆ Winiarski (1991) has written,

. . . while we may have some religious or ethical considerations regarding suicide, we may be confused about whether to apply these in therapy. One therapist, working with a Catholic patient considering suicide, may attempt to dissuade him or her by raising the issue of mortal sin. Another practitioner may feel more comfortable steering clear of religious issues. (p. 123)

◆ Finally, would you kill yourself in this situation? Do you reveal that to the client?

7. Since I can't be cured, wouldn't it be better to give up?

◆ Do you believe a person's life—even a disfigured or terminally ill person's life—is worth fighting for? Is each life equal to the next?

◆ If you believe in rational suicide, would you elect not to intervene with a passive suicide (e.g., noncompliance with medical regimens, signing out of a hospital against medical advice, or refusing emergency treatment)? Deferring intervention may involve avoiding certain questions because you would rather not hear the answers.

8. Is there a God?

9. Why would God put me through this?

◆ Winiarski (1991) has written,

In therapist and [patient] alike, the asking and responding to this question raises profound questions of life's meaning and possibilities of connections with larger realities. This is the same question that arises during any tragedy. In the face of tragedy, can we believe in a benevolent deity? What role does the concept of God have in our lives? Is he or she a rescuer, or a fellow sufferer whose divine presence gives us courage? If God is a rescuer and we are not rescued, are we undeserving? (p. 123)

◆ Do you restrict yourself to exploring the psychodynamics of this question? attempt to address it on a religious level? collaborate with a member of the clergy? How self-revealing is it appropriate to be?

10. Am I forgiven?

◆ If there is the need for forgiveness, what is the transgression?

◆ Who is that eventually forgives? Are you in a position to offer forgiveness? Are you angry at the patient for being sick? Does the patient sense this? Do you need to be forgiven for some of your feelings regarding the patient?

11. What will happen to my family?

Countertransference reactions to this question can be particularly difficult with HIV-infected patients. Winiarski (1991) has stated,

> This question can raise feelings of punitiveness in the therapist, due to a sense that the client may be responsible for his or her own plight and, especially, the plight of family members, including children. Therapists who have lost parents or friends due to per-

ceived "carelessness" may have difficulty empathizing with a person who has been careless about his or her health and therefore has "caused" others' suffering. (p. 124)

12. Why should I tell anyone?

◆ Think through your stance on this issue, especially with HIV patients or patients whose cancer has metastasized. Do you believe that no secrets should be kept? Can there be exceptions? Why confide in a family member who has always been rejecting or untrustworthy?

◆ Be alert to potential incongruity between the patient's goals for comfort and your goals for communication and reunion.

◆ With HIV-infected individuals, what is your reaction to the person who insists on maintaining the secret, although others may be injured? What of the man who continues to have unsafe sex or share needles, thus spreading HIV? What about the HIV-positive woman who chooses to bring the fetus to term, with the possibility that the child may be HIV-positive? What do you do about warning the partner?

Source.   Adapted from Winiarski M: *AIDS-Related Psychotherapy.* Elmsford, NY, Pergamon, 1991, pp. 121–124.

Appendix M. Effects of Psychotropics During Pregnancy

Source. Adapted from Briggs GG, Freeman RK, Yaffe SJ: *Drugs in Pregnancy and Lactation*, 4th Edition. Baltimore, MD, Williams & Wilkins, 1994.

(*Note.* This table is meant to be a quick-reference guide, not a substitute for clinical judgment.)

Category A: Controlled studies have failed to demonstrate a risk to the fetus in the first trimester; there is no evidence of risk in later trimesters; the possibility of fetal harm appears remote.

Category B: Either animal-reproduction studies have not demonstrated a fetal risk but there are no controlled studies in pregnant women, or animal-reproduction studies have shown an adverse effect (other than a decrease in fertility) that was not confirmed in controlled studies in women in the first trimester (and there is no evidence of risk in later trimesters).

Category C: Either studies in animals have revealed adverse effects on the fetus (teratogenic or embryocidal or other) and there are no controlled studies in women, or studies in women and in animals are not available. The drug should be given only if the potential benefit justifies the potential risk to the fetus.

Category D: There is positive evidence of human fetal risk, but the benefits of use in pregnant women may be acceptable despite the risk (e.g., if the drug is needed in a life-threatening situation or for a serious disease for which safer drugs cannot be used or are ineffective).

Category X: Studies in animals or humans have demonstrated fetal abnormalities, or there is evidence of fetal risk based on human experience, or both of these conditions apply, and the risk of drug use in pregnant women clearly outweighs any possible benefit. The drug is contraindicated in women who are or who may become pregnant.

m: Manufacturer's rating (1995 Physicians' Desk Reference).
m*: Manufacturer's rating (1994 Physicians' Desk Reference).

Medication	Risk rating	Effects on fetus	Effects on neonate and on breast feeding
Alprazolam (Xanax)	Dm	Although no congenital anomalies have been attributed to the use of alprazolam in human pregnancies, other benzodiazepines (e.g., diazepam) have been suspected of producing fetal malformations after first-trimester exposure.	The neonate may be at risk for withdrawal symptoms, neonatal flaccidity, and respiratory problems during the postnatal period. Infant lethargy and weight loss have been reported in infants whose nursing mothers received chronic benzodiazepines. According to manufacturer, nursing should not be undertaken by mothers who must use alprazolam.
Amantadine (Symmetrel)	Cm*	In a 1985–1992 surveillance study, 51 newborns had been exposed during the first trimester. A total of 5 (9.8%) major birth defects were observed (2 expected). Although this is high, the number of exposures is too small to draw any conclusions.	Excreted into breast milk in low concentrations. The manufacturer recommends that it be used with caution in nursing mothers because of the potential for urinary retention, vomiting, and skin rash.

(continued)

Appendix M. Effects of Psychotropics During Pregnancy (*continued*)

Medication	Risk rating	Effects on fetus	Effects on neonate and on breast feeding
Amitriptyline (Elavil)	D	Although occasional reports have associated the therapeutic use of amitriptyline with congenital malformations, the bulk of the evidence indicates that tricyclic antidepressants are relatively safe during pregnancy.	Neonatal withdrawal has been described after in utero exposure to other tricyclics, but not with amitriptyline. The potential for this side effect exists, however, because of the similarities among these compounds. Neonatal urinary retention has been associated with nortriptyline, an amitriptyline metabolite. Amitriptyline is excreted into the breast milk; the American Academy of Pediatrics classifies it as a drug whose effects on the nursing infant are unknown but of potential concern.
Amobarbital	D**	Crosses the placenta, achieving levels in cord serum equivalent to mother's serum. Increased incidence of congenital defects reported in 95 of 273 patients receiving amobarbital in first trimester. Defects associated with barbiturates: anencephaly, congenital heart disease, severe limb deformities, cleft lip and palate, intersex, papilloma of the forehead, hydrocele, congenital dislocation of the hip, soft tissue deformity, of the neck, hypospadias, accessory auricle, polydactyly, and nevus. Of 298 patients with first-trimester exposure to amobarbital, only 25 showed a possible association between use of the drug and abnormalities (7 cardiovascular malformations; 2 polydactyly, 3 genitourinary malformations other than hypospadias, 9 inguinal hernia, 4 clubfoot).	Prolonged half-life in the newborn (2.5 times maternal) when mother is dosed near term. No data available on use in breast feeding.

**Presents different risks to the fetus depending on when and for how long it is used.

Drug	Category		
Amoxapine (Asendin)	Cm	No reports linking the use of amoxapine with congenital defects have been found, but the number of exposures is too small to draw a conclusion. Animal studies showed embryotoxicity and fetotoxicity but no teratogenic effects.	Excreted into the breast milk; the American Academy of Pediatrics classifies amoxapine as a drug whose effects on the nursing infant are unknown but of potential concern.
Amphetamines (e.g., Dexedrine)	Cm	The literature is complicated and varied in its results; be sure to review Briggs et al. (1994) directly before prescribing. Briefly summarized, its seems that using amphetamines for medical indications does not pose a significant risk to the fetus for congenital anomalies; amphetamines do not appear to be human teratogens. Illicit maternal use of these drugs, however, presents significant risks to the fetus and newborn. These poor outcomes are probably multifactorial in origin, involving multiple drug use, lifestyles, and poor maternal health.	When used for medical indications, mild withdrawal symptoms may be observed in the newborns, but long-term sequelae have not so far been demonstrated; more studies are needed. Excreted into the breast milk; the American Academy of Pediatrics classifies amphetamines as contraindicated during breast feeding.
Atenolol (Tenormin)	Cm	In utero exposure apparently has no effect on infant growth or behavior. It has been safely used for the treatment of hypertension in pregnant women.	Infants exposed near delivery should be closely monitored for signs of beta-blockade during the first 24–48 hours. The long-term effects of in utero exposure are not known. The American Academy of Pediatrics considers drug to be compatible with breast feeding, but infants should be monitored for signs of beta-blockade.
Benztropine (Cogentin)	C	A possible association exists between first-trimester exposure and cardiovascular defects.	Two newborns exposed to chlorpromazine and benztropine at term developed paralytic ileus. The small-left-colon syndrome was characterized by decreased intestinal motility, abdominal distention, vomiting, and failure to pass meconium. No data available on use in breast feeding.

(continued)

Appendix M. Effects of Psychotropics During Pregnancy (*continued*)

Medication	Risk rating	Effects on fetus	Effects on neonate and on breast feeding
Bupropion (Wellbutrin)	Bm	In a 1985–1992 surveillance study, 3 newborns had been exposed during the first trimester. No major birth defects were observed (0 expected). Although this is encouraging, the number of exposures is too small to draw any conclusions.	The one reported case of breast feeding showed no adverse effects in the infant. The American Academy of Pediatrics considers antidepressants a drug class whose effects on the nursing infant are unknown but of potential concern.
Buspirone (BuSpar)	Bm	Not listed in Briggs et al. (1994). According to manufacturer, no adverse effects were demonstrated in animal studies, but human studies do not exist.	Because the extent of excretion in human milk is unknown, the manufacturer recommends that buspirone be avoided in nursing women.
Carbamazepine (Tegretol)	Cm	The literature is complicated and varied in its results; be sure to review Briggs et al. (1994) directly before prescribing. Probably a human teratogen; carbamazepine has been associated with cardiovascular defects, spina bifida, and other malformations.	Drug is excreted into the breast milk; the American Academy of Pediatrics classifies carbamazepine as compatible with breast feeding.
Chloral hydrate	Not rated	No reports linking chloral hydrate with congenital defects.	Administered during labor, with cord blood concentrations similar to maternal levels. The sedative effects on the newborn have not been studied. Drug is excreted into the breast milk; the American Academy of Pediatrics classifies chloral hydrate as compatible with breast feeding.
Chlordiazepoxide (Librium)	D	Data are variable; older studies concluded that it was associated with higher than expected rates of congenital defects; the 1985–1992 surveillance study of 788 newborns with first trimester exposure showed no greater than expected incidence of congenital anomalies. A 1992 study suggested that co-ingestion of alcohol and abuse of other substances may confound results of benzodiazepine studies.	Neonatal withdrawal may consist of severe tremulousness and irritability. Unresponsiveness, hypotonicity, and poor feeding were observed in neonates whose mothers received chlordiazepoxide within a few hours of delivery. No data available on use in breast feeding.

Drug	Category		
Chlorpromazine (Thorazine)	C	Has been used since the mid-1950s for control of nausea and vomiting during pregnancy. Unpredictable hypotension is the main adverse side effect. Although one survey found an increased incidence of defects and a report of ectromelia exists, most studies have found chlorpromazine to be safe for both mother and fetus if used occasionally in low doses. Near-term use should be avoided due to danger of maternal hypotension and adverse effects in the newborn.	When used in large doses by the mother near term, has been associated with hypotonicity, lethargy, depressed reflexes, and jaundice in the neonate. Extrapyramidal syndrome, which may persist for months, has been observed in some infants whose mothers received chlorpromazine near term. Paralytic ileus has also been described, although most reports have concluded that the medication does not adversely affect the fetus or newborn. Excreted into the breast milk in small doses; the American Academy of Pediatrics classifies chlorpromazine as a drug whose effects on the nursing infant are unknown but of potential concern because of the reports of drowsiness and lethargy.
Clomipramine (Anafranil)	Cm	Does not appear to be teratogenic in animals or humans, but the number of known exposed human fetuses is too small to determine actual risk.	Significant newborn toxicity may occur, apparently due to drug withdrawal. No long-term effects of in utero exposure and newborn withdrawal have been observed, but follow-up has not been beyond 6 months of age. Although the American Academic of Pediatrics classifies other antidepressants as agents to be used with caution because of unknown effects on the infant's central nervous system, it considers clomipramine to be compatible with breast feeding. However, Briggs et al. (1994) advise caution because of the potential for toxicity in the infant.
Clonazepam (Klonopin)	C	No reports linking clonazepam with congenital defects have been located, but there is the risk of neonatal toxicity (e.g., apnea, lethargy, hypotonia).	Excreted into breast milk, and may be associated with central nervous system depression or apnea. Because of prolonged half-life, it is recommended that infants exposed in utero or during breast feeding have serum levels determined and be closely monitored for CNS depression or apnea.

(continued)

Appendix M. Effects of Psychotropics During Pregnancy (*continued*)

Medication	Risk rating	Effects on fetus	Effects on neonate and on breast feeding
Clozapine (Clozaril)	Not listed	—	—
Desipramine (Norpramin)	C	No reports linking desipramine's use with congenital defects have been located. In a 1985–1992 surveillance study, 31 newborns had been exposed to first trimester desipramine. One major birth defect was observed (one expected); no anomalies were observed in other defect categories. The number of exposures was too small for conclusions.	Neonatal withdrawal symptoms have been observed, including cyanosis, tachycardia, diaphoresis, and weight loss after desipramine was taken throughout pregnancy. Drug is excreted into the breast milk; the American Academy of Pediatrics classifies desipramine as a drug whose effect on the nursing infant is unknown but of potential concern.
Dextroamphetamine	Cm	See Amphetamines.	See Amphetamines.
Diazepam (Valium)	D	Freely crosses the placenta and accumulates in the fetal circulation with newborn levels 1 to 3 times greater than maternal serum levels. Although a 1989 study concluded that exposure to benzodiazepines produced a teratogenic syndrome, subsequent research has not corroborated these findings. (See Chapter 8 text for further discussion.)	Plasma half-life in newborns is significantly increased due to decreased clearance of the drug. When doses during labor exceed 30–40 mg or drug is taken for extended periods by the mother, diazepam has been associated with floppy infant syndrome and a withdrawal syndrome. Not recommended for use in lactating women. Drug is excreted into the breast milk; the American Academy of Pediatrics classifies diazepam as a drug whose effect on the nursing infant is unknown but of potential concern.

Drug		Pregnancy	Lactation
Diphenhydramine (Benadryl)	C	Evidence linking this medication to a variety of malformations has been variable, with some studies showing possible association, while others do not. The data are poor, marked by exposure to other concurrent drugs that may be contaminating the findings. Conclusions are not possible at present. Potential interaction between diphenhydramine and temazepam has been described which resulted in violent intrauterine fetal movements, then subsequent birth of a stillborn infant. There may be an association between exposure to antihistamines in the last 2 weeks of pregnancy and retrolental fibroplasia in premature infants.	Withdrawal (generalized tremulousness and diarrhea) was reported in a newborn whose mother had taken 150 mg/day during pregnancy. Considered contraindicated in nursing mothers by manufacturer, secondary to increased sensitivity of newborn or premature infants to antihistamines.
Doxepin (Sinequan)	C	No reports linking the use of doxepin with congenital defects have been located. The 1985–1992 surveillance study reported that of 118 newborns exposed to this medication, a higher than expected incidence of major birth defects was found, especially polydactyly. However, other factors, including concurrent drug use and chance, may be involved.	Paralytic ileus was reported in an infant exposed to doxepin at term, which may have been synergistic with anticholinergic effects of chlorpromazine. Drug is excreted into the breast milk; the American Academy of Pediatrics classifies doxepin as a drug whose effects on the nursing infant are unknown but of potential concern. Serious and potentially fatal effects were observed in one infant (near respiratory arrest), leading to the recommendation that doxepin be taken with caution, if at all, during breast feeding.
Fluoxetine (Prozac)	Bm	Extant studies do not support an association between fluoxetine and congenital defects. The higher than expected number of spontaneous abortions on fluoxetine also occurred on tricyclics; it is unclear whether this is an effect of the drug or the psychiatric condition.	One case report has shown no adverse drug-related effects in a nursing infant, except perhaps increased irritability. As with other antidepressants, the American Academy of Pediatrics classifies fluoxetine as a drug whose effects on the nursing infant are unknown but of potential concern.

(continued)

Appendix M.   Effects of Psychotropics During Pregnancy (*continued*)

Medication	Risk rating	Effects on fetus	Effects on neonate and on breast feeding
Fluphenazine (Prolixin)	C	See also Chlorpromazine. Although phenothiazines are relatively safe during pregnancy, an infant with multiple anomalies was born to a mother treated with fluphenazine and Debendox during the first trimester. In the 1985–1992 surveillance study, 13 newborns had been exposed to it in the first trimester; 1 major birth defect was observed (cardiovascular); 0 expected. The number of exposures is too small for comment.	Extrapyramidal symptoms reported in newborns exposed in utero. No data available on use in breast feeding.
Flurazepam (Dalmane)	Xm	A member of the benzodiazepine class, which has been found to cause congenital defects. (See Diazepam.) Although not specifically linked to major birth defects, the manufacturer considers flurazepam to be contraindicated during pregnancy.	It should be expected that, like diazepam, this agent and its active, long-acting metabolites pass into breast milk and may adversely affect the infant. Like other benzodiazepines, the American Academy of Pediatrics classifies it as a drug whose effect on the nursing infant is unknown but of potential concern.
Haloperidol (Haldol)	Cm	Two cases of limb-reduction malformations has been described after first-trimester use. In one case, high doses (15 mg/day) were used. In 98 of 100 patients treated with haloperidol for hyperemesis gravidarum in the first trimester, no adverse side effects were reported. Has been used for control of chorea gravidarum and manic-depressive illness during second and third trimester without adverse effects on the newborn. In the 1985–1992 surveillance study, of 56 newborns exposed to haloperidol during the first trimester, 3 major birth defects were observed (2 expected), 2 of which were cardiovascular (0.6 expected).	Drug is excreted into the breast milk; the American Academy of Pediatrics classifies haloperidol as a drug whose effects on the nursing infant are unknown but of potential concern. Haloperidol has been safely used during labor.

Drug		
Hydroxyzine (Atarax/Vistaril)	C	The manufacturer considers hydroxyzine to be contraindicated in early pregnancy because of the lack of clinical data; some studies have suggested an association with congenital defects, while others have not.	Safe and effective for the relief of anxiety during labor. No data available on use in breast feeding.
Imipramine (Tofranil)	D	Although early studies suggested an association between first-trimester exposure and limb-reduction defects, they have not been corroborated by subsequent work. The 1985–1992 surveillance study showed that of 75 newborns exposed during the first trimester, there was a suggestion of an association with cardiovascular defects, but other factors, including the mother's disease, concurrent drug use, and chance, were cited as possibly involved.	Neonatal withdrawal symptoms have been reported (e.g., colic, cyanosis, rapid breathing, irritability). Drug is excreted into the breast milk; the American Academy of Pediatrics classifies imipramine as a drug whose effects on the nursing infant are unknown but of potential concern.
Lithium	D	Lithium has been related to increased incidence of congenital defects, particularly of the cardiovascular system (including, but not limited to, Ebstein's anomaly). It is the magnitude of the risk that is controversial. Larger sample sizes are needed to define the actual magnitude of the risk. (See discussion in Chapter 8 text of Ms. Sawyer.) Fetal red blood cell choline levels are elevated during maternal therapy with lithium; the clinical significance of this effect is unknown.	Serum half-life in newborns is prolonged: 68–96 hours (adult: 10–20 hours). Infants exposed to lithium in utero may be born with signs of lithium toxicity. Breast-milk levels average 40% of maternal serum concentration. Although no toxic effects in the nursing infant have been reported, the long-term effects have not been studied. The American Academy of Pediatrics considers lithium to be contraindicated during breast feeding because of the potential for lithium-induced toxicity in the nursing infant.

(continued)

Appendix M. Effects of Psychotropics During Pregnancy (*continued*)

Medication	Risk rating	Effects on fetus	Effects on neonate and on breast feeding
Lorazepam (Ativan)	Dm	No reports linking the use of lorazepam with congenital defects have been located. Other benzodiazepines, however, have been variously implicated in causing fetal malformations. (See Diazepam.) Crosses the placenta, achieving cord levels similar to maternal serum concentrations.	High intravenous doses in the mother may produce the "floppy infant" syndrome. Has been used in labor to potentiate the effects of narcotic analgesics; although not statistically significant, a higher incidence of respiratory depression occurred in these newborn infants. Drug is excreted into breast milk in low concentrations. No effects on the nursing infant have been reported, but the slight delay in establishing feeding in one study was cause for concern. The American Academy of Pediatrics classifies lorazepam as a drug whose effects on the nursing infant are unknown but of potential concern.
Loxapine (Loxitane)	C	No data available.	No data available on use in breast feeding.
Maprotiline (Ludiomil)	Bm	No reports linking the use of maprotiline with congenital defects have been located. The 1985–1992 surveillance study of 13 newborns exposed to first-trimester maprotiline showed a possible association with oral cleft, but the number of exposures is too small to draw any conclusions.	Drug is excreted into breast milk in low concentrations. No information was reported on breast feeding from the American Academy of Pediatrics.
Methylphenidate (Ritalin)	C	No reports linking the use of methylphenidate with congenital defects have been located, although the number of cited cases is small.	No data available on use in breast feeding.
Molindone (Moban)	C	Only one reported use in pregnancy was in a woman who had ingested at total of 9800 mg during her 9-month pregnancy and gave birth to normal twin boys. No physical or mental developmental abnormalities were noted in their first 20 years of life.	No data available on use in breast feeding.

Drug			
Nortriptyline (Pamelor)	D	Although there has been some association with limb-reduction abnormalities, data do not support nortriptyline as a major cause of congenital defects.	Urinary retention in the neonate has been associated with maternal use. Nortriptyline is excreted into breast milk in low concentrations. It was not detected in the serum of other breast-fed infants whose mothers took the drug. The American Academy of Pediatrics classifies antidepressants as drugs whose effects on the nursing infant are unknown but of potential concern, especially after prolonged exposure.
Oxazepam (Serax)	D	Oxazepam is an active metabolite of diazepam. (See also Diazepam.) Although not consistently corroborated, a 1989 study concluded that exposure to either diazepam ($\geq$ 30 mg/day) or oxazepam ($\geq$ 75 mg/day) produced a teratogenic syndrome in 8 infants. The mothers did not use alcohol or street drugs and had regular prenatal care. Major problems included craniofacial defects, mental retardation, and gross disability, to name a few. (See Chapter 8.)	No specific data relating to oxazepam usage in lactating women are available.
Perphenazine (Trilafon)	C	The phenothiazines readily cross the placenta. Although occasional reports have linked various phenothiazines with congenital malformations, the bulk of the evidence indicates that these drugs are safe.	Has been used as an antiemetic during normal labor without observable effects on the newborn. The American Academy of Pediatrics considers the effects of perphenazine on the nursing infant to be unknown but of potential concern.
Phenelzine (Nardil)	C	In 21 mother-child pairs exposed to monoamine oxidase inhibitors (MAOIs) in the first trimester, 3 of which were exposed to phenelzine, an increased risk of malformations was found (details of these 3 cases not available).	No data available on use in breast feeding.

(continued)

Appendix M.   Effects of Psychotropics During Pregnancy *(continued)*

Medication	Risk rating	Effects on fetus	Effects on neonate and on breast feeding
Propranolol (Inderal)	Cm	Has been used safely during pregnancy for maternal and fetal indications. It is apparently not a teratogen, but does produce fetal and neonatal toxicity, mainly due to the effects of beta-blockade. Daily doses of >160 mg produce the most serious complications. Other effects have included respiratory depression in the neonate, and fetal bradycardia. Intrauterine growth retardation has also been attributed to propranolol. Oxytocic effects have been demonstrated following intravenous, extraamniotic injections and high oral dosing.	Although beta-blockers are considered relatively safe during pregnancy, newborns of women taking the drug near delivery should be closely observed during the first 24–48 hours after birth for bradycardia, hypoglycemia, and other symptoms of beta-blockade. The American Academy of Pediatrics considers propranolol to be compatible with breast feeding, although nursing infants should be closely observed for symptoms of beta-blockade. Long-term effects of exposure to beta-blockers from breast milk have not been studied.
Sertraline (Zoloft)	Bm	No available reports exist describing the use of sertraline in human pregnancy.	No data available on use in breast feeding.
Temazepam (Restoril)	Xm	The manufacturer considers temazepam to be contraindicated during pregnancy. A potential drug interaction with diphenhydramine is toxic to the fetus (see Diphenhydramine).	The American Academy of Pediatrics considers the effects of temazepam on the nursing infant to be unknown but of potential concern.
Thioridazine (Mellaril)	C	No anomalies found in the offspring of 23 patients exposed throughout gestation. (Twenty of the infants were evaluated for up to 13 years.) One case of a congenital defect has been described. Although occasional reports have linked various phenothiazines with congenital malformations, the bulk of the evidence indicates that these drugs are safe. (See Chlorpromazine.)	No data available on use in breast feeding.

Thiothixene (Navane)	C	Few data are available. In a 1985–1992 surveillance study, 38 newborns had been exposed to first-trimester thiothixene. Anomalies were no greater than expected by chance.	No data available on use in breast feeding.
Tranylcypromine (Parnate)	C	In 21 mother-child pairs exposed to MAOIs in the first trimester, 13 of which were exposed to tranylcypromine, an increased risk of malformations was found. Details of these 13 cases are not available.	No data available on use in breast feeding.
Trazodone (Desyrel)	Cm	There are anecdotal case reports of using this medication during pregnancy, but no conclusions can be drawn. In the 1985–1992 surveillance study, 100 newborns had been exposed to first trimester trazodone. No greater than chance numbers of defects were observed.	Trazodone is excreted into human milk. The American Academy of Pediatrics considers the effects of trazodone on the nursing infant to be unknown but of potential concern.
Triazolam (Halcyon)	Xm	The manufacturer considers this medication contraindicated during pregnancy, even though there are no data that consistently support an association with congenital defects.	No data available on use in breast feeding.
Trifluoperazine (Stelazine)	C	Has been safely used for the treatment of nausea and vomiting of pregnancy. In 1962, the Canadian Food and Drug Directorate warned that 8 cases of congenital defects were associated with trifluoperazine. drug. This correlation was later refuted in a series of articles from the medical staff of the manufacturer. In 480 pregnant women, the incidence of congenital malformations was no higher than in control subjects. Two cases of phocomelia and a case of congenital heart defect were described, but there was no clear relationship between drug and defect.	Extrapyramidal symptoms have been described in a newborn exposed to this medication in utero, but the reaction was probably due to chlorpromazine. (See Chlorpromazine.) No data available on use in breast feeding.

(continued)

Appendix M. Effects of Psychotropics During Pregnancy (*continued*)

Medication	Risk rating	Effects on fetus	Effects on neonate and on breast feeding
Trifluoperazine (Stelazine) (*continued*)	C	Another study of 42 patients with first-trimester exposure showed no evidence of malformations and no effects on perinatal mortality rate, birth weight, or IQ scores at 4 years of age. Although occasional reports have linked various phenothiazines with congenital malformations, the bulk of the evidence indicates that these drugs are safe. (See Chlorpromazine.)	
Trihexyphenidyl (Artane)	C	A possible association has been found between trihexyphenidyl and minor malformations.	No data available on use in breast feeding.
Valproic acid (Depakene)	D	Valproic acid and the salt form, sodium valproate, should be considered human teratogens. The absolute risk of producing a child with neural tube defects when these agents are used between the 17th and 30th days after fertilization is 1%–2%. A characteristic pattern of minor facial defects is also associated with valproic acid. Other major and minor abnormalities may be related to valproic acid therapy, but given that an epileptic woman has a 2–3 times greater risk for delivering a child with defects compared with the general population, these associations are difficult to establish. A distinct constellation of defects has been suggested for infants exposed in utero; these involve the head, face, digits, urogenital tract, and mental and physical growth. Other problems, such as intrauterine growth retardation, hyperbilirubinemia, hepatotoxicity, and fetal/newborn distress, need additional investigation.	The American Academy of Pediatrics considers valproic acid to be compatible with breast feeding.

Appendix N. Guidelines for Using Psychotropics During Pregnancy (adapted with permission from [2–4])

Depression

1. Medical differential diagnosis.
2. Withhold medication in trimester 1 if possible.
3. Inability to care for self or to provide prenatal care indicates need for somatic therapy.
4. Despite early reports linking tricyclics with limb reduction abnormalities, many experts feel that this literature is extremely weak and anecdotal at best. Secondary-amine tricyclics preferred over tertiary-amine tricyclics because of their more favorable side-effect profile.
5. Of the "newer" antidepressants, fluoxetine seemed safe in one small study.
6. ECT for delusional depression.
7. Antidepressants are secreted in breast milk.

Anxiety Disorders

1. Medical differential diagnosis.
2. Withhold medication in trimester 1 if possible.
3. Use cognitive/behavioral and supportive psychotherapy in lieu of medications for as long as possible.
4. Attempt to taper benzodiazepine therapy prior to conception.
   a. Former recommendation: For panic disorder, consider changing to tricyclics if cannot discontinue medications entirely.
   b. Current recommendation: If unable to taper short-acting benzodiazepines, consider changing to clonazepam.
5. If patient is on anxiolytics when pregnancy is confirmed, attempt to taper.
6. Avoid additional drug introduction, particularly in trimester 1.
7. Benzodiazepines are secreted in breast milk.

Psychosis

1. Maintenance low dose antipsychotic therapy for chronically psychotic patients may offset risk of relapse and need for higher doses.
2. Medical differential diagnosis and workup for new-onset psychotic states. (e.g., rule out thyroid disease, systemic lupus erythematosus.)
3. Phenothiazines originally thought to be relatively low in teratogenicity,[1] but with some later evidence of teratogenicity.
4. High-potency neuroleptics are preferred.[2]
5. Consider clonazepam as an adjuvant.
6. Medication is present in breast milk.

Mania

1. Medical differential diagnosis and workup for new-onset manic symptoms.
2. Careful contraceptive history.
3. Evaluate need for prophylaxis.
4. **Trimester 1:**
   a. Try to avoid lithium carbonate.
   b. If exposure to lithium before week 12: fetal cardiac ultrasound at weeks 18–20.
   c. If clear need for antimanic prophylaxis: discontinue lithium only at documentation of pregnancy
5. For brittle bipolar patients requiring antimanic prophylaxis:
   a. Use high-potency neuroleptics until trimester 2, when lithium can be reinstituted; for very vulnerable patients, continue lithium even during trimester 1. Perform cardiac ultrasound at weeks 18–20 for those patients exposed to lithium before week 12.[2]
   b. Given its lack of proven efficacy as monotherapy for bipolar disorder, former recommendations to use carbamazepine have been modified, except in those patients demonstrating a specific requirement for this agent.[2]
   c. **Valproic acid controversy:**
   Pro: Consider valproic acid for bipolar patients willing to have ultrasound, alpha fetoprotein, and possible therapeutic abortion for neural tube defects at week 20.[5]
   Con: 1% incidence of spina bifida; "valproic acid is not a thoughtful intervention for the majority of bipolar patients, perhaps with the exception of those who have not responded whatsoever to any other antimanic treatment."[2]
   d. **Carbamazepine:** Newly described association with spina bifida
6. **Trimesters 2 and 3:**
   a. After week 12 and with need for treatment, consider lithium carbonate re(introduction), administered in small divided doses.[3,4]
   b. Alternatively, consider valproic acid[5] (see **controversy** above).
   c. **Former recommendations:** Discontinue lithium before delivery date.
   Current recommendations: Decrease dose by 30%–50% prior to delivery.[2]
   Postpartum lithium prophylaxis for high-risk women reduces psychiatric morbidity.

7. Lithium secreted into breast milk. It is considered contraindicated during breast feeding by the American Academy of Pediatrics.

References

1. Briggs G, Freeman R, Yaffe S: Drugs in Pregnancy and Lactation, 4th Edition. Baltimore, MD, Williams & Wilkins, 1994

2. Cohen L: Personal communication, March 12, 1992

3. Cohen L, Heller V, Rosenbaum J: Treatment guidelines for psychotropic drug use in pregnancy. Psychosomatics 30:25–33, 1989

4. Cohen L, Rosenbaum J, Heller V: Psychotropic drug use in pregnancy, in The Practitioner's Guide to Psychoactive Drugs, 3rd Edition. Edited by Gelenberg A, Bassuk E, Schoonover S. New York, Plenum Medical Book, 1991, pp 389–405

5. Markovitz P, Calabrese J: On the use of anticonvulsants for manic depression during pregnancy (letter). Psychosomatics 31:463–4, 1990

Appendix O. Notes on the "New" Antidepressants in the Medical Setting

| | SSRIs | | | Bupropion (Wellbutrin) | Venlafaxine (Effexor) | Nefazodone (Serzone) |
	Fluoxetine (Prozac)	Paroxetine (Paxil)	Sertraline (Zoloft)			
Mechanism	Selectively inhibit neuronal re-uptake of serotonin			Mechanism of action not well understood; presumed to act by inhibiting dopamine reuptake and with weak effects on norepinephrine reuptake Does not act at 5-HT$_2$, histaminic, cholinergic, and alpha-adrenergic receptors.	Like TCAs, exhibits both serotonergic and noradrenergic presynaptic reuptake blockade No significant postsynaptic effects on histaminic, cholinergic, and alpha-adrenergic receptors	Inhibits postsynaptic sero-tonin reuptake Weak effects on presynaptic norepinephrine reuptake
Half-life	Norflu-oxetine: 8–12 days	Approx. 24 hours	Approx. 24 hours	Approximately 14 hours (range 8–24 hours)	Parent compound: 4.1 ± 1.3 hours Desmethyl-venlafaxine 10.4 ± 1.7 hours	Approximately 2–4 hours
Common side effects	Nausea, headache, anorexia, anxiety, insomnia			Nausea, anxiety, insomnia, tremor, agitation, dry mouth, headache, constipation	Nervousness, nausea, sweating, anorexia, dry mouth, dizziness, headache	Asthenia, dizziness, light-headedness
Cardiac effects	Cardiotoxicity: no adverse effects on conduction in healthy patients, but not extensively studied in the setting of severe cardiac disease Prozac: rare bradycardia			Cardiotoxicity: no adverse effects on conduction found in patients with conduction disease Can elevate blood pressure; monitor patients with hypertension	Cardiotoxicity: no adverse effects on conduction in healthy patients, but not extensively studied in the setting of severe cardiac disease Can elevate blood pressure; monitor patients with hypertension	Cardiotoxicity: no adverse effects on conduction in healthy patients, but not extensively studied in the setting of severe cardiac disease May cause sinus bradycardia

(continued)

Appendix O.   Notes on the "New" Antidepressants in the Medical Setting *(continued)*

	SSRIs			Bupropion (Wellbutrin)	Venlafaxine (Effexor)	Nefazodone (Serzone)
	Fluoxetine (Prozac)	Paroxetine (Paxil)	Sertraline (Zoloft)			
Anticholinergic effects	Anticholinergicity: none	Paxil: weak, but at times signif- icant anticholinergic properties		Anticholinergicity: none	Anticholinergicity: none	Mild anticholineric and anti- histaminic effects
Hepatic effects	Inhibits cytochrome CyP450-2D6 (which metabolizes most other psychotropics, beta-blockers, antiarrhythmics, vinblastine), causingserum elevations of these medications Paxil: the most potent CyP450-2D6 inhibitor of all the SSRIs Also: oxidative interference of certain benzodiazepine metab- olism, e.g., diazepam, alprazo- lam (no effect on clonazepam) Reduce starting doses in cirrhotic patients			In cirrhotic patients, half-life of metabolites were pro- longed; metabolites accu- mulate to 2–3 times those of healthy indivduals Start these patients at re- duced dosages Drugs that induce or inhibit hepatic enzymes may alter its metabolism	In cirrhotic patients, half- life of parent compound increased by one-third, and principal metabolite by 60%. Start these patients at re- duced dosages (50%). May interact with other drugs that inhibit cyto- chrome CyP450-2D6.	Inhibits cytochrome CyP450- 3A isoenzyme, thereby increasing serum levels of alprazolam and triazolam. No information yet available on use in cirrhotic patients.

Renal effects	Patients with renal disease should initiate treatment at reduced dosages	Patients with renal disease should initiate treatment at reduced dosages	In renal disease, half-life is also increased (and clearance creased). Reduce total daily dose by 25% in patients with mild to moderate renal impairment. Reduce total daily dose by 50% in hemodialysis patients; also, withhold daily dose until dialysis treatment is completed.	No information yet available on use in renal disease.
Miscellaneous effects	Prozac: increases bleeding times by diminishing granular storage of serotonin in platelets ⇒ petechiae, ecchymoses	Obligate 3-times-daily dosage regimen is cumbersome	Incidence of sexual dysfunction comparable to that of placebo in men and women	
	Paxil, Zoloft: increase prothrombin times when coadministered with warfarin (Coumadin)	Fewer sexual side effects than the SSRIs, tricyclics, venlafaxine, and MAOIs	CONTRAINDICATED with the following medications (used for seasonal allergic rhinitis): ◆ astemizole (Hismanal) ◆ terfenadine (Seldane)	
	Hyponatremia has been reported with the SSRIs, possibly due to SIADH; at risk are older patients and those who are taking diuretics or who are otherwise volume depleted			

(continued)

Appendix O. Notes on the "New" Antidepressants in the Medical Setting (*continued*)

	SSRIs Fluoxetine (Prozac) Paroxetine (Paxil) Sertraline (Zoloft)	Bupropion (Wellbutrin)	Venlafaxine (Effexor)	Nefazodone (Serzone)
Neurological effects	Extrapyramidal effects (including akathisia, dyskinesias, dystonias, parkinsonism): ◆ likely due to inhibition of dopamine production, and/or ◆ release by dopaminergic neurons caused by increases in synaptic serotonin	Propensity for seizures may be enhanced by bupropion, so use with care in the setting of: ◆ prior seizure activity ◆ head trauma ◆ epileptiform EEG activity ◆ bulimia, anorexia ◆ benzodiazepine or alcohol withdrawal ◆ other neurological illnesses that lower seizure threshold In Parkinson's disease, co-administration with L-dopa may lead to synergistic dopaminergic action		

Notes. MAOI = monoamine oxidase inhibitor; SIADH = syndrome of inappropriate antidiuretic hormone; SSRI = selective serotonin reuptake inhibitor.
Sources. Stoudemire A: Expanding psychopharmacologic treatment options for the depressed medical patient. *Psychosomatics* 36:S19–S26, 1995.
Information for Prescribers: Bristol-Myers Squibb Company (Serzone; 12/94), Burroughs Wellcome Co. (Bupropion hydrochloride; PDR 1995), Dista Products Company (Fluoxetine; PDR 1995), Roerig Division—Pfizer (Sertraline; 1/94), SmithKline Beecham Pharmaceuticals (Paroxetine; 7/94), Wyeth-Ayerst Laboratories (Venlafaxine; 8/94).

Appendix P.   Practical Suggestions for Bedside Manner in the General Hospital Setting

1. **Sit down.**
   - ◆ Ideally, pull up a chair up to the bedside and conduct the interview sitting down.
   - ◆ Sitting reduces the status difference between physician and patient; it also conveys to the patient that the consultant has some time to spend and is not going to quickly dash off.
   - ◆ Physicians who sit with patients are usually perceived by the patient to have been present for much longer than those who remain standing.

2. **Do something tangible for the patient.**
   - ◆ Helpful gestures further rapport, such as offering a drink of water or adjusting a pillow. For someone who is ill, supportive, concrete attempts to help convey compassion and are much appreciated.

3. **Shake hands.**
   - ◆ Don't forget the comforting power of touch. A warm handshake at the opening and close of the consultation conveys friendliness and humane caring.
   - ◆ Severely ill patients, particularly the elderly or those with cancer or AIDS, frequently receive far less physical touch than ever before in their lives and probably less than other patients. This situation intensifies the feeling of alienation and isolation. When appropriate, a light touch on the patient's arm or shoulder can be enormously comforting and humanizes an often frightening medical environment.

4. **Smile at the patient.**
   - ◆ "Even if you are not usually a warm person, act as if you were!" Unless clinically inappropriate, a smile can reduce interpersonal distance, convey a benevolent intention, and may reduce the sense of threat that a patient may feel when seeing a psychiatrist.

5. **Begin by telling the patient what you know about his or her situation.**
   - ◆ Rather than ask the patient to tell the story from the beginning, start by summarizing in simple language the key elements in the patient's history. It might even be possible to offer a preliminary formulation. Ask the patient to correct any misinformation or misperceptions.
   - ◆ This spares the patient the ritual of once again repeating information, and provides a platform for the patient to correct misperceptions, amplify on certain matters, and provide new information.
   - ◆ It also indicates that the consultant has been thinking about their problems prior to the meeting, and lets them assess the consultant's level of understanding and concern.
   - ◆ Don't take for granted that a preliminary formulation, however rudimentary, may offer the patient a first-ever insight into the situation.

6. **Find out the patient's most pressing immediate concerns.**
   - ◆ If the patient is preoccupied by an undisclosed fear or concern, their full attention and cooperation will not be with the consultant.
   - ◆ Eliciting and dealing with the patient's major concern clears the air so that other necessary information can be used more effectively.

7. **Ask what the patient thinks about the illness.**
   - ◆ Ask in detail about the patient's understanding regarding the nature, cause, and prognosis of the illness or injury. Find out the patient's specific concerns about pain, disability, disfigurement, or death.
   - ◆ This strategy enables the consultant to tap the patient's perspective and expectations. It also creates opportunities to correct misimpressions and provide information that may ease the patient's cooperation with treatment.
   - ◆ For example,
     - • "Even though your doctors are still trying to find out exactly what your problem is, and neither we nor you know for sure, what have you thought yourself about what is making you sick?"

8. **Ask about the patient's life and family.**
   - ◆ Find out the details about the patient's family, major social roles such as occupation, and the impact of the current illness on those relationships and roles.
   - ◆ These questions might be phrased as follows:
     - • "Who are the important people in your family and the rest of your life, and how are they coping with your being in the hospital?"

- "What are your major concerns about the impact that your illness is having outside the hospital?"

9. **Ask about the patient as "a person."**
   - ◆ What are the specific personal characteristics, activities, and attainments that the patient has achieved in life in which he or she takes pride? Find appropriate (not forced) opportunities to acknowledge these achievements.
   - ◆ The patient role can be demoralizing. Many seriously ill patients feel themselves to be useless to their families, jobs, and communities. Many also feel that their caregivers are ignorant about their personal lives and do not appreciate their worth or the contributions that they have made.
   - ◆ Allowing the patient to speak about their gratifying past bolsters self-esteem, and allows the patient to feel appreciated as a whole person, rather than a sick body.

10. **Acknowledge the patient's plight.**
    - ◆ It can be enormously comforting to hear from an authority figure that if the consultant were faced with similar circumstances, he or she might well have similar psychological reactions. The patient should be told that it is very human—and expected—to lose emotional control when bearing severe pain, confronting death, experiencing major physiological upheavals, suffering cognitive deficits, or contending with physical and social disabilities.
    - ◆ The consultant's acknowledgment helps validate the patient's feelings, and encourages an atmosphere of support and rapport.

11. **Involve the patient as an ally and coinvestigator in the mental status examination.**
    - ◆ Fully explain the need for and purposes of a mental status examination in an informative way.
    - ◆ Too often there is an abrupt shift in the interview from history-gathering to the embarrassed statement, "I just need to ask you a few questions that we ask everybody." Many patients interpret the mental status exam as a search for serious mental problems, or as an indication that the consultant thinks they may be crazy.
    - ◆ Instead, try to cull as much as you can from naturalistic observations made during the course of the interview.
    - ◆ If specific aspects of formal testing are required, try to enlist the patient as an investigative participant, with a clear explanation as to how the patient stands to benefit by cooperating. This frees the patient from feeling like a passive "specimen," and removes the consultant from the role of inquisitor. For example,
      - "Please give me a hand in figuring out whether your condition is causing any subtle thinking problems. If there are some problems, we'll do our best to figure out what's causing them and do something about them. I would appreciate your helping me with some tests to see how well you can concentrate, remember, and think about things. As we go along in your treatment, we can follow these tests, just as we do with blood tests."

12. **Leave the patient with something concrete.**
    - ◆ Give the patient feedback. Convey a revised formulation, or confirmation that the original one was correct.
    - ◆ Indicate what you intend to do with the information: e.g., share it with the primary physician, recommend certain diagnostic or treatment interventions, return for further interviews, suggest medications, etc.
    - ◆ Once again ask the patient for feedback. This allows the consultant to assess what the patient has heard and retained, and also accesses the patient's opinion about the plan.
    - ◆ Although in some cases it is not appropriate to share every detail (e.g., for the patient who requires involuntary hospitalization and is an elopement risk,) the patient should know something about what to expect.
    - ◆ If you intend to return, try to be specific about when the patient should expect you. When possible, calling the patient to find out when a follow-up visit can be conveniently scheduled for both parties is another humanizing act.

Source. Adapted from Yager J: Specific components of bedside manner in the general hospital psychiatric consultation: 12 concrete suggestions. *Psychosomatics* 30:209–212, 1989.

⚑ INDEX ⚑

⚑ A

Acetazolamide, 56
Acid-base imbalance, 409–411
Acquired QT syndrome, 43, 54, 79
Acute intermittent porphyria, 283–284
Acyclovir, 177
Addisonism, 205
Adjustment disorders, HIV infection, 261
Advance directives, 407
African Americans, HIV risk, 257–259
Agitation. *See* Psychomotor agitation.
AIDS anxiety, 226, 261
AIDS dementia complex (ADC), 216–226
    versus Alzheimer dementia, 222
    assessment, 222–223
    and asymptomatic seropositive persons, 222
    clinical course, 221
    definitional criteria, 216, 415
    differential diagnosis, 221–222
    epidemiology, 220
    features, 220–221
    laboratory studies, significance of, 225
Neuropathology, 225
    nonpharmacological management, 224–225, 417
    in older patients, 222
    pharmacological treatment, 223–224
    proposed pathophysiological mechanisms, 225–226
AIDS phobia, 226
AIDS-related complex, 220
AIDS. *See* HIV infection.
Akathisia
    management in pregnancy, 332
    and nonpsychiatric drugs, 82
Albumin binding, in renal failure, 150
Alcohol withdrawal, 124–126

    differential diagnosis, 403
Alcohol withdrawal delirium. *See* Delirium tremens.
Alcohol withdrawal seizures, 126
Alcoholic hallucinosis, 124–125
    differential diagnosis, 403
Alcoholism, 117–139
    and liver disease, 117–139
    and liver transplantation, 134
Alpha interferon, 177
Alprazolam
    in cardiac disease, 17
    and chemotherapy-related nausea, 80
    and delirium, 76
    in hepatic failure, 134
    in HIV infection, 230
    in irritable bowel syndrome, 290
    and isoenzyme-3A4, 19
    in kidney transplantation, 179
    in pregnancy, 314, 421
    respiratory effects, 104
    in renal failure, 172, 412
    teratogenicity, 314
Alternate-day steroids, 205–206
Aluminum intoxication, and dialysis, 149
Amantadine
    in AIDS patients, 263
    teratogenicity, 332
Amiloride, 56
Amitriptyline
    in HIV infection, 229
    in irritable bowel syndrome, 290
    and isoenzyme-2D6, 19
    in pregnancy, 422
    in renal failure, 412
    suppositories, 85

Ammonia levels, hepatic encephalopathy, 129, 133

Amnestic disorder. *See also* Korsakoff's syndrome.
  DSM-IV coding for, 392–393

Amoxapine, cardiovascular effects, 44

Amphotericin B, 177, 264

Anabolic steroids, 207–208

Androgen deficiency syndrome. *See* Female androgen
  deficiency syndrome.

Anger
  and breast cancer outcome, 379
  and heart disease, 11–12, 14
  hypertension association, 56–57

Angina pectoris, and depression, 8

Antianxiety drugs. *See* Anxiolytics.

Antiarrhythmics
  as delirium precipitators, 76
  and isoenzyme metabolism, 19
  psychiatric side effects, 45–46
  and tricyclic antidepressants, 39

Antibiotics, and delirium, 76

Antibody testing, HIV, 251–253

Anticholinergic drugs
  prenatal exposure, 332
  and sundowning, 81

Anticipatory nausea, 84

Antidepressants. *See also* Tricyclic antidepressants.
  in cancer patients, 84–85
  and kidney transplantation, 179
  and pulmonary disease, 105–106
  and renal failure, 171
  and steroid-induced psychosis, 206

Antiemetics, 82

Antifungals. *See* Fluconazole; Itraconazole;
  Ketoconazole; Metronidazole.

Antihistamines. *See* Diphenhydramine; Hydroxyzine.

Antihypertensive drugs
  antidepressant drug interactions, 58
  as delirium precipitators, 76
  depression association, 57

Antiparkinsonian medication
  in AIDS patients, 263
  and renal failure, 151

Antipsychotic drugs. *See* Neuroleptics.

Antituberculosis drugs, 229

Anxiety
  and asthma, 97
  in dialysis patients, 167–168
  in irritable bowel syndrome, 288–289

Anxiety disorder due to a general medical condition,
  DSM-IV coding for, 394–395

Anxiety disorders

and chronic obstructive pulmonary disease, 102
and heart disease, 9–11
and HIV infection, 261–262

Anxiolytics. *See also* Benzodiazepines.
  irritable bowel syndrome, 290
  kidney transplantation, 179
  and respiration, 103–105
  teratogenicity, 312–314

Astemizole, 19, 439

Asterixis, 128

Asthma, 93–115
  and anxiety disorders, 102
  and bronchodilators, 102
  and depression, 102–103
  and ECT, 106–107
  and family factors, 98–99
  medication psychotoxicity, 101–102
  neuropsychiatric effects of hypoxia, 99–100
  and physician assessment factor, 101
  psychodynamics, 107
  psychological precipitants, 97–99, 107
  psychopharmacology, 103–106
  psychotherapy, 107–108
  and sexuality, 99
  sleep disruption, 103
  and somatization, 102

Asymptomatic HIV seropositivity
  cognitive changes, 222
  psychosocial distress, 227

Atenolol, 55, 332

Atrial fibrillation
  fluoxetine risk, 20
  tricyclic antidepressant risk, 42, 44

Auditory Verbal Learning Test, 223

Autoimmune thyroiditis, 310

Azathioprine, 178

AZT. *See* Zidovudine.

◆ B

Barbiturates
  in renal failure, 172, 412
  teratogenicity, 314

Bedside manner, 383, 441–442

Bedside tests
  AIDS dementia complex, 223
  delirium, 77–78

Behavioral techniques, and dialysis, 169–170

Benzodiazepines
  in cardiac disease, 17
  in chemotherapy patients, 84
  in chronic pulmonary disease, 103–104

in delirium, 80
in delirium tremens, 127
in hepatic failure, metabolism, 134–135
in HIV infection, 261
in irritable bowel syndrome, 290
and isoenzyme-3A4, 19
in kidney transplantation, 179
in pregnancy, 312–314
in renal failure, 150, 171–172, 412–413
and respiratory depression, 103
in steroid-induced mood disturbance, 207
teratogenicity, 313–314
withdrawal, 264
Benztropine
prenatal use, 332
in HIV infection, 263
in kidney transplantation, 179
in renal failure, 151, 414
Bepridil hydrochloride, 46
Beta-blockers
cardiac disease contraindication, 17
depression association, 57
and fluoxetine, 20
and isoenzyme-2D6, 19
HIV infection contraindication, 261
lithium interactions, 55
lung disease contraindication, 104
in pregnancy, 332
in renal failure, 414
Bipolar disorder, HIV risk, 231
Bisexuals, HIV risk, 258–259
Blood urea nitrogen, 148
Borderline personality disorder, 232
Bound drugs, and renal failure, 150
Brain metastases, 82–83
Breast cancer, 370–389
adjuvant chemotherapy, 377
coping styles of patients, 374–375, 379
mastectomy versus limited resection, 375–376
medical decision making, 373–374
posttreatment adjustment, 377
prognosis, 381
psychological effects, 378–381
psychotherapy guidelines, 381–383
and sexuality, 377–378
Breast feeding
and HIV transmission, 260
and lithium, 336
and medication effects, 316–318
and neuroleptics, 332
Breast reconstruction, 376–377

Breast-conserving surgery, 375–376
Breathlessness, 100–101. *See also* Dyspnea.
Briquet's syndrome, 361
Bromocriptine, and pregnancy, 332
Bronchodilators, psychotoxicity, 102
Bundle branch block, 42–43
Bupropion, 437–440
cardiac effects, 20–21
in dialysis patients, 171
in HIV infection, 230
in kidney transplantation, 179
in Parkinson's disease, 440
in pregnancy, 315, 424
in renal failure, 171, 412
and seizures, 230, 440
Burnout. *See also* Countertransference.
in HIV caregivers, 234
Buspirone
in cardiac disease, 17
in HIV infection, 261
in kidney transplantation, 179
in pulmonary disease, 104
in renal failure, 172, 412
in sleep apnea, 104

C

Cadaver organ recipients, 176
Calcium channel blockers, 56
Cancer. *See also* Breast cancer; Lung cancer.
and benzodiazepines
for chemotherapy, 84
for anticipatory nausea, 84
breast, 370–389
and delirium, 84
disease progression
and psychological factors, 378–381
and psychosocial treatment, 379–381
doxorubicin-tricyclic cardiotoxicity, 84
intracranial metastases, 82
Karnofsky Scale, 84
and lithium, 85
lung, 73, 82–85
meningeal carcinomatosis, 83
neuropsychiatric effects of antiemetics, 82
neuropsychiatric presentations, 82–83
pancreatic, 283
paraneoplastic syndromes, 83–84
parenteral and rectal antidepressants, 84–85
psychotherapy, 73–74, 381–382
Capacity. *See* Competency.
Capgras' syndrome, 330

Captopril, 55, 56
Carbamazepine
    cardiovascular toxicity, 56
    in HIV-related mania, 262
    and isoenzyme-3A4, 19
    in kidney transplantation, 179
    in pregnancy, 334–335, 424
    in renal failure, 154, 414
    in steroid-induced mania, 207
    teratogenesis, 334–335
Cardiac conduction disturbances, and tricyclics,
        39–40, 42–43
Cardiac disease. See Cardiovascular disorders.
Cardiac surgery, and delirium, 58–59
Cardiovascular disorders, 1–63
    and anxiety disorders, 9–11
    and depression, 4–9, 35–50
    failure-to-treat consequences, 8
    hostility relationship, 11–12
    pharmacotherapy, 16–23, 39–46, 54–59
    psychotherapy dilemma, 13
    stress effects, 11–14
Cardiovascular malformations, and lithium,
        333–334
Caregivers, of HIV patients, 233–234, 259, 417
Catastrophic reaction, 132
Catatonic disorder due to a general medical
        condition
    DSM-IV coding for, 394
    and HIV infection, 263
    and paraneoplastic syndromes, 83
    and steroid withdrawal, 205
Cephalosporins, 177
Characterological panic-fear, 97–98
Chemical restraint, 331
Chemotherapy-induced emesis, 82, 84
Chemotherapy
    and benzodiazepines, 84
    and breast cancer, 377
    sexual side effects, 377–378
Chest pain, 9–10
Childhood sexual abuse survivors
    and chronic pelvic pain, 359
    and HIV infection, 254–255
    and irritable bowel syndrome, 288
Children, and HIV infection, 259–261
Chloral hydrate
    in delirium, 81, 402
    in pregnancy, 424
    in renal failure, 172, 412
Chloramphenicol, 76

Chlordiazepoxide
    in alcohol withdrawal, 126
    in hepatic encephalopathy, 124
    in hepatic failure, 134
    in pregnancy, 424
    in renal failure, 172, 413
    respiratory-depressant effects, 103
Chlorpromazine
    cardiovascular effects, 54
    cirrhosis contraindication, 135
    in delirium, 81
    in hepatic failure, 134, 135
    in pregnancy, 425
    in pulmonary disease, 105
    in renal failure, 413
    teratogenicity, 331
Cholestyramine resin, 46
Chronic obstructive pulmonary disease.
        See Asthma; Pulmonary disease.
Chronic pelvic pain, 358–360
Cimetidine, 19, 76, 178–179
Ciprofloxacin, 76, 177
Cirrhosis. See Liver disease.
Climacteric, 351
Clock-drawing task, 77
Clomipramine, 19, 316, 425
Clonazepam
    adjuvant use, in pregnancy, 332
    in cardiac disease, 17
    in delirium, 80
    in HIV infection, 262
    in kidney transplantation, 179
    in pregnancy, 425
    in renal failure, 172, 413
    in steroid-induced mania, 206–207
    teratogenicity, 314
Clonidine, 55, 57
Clorazepate, 134, 172, 413
Clozapine
    cardiovascular effects, 54
    pregnancy use, 332
    respiratory side effects, 105
Cobalamin deficiency, 284–285
Cognitive changes
    in asymptomatic HIV patients, 222
    and hypoxemia, asthma, 99–100
    and steroids, 203–204
Competency
    guidelines, 405–408
    in HIV patients, 227–229
    mini-outline of requirements, 404

Compliance with medical care
    Health Belief Model, 170
    Health Locus of Control, 253
    in kidney transplantation, 176–177
    in renal failure, 169–170
    and safer sex strategies, 252–253
Condoms, 252, 254
Conduction disease
    and bupropion, 20–21
    and carbamazepine, 56
    and ECT, 23
    and heart block, 42–43
    and neuroleptics, 54–55
    and tricyclic antidepressants, 39–40
Confabulation, and Korsakoff's syndrome, 130, 131
Congenital malformations. See Teratogenicity.
Congestive heart failure
    lithium effects, 55
    and tricyclic antidepressants, 43
Consciousness states, and delirium, 75
Constructional ability, 77
Continuous abdominal peritoneal dialysis, 166
Cook-Medley Hostility Inventory, 12
Coping styles, in breast cancer patients, 374–375, 379
Coronary artery disease
    and depression, 8–9
    and anxiety disorders, 9–11
    hostility relationship, 11–12
    pharmacotherapy, 16–23
    stress relationship, 11–14
Coronary artery bypass graft (CABG) surgery. See
    Cardiac surgery.
Coronary bypass, and delirium, 58–59
Coronary-prone behavior, 11–12, 14–16
Corticosteroids. See Steroids.
Countertransference
    and breast cancer patients, 383
    and cancer patients, 74, 381–384
    and cardiac patients, 15–16
    and dialysis patients, 168–169
General guidelines, 418–420
    and HIV patients, 234–235, 253, 256
    and physician objectivity, 101
    pretest for clinicians, 418–420
    and respiratory disease patients, 101
    and sexuality, 354
Creatinine clearance
    lithium effects, 151–152
    in renal failure, 148–149
Crohn's disease, 287–288
Cyclic AMP, in postpartum elation, 311

Cyclosporine
    and fluoxetine, 19, 20, 179
    and lithium, 180
    neuropsychiatric complications, 178
Cytochromes
    and antifungals, 229
    in hepatic failure, 134
    and SSRIs, in cardiac disease, 17–19
    and tricyclic antidepressants, 41–42
Cytomegalovirus encephalitis, 221

D

Dantrolene, in pregnancy, 332
Decision making
    in breast cancer patients, 373–374
    in renal failure patients, 168–169
Delirium of hepatic insufficiency, 124
Delirium, 74–81, 400–403
    in AIDS patients, 263–264
    and acute intermittent porphyria, 283–284
    and anticholinergic effects, 76, 81, 206, 262
    bedside assessment of, 77–78
    and cancer, 84
    and cardiac surgery, 58–59
    in cirrhosis, 132
    versus dementia, 75–76
    diagnostic pitfalls, 75–76
    in dialysis patients, 149
    drug induced, 76
    DSM-IV coding for, 392–393
    environmental management, 78
    etiology, 76
    haloperidol treatment, 78–80, 400–401
    and hepatic encephalopathy, 130
    and kidney transplantation, 177–179
    and Korsakoff's syndrome, 131–132
    management strategies, 78–81, 400–402, 417
    and paraneoplastic syndromes, 83
    presenting features, 74–75
    and postpartum psychosis, 328
    in renal failure, 148–149
    risk factors and outcome, 74–75
    steroid induced, 202–204
    and sundowning, 81
    and vitamin B_{12} deficiency, 284
    and Wernicke's encephalopathy, 130
Delirium tremens
    differential diagnosis, 124, 403
    DSM-IV criteria, 127
    presenting symptoms, 126–127
    treatment, 127

Dementia
    AIDS dementia complex (ADC), 216–226
    versus delirium, 75–76
    and meningeal carcinomatosis, 83
Denial
    and AIDS, 255
    and asthma, 97–98
    and coping
        with dialysis, 164
        with medical illness, 73–74, 381–382
    as HIV risk factor, 233
    and silent ischemia, 12
Depression
    antihypertensive induced, 57–58
    and breast cancer, 374–381
    in cardiovascular disease, 1–9, 35–50
    in chronic obstructive pulmonary disease,
        102–103
    and coronary disease outcome, 8
    diagnostic criteria for, in medically ill, 8–9
    in dialysis patients, 167–168
    and dyspnea perceptions, in asthma, 100–101
    failure-to-treat consequences, 8
    in hepatic encephalopathy, 125, 128
    and hysterectomy, 360–364
    in HIV infection, 226–231
    in irritable bowel syndrome, 288–289
    in menopause, 350–357
    and oral contraceptives, 307
    in pancreatic cancer, 283
    and paraneoplastic syndromes, 83
    in pregnancy, 307–318, 435
    and pulmonary function, 100–101
    in renal disease, 166–168, 171–172
    steroid induced, 203–205, 207
    and vitamin B_{12} deficiency, 284–285
Desipramine
    cardiotoxicity, cytochromes, 41–42
    in HIV infection, 229
    in irritable bowel syndrome, 290
    and isoenzyme-2D6, 19
    in kidney transplantation, 179
    in pregnancy, 315, 316, 426
    in renal failure, 171, 412
Dexamethasone. See Steroids.
Dextroamphetamine
    in cardiac disease, 21–22
    in HIV infection, 230
    suppositories, 85
Dextromethorphan, 19
DHPG. See Ganciclovir.

Dialysis, 144–156
    coping, 164–167
    dementia syndrome, 149
    depression and anxiety, 167–168
    disequilibrium syndrome, 149
    hemodialysis versus peritoneal dialysis, 166
    and lithium, 153–154
    psychodynamic factors, 170
    psychopharmacology, 171–172
    psychosocial survival factors, 166–167
    psychotherapy, 168–170
    psychotropic drug removal, 150
    rational treatment withdrawal, 168
    quality-of-life differences, 166
Diazepam
    in delirium, 80, 81
    in delirium tremens, 127
    in hepatic failure, 134, 135
    in irritable bowel syndrome, 290
    in pregnancy, 426
    in renal failure, 172, 413
    respiratory-depressant effects, 103
    teratogenicity, 313
Didanosine, and mania, 262
Digoxin, 45–46, 55, 76
Diltiazem, 19, 46, 55, 56
Diphenhydramine
    anxiolytic use, in pulmonary patients, 104
    delirium contraindication, 81
    hazards in pregnancy, 314, 332
    HIV infection contraindication, 262
    in pregnancy, 314, 332, 427
    in renal failure, 151, 414
Disability insurance, 164–165
Diuretics
    depression association, 57
    and lithium, 154
    tricyclic antidepressant interactions, 58
Do-not-resuscitate orders, 407–408
Dothiepin, neonatal toxicity, 316
Doxepin
    and breast feeding, 317
    bronchodilator effects, 105
    cardiovascular effects, 40
    in HIV infection, 229
    in kidney transplantation, 179
    in pregnancy, 427
    in renal failure, 171, 412
    suppositories, for cancer patients, 85
Doxorubicin, 84
Droperidol, delirium treatment, 80

Drug absorption, in renal failure, 150
Drug clearance, in renal failure, 150–151
DSM-IV
    coding, with medical conditions, 392–397
    and mental illness, 8–9
    "organic versus functional," 9
Durable power of attorney, 407
Dysgraphia, and delirium, 78
Dysmenorrhea, 358
Dyspareunia, 354, 358
Dyspnea
    and depression, 100–101
    and lung cancer, 82
    psychotherapy, 107
    subjective perceptions, 100–101

E

Ebstein's malformation, 333–334
Educational techniques, for dialysis patients, 170
Electrocardiogram (ECG), and tricyclic
    antidepressants, 40–41
Electroconvulsive therapy (ECT)
    in cardiac disease, 22–23
    in chronic pulmonary disease, 106–107
    in HIV infection, 231
    in kidney transplantation, 179
    pacemaker effects, 23
    in pregnancy, 315–316, 331
    in renal failure, 171
    in steroid-induced depression, 206
    theophylline interactions, 106
Electroencephalogram
    and hepatic encephalopathy, 133
    and renal failure, 148
Electrolyte imbalance, 409–411
Employment, dialysis patients, 164
Encainide, 19
End-stage renal disease. See Renal failure.
Erythromycin, 19, 177
Erythropoietin, in dialysis patients, 166
Estradiol, 355
Estrogen deficiency, 353–355
Estrogen replacement therapy, 355
Estrogen
    and chemotherapy, 378
    deficiency symptoms, 353–355, 378
    menopausal levels, 351
    for postmenopausal depression, 353
    and postpartum depression, 310
Ethical issues, 227–228, 404–408

Ethnic minorities, HIV risk, 258–259
Ethylmorphine, 19
Etomidate, 81
Extrapyramidal side effects (EPS)
    in AIDS patients, 263
    management in pregnancy, 332

F

Families
    of asthma patients, 98–99
    and cardiac care, 15
    of HIV patients, 233, 259, 417
    of renal failure patients, 165
Felodipine, 19
Female androgen deficiency syndrome, 378
Fertility, and HIV seropositivity, 260–261
Fetal valproic syndrome, 335
Filicide, 328
Finger-tapping test, 223
FK506, neuropsychiatric complications, 178
Flecainide, 19
Fluconazole, nortriptyline interactions, 229
Flumazenil
    delirium management, 81
    in hepatic encephalopathy, 129
Fluoxetine, 437–440
    and bleeding time, 439
    and breast feeding, 317
    cardiac side effects, 18, 20
    and cyclosporine, 20, 179
    and drug interactions, 20
    and EPS, 440
    in hemodialysis patients, 171
    and hepatic metabolism, 135
    in HIV infection, 230–231
    and isoenzyme-2D6, 19
    in kidney transplantation, 179
    neonatal toxicity, 316
    in pregnancy, 315, 427
    pulmonary damage, 106
    in renal failure, 171, 412
    in steroid-induced depression, 206
    And zidovudine, 231
Flurazepam, 134, 172, 413, 428
Fluvoxamine, 106
Follicle-stimulating hormone, 351
Free drug levels, and renal failure, 150
Free estriol, and postpartum depression, 310
Fregoli syndrome, 330
Functional disorders, 9

Furosemide
    depression association, 57
    and lithium, 154

G

Gamma-aminobutyric acid (GABA), 129
Ganciclovir (DHPG), 177, 264
Gastrointestinal symptoms, 275–297
Gay men, AIDS caregiving, 259
Generalized anxiety. See Anxiety.
Gentamicin, 76, 177
Glomerular filtration rate, of lithium, 151–153
Grooved Pegboard test, 223
Gynecology, 344–369. See also Breast cancer; Chronic
    pelvic pain; Hysterectomy; Menopause.

H

H₂ antagonists, 76
Halazepam, 134, 172
Haloperidol
    in AIDS delirium, 264
    cardiovascular effects, 54, 79–80
    for delirium, 78–80, 400–401
        intravenous use, 79–80
    in hepatic encephalopathy, 129
    and hepatic failure, metabolism, 135
    in HIV infection, 264
    and isoenzyme-2D6, 19
    in kidney transplantation, 179
    lorazepam combination, for delirium, 80
    in pregnancy, 331–332, 428, 435
    in pulmonary disease, 105
    in renal failure, 150, 151, 413
    in steroid-induced psychosis, 206
Health belief model, 170
Health Locus of Control, 253
Heart block, and tricyclics, 42–43
Heart disease. See Cardiovascular disease.
Heart rate, and tricyclics, 39–41
Hemodialysis. See Dialysis.
Hepatic coma, 128
Hepatic encephalopathy, 127–129
    and alcoholism, 117–139
    clinical stages, 128
    diagnostic workup, 133
    differential diagnosis, 124–125, 403
    etiology, 128–129
    motor symptoms, 128
    personality changes, 125, 128
    treatment, 129

Hepatic failure, psychopharmacology, 134–135
Heterosexual HIV transmission, 259–260
Hispanics, HIV risk, 258–259
Histamine blockers, and delirium, 76
HIV infection, 213–273. See also AIDS dementia
        complex (ADC).
    antibody testing, 251–253
    anxiety and adjustment disorders, 261–262
    bisexual behavior, risk, 258–260
    and burnout, 234–235
    and caregiver issues, 233–235
    and catatonia, 263
    classification, 220, 416
    and competency, 227, 404–408
    cultural aspects, 233, 257–258
    and delirium, 263–264
    and depression, 226–231
        differential diagnosis, 228
        treatment, 229–231
    and ethical issues, 228
    and ethnic minorities, 258–259
    and gay men, 259
    and health care workers, 233–235
    heterosexual transmission, 259–260
    and intravenous drug users, 232–233
    and knowledge-behavior gap, 252–253
    and manic symptoms, 262
    maternal HIV transmission, 260
    and monosymptomatic hypochondriacal psychosis,
        263
    and Munchausen syndrome, 232
    and neuroleptics, adverse effects of, 263
    and obsessional disorders, 232, 261
    in other psychopathology, 232
    and perception of risk, 233, 252–253
    and postpartum psychosis, 330
    prodromal symptoms, 226
    in psychiatric patients, 231–233
    psychological adaptation stages, 255–256
    psychoneuroimmunology, 256–257
    and psychopathological risk, 252
    psychopharmacology, 229–231, 261–264
    and psychosis, 262–263
    and psychostimulants, 229–230
    and psychotherapy, 253–257
    safer sex guidelines, 253–254
    and suicide risk, 227–228
    and tricyclic antidepressants, 229
    in women and children, 259–261
HIV seropositivity, 251–253
HIV testing, 251–253

Homicidal ideation
    and anabolic steroids, 207
    in postpartum psychosis, 328
Homosexual men, AIDS caregiving, 259
Hormone replacement therapy, 355
Hospital staff, HIV caregiving, 233–235
Hostility, and heart disease, 11–12, 14
Hot flashes, 355
Hydrochlorothiazide, 154
Hydrophilic psychotropic drugs, 150
Hydroxyzine, 104, 262
Hypertension
    in manic patients, 51–59
    psychological mediators, 56–57
Hyperventilation, 102
Hypnotherapy, kidney transplantation, 177
Hypomania, and postpartum depression, 310
Hyponatremia, and SSRIs, 439
Hypothyroidism, 330
Hypoxia
    and benzodiazepines, 103
    and mental status, 76–77, 99–100
    neuropsychiatry of, 76–77, 99–100
    and *P. carinii* pneumonia, 264
Hysterectomy
    and oophorectomy, 362–363
    psychiatric evaluation before and after, 363
    psychiatric sequelae, 361
    psychological meanings of uterus, 360–361
    risk factors for adverse psychiatric sequelae, 363
    sexuality effects, 362
    symbolic meanings, 362

I
"ICU psychosis," 58, 77
Illness behavior, 288–289
Illness intrusiveness, 165
Imipramine. *See also* Tricyclic antidepressants.
    cardiac effects, 39–40, 43
    in chest pain patients, 10
    in HIV infection, 229
    in irritable bowel syndrome, 290
    and isoenzyme-2D6, 19
    in pregnancy, 429
    in renal failure, 412
Immune function, in HIV infection, 256–257
Immunosuppressants, 178
Implantable cardioverter-defibrillators, 11
Impotence, and renal failure, 165–166
Incontinence, as delirium marker, 75
Indapamide, 56

Indomethacin, 76
Infection, neuropsychiatric complications, 177
Informed consent
    guidelines, 405–408
    in HIV patients, 227–228
    mini-outline of requirements, 404
    in pregnant patients, for medication, 312
Insight-oriented psychotherapy
    cardiac disease dilemma, 13
    in medically ill, 73
Insomnia. *See* Sleep disturbance due to a general
        medical condition.
Interview techniques, with medical patients, 383,
        441–442
Intraaortic balloon pump, 59
Intracranial metastases, 82–83
Intravenous drug use, 232–233
Intravenous haloperidol, 79–80
Involutional melancholia, 351–352
Irritable bowel syndrome
    and childhood sexual abuse, 286, 288
    definition, 285–286
    epidemiology, 286
    and illness behavior, 288–289
    methodological problems, 289
    objective findings, 286–287
    and personality, 289
    and psychiatric comorbidity, 287–290
    psychological treatments, 290–291
    psychopharmacology, 290
    and sexual dysfunction, 286
    stress and emotions in, 287
Isaacs Set Test, 77–78
Ischemia. *See* Myocardial ischemia.
Isoenzymes, and SSRIs, in cardiac patients, 17–19
Isoflurane, 81
Isoniazid, 229, 263, 264
Itraconazole, 19, 261

J
Job strain, and coronary risk, 14

K
Karnofsky Scale, 84
Ketoconazole, 19, 177, 261
Kidney disease. *See* Renal failure.
Kidney donors, 174
Kidney transplantation, 172–180
    cadaver versus family organ recipients, 176
    candidates for, 172–173
    decision making, 168–169

Kidney transplantation (*continued*)
    and differential diagnosis of tremor, 179
    and ECT, 179
    and lithium, 179–180
    medical risks, 173–174
    neuropsychiatric complications, 177–178
    organ donation, 174
    psychopharmacology, 179
    psychosocial predictors, of graft survival, 173
    psychotherapeutic issues, 174–177
    return to work after, 174
    and suicide, 176–177
Korsakoff's syndrome, 131–132
    catastrophic reaction in, 132
    differential diagnosis, 124, 131, 403
    DSM-IV criteria, 131
    neuropsychology, 131–132
Kupperman menopausal index, 353–354

L

Laparoscopy, 359–360
Laryngeal dystonia, 81
"Latent" encephalopathy, 132
Latex condoms, 254
Latinos, HIV risk, 257–259
Left-right tasks, 78
Lidocaine, 19, 45
Life event stress
    and breast cancer outcome, 379
    and sudden cardiac death, 13
Limbic encephalitis, 83–84
Limited breast resection, 375–376
Lipid-lowering agents, 46
Lipophilic drugs, and renal failure, 150
Lisinopril, 56
Lithium Baby Register project, 333
Lithium
    and breast feeding, 336
    in cancer patients, 85
    cardiovascular effects, 55–56
    childhood developmental effects, 336
    controversial renal effects, 151–152
    dialyzability, 153–154
    distal-nephron lesions, 153
    and diuretics, 154
    drug interactions, in cardiac patients, 55–56
    and Ebstein's malformation, 333–334
    and hepatic failure, metabolism, 135
    and HIV infection, 262
    and kidney transplantation, 179–180
    maintenance

    before conception, 332–333, 435
    during pregnancy, 333–334, 435
    after childbirth, 335–336, 435
    in renal failure, 153
    neonatal toxicity, 336
    and pregnancy, 332–336, 429, 435–436
        pharmacokinetics, 334
    and renal failure, 150, 151–154, 414
    in steroid-induced mania, 206–207
    teratogenicity, 333–334, 429
Liver disease, 117–139, 403. *See also* specific syndromes.
    differential diagnosis, 403
Psychopharmacology in, 134–135
Liver transplantation, 134
Living alone, and cardiac events, 14
Living will, 407
Lorazepam
    in chemotherapy patients, 84
    delirium treatment, 400–401
    haloperidol combination, for delirium, 80
    in hepatic encephalopathy, 124, 129
    in hepatic failure, 134
    in HIV infection, 261, 264
    in insomnia, 81, 402
    in irritable bowel syndrome, 290
    in kidney transplantation, 179
    in pregnancy, 314, 430
    in renal failure, 172, 413
    respiratory effects, 103–104
    in steroid-induced anxiety, 207
    teratogenicity, 314
Lumpectomy, 375–376
Lung cancer, 68–74, 82–85. *See also* Cancer.
    and antiemetic side effects, 82
    and intracranial metastases, 82–83
    and Karnofsky Scale, 84
    paraneoplastic syndromes, 83–84
    psychotherapy, 73–74
Lung disease. *See* Asthma; Lung cancer; Pulmonary disease.

M

Macrocytosis, 285
Malignant melanoma, 379
Mania, 51–59
    in cardiac disease, 51–59
    in HIV infection, 262
    and lithium, in kidney disease, 144–156
    in pregnancy, 328–336, 435
    and steroids, 206–207

Maprotiline
    cardiovascular effects, 44
    in pregnancy, 430
    in renal failure, 412
Marie Three Paper Test, 77
Marital conflict, and cardiac events, 14
Mastectomy, 375–376, 378
Masturbation, in dialyzed men, 167
Maternal HIV transmission, 260–261
Memory. *See also* AIDS dementia complex (ADC);
        Korsakoff's syndrome.
    and hypoxia, 99–100
    and steroids, 101, 203–204
Meningeal carcinomatosis, 83
Menopause, 346–358
    cultural factors, 356
    definition, 351
    estrogen deficiency symptoms, 353–355
    hormone replacement therapy, 355
    psychiatric morbidity, 350–353
    psychodynamics, 355–357
Menorrhagia, 358
Menorrhalgia, 358
Mental disorder due to a general medical condition,
        DSM-IV coding for, 392–397
Mental illness. *See* Psychiatric patients.
Meperidine, 264
Methyldopa
    and delirium, 76
    and depression, 57
    and haloperidol, 57
    and lithium toxicity, 55
Methylphenidate
    in cardiac disease, 21–22
    in HIV infection, 230
    in pregnancy, 430
    in renal failure, 179
Methymalonic acid, serum, 285
Metoclopramide, 82
Metoprolol, 19, 76
Metronidazole, 76, 177
Mexiletine, 19
Midazolam
    adverse antifungal interaction, 261
    and chemotherapy-related nausea, 80
    and delirium, 80
    in HIV infection, 261
    and isoenzyme-3A4, 19
Mini-Mental State Exam, 398
    AIDS dementia complex assessment, 222
    delirium assessment, 77

Mitral valve prolapse, 10
Molindone, in AIDS patients, 263
Monoamine oxidase inhibitors
    and antihypertensives, 58
    and asthma, 105
        drug interactions, 106
    cardiovascular effects, 44–45
    in HIV infection, 230
    and isoenzyme-2D6, 19
    in pregnancy, 315
    and psychostimulants, 22
    and renal failure, 171, 412
    in transplant patients, 179
Monoamine oxidase levels
    in depressed women, 353
    and postpartum depression, 311
Monosymptomatic hypochondriacal psychosis,
        263
Mood disorder due to a general medical condition,
        DSM-IV coding for, 394–395
Moricizine, 39
Motor symptoms, of hepatic encephalopathy, 128
Myocardial infarction
    and countertransference, 15–16
    and depression, 8
    and ECT, 22–23
    and hostility/anger, 11–12
    and lithium, 55
    problems in psychotherapy, 13
    psychotherapy and cardiac morbidity, 14–15
    and silent ischemia, 12–13
    social support and cardiac morbidity, 15–16
    and stress, 13–14
    and sudden death, 13–14
    and tricyclic antidepressants, 39–40, 42
    and type A behavior, 11–12
Myocardial ischemia
    antidepressant drug guidelines, 40
    stress effects, 11
Myxedema, 330

N

Narcotic analgesics, and delirium, 76
Naproxen, 76
Needle sharing, 233
Nefazodone, 19, 437–440
Neonatal toxicity
    of anticholinergics, 316
    of benzodiazepines, 317
    of fluoxetine, 316–317
    of lithium, 336

Neonatal toxicity (*continued*)
    of tricyclics, 316–317
    and tricyclic withdrawal, 316
Nephrotic syndrome, and lithium, 153
Neuroleptic malignant syndrome
    in AIDS patients, 263
    management in pregnancy, 332
Neuroleptics
    for anxiolysis, 105, 261
    in AIDS patients, 263
    antidepressant interactions, 55
    cardiovascular effects, 54–55
    and isoenzyme-3A4, 19
    in kidney transplantation, 179
    in pregnancy, 331–332
    in pulmonary disease, 105
    in renal failure, 151, 413
    respiratory effects, 81
    in steroid-induced psychosis, 206
    teratogenicity, 331–332
Nifedipine, 57
Nonsteroidal antiinflammatory agents, 76
Norfloxacin, 76
Norplant, 307
Nortriptyline
    adverse interactions, 229
    and congestive heart failure, 43
    fluconazole interactions, 229
    and heart block, 42
    in HIV infection, 229
    and orthostatic hypotension, 41, 43
    in pregnancy, 315, 316, 317, 431
    in renal failure, 151, 171, 412
    respiratory effects, 105

⚜ **O**

Obsessive-compulsive disorder
    in acute intermittent porphyria, 284
    in HIV infection, 226, 232
    in pregnancy, 311
Obstetrics, 299–342
Occupational stress, and cardiac disease, 14
Ofloxacin, 76
OKT3, neuropsychiatric complications, 178
Ondansetron, 82
Oophorectomy, 362–363
Open-heart surgery, and delirium, 58–59
Ophthalmoplegia, 130
Oral contraceptives, and depression, 307
Organ donation, 174
"Organic" mental disorders, 9

Orthostatic hypotension
    and neuroleptics, 54
    and tricyclic antidepressants, 41
Oxazepam
    in delirium, 80, 402
    in hepatic encephalopathy, 129
    in hepatic failure, 135
    in HIV infection, 261
    in kidney transplantation, 179
    in pregnancy, 313–314, 431
    in renal failure, 172, 413
    respiratory effects, 103
    in steroid-induced anxiety, 207
    teratogenicity, 313–314

⚜ **P**

Pacemaker syndrome, 10–11
Pacemakers, and ECT, 23
Pain, 286
Pancreatic cancer, 283
Panic disorder
    as asthma precipitator, 97–98
    in chronic obstructive pulmonary disease, 102
    and estrogen replacement therapy, 355
    in heart disease, 9–11
    in irritable bowel syndrome, 288
    pacemaker syndrome overlap, 10–11
    in pregnancy, 311
Paralytic agents, in delirium, 80–81
Paraneoplastic syndromes, 83–84
Parenteral antidepressants, for cancer patients, 84–85
Paroxetine, 437–440
    cardiovascular side effects, 20
    and EPS, 440
    and isoenzyme-2D6, 19
    in kidney transplantation, 179
    and prothrombin time, 439
    in renal failure, 171
Pemoline
    in cancer patients, 85
    in cardiac patients, 22
    in HIV patients, 230
Pemphigus, 202
Penicillin, psychiatric side effects of, 76, 177
Pernicious anemia, 284–285
Personal psychiatric consultation, 383
Personality change due to a general medical condition
    DSM-IV coding for, 396
    and hepatic encephalopathy, 128
    and HIV as "great imitator," 262
    and paraneoplastic syndromes, 83

and steroids, 207
and vitamin B$_{12}$ deficiency, 284
Personality disorders, in HIV infection, 231–232
Phase I metabolism, 134
Phase II metabolism, 135
Phenothiazines
cardiovascular effects, 54–55
and renal failure, 150–151
teratogenicity, 331–332
Physical restraints, 330–331
Physician effects, 101
Physostigmine, as bronchospasm precipitator, 106
Pimozide, cardiac effects, 54
"Pink puffers," 103
Polyuria, and lithium, 152–153
Postcardiotomy delirium, 58–59
Postmenopausal depression, 346–358
Postpartum blues, 307–308
Postpartum depression, 308–311
effects on infant, 309
incidence, 308–309
physiological correlates, 310–311
risk factors, 309–310
suicide risk, 309
Postpartum psychosis, 324–342
definitions, 328
differential diagnosis, 330
and ECT, 331
features, 328
and homicidal ideation, 328
prognosis, 329–330
and prophylactic lithium, 335
psychopharmacology, 331–336
Posttraumatic stress disorder, 10
Postural hypotension. See Orthostatic hypotension.
Pravastatin, 46
Prazepam, 134, 172, 413
Pre-renal azotemia, and lithium, 55
Prednisone, 201–207
and kidney transplantation, 178
psychotoxicity, 201–205
withdrawal syndrome, 204–205
Pregnancy
and breast feeding on psychotropics, 316–318, 336
in chronically mentally ill, 330
and depression, 307–311, 314–316, 435
and EPS-management guidelines, 332
and HIV transmission, 260–261
and light therapy, 316
and neonatal psychotropic toxicity, 316
and obsessive-compulsive disorder, 311

and panic disorder, 311, 435
and psychopharmacology, 311–315, 331–336, 421–437
and sleep-deprivation therapy, 316
and suicide risk, 309
and teratogenic factors, 312–315, 331–336, 421–437
and tricyclic antidepressant dosage, 314–315
and violence management, restraints, 330–331
Premenstrual dysphoria, 310
Primary mental disorder, 9
Problem solving, in progressive hypoxemia, 100
Procedural memory, 131
Profile of Mood States, 223
Progesterone, in postpartum depression, 310
Progestin, 307, 355
Prolonged QT interval. See Acquired QT syndrome.
Prolactin, in postpartum depression, 310
Propafenone, 19, 46
Propofol, delirium management, 81
Propranolol. See also Beta-blockers.
as delirium precipitator, 76
depression-inducing effect, 57
and HIV infection, 261
lithium interactions, 55
in pregnancy, 332
psychosis-inducing effect, 57
Protein binding, in renal failure, 150
Proteinuria, and lithium, 153
Psychiatric patients
and HIV infection, 231–233
and pregnancy, 330
"Psychodynamic life narrative," 73
Psychodynamics
in chronic pulmonary disease, 107
in dialysis patients, 170
in kidney transplantation, 174–175
in postmenopausal women, 355–357
Psychomotor agitation
delirium relationship, 75
pharmacotherapy, 80–81
Psychoneuroimmunology, and HIV infection, 256–257
Psychopharmacology
in alcohol withdrawal, 126
in cardiovascular disease, 16–22, 39–46, 54–58
in cancer, 82–85
in delirium, 78–82
in delirium tremens, 127
in hepatic failure, 134–135, 150
in HIV infection, 228–231, 261–263
in irritable bowel syndrome, 290
and isoenzyme inhibition, 19

Psychopharmacology (continued)
    in kidney transplantation, 179–180
    and the neonate, 316–317, 336
    in pregnancy, 311–315, 331–336, 421–434, 435–436
    in pulmonary disease, 103–106
    in renal failure, 149–154, 412–414, 171–172
    in steroid-induced mental disturbance, 206–207
Psychosis
    and HIV infection, 262–263
    and propranolol, 57
    and renal failure, 151
Psychostimulants
    in cardiac disease, 21–22
    dextroamphetamine suppositories, 85
    dosages, 22, 230
    drug interactions, 22
    in HIV infection, 229–230
    indications, 21, 230
    in kidney transplantation, 179
    relative contraindications, 22
    side effects, 21–22, 230
Psychotherapy
    and cardiac disease dilemma, 13
    for cancer patients, 73–74, 381–383
    for chronic pulmonary disease patients, 107–108
    for HIV patients, 253–257
    for irritable bowel syndrome patients, 290–291
    for kidney transplantation patients, 174–177
    for medically ill patients, 73–74
    "psychodynamic life narrative," 73
    for renal failure patients, 168–170
    for type A behavior, 15–16
Psychotic disorder due to a general medical condition
    or substance induced, DSM-IV coding for,
    394–395
Pulmonary disease. See also Asthma; Lung cancer.
    and antidepressants, 105–106
    and anxiety disorders, 102
    and anxiolytics, 105
    and benzodiazepines, 103
    and bronchodilators, 102
    and buspirone, 104
    and drug interactions, 106
    dyspnea and mood, 100–101
    and ECT, 106–107
    and family factors, 98–99
    and major depression, 102–103
    and neuroleptics, 105
    neuropsychiatric effects of hypoxia, 99–100
    psychological precipitants, 97–98
    and psychosocial dysfunction, 98

    psychotherapy, 107–108
    and sexuality, 99
    and somatization, 102
    and steroids, 101–102, 193–211
    and tartrazine dye, 106
    and theophylline, 76, 102, 106
Pyridoxine, 307

Q
QRS complex, 165
QT interval, 41–43, 79. See also Acquired QT
    syndrome.
Quality of life, 165
Quinidine, 19, 45

R
Radical mastectomy, 375–376
Ranitidine, 76
Rapport, establishing with medical patients, 383,
    441–442
Rational suicide, in HIV patients, 228
Rational treatment withdrawal, 168
Reach to Recovery, 375
Recombinant erythropoietin, 166
Reitan-Indiana Aphasia Screening Test, 77
Relaxation techniques
    as asthma-attack precipitator, 108
    for cardiac rehabilitation, 15–16
    for chemotherapy-related nausea, 80
    for irritable bowel syndrome, 290
    for ventilator weaning, 82
Renal clearance, and psychotropic drugs, 150–151
Renal failure, 144–191. See also Dialysis.
    and compliance with medical care, 169–170
    coping, in patients, 164–167
    depression and anxiety in, 167–168
    and disability insurance, 164–165
    and drug dosage adjustment, 149–150
    and lithium use, 153–154
    and medical decision making, pitfalls, 168–169
    neuropsychiatric presentations, 148–149
    and psychopharmacology, 149–151, 171–172,
        412–414
    psychosocial survival factors, 166–167
    and psychotherapy, 168–170
    and restless leg syndrome, 168
    and sleep disturbance, 168
    and suicide, 168
Renal function, and lithium, 151–153
Renal transplantation. See Kidney transplantation.
Repressive coping style, 379

Reserpine
   and delirium, 76
   and depression, 57
Respiratory effects, of neuroleptics, 81
Restraints, and violent pregnant patients, 331
Return to work, dialysis patients, 164
Reverse anorexia nervosa, 208
Rifampin, nortriptyline interaction, 229
Risperidone, in AIDS patients, 263
Rule of two-thirds, 149–150, 171–172
"Rum fits," 126

S

Safer sex, 252–254
Schilling Test, 285
Schizophrenia
   and HIV risk, 232
   and pregnancy, 330
Secondary adrenocortical insufficiency, 205
Seizures, alcohol withdrawal, 126
Selective serotonin reuptake inhibitors (SSRIs),
     437–440. *See also* Fluoxetine; Paroxetine;
     Sertraline.
   in cardiac disease, 17–20
   in HIV infection, 230–231
   and hyponatremia, 439
   isoenzyme effects, 17–20
   in medical setting, 437–440
   and SIADH, 439
   in steroid-induced psychosis, 206
   and warfarin, 18
Semantic distancing strategy, 381
Senile dementia of the Alzheimer type, 220
Sertraline, 437–440
   cardiovascular side effects, 20
   and EPS, 440
   in HIV infection, 231
   and isoenzyme-2D6, 19
   in kidney transplantation, 179
   in pregnancy, 432
   and prothrombin time, 439
   in renal failure, 412
Serum levels, in renal failure, 151
Sexual risk behavior, 252–254
Sexual-abuse survivors, 254–255, 288
Sexual dysfunction due to a general medical condition
   and asthma, 99
   and breast cancer, 377–378
   and chemotherapy, 378
   DSM-IV coding for, 396
   and female androgen deficiency syndrome, 378

   and hysterectomy, 362
   and menopause, 354
   and renal failure, 165–166
SHARE, 375
Sick sinus syndrome, 44
Silent myocardial ischemia, 12–13
Simvastatin, 46
Sinus bradycardia, 20
Sleep apnea, 103–104
Sleep deprivation, and postpartum depression, 316
Sleep disturbance due to a general medical condition
   and delirium, pharmacotherapy, 81, 402
   DSM-IV coding for, 396
   estrogen effects, 355
   and menopause, 355
   and postpartum depression, 310–311
Social network, and cardiac morbidity, 14
Social support, and cardiac morbidity, 14–15
Somatization, asthma, 102
Spina bifida
   and carbamazepine, 334
   and valproic acid, 335
"Steroidphobia," 101, 206
Steroid-induced mental disturbance, 193–211
   alternate-day administration, 205–206
   and cognitive difficulties, 101, 203–204
   and delirium, 76
   dosage factors, 201
   incidence, 202–203
   and lithium, 180
   and patient education, 206
   presentation and course, 203
   and prior psychiatric history, 202
   prodrome, 203
   and pulmonary disease, 101
   risk factors, 201–202
   in transplant patients, 178, 180
   treatment, 206–207
   and tricyclic antidepressants, 206
   withdrawal syndromes, 204–205
Stokes-Adams attacks, 43
Stress-reduction programs, 15–16
Stress
   and asthma, 97
   and breast cancer outcome, 379
   and irritable bowel syndrome, 287
   and myocardial ischemia episodes, 1119612
   and sudden cardiac death, 13–14
Subclinical encephalopathy, 132
Substance abusers, HIV risk, 232–233

Substance-induced disorders, DSM-IV coding for, 392–397

Substance-induced persisting amnestic disorder, 131

Sudden cardiac death, 10, 13–14

Suicide
    in dialysis patients, 168
    in AIDS patients, 227–228
    as reaction to HIV seropositivity, 251
    in kidney transplantation, 176–177
    in pregnancy, 309

Sulfamethoxazole, 264

Sulfonamide antibiotics, 177

Sulindac, and delirium, 76

Sundowning, 81

Supine hypotensive syndrome (of pregnancy), 330

Support groups, for breast cancer patients, 381

Supportive psychotherapy, 73

Suppository antidepressants, 84–85

Surgery, psychological preparation and outcome, 175–176

Surgical menopause, 353

Syndrome of inappropriate antidiuretic hormone (SIADH), 284, 439

Syringe sharing, 233

Systemic lupus erythematosus
    versus postpartum psychosis, 330
    and steroid psychosis, 202

T

T-wave abnormalities, 55

Tachycardia, 40–41

Tamoxifen, 19, 377–378

Tardive dyskinesia, in AIDS patients, 263

Tardive respiratory dyskinesia, 81

Tartrazine dye, 106

Temazepam
    in delirium, 80, 402
    hazards in pregnancy, 314, 432
    in hepatic failure, 135
    in HIV infection, 261
    in renal failure, 172, 413
    and respiratory depression, 103
    Teratogenic effects
    of benzodiazepines, 312–314
    of ECT, 315–316, 331
    of fluoxetine, 315
    of lithium, 333–334
    of neuroleptics, 331–332
    risk factors, 312
    of tricyclic antidepressants, 314–315

Terfenadine, 19, 439

Testosterone
    chemotherapy effects, in women, 378
    in postmenopausal women, 354–355

Theophylline, 76, 102, 106

Thiamine deficiency, 130

Thiazide diuretics
    depression association, 57
    and lithium, 154

Thioridazine
    for anxiolysis, 105
    and cardiotoxicity, 43, 54
    and isoenzyme-2D6, 19
    in pregnancy, 432
    in pulmonary disease, 105
    for steroid-induced psychosis, 206

Thyroid disease, 330

Thyroid hormones, in postpartum depression, 310

Timed Gait test, 223

Tobramycin, 76

Torsade de pointes
    and haloperidol, 79
    and psychotropics, 43
    and thioridazine, 54

Trail Making Tests
    age distribution, of scores, 399
    AIDS dementia complex assessment, 223
    delirium assessment, 77

Transference
    and cancer patients, 73–74
    and dialysis patients, 170
    and HIV patients, 256
    and gynecology patients, 350
    and sexual-abuse survivors with HIV, 256

Transplantation. See Liver transplantation; Kidney transplantation.

Trazodone
    cardiovascular profile, 44
    in hepatic failure, 135
    in HIV infection, 229, 261–262
    for insomnia of delirium, 81
    in kidney transplantation, 179
    in pregnancy, 433
    in renal failure, 171, 412

Triamterene, 56

Triazolam
    adverse antifungal interaction, 261
    and delirium, 76, 80, 402
    in hepatic failure, 134, 135
    in HIV infection, 261
    and isoenzyme-3A4, 19
    postoperative use, 80

in pregnancy, 314, 433
pregnancy contraindication, 314
in renal failure, 413
Tricyclic antidepressants
additive toxicity
with carbamazepine, 56
with class I antiarrhythmics, 39–40
with doxorubicin, 84
with neuroleptics, 55
antihypertensive drug interactions, 58
and breast feeding, 317
cardiovascular side effects, 39–44, 55
in hepatic failure, metabolism, 135
in HIV infection, 229
in irritable bowel syndrome, 290
in kidney transplantation, 179
neonatal toxicity, 316
neuroleptic interactions, 55
parenteral and rectal administration, 84–85
pregnancy dose changes, 314
in pulmonary disease, 105–106
adverse drug interactions, 106
in renal failure, 150, 171, 412
in steroid-induced psychosis, 206
teratogenicity, 314–315
Trihexyphenidyl
in HIV infection, 263
in pregnancy, 332, 434
in renal failure, 414
Trimethoprim, 264
Tryptophan
and postmenopause estrogen treatment, 353
and postpartum depression, 311
Tuberculosis. *See* Isoniazid; Rifampin.
Type A behavior
and cardiac disease, 11–12, 14
counseling for, 15–16

U

Ulcerative colitis, 287–288

Unsafe sex, 252–254

V

Vaginitis, 354
Valproate, 154. *See also* Valproic acid.
in renal failure, 414
in steroid-induced mania, 207
Valproic acid
cardiac effects, 56
side effects, 56
teratogenesis, 335
Venlafaxine, 171, 437–440
Ventilator weaning, 81–82
Ventricular arrhythmias, 8, 13
Verapamil, 19, 46, 56, 335
Vitamin B$_{12}$ deficiency, 284–285
Volume of distribution, 43, 150, 314

W

Warfarin, 18, 76
Wernicke's encephalopathy, 124, 130
differential diagnosis, 403
White-matter lesions, in HIV infection, 225
Wisconsin Card Sorting Test, 78
Women
cardiac disease risk, 14
and HIV infection, 259–261
Work stress, and cardiac disease, 14
"Worried well," 226
Writing impairment, and delirium, 78

Z

Zidovudine (AZT)
in AIDS dementia complex, 223–224
and antidepressants, 231
and delirium, 264
mania-inducing effect, 262
and maternal HIV transmission, 260
neuropsychiatric side effects, 224